Histopathology

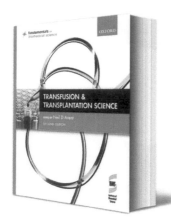

TRANSFUSION & TRANSPLANTATION SCIENCE

Edited by Neil D Avent

SECOND EDITION

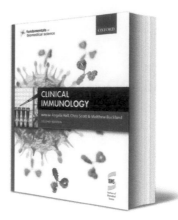

CLINICAL IMMUNOLOGY

Edited by Angela Hall, Chris Scott & Matthew Buckland

SECOND EDITION

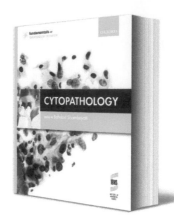

CYTOPATHOLOGY

Edited by Behdad Shambayati

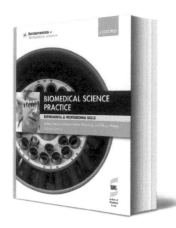

BIOMEDICAL SCIENCE PRACTICE

EXPERIMENTAL & PROFESSIONAL SKILLS

Edited by Sheelagh Heugh, Nisha Sharma, and Glenn Walker

SECOND EDITION

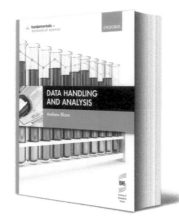

DATA HANDLING AND ANALYSIS

Andrew Blann

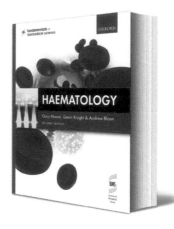

HAEMATOLOGY

Gary Moore, Gavin Knight & Andrew Blann

SECOND EDITION

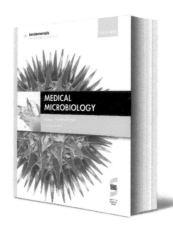

MEDICAL MICROBIOLOGY

Edited by Nicholas Eigel

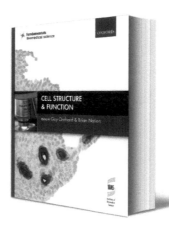

CELL STRUCTURE & FUNCTION

Edited by Gary Orchard & Brian Nation

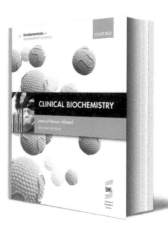

CLINICAL BIOCHEMISTRY

Edited by Nessar Ahmed

SECOND EDITION

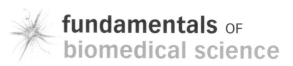

fundamentals OF
biomedical science

Histopathology

Second Edition

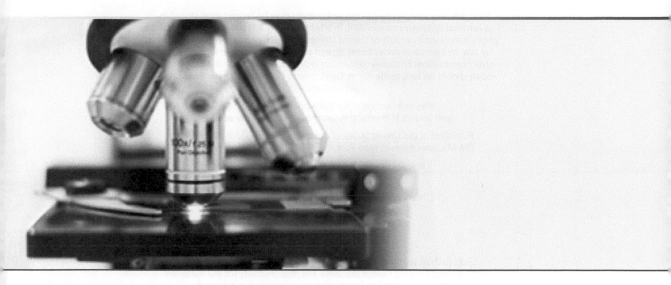

Edited by

Guy Orchard

*Consultant Grade Biomedical Scientist and
Laboratory Manager, Viapath,
St. John's Institute of Dermatology, London*

Brian Nation

Editor, Institute of Biomedical Science

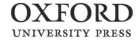

OXFORD

UNIVERSITY PRESS

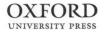

OXFORD
UNIVERSITY PRESS

Great Clarendon Street, Oxford, OX2 6DP,
United Kingdom

Oxford University Press is a department of the University of Oxford.
It furthers the University's objective of excellence in research, scholarship,
and education by publishing worldwide. Oxford is a registered trade mark of
Oxford University Press in the UK and in certain other countries

Published in the United States of America by Oxford University Press
198 Madison Avenue, New York, NY 10016, United States of America

British Library Cataloguing in Publication Data
Data available

Library of Congress Control Number: 2017951000

ISBN 978-0-19-871733-1

Printed in Great Britain by
Bell & Bain Ltd., Glasgow

Acknowledgments

We would like to thank the contributors in this the second edition for all their hard work in the preparation of the chapters that comprise this textbook, and we also would like to acknowledge those authors from the first edition, who no longer appear in this edition, for their original contributions. In addition, we would like to thank the staff at Oxford University Press, in particular Lucy Wells, for their help and support throughout this project.

Special thanks also are due to our respective families, specifically Sarah, Ross, and Kim, for their understanding and forbearance during the many hours devoted to the completion of this the second edition of *Histopathology*.

Guy Orchard
Brian Nation

Foreword

As students, we revelled in the pleasure of reading and dipping into well-constructed textbooks on histopathology technique. At the time, these books, which were owned by laboratories, were relatively few in number but highly regarded. They represented highly informative insights into very specific areas of histopathology investigation. These books gave the reader an understanding of how techniques worked and how they should be used in any given situation to investigate pathological states. In essence, they aimed to provide the reader with the support to perform these methods in their own working environment.

So, what is new? In what way does this book differ from the traditional textbooks we have known and used for so long? The answer lies in how our needs have changed and how the professional demands have dictated changes in our educational and professional training. In modern education, there is much greater need to link themes in order to comprehend and develop an understanding of concepts. There is also the growing encouragement to question theory and practice and to develop a more individualistic approach to problem solving.

The second edition of this book continues to reflect these changing needs, and aims to complement much-valued traditional textbooks. It highlights learning objectives and maps out the key information as it guides the reader from chapter to chapter, linking concepts throughout the entire text. The second edition contains an additional six new chapters and expands the student's knowledge base for learning.

Finally, we are drawn to one undeniable fact that has stood firm for the past century. On the coat of arms of the Institute of Biomedical Science is the Latin motto *Disce ut proficias*, which translates as 'Learn, that you may improve'. We hope that the second edition of this book will go some way to providing the reader with the opportunity to do exactly that!

'Education is the great engine of personal development'
Nelson Mandela

Guy Orchard
Brian Nation

An introduction to the Fundamentals of Biomedical Science series

Biomedical scientists form the foundation of modern healthcare; from cancer screening to diagnosing HIV, from blood transfusion for surgery to food poisoning and infection control. Without biomedical scientists, the diagnosis of disease, the evaluation of the effectiveness of treatment, and research into the causes and cures of disease would not be possible.

However, the path to becoming a biomedical scientist is a challenging one; trainees must not only assimilate knowledge from a range of disciplines, but must understand—and demonstrate—how to apply this knowledge in a practical, hands-on environment.

The *Fundamentals of Biomedical Science* series is written to reflect the challenges of biomedical science education and training today. It blends essential basic science with insights into laboratory practice to show how an understanding of the biology of disease is coupled to the analytical approaches that lead to diagnosis.

The series provides coverage of the full range of disciplines to which a biomedical scientist may be exposed; from microbiology to cytopathology to transfusion science. Alongside volumes exploring specific biomedical themes and related laboratory diagnosis, an overarching *Biomedical Science Practice* volume provides a grounding in the general professional and experimental skills with which every biomedical scientist should be equipped.

Produced in collaboration with the Institute of Biomedical Science, the series:

- understands the complex roles of biomedical scientists in the modern practice of medicine
- understands the development needs of employers and the Profession
- places the theoretical aspects of biomedical science in their practical context.

Learning from this series

The *Fundamentals of Biomedical Science* series draws on a range of learning features to help readers master both biomedical science theory and biomedical science practice.

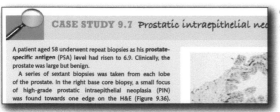

CASE STUDY 9.7 Prostatic intraepithelial neo

A patient aged 58 underwent repeat biopsies as his prostate-specific antigen (PSA) level had risen to 6.9. Clinically, the prostate was large but benign.

A series of sextant biopsies was taken from each lobe of the prostate. In the right base core biopsy, a small focus of high-grade prostatic intraepithelial neoplasia (PIN) was found towards one edge on the H&E (Figure 9.36).

Case studies illustrate how the biomedical science theory and practice presented throughout the series relate to situations and experiences that are likely to be routinely encountered in the biomedical science laboratory.

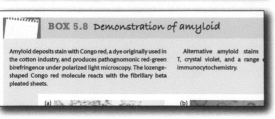

BOX 5.8 Demonstration of amyloid

Amyloid deposits stain with Congo red, a dye originally used in the cotton industry, and produces pathognomonic red-green birefringence under polarized light microscopy. The lozenge-shaped Congo red molecule reacts with the fibrillary beta pleated sheets.

Alternative amyloid stains T, crystal violet, and a range immunocytochemistry.

(a)   (b)

Additional information to augment the main text appears in **boxes**.

METHOD 4.2 *Urgent frozen sections*

- On arrival, the time is noted, the tissue is described and a small representative piece is placed on a labelled chuck. The specimen is frozen down.
- Frozen sections are cut at 5 μm, usually two per slide.
- The slide is labelled with patient details.

Method boxes walk through the key protocols that the reader is likely to encounter in the laboratory on a regular basis.

HEALTH & SAFETY 3.1

Known infected specimens should be identified to the laboratory with Danger of Infection labels and handled appropriately, but all tissue submitted is potentially hazardous. Hepatitis viruses, mycobacteria and HIV are some of the infective agents that you may be required to deal with. Adequate formalin fixation (24 hrs) will render most tissues safe to handle, but Category III cabinets are required to deal with pathogen 4 specimens, therefore most laboratories will not accept fresh tissue from known infected patients.

Health and safety boxes raise awareness of key health and safety issues related to topics featured in the series, with which the reader should be familiar.

CLINICAL CORRELATION

Appendicitis is a common condition with approximately 50,000 people admitted to hospital with appendicitis each year in the UK; around one in every 13 people develop it at some point in their life. It can develop at any age, but it is most common in younger people (10 to 20 years old). The appendix is a tubular structure extending from the caecum with no known specific function. It has a lumen which is continuous with that of the caecum, together with

Clinical correlations bring relevance to the material by placing it in its clinical context.

Key Point

Probe preparation

A probe is composed of two elements: a nucleic acid sequence that has a complementary base sequence to the target and a label to allow visualization of the nucleic acid hybrid.

Key points reinforce the key concepts that the reader should master from having read the material presented, while **Summary** points act as an end-of-chapter checklist for readers to verify that they have remembered correctly the principal themes and ideas presented within each chapter.

---

e used in immunocytochemistry for **antigen retrieval**. It is oteolytic effect by cleaving peptides at the carboxyl side of residues—three amino acids containing phenyl rings. Used agent than trypsin, but many commercial trypsin products trypsin to offer a wider spectrum of digestive activity.

e approach more selective by utilizing specific families of n. Many of the ready-to-use solutions available commernufactured for use on automated staining platforms. These

Antigen retrieval
A series of techniques that permit the controlled unmasking of antigenic epitopes, following the fixation of tissue and prior to subsequent demonstration of final reaction products with labelled antibodies. Conventionally, this relies on the application of heat (HIER) using a waterbath, microwave oven, or

Key terms provide on-the-page explanations of terms that the reader may not be familiar with; in addition, each title in the series features a **glossary**, in which the key terms featured in that title are collated.

SELF-CHECK 3.6

Can you list the common benign and malignant lesions that occur in the breast? Do you know what surgical procedures are used to treat these conditions?

CASE STUDY 3.2 *Benign breast lump*

Self-check questions throughout each chapter and extended questions at the end of each chapter provide the reader with a ready means of checking that they have understood the material they have just encountered. Answers to these questions are provided in the book's accompanying website; visit **www.oup.com/uk/orchard2e**

---

ot being linked correctly to the right patient?

Cross reference
See Chapter 17 where audit trails and quality issues are discussed in greater detail.

Cross references help the reader to see biomedical science as a unified discipline, making connections between topics presented within each volume, and across all volumes in the series.

Online learning materials

online resource centre

The *Fundamentals of Biomedical Science* series doesn't end with the printed books. Each title in the series is supported by an Online Resource Centre, which features additional materials for students, trainees, and lecturers.

www.oxfordtextbooks.co.uk/orc/fbs/

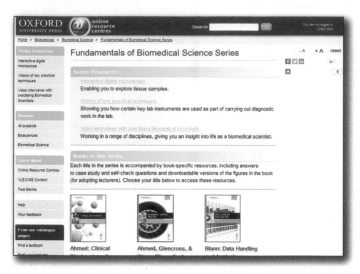

Guides to key experimental skills and methods

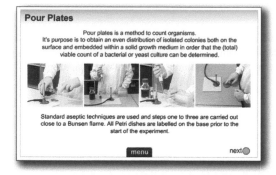

Multimedia walk-throughs of key experimental skills—including both animations and video—to help you master the essential skills that are the foundation of biomedical science practice.

Biomedical science in practice

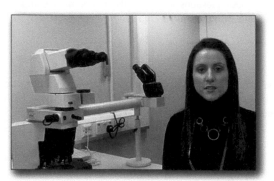

Interviews with practising biomedical scientists working in a range of disciplines, to give you valuable insights into the reality of work in a Biomedical Science laboratory.

Digital Microscope

A library of microscopic images for you to investigate using this powerful online microscope, to help you gain a deeper appreciation of cell and tissue morphology.

The Digital Microscope is used under licence from the Open University.

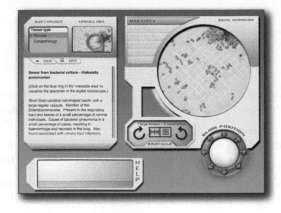

Answers to self-check, case study, and end-of-chapter questions

Answers to questions posed in the book are provided to aid self assessment.

Lecturer support materials

The website for each title in the series also features figures from the book in electronic format, for registered adopters to download for use in lecture presentations, and other educational resources.

To register as an adopter visit **www.oxfordtextbooks.co.uk/orc/ fbs/** and follow the on-screen instructions.

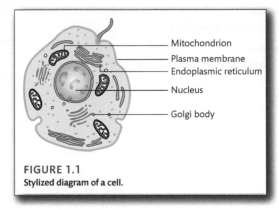

FIGURE 1.1
Stylized diagram of a cell.

Any comments?

We welcome comments and feedback about any aspect of this series.
Just visit www.oxfordtextbooks.co.uk/orc/feedback/ and share your views.

Contributors

Sue Alexander
Royal Marsden NHS Foundation Trust

Patricia Fernando
Viapath, St. John's Institute of Dermatology

David Furness
School of Life Sciences, Keele University

Ishbel Gall
Fosterhill, NHS Grampian

Chantell Hodgson
UK NEQAS CPT Scheme Manager, Queen Elizabeth Hospital

Merdol Ibrahim
UK NEQAS ICC Scheme Manager

Vanda McTaggert
University Hospital Crosshouse

David Muskett
Salford Royal Foundation Trust

Brian Nation
Editor, Institute of Biomedical Science

Guy Orchard
Consultant Grade Biomedical Scientist and Laboratory Manager, Viapath, St. John's Institute of Dermatology

Brendan O'Sullivan
University Hospitals Birmingham NHS Foundation Trust

Susan Pritchard
University Hospital South Manchester

Mohammad Shams
Viapath, St. John's Institute of Dermatology

Philippe Taniere
University Hospitals Birmingham NHS Foundation Trust

Emanuela Volpi
University of Westminster

Chris Ward
Head of Examinations, Institute of Biomedical Science

Anthony Warford
University of Westminster

Anne Warren
Cambridge University Hospitals NHS Foundation Trust

Contents

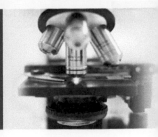

1

What is histopathology?

David Muskett, Guy Orchard and Anne Warren

Learning objectives

After studying this chapter, you should be able to:

- Describe the role of histopathology in the diagnosis of disease.
- List the different types of biopsy submitted to the histopathology laboratory.
- Outline the specimen journey through the laboratory.
- List the special staining techniques that can be used to aid diagnosis.
- Discuss the concept of consent.
- Understand the principles of the Human Tissue Act 2004.
- Outline the laboratory management systems that support an effective histopathology service.

1.1 Introduction

SELF-CHECK 1.1

What made you first consider histopathology?

Welcome! You are lucky enough to have stumbled upon histopathology, a subject of huge content and never-ending interest. Histopathology is a wonderful mix of cell biology, biochemistry, chemistry, and genetics. It is a subject pertinent to each family and appears in the news in all advanced and advancing countries. Practitioners of histopathology carry out a valuable service to their fellow men and women.

Histopathology is a broad subject with many nooks and crannies of interest, and offers a valuable and rewarding career to many thousands of individuals across the globe. For students to whom this subject is just a module, please take time to enjoy this subject. For students who are looking to work or do work in another subject area, it is interesting to see how the differing medical disciplines complement each other in delivering the healthcare we all recognize.

As a laboratory-based subject handling small pots of tissue and microscope slides it is easy to forget the patient; however, they are the reason we are here.

Key Point

The patient is the centre of the histopathology process

Cross reference

You will read more about the morphology of histopathology specimens in the reporting chapter (Chapter 13).

It is interesting to note that each one of our organs shows the same general histology as the next person (Box 1.1, Figure 1.1), and possibly more importantly, each pathology of the same type has a characteristic morphology and pattern. It is the manual visual interpretation of these things that forms the basis of histopathology.

BOX 1.1 Cells are the functional unit of the body and each one has a number of key features:

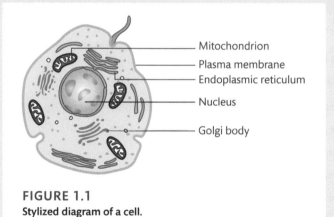

Mitochondrion
Plasma membrane
Endoplasmic reticulum
Nucleus
Golgi body

FIGURE 1.1
Stylized diagram of a cell.

1.2 What is pathology?

SELF-CHECK 1.2

Of what does the word pathology make you think?

Pathology is the study of disease. More precisely, it is the study (*logos*) of suffering (*pathos*). It is a form of science and a branch of medicine that involves testing patient samples (blood, urine, tissue, etc.) in order to aid or provide a diagnosis. As a form of science it is dedicated to the evaluation of structural and functional changes in cells, tissues and organs. Broadly speaking there are four facets to pathology, helping to define cause (aetiology), mechanism of effect (pathogenesis), structural changes to cells, tissues

TABLE 1.1 Components of disease

Characteristic	Definition	Example
Incidence	How often the disease is seen. This is usually described as the number of cases per 100,000 of the population per year.	About one in eight US women (about 12%) will develop invasive breast cancer over the course of their lifetime.
Aetiology	What causes the disease.	Human papillomavirus is a causative agent of cervical cancer.
Pathogenesis	The mechanism by which the disease is caused.	The interaction of *Helicobacter pylori* with the gastric epithelium, resulting in cytotoxin production, inflammation and neoplastic change.
Pathology	The nature of the disease itself.	A benign or malignant tumour.
Sequelae	The consequences that happen because of the disease.	Small lesions showing cervical intraepithelial carcinoma grade 3 (CIN3) if left will develop into invasive carcinoma.
Outcome	The endpoint of the disease.	For malignant melanoma, this would be metastatic melanoma leading to death, whereas a basal cell carcinoma does not metastasize and leads to an increasingly large ulcer.
Treatment	How the disease is managed.	This could be by surgery and chemotherapy for invasive colonic carcinoma, or acid control therapy for Barrett's oesophagus.

and organs (morphology), and finally changes to functional activity (clinical significance) (see Table 1.1). Effective healthcare is underpinned by information that pathology services provide to clinicians. It is estimated that in developed countries 70–80% of diagnoses and clinical decisions are facilitated by the information generated by laboratory-based medical specialties. This fact is often not appreciated by the general public or even healthcare professionals. Furthermore, pathology services work at the laboratory–clinic interface and have been instrumental in the development of new diagnostic tests and treatments, and hopefully the 'cure', which reflects the contributions of the discipline of pathology at the forefront of medical advances. Increasingly, pathology is termed laboratory medicine and comprises specific disciplines that include haematology, clinical biochemistry, microbiology, immunology and histopathology.

1.3 **What is histopathology?**

Histopathology is the study of the pathology of cells and tissues. This laboratory-based discipline differs from cytopathology, which deals with cells in solution. Cells are the building blocks of human life and come in many varied and specialized types (see Box 1.1). Tissues are defined as an organized mass of cells working as a common function. Histopathology is different yet complementary to cytopathology, which looks at cells received in fluids or washing, and both disciplines are part of the branch of science known as cellular pathology. Cellular pathology also complements the blood and infective sciences that form part of the larger family of biomedical science.

Histopathology is the discipline concerned with producing accurate diagnostic information from patient tissue samples presumed abnormal in nature. Diseases such as infection, inflammation and cancer are recognized by typical microscopic changes in tissues. In some circumstances, these changes can be identified in the absence of obvious clinical signs and symptoms of disease. Recognizing and understanding changes in the architecture of tissue and changes in individual cells is a highly skilled but at times a rather subjective process. Here lies one of the key differences between histopathology and other laboratory specialties; the histopathology report is based on the interpretive skill of a

Cross reference
You will read more about the microscope in Chapter 14.

medically qualified practitioner (histopathologist), whereas the majority of test results generated by other scientific disciplines (e.g. clinical biochemistry and haematology) rely on information generated by highly complex, calibrated pieces of equipment.

Cytopathology is closely allied to histopathology but is distinct because the diagnostic information is acquired following analysis of cell preparations—typically the cells are disaggregated and lack the architectural features present in tissue samples (see the *Cytopathology* volume in the *Fundamentals of Biomedical Science* series).

The majority of histopathology examinations are undertaken on tissue obtained from patients undergoing a tissue biopsy for diagnostic purposes. Some patients will be referred for biopsy as a result of a national cancer screening programme (e.g. breast, cervical or colorectal). If a disease requires surgical intervention, often the operation will involve removal of a tissue specimen for further histopathological analysis. Histopathology is also used to help the establishment of cause of death as part of a post-mortem examination (see Chapter 16, Mortuary practice).

1.4 Histopathology specimens

Laboratory management should also review and audit specimen collection services to ensure that specimens are delivered in a timely manner, as well as safely and securely (you will read more about laboratory management in Chapter 17). The majority of samples received in histopathology come from the hospital in which the department is located, but it is not uncommon for histopathology to receive samples from further afield. The majority of these samples will be in a formalin-based fixative, and containers should all be labelled with appropriate hazard warning labels. Laboratory management should ensure that those transporting the samples are aware of the hazards of formalin, that they are trained to know what to do in the event of spillage, and, if necessary, have spillage containment equipment and personal protective equipment (PPE) available. Laboratory management should also ensure that the systems for conveying samples are safe and secure. Most histopathology samples are irreplaceable and a lost sample can have serious consequences for the patient. There should also be measures in place to protect the patient information contained on an accompanying request form from unauthorized access (see Box 1.2).

BOX 1.2 Data Protection Act

The Data Protection Act 1998 applies to personal information and ensures that it is handled properly. The Act works in two ways. First, it helps to protect the interests of members of the public by obliging organizations to manage the information they hold in a proper way. It states that anyone who processes personal information must comply with eight principles. These are designed to ensure that data are:

- fairly and lawfully processed
- processed for limited purposes
- adequate, relevant and not excessive
- accurate and up to date
- not kept for longer than is necessary
- processed in line with an individual's rights
- secure
- not transferred to other countries without adequate protection.

The second area covered by the Act gives members of the public certain rights about personal information kept by organizations, including the right to know what information is held and the right to correct information that is wrong. Members of the public also have the right to claim compensation through the courts if an organization breaches the Act and this causes damage (e.g. financial loss). Similar pieces of legislation exist in most other countries. Further information can be found at www.ico.gov.uk/

Key Point

Patient information accompanying a specimen is covered by the Data Protection Act. Laboratory personnel must be aware of their obligations under this Act.

The majority of biopsies submitted for histological examination are taken for diagnostic purposes. Typically, these are small biopsies and they are placed into a fixative in order to preserve the tissue by preventing autolysis and bacterial decomposition (putrefaction). Various methods can be used to obtain the sample and the biopsy method is often used to describe the type of sample. Surgical treatment of disease aims to remove all diseased tissue and include a margin of unaffected, healthy tissue. Surgical specimens are usually complex and require systematic examination and selection of areas for microscopic examination.

Cross reference

You will read more about fixation in Chapter 2.

You will read more about histopathology specimens in Chapter 3, in which dissection is discussed.

You will read more about the various specimens received in the laboratory in Chapter 3.

Key Point

Fixation is the bedrock of effective routine histopathology; it is the process of preserving tissue in a lifelike manner and allows subsequent tests to be carried out.

The most common fixative employed in histopathology is 10% neutral buffered formalin, which is a hazardous substance.

Key Point

The type of specimen a clinician selects to send to the laboratory is informed by the purpose of the procedure, which can be divided up into screening (without symptoms), diagnostic (with symptoms but the cause uncertain), and therapeutic (the diagnosis is clear and the specimen is taken to remove the pathology in its entirety).

1.5 Histopathology service users

Users of the histopathology service are the clinicians who assess the patients and take various tissue samples. Clinicians and surgeons act in the best interests of their patients. The expectation from providing tissue samples for histopathological examination is that it will enable the production of a histopathology report that will include interpretive information on:

- Histological features seen under the light microscope.
- Information regarding the pathological processes evidenced from reviewing the material under the microscope.
- Some guidance about the possible diagnosis, which will often confirm or refute the clinically suggested diagnosis.
- Some guidance in the case of tumours about whether or not the margins of excision are cleared, and any suggested further tests required to confirm or support the proposed diagnosis. These may be molecular-based tests or tests performed in the other laboratory disciplines (i.e. haematology, microbiology or clinical biochemistry). Results from such additional investigations may take some time to produce, but will be incorporated into the final report as a 'supplementary report', which follows the first report issued by the histopathologist.

Cross reference

You will read more about understanding service users' requirements in Chapter 13.

Key Point

Regular dialogue and communication with service users is essential for the smooth running of the laboratory service. It is important that the laboratory is open to service users so that they can see what goes on and thereby understand what is involved in providing the service.

1.6 Patients

SELF-CHECK 1.3

What information would you need to give your consent for histopathological analysis?

Key Point

Surgical specimen/sample information

Patient information accompanying a specimen is covered by the Data Protection Act. Laboratory personnel must be aware of their obligations under this Act. All information accompanying patient tissues should be regarded as strictly confidential and only those qualified and directly involved in the patient management pathway should have access to this information.

SELF-CHECK 1.4

What information would you need as a patient to understand what was happening to your specimen following an operation or procedure?

Organs, tissues, and body fluids from patients (including surgical biopsy and resection specimens) do not fall under the terms of the Act if diagnosis is the primary purpose for removal and storage. This would apply to the vast majority of surgical specimens entering most histopathology departments. Consequently, specific consent from the patient is not required for that purpose, nor is it essential to obtain consent for a range of other purposes associated with clinical care, including:

- clinical audit
- quality assurance
- public health monitoring
- reference range evaluation
- method comparison
- assay development
- validation of new methodology.

However, it is good practice for consent forms to include a section on consent for the use of surplus tissue to be stored and used for approved research, either within an NHS trust or by external organizations. It should be noted that any conditions laid down by the patient at this point (e.g. exclusion of the use of samples for research) should be respected. Laboratories must have systems in place to capture and record these conditions, and ensure that they are followed when selecting tissue for research purposes.

1.6.1 Consent

Patients must give their consent to treatment. It is the principle that a person must give their consent/permission before they can receive any type of medical treatment or examination. This is most often a part of the basis of the preliminary explanation by any given clinician. It is also the case that consent is required even if the patient does not require invasive tests. In other words, consent is required if the patient is simply having a physical examination or an extensive invasive procedure such as organ transplantation.

Consent can be:

- Verbal (e.g. agreeing by saying they are happy to have an X-ray).
- Written (e.g. by signing a pre-prepared consent form for surgery).

Consent is not required in some instances, such as:

- Treatment required in an emergency and the patient is unable to give consent.
- During an operation when it becomes obvious that a patient requires unplanned and immediate additional procedures to treat life-threatening problems which were not included in their original consent.
- The patient has a severe mental health condition such as schizophrenia, bipolar disorder or severe dementia. However, in these cases, treatment for unrelated physical conditions still requires consent, which the patient may be able to provide despite their mental health condition.

Key Point

Clinical teams make great use of information leaflets about the procedures they carry out to inform patients about treatment. This is part of the informed consent pathway.

1.7 Post-mortem specimens

SELF-CHECK 1.5

Why is sample handling from the deceased considered differently?

Under the Human Tissue Act 2004, consent is needed for the removal, storage and use of material from the deceased for all scheduled purposes as listed below:

- Anatomical examination.
- Determining the cause of death.
- Establishing, after a person's death, the efficacy of any drug or other treatment administered.
- Obtaining scientific or medical information, which may be relevant to any person (including one yet to be born).
- Public display.
- Research in connection with disorders or the functioning of the human body.
- Transplantation patient information accompanying a specimen is covered by the Data Protection Act. Laboratory personnel must be aware of their obligations under this Act.
- Clinical audit.
- Education or training relating to human health.
- Performance assessment.

Cross reference

You will read more about the role of the coroner in Chapter 16.

- Public health monitoring.
- Quality assurance.

Although consent is not required to undertake a coroner's post-mortem, consent is required under the Act for the continued storage or use of tissue, for 'scheduled purposes', once the coroner's purposes are complete.

1.8 Human Tissue Authority

The Human Tissue Authority (HTA) was established in 2005 under the 2004 Act and is the regulatory authority for human tissues. Governance of these practices is achieved by licensing organizations engaged in the activities described above. It is responsible for the implementation of the Act and ensuring compliance by licensing and inspection. The HTA has produced codes of practice relating to the licensed activities in pathology (and in other areas including anatomy, transplantation, and public display), which are the product of extensive consultation with professional and lay bodies and individuals. Departments complete an online Compliance Report application form, available on the HTA's website (www.hta.gov.uk), which requires information on the proposed licence holder for each organization (e.g. a chief executive of an NHS trust), and the designated individual in that organization who is responsible for compliance with the terms of the licence (generally a head/clinical lead of a pathology department). The impact of the HTA guidelines has set the path for how modern-day histopathology is conducted in terms of diagnostic teaching, training and research.

Cross reference

You will read more about post-mortem examinations in Chapter 16.

Key Point

Consent is the fundamental principle of the Human Tissue Act 2004. There are different consent requirements for dealing with tissue from the deceased and the living.

Consent is required to remove tissue from the deceased for histological examination in order to determine the cause of death (and for other purposes such as research or teaching).

Consent is not required to remove tissue samples from living patients if the primary purpose is diagnosis.

1.9 Clinical trials

Ethics

Ethics is the branch of medicine that deals with establishing the rights and wrongs of clinical practice. Sometimes known as medical ethics, the values expressed as right and wrong are not static, and public opinion about what is acceptable does change over time. Biomedical practitioners need to be sensitive to these changes. In the UK, biomedical scientists are registered with the HCPC and they must adhere to its ethical code. Similar ethical codes exist in other countries for registered histotechnologists, medical and biomedical scientists.

Clinical trials are controlled experiments in which patients are put on new drugs or treatments. This has potential to be very hazardous and clinical trials are managed by the organization's ethics committees, which review the risks and benefits to patients. Once trials have been approved, informed patient consent is required. Prior to agreeing to participate, every volunteer/patient has the right to know and understand what will happen in any given clinical trial in which they may take part. This is often an additional component of the informed consent procedures. In brief, if you have given consent to participate in a clinical trial or if you have given consent on behalf of another person, both parties are entitled to the following rights:

- To be told the purpose of the clinical trial.
- To be told about the risks and side-effects.
- To be informed of any benefits that can be expected.
- To be informed of what will happen in the trial and whether any procedures, drugs or devices being used are different from those used in any standard treatment.
- To be informed of any options that may be available and whether they may be better or worse than being in a clinical trial.
- To be allowed to ask questions about the trial prior to consenting and throughout the trial period.

- To be given ample time to decide without any additional pressure whether or not to consent to participation in the trial.
- To refuse to participate for any reason before and after the trial has started.
- To receive a signed and dated copy of the consent form.
- To be informed of any medical treatments should complications occur during the trial.

Key Point

Clinical trials offer a way of developing new and innovative forms of patient drug therapy and treatment.

1.10 Laboratory processing

The workflow through the laboratory is tightly regulated to ensure that the tissue submitted (input) emerges with the correct diagnostic information (output). The process is undertaken by a dedicated team of medical laboratory assistants, biomedical scientists, medical secretaries and histopathologists.

From a patient's perspective, histopathology services probably appear straightforward. The patient gives consent (see Box 1.3) to have a biopsy and for the report to be communicated to them by the attending clinician. However, histopathology is a complex process that involves multiple steps, from the acquisition of tissue to diagnosis (Figure 1.2). The majority of diagnoses are based on the assessment of haematoxylin and eosin (H&E)-stained sections of formalin-fixed, paraffin wax-embedded tissue.

Owing to the presence of formalin, histopathology specimens are not normally considered infectious, but are often collected with other samples that may be infectious. If specimens are transported for any distance over the public highway, by hand, or in vans/cars, it is important that they should

---

BOX 1.3 Human Tissue Act (2004)

'Sixteen doctors reported to GMC in organs scandal'
Independent, 15 March 2001
'Relatives win right to launch mass action over organ removal'
Guardian, 12 May 2001
'Organ scandal parents get £5m payout'
The Times, 1 February 2003
'Doctors who "steal" organs face jail'
The Times, 5 December 2003
'NHS negligent in removing baby organs'
The Independent, 27 March 2004

The headlines above are just some of the many examples of media attention in the early years of the twenty-first century on the subject of human tissue samples. There was general outrage at the practice of removing and storing organs from post-mortems without the informed consent of the relatives. Such was the public outcry that the government of the time was compelled to introduce an act making such practices illegal. The Human Tissue Act 2004, which covers England, Wales, and Northern Ireland, established the Human Tissue Authority (HTA) to regulate activities concerning the removal, storage, use,

and disposal of human tissue. Consent is the fundamental principle of the legislation and underpins the lawful removal, storage, and use of body parts, organs, and tissue. Different consent requirements apply when dealing with tissue from the deceased and the living. The Act lists the purposes for which consent is required (these are called 'scheduled purposes') and include:

- determining the cause of death
- obtaining scientific or medical information about a living or deceased person which might be relevant to any other person (including one yet to be born)
- research in connection with disorders, or the functioning, of the human body
- clinical audit
- quality assurance
- establishing after a person's death the effects of any drug or other treatment administered to them
- education or training relating to human health
- public health monitoring.

Consent for histopathology specimens

Surgical specimens (samples removed from living patients)

Organs, tissues and body fluids from living patients (including surgical biopsy and resection specimens) do not fall under the terms of the Act if diagnosis is the primary purpose for removal and storage. This would apply to the vast majority of surgical specimens entering most histopathology departments. Consequently, specific consent from the patient is not required for that purpose, nor is it essential to obtain consent for a range of other purposes associated with clinical care, including:

- clinical audit
- quality assurance
- public health monitoring
- reference range evaluation
- method comparison
- assay development
- validation of new methodology.

However, it is good practice for consent forms to include a section on consent for the use of surplus tissue to be stored and used for approved research, either within an NHS trust or by external organizations. It should be noted that any conditions laid down by the patient at this point (e.g. exclusion of the use of samples for research) should be respected. Laboratories must have systems in place to capture and record these conditions, and ensure that they are complied with when selecting tissue for research purposes.

Post-mortem specimens (samples removed from the deceased)

Under the Act, consent is needed for the removal, storage and use of material from the deceased for all scheduled purposes as listed below:

- anatomical examination
- determining the cause of death
- establishing, after a person's death, the efficacy of any drug or other treatment administered to them
- obtaining scientific or medical information, which may be relevant to any person (including one yet to be born)
- public display
- research in connection with disorders, or the functioning, of the human body
- transplantation
- clinical audit
- education or training relating to human health

- performance assessment
- public health monitoring
- quality assurance.

Although consent is not required to undertake a coroner's post-mortem, consent is required under the Act for the continued storage or use of tissue, for 'scheduled purposes', once the coroner's purposes are complete.

Licensing

The Act requires that departments engaged in the following activities should be licensed:

- undertaking a post-mortem examination
- storing the body of a deceased person, or 'relevant material' from a human body, for a scheduled purpose
- removal from the body of a deceased person material of which the body consists or which it contains for use for a 'scheduled purpose' other than post-mortem examination or transplantation.

A licence is not required for organs, tissues and body fluids from living patients (including surgical biopsy and resection specimens) if diagnosis is the primary purpose for removal and storage.

The Act describes 'relevant material' as anything that contains cells and has come from a human body (apart from hair, nail, gametes, and embryos created outside the body). This means that, in addition to solid organs and tissues, body fluids (if stored) also come under the scope of the Act.

Human Tissue Authority

The HTA was established in 2005 under the Act and is a watchdog that supports public confidence by licensing organizations engaged in the activities described above. It is responsible for the implementation of the Act and ensuring compliance by licensing and inspection. The HTA has produced codes of practice relating to the licensable activities in pathology (and in other areas including anatomy, transplantation and public display), which are the product of extensive consultation with professional and lay bodies and individuals.

Licensing of pathology departments commenced on 1 September 2006. Departments complete an online Compliance Report application form, available on the HTA's website (www.hta.gov.uk), which requires information on the proposed licence holder for each organization (e.g. a chief executive of an NHS trust), and the designated individual in that organization who is responsible for compliance with the terms of the licence (generally a head/clinical lead of a pathology department). The impact of the HTA guidelines has set the path for how modern-day histopathology is now conducted in terms of diagnostic teaching, training and also research.

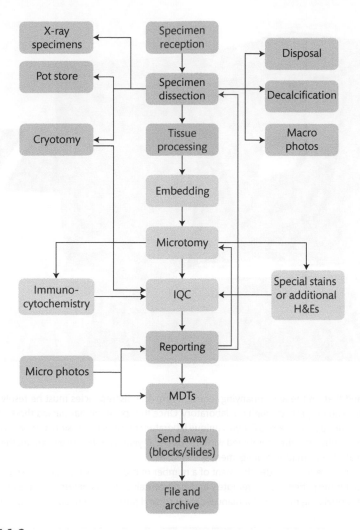

FIGURE 1.2

Histopathology is a complex process that involves multiple steps, both forward (black arrows) and backwards (red arrows), from the acquisition of tissue to diagnosis. In most cases, tissues follow the same route through the department as outlined above.

be in designated leakproof, washable, closed boxes. The boxes should bear the labelling 'Danger of Infection' and a formalin hazard notice, together with the address and telephone number of the laboratory to which they are being sent.

The transport boxes should be inspected and cleaned regularly and immediately in the event of a spillage of specimen material.

In the UK it is possible to post small histopathology specimens provided that the packaging complies with UN3373 standards, and the volume of formalin does not exceed 50 mL (Figure 1.3). However, it is advisable to check the most recent Post Office regulations before sending specimens by post (www.royalmail.com). Separate regulations exist for sending samples overseas.

Following receipt of the specimen in the laboratory, the sample is checked systematically. It is important that the laboratory defines a specimen acceptance policy which determines the minimum amount of patient information that the department will accept (minimum acceptance criteria). This normally encompasses checks to ensure the patient details correlate on specimen pot and request form. There should be concordance with regard to patient name, hospital number and date of birth, and also all requests should be signed by the requesting clinician. The laboratory will have actions to be taken if any of it is missing or if there is any discrepancy between the information on the specimen

Cross reference

You will read more about specimen transport and reception in Chapter 2.

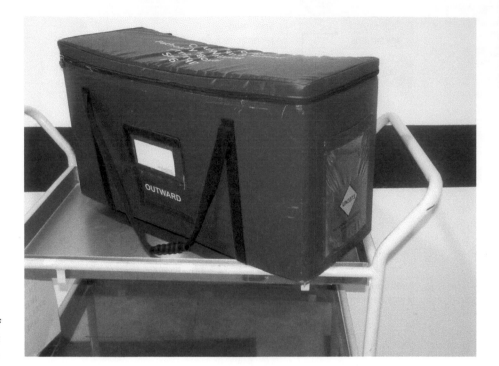

FIGURE 1.3
A pathology transport box used between hospital sites via dedicated transport. Note the yellow rhombus on the side (UN 3373), which is the transport code for diagnostic samples. The transport box is labelled with contact details of the laboratory and the current direction of travel (outbound).

Cross reference
You will read more about the sequences of tissue fixation, processing, embedding, staining, and the principles and reporting in subsequent chapters.

container and that on the accompanying request form. Any discrepancies must be resolved before the specimen can progress through the laboratory. Once the specimen has passed these checks, the request form and specimen are assigned a unique laboratory number (accession number), which typically is a consecutive number combined with the calendar year. The data provided are then entered on the laboratory information management system (LIMS).

Recent years have seen the development of a number of order-communication systems whereby the user submits the patient details remotely and electronically. This system updates the department's LIMS, thereby obviating the need for manual data entry and possibly the need for a request form.

Key Point

Patient information accompanying a specimen is covered by the Data Protection Act. Laboratory personnel must be aware of their obligations under this Act.

SELF-CHECK 1.6

What are the standard minimum acceptance criteria for the receipt of a sample in a histopathology laboratory?

Key Point

Correct specimen labelling and the provision of accurate and relevant clinical details are essential for a safe and effective laboratory service. Measures such as a specimen acceptance policy are essential. There is no benefit in a laboratory that can produce perfect results but reports them on the wrong patient or sample.

1.11 Reporting results

Diagnostic histopathology is a relatively slow process and does not normally produce reports in a matter of minutes (with the exception of intraoperative frozen sections). There are a number of factors that affect the time taken to produce a report (e.g. size of the tissue, presence of calcium, complexity of the case, etc.). However, as a general rule, the majority of cases should be reported within seven days. Patients and their relatives are understandably anxious to know the result of their biopsy and laboratories make every effort to reduce turnaround time. While timely results are important, quality assurance is paramount as mistakes have potentially serious consequences for the patient, and safety and accuracy must be the prime concerns of the laboratory. Consequently, checking specimen identification throughout the specimen journey is of great importance. The right result on the right patient at the right time requires good management and effective teamwork. The provision of healthcare is not immune from financial pressures and histopathology is no exception. In the UK, most histopathology services are provided by publicly funded laboratories and are consequently under pressure to maximize scarce resources. In the UK the NHS embarked on a Quality, Innovation, Productivity, and Prevention (QIPP) agenda, which can be summarized as a commitment to providing high-quality services at less cost, and similar initiatives can be found worldwide. In an attempt to address this challenge, many histopathology departments around the world have turned to modern management techniques to improve their quality of service and at the same time reduce cost. Most commonly, the Toyota Production System, often referred to as 'Lean', has been adopted (see Box 1.4). In the UK, the NHS has set up the NHS Improvement Agency with a specific division devoted to help improve diagnostics (pathology and radiology). In recent years the NHS Improvement Diagnostics Team has been working with a number of pathology pilot sites to test Lean methodology, to demonstrate the benefits to pathology and the impact on the wider healthcare system. The approach has been extremely successful and is being adopted widely in many pathology laboratories and clinical settings.

The final histopathology report serves to provide a record of the specimen received in the laboratory and to provide a pathological diagnosis. It should include the precise clinical information on the request form that was provided by the clinician submitting the sample. This may be typed onto the laboratory system on receipt, or ideally, where electronic requesting is available, entered directly onto the hospital computer system by the clinician. The latter reduces the risk of transcription errors or misinterpretation. There follows a macroscopic description of the specimen, to include measurements, gross appearance, and details of the blocks taken for histological assessment. Following systematic assessment of the haematoxylin and eosin (H&E)-stained sections, the histopathologist writes a description of the microscopic findings, recording the tissue type, the pathological features, and a final interpretation of the findings. Additional special techniques such as immunocytochemistry (ICC, see Chapter 8) or special stains (see Chapters 2, 3, and 4) may be required before a definitive diagnosis can be given and will also be recorded on the report (you will read more about these investigations later in this book). For cancer diagnoses, it is important that the histopathology report provides the detailed pathological information that enables appropriate treatment to be selected (following discussion at the multidisciplinary team meetings) and to provide information on prognosis. Guidance is provided in The Royal College of Pathologists (RCPath) datasets, available for all cancer sites. These aim to standardize pathology reports by specifying how specimens should be handled and detailing items of information that must be included in reports, such as tumour size, type and stage, and assessment of surgical margins, and other information that is recommended but not essential. The datasets serve as a helpful aide memoire for pathologists and facilitate the adoption of proforma style electronic reporting instead of free text, which can make the information more easily accessible and

BOX 1.4 Lean production methodology

Lean methodology is a way of improving practice and being more effective with fewer resources, be that staff or consumables. Lean involves analyzing current practice and looking for activities that are wasteful and inefficient, and looking to remove them or adjust to gain efficiency.

Cross reference
You will read more about accreditation in Chapter 17.

electronically transferable. The RCPath Tissue Pathway documents also give guidance for handling non-cancer specimens. Information required for the national Cancer Outcomes and Services Dataset is similar to that specified in the RCPath datasets.

Many of the practices advocated by Lean found a common link with those already established in laboratories following the introduction of a system of laboratory accreditation (see Box 1.5).

BOX 1.5 Accreditation systems

Accreditation is the process of an external body measuring the compliance of a laboratory with an agreed set of standards. The international standard for laboratories is known as ISO 15189. This published standard lists about 900 criteria that laboratories should follow. The standards are categorized into management and technical standards. Laboratory accreditation is not mandatory but is good practice. Would you want your specimen handled by a laboratory which did not review its practices?

It is the responsibility of the laboratory manager to comply with any scheme the laboratory is enrolled in and establish systems of work which meet the standards.

Cross reference
Read more about electron microscopy in Chapter 15.

Needless to say, whichever standards you are working towards, the importance of standard operating procedures (SOPs; e.g in electron microscopy [see Box 1.6]), document control, and the implementation of a quality management system all have a place in a Lean laboratory.

BOX 1.6 Electron microscopy

The majority of histopathology reports are produced with the aid of the light microscope. However, the resolution of the light microscope is insufficient for the histological diagnosis of some conditions (e.g. minimal change glomerulopathy). The maximum resolution obtainable with the light microscope is approximately 200 nm, and radiation with a shorter wavelength is required to achieve higher resolution, such as that needed to visualize skeletal muscle striations (Figure 1.4). An electron beam can achieve a resolution of 0.2 nm. However, tissue sections for electron microscopy must be much thinner than for light microscopy; consequently, different embedding media (i.e. acrylic, epoxy or polyester resins) must be employed. In addition to the microscope itself, electron microscopy requires highly specialized equipment (e.g. ultramicrotome, glass knife maker). As a result of this costly equipment and limited application, such a facility is usually found only in specialist centres. You will read more about electron microscopy in Chapter 15.

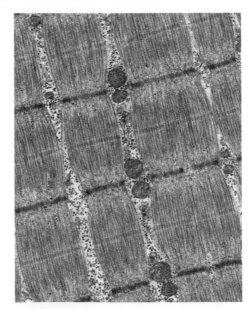

FIGURE 1.4
Electron micrograph of skeletal muscle tissue showing the characteristic striations.

1.12 Reporting

1.12.1 Slide review by the histopathologist

The request form and slides are then delivered to the histopathologist for examination. They will check to ensure that the request form and slides match. The H&E-stained section is examined and assessed for adequacy of sectioning and staining. The tissue type is identified and should match the details given on the request form. The biopsy is assessed for adequacy of sampling, its size, and preservation of the tissue. It is not uncommon to receive tiny biopsies that show crush and stretch artefact. The use of cauterizing instruments and laser equipment introduce thermal damage to the tissues. All these factors can hamper accurate interpretation of the material. (You will read more about this in the chapter on artefacts, Chapter 6.)

Next, the histopathologist will identify the tissue type to ensure that it matches the site of the biopsy indicated on the request form. Careful inspection of the tissue is carried out using low magnification (2–4× objective lens), medium-power magnification (10–20× objective lens) and high power (40–60× objective lens). Occasionally, a 100× objective lens is employed, but this requires the use of immersion oil between the lens surface and the slide to obtain an optimal image.

The histopathologist will adopt a systematic approach to analysis of the tissue depending on the tissue type and the disease process. For example, a skin biopsy is assessed by looking at the overall architecture of the tissue, inspecting the epidermis, the epidermal–dermal interface, the dermis, and the subcutaneous tissue. They will then assess the cellular composition of the tissues and identify any pathological changes. The assessment of individual parameters is then synthesized to form an impression of the disease process involved and render a diagnosis. The two main disease processes that may be encountered in tissues are inflammation and neoplasia. You can read more about these pathological processes in the chapter on reporting (Chapter 13).

In about 80–90% of histopathology requests, a diagnosis can be achieved on H&E stains alone. In the remaining cases, extra tests are required to establish the nature of the disease. Many of the following chapters discuss supplementary laboratory tests. See Box 1.7 for a brief summary of report content.

The histopathology report will contain:

- Patient details.
- Specimen type, site and date collected.

BOX 1.7 Supplementary laboratory work

Supplementary work	Description
Levels	The biomedical scientist will cut deeper into the block, typically producing three further levels that are spaced 50 μm apart. These are mounted on a single slide and stained with H&E.
Serial sections	The biomedical scientist will produce a ribbon of sequential sections mounted across multiple slides. The technique is usually used for very small diagnostic samples to yield the maximum amount of diagnostic material.
Histochemistry (special stains)	Histochemistry is used to highlight various biological materials in the tissue by different staining techniques (see Chapters 2, 3 and 4 for more information). Periodic acid Schiff (PAS): carbohydrates Diastase PAS: epithelial mucin Elastic van Gieson: elastin fibres and collagen Grocott: fungal hyphae Ziehl-Neelsen: acid–alcohol-fast bacilli

Immunocytochemisty	Immunocytochemistry employs specific antibodies to detect the location of antigens in tissue sections. The location of the bound antibody is visualized using a chromogen, typically producing a brown product. In tumour pathology the detection of specific antibodies aids diagnosis by providing information about the differentiation of the malignant cells. Most histopathology laboratories have a broad range of antibodies available (see Chapter 8 for more details).
	Cytokeratin (CK): epithelial cells **CD45: lymphoid cells** **S100: melanocytes and neural elements** **Desmin: muscle cells** **Vimentin: mesenchymal cells**
In situ hybridization	*In situ* hybridization is a method to detect nucleic acids (i.e. DNA and RNA) using a labelled DNA probe that hybridizes (joins) to complementary nucleic acid sequences in the tissue section.
	Kappa and lambda immunoglobulin light chains **HER2 (a growth factor receptor)** **Epstein–Barr virus** **Human papillomavirus**
Polymerase chain reaction	The polymerase chain reaction (PCR) is a method of amplifying short lengths of DNA from tissue samples. The PCR products are separated by agarose gel electrophoresis. The DNA bands can be visualized by staining with ethidium bromide and viewing the gel under ultraviolet light (see Chapter 11 for more information on molecular procedures).
	Kappa and lambda immunoglobulin light chains **T-cell receptor rearrangements**

- Date received.
- A macroscopic description—details of what the specimen looks like to the naked eye.
- A microscopic description—details of what the specimen looks like under the microscope.
- A conclusion.
- Occasionally advice about repeat specimens or treatment.
- The report will also be coded using SNOMED codes or ICD10 codes.
- Name of the person reporting the case.
- Name of the person authorizing the case.
- Date of authorization.
- Date of printing (if relevant).

1.12.2 Histopathology within the multidisciplinary team

Key Point

The multidisciplinary team is a group of healthcare professionals from different specialties (commonly medicine, surgery, radiology, pathology and oncology) who come together to discuss patient results and clinical history and plan what is the best treatment for them.

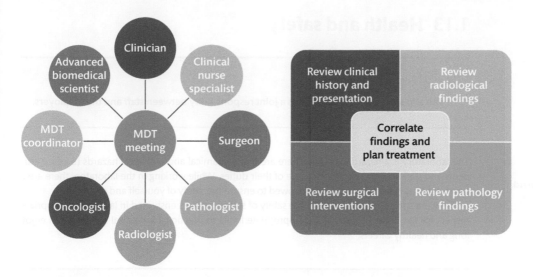

FIGURE 1.5
The multidisciplinary team (MDT) meeting is usually a weekly meeting where the clinical team involved in patient management and treatment come together. The teams focus on a single body system such as skin or upper GI tract. The meeting will discuss new patients and those where diagnostic interventions and treatments are ongoing. Bringing different healthcare professionals together facilitates the review of information and results in a better outcome for the patient. The introduction of MDT meetings over 20 years ago has improved patient outcomes through the simple sharing of patient information.

Histopathology services are most effective when the tissue is examined in the context of a patient's clinical signs and symptoms. In some instances an accurate diagnosis can only be achieved by the synthesis of information from sources such as the clinical examination, imaging modalities (ultrasound, X-ray, computed tomography [CT], magnetic resonance imaging [MRI]), and other laboratory tests. This highlights the importance of communication between clinicians and those providing diagnostic information. In modern-day cancer patient management, the involvement of multiple healthcare professionals forms the basis of regular weekly meetings to discuss individual cases. These meetings are termed multidisciplinary team (MDT) meetings. You will read more about the role of these meetings later on in this chapter and throughout this book. Needless to say histopathology reports play an integral part in overall patient management. The important point to remember is that no biomedical discipline stands on its own but is invariably interlinked with several others, providing information that combines to make the whole interpretive exercise of patient diagnosis complete. It's a bit like pieces of a jigsaw that come together and fit neatly to show us the overall features of any given pathological disease process. Thus all the biomedical disciplines, although unique in many ways, are all either directly or indirectly linked. A review of all the patient's investigative tests performed in several biomedical disciplines is often explored at these important MDT meetings (Figure 1.5). The end result is planned patient treatment and management regimes agreed by a wide cross section of experts from a pool including general clinicians, nursing staff, surgeons, radiographers, pathologists, biomedical scientists and oncologists.

SELF-CHECK 1.7

Which professionals are involved in the decisions upon which patient treatment is based?

1.13 Health and safety

> **Key Point**
>
> Health and safety in the laboratory is a joint responsibility between staff and the employers.

Cross reference

For further information on risk assessments, see Chapter 17.

The laboratory is a hazardous place. There are many chemical and biological hazards to which students and staff are exposed in the course of their duties. While working in the laboratory there are a number of key rules that need to be followed to ensure the safety of yourself and of others.

There is a shared responsibility for the safety of self and others enshrined in law. With appropriate respect for the hazards (Box 1.8) and appropriate limits to practice, biomedical scientists can enjoy long and healthy careers.

> **Key Point**
>
> **Error logging**
>
> **Major errors would include:**
>
> An incorrect report sent out and the patient treated incorrectly.
>
> Harm that requires time off work from a staff member.
>
> **Minor errors would include:**
>
> Quality control failures picked up before the tests are authorized.

> **Key Point**
>
> **Why log errors?**
>
> Understanding how errors occur is the first stage in helping them to be prevented. Use of IT is important to record all aspects of errors and be clear about the corrective actions.

Important general health and safety factors to consider include:

- **Hazards associated with chemicals**. A wide range of chemicals which are potentially dangerous are employed in pathology laboratories. The risks associated with hazardous chemicals may be controlled by having adequate knowledge of the properties of these substances and protective equipment and preventive measures available.

- **Health hazard effects of chemicals**. Nearly all the chemicals can be irritants, given sufficient exposure to tissue, and can cause reversible inflammation especially to eyes, skin, and respiratory passages. The alkaline substances, strong acids, and dehydrating and oxidizing agents are particularly corrosive and can damage or destroy living tissues. Chemicals that are sensitizers cause allergic reactions in a substantial proportion of exposed subjects. Sensitization may occur at work because of the high exposure level, formaldehyde being a prime example. Chemicals including chloroform, chromic acid, dioxane, formaldehyde, nickel chloride and potassium dichromate, and dyes such as auramine O, basic fuchsin and Congo red, are carcinogenic.

- **Toxic materials**. These are capable of causing death by ingestion, skin contact, or inhalation at certain specified concentrations. Mercury, lead, arsenic, and a number of organic substances are cumulative poisons and are injurious to health on long exposure. Methanol is toxic; chromic acid, osmium tetroxide, and uranyl nitrate are highly toxic. Chemicals causing specific harm to select anatomical or physiological systems are said to have target organ effects. These are not immediately evident, but are cumulative and frequently irreversible. Xylene and toluene have neurotoxic effects and benzene can affect the blood.

- **Physical risks of chemicals/risk from fire and explosion**. Many of the commonly used organic solvents like diethyl ether, ethyl alcohol, methyl alcohol and acetone have flash points below 21°C and are highly flammable. Some have very low ignition temperatures and can even be ignited on contact with surfaces below red heat. Explosive chemicals are rare in histopathology, the primary example being picric acid. Certain silver solutions may become explosive upon ageing and they should never be stored after use. Oxidizers can initiate or promote combustion in other materials and may present a serious fire risk when in contact with suitable substances. Sodium iodate, mercuric oxide and chromic acid are some examples for oxidizers.

Actions to consider:

- **Safety measures while handling hazardous chemicals**. Even for substances with no known significant hazard, exposure should be minimized. Unless known to the contrary, assume that any mixture will be more toxic than its most toxic component and all substances of unknown toxicity are hazardous. The permissible exposure limits (PEL) of the Occupational Safety and Health Administration (OSHA) should be observed.

- **Control measures**:

  a) Minimize all chemical exposure by taking precautions. Seek replacements of less toxic equivalents (e.g. xylene substitute).

  b) Laboratory staff should have information on correct handling and disposal.

  c) Personal hygiene should be followed at all times (e.g. no eating and drinking in clinical areas).

  d) Personal protective equipment (PPE; e.g. goggles, laboratory coats, aprons [Figure 1.6]) should be worn at all times in clinical areas.

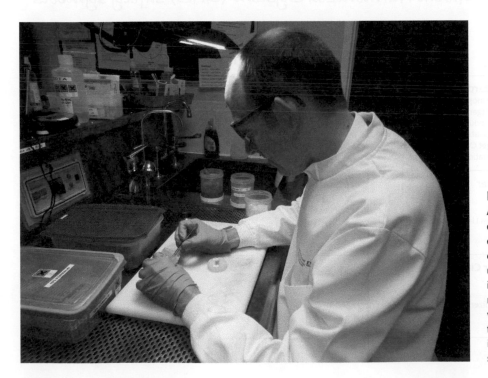

FIGURE 1.6

A biomedical scientist dressed in personal protective equipment working in a containment level 2 laboratory, undertaking specimen transfer in the specimen dissection room. The metal bench is ventilated to allow extraction of formalin fumes that accumulate in the environment when specimen pots are opened.

e) Labels and signage should be evident wherever there are risks.

f) Ventilation should be adequate and monitored regularly.

g) First aid should be available and adequate for the number of staff working in any given laboratory. This should be monitored.

h) Eye wash irrigation bottles should be available and checked to ensure they are in date for use.

i) Storage of hazardous chemicals (e.g. acids).

j) Spill kits and spill containment equipment should be provided (e.g. formalin and acids).

k) Waste disposal and recycling provision should be provided and be adequate.

1.13.1 Use of formalin

When using formalin always:

- Wear appropriate PPE. In situations where large volumes are used, some form of environmental control may be required (e.g. downdraft fume extraction and/or respirators). Environmental monitoring should be undertaken where formalin is in regular use.
- Read COSHH data sheets and local risk assessments.
- Adhere to local health and safety policies and procedures.

1.13.2 Use of solvents

- The solvents employed in tissue processing are hazardous. Check COSSH documentation.
- Fire is a major risk associated with industrial methylated spirit (alcohol). Be aware of local fire regulations.
- Wear PPE when handling tissue-processing solvent.
- Ensure that you adhere to local regulations on waste disposal.

BOX 1.8 Global Harmonized System (GHS) safety symbols

Hazard Communications Pictograms

Health Hazard	Flame	Exclamation Point
• Carcinogen • Mutagenicity • Reproductive Toxicity • Respiratory Sensitizer • Target Organ Toxicity • Aspiration Toxicity	• Flammables • Pyrophorics • Emits Flammable Gas • Self-Reactive • Organic Peroxides	• Irritant (skin & eye) • Skin Sensitizer • Acute Toxicity • Narcotic Effects • Respiratory Tract Irritant
Gas Cylinder	**Corrosion**	**Exploding Bomb**
• Gases Under Pressure	• Skin Corrosion/Burns • Eye Damage • Corrosive to Metals	• Explosives • Self-Reactives • Organic Peroxides
Flame Over Circle	**Environmental**	**Skull & Crossbones**
• Oxidizers	• Non-Mandatory • Aquatic Toxicity	• Acute Toxicity (fatal or toxic)

> ## Key Point
> Control of substances hazardous to health (commonly known as COSHH) is the process of managing risk to staff and the public through the selective and controlled use of chemicals. Where possible, safer alternatives are substituted.

Risk assessments are used in order to provide addition insight into potential risks and how to prevent harm to staff and others working in the laboratory environment. These are a form of audit of potentially harmful issues in any given environment or with any given procedural activity. They highlight the risks and then help to identify corrective and informative preventative actions. In addition, error-logging procedures record events that result in errors within the laboratory, some of which may be potentially harmful to patient samples or staff. These help to identify consistent errors and the sources of such errors, and in so doing they can help identify trends and pinpoint the cause of errors. You will read more about these issues in Chapter 17.

1.14 Public health considerations

Histopathology has a role to play in supporting public health, which is the branch of medicine concerned with the prevention of disease.

1.14.1 Screening

This is the process of identifying healthy people who may be at increased risk of disease. The screening provider then offers information, further tests, and treatment. This is to reduce associated risks or complications. At each stage of the screening process, people can make their own choices about further tests, treatment, advice or support.

Because the NHS invites apparently healthy people for screening, healthcare professionals have to ensure individuals receive guidance to help make informed choices and support throughout the screening process.

However, members of the public should have realistic expectations of what a screening programme does. Screening can:

- save lives or improve quality of life through early risk identification
- reduce the risk of developing a serious condition or its complications.

Screening does not guarantee protection. Receiving a low-risk result does not prevent the person from developing the condition at a later date.

In any screening programme there are false-positive and false-negative results:

- false positive can indicate: wrongly reported as having the condition
- false negative can indicate: wrongly reported as not having the condition.

The main purpose of national screening programmes is to detect diseases before they become clinically apparent, thus allowing early treatment, or to detect risk factors for a disease where early intervention may prevent its development. Some existing screening programmes are for non-malignant conditions such as tests performed during pregnancy (e.g. for infectious disease, Down's syndrome) or in the newborn (e.g. the bloodspot tests for sickle cell disease, cystic fibrosis, congenital hypothyroidism, and other conditions) and for the detection of abdominal aortic aneurysms. Histopathology has a particular role in the national cancer screening programmes for breast cancer and bowel cancer. Participation in breast screening is offered to women aged 50–70 years where mammography is the screening tool, and bowel screening uses faecal occult blood (FOB) detection for those aged 60–74 years (or the more recently introduced bowel scope screening in those over 55 years) as the trigger for further investigation. Suspected premalignant or cancerous lesions are biopsied and/or resected and these specimens are sent for histological analysis. In both programmes, the aim is to detect and treat cancers before they are symptomatic and to treat premalignant lesions before they become invasive. Both generate considerable workloads for histopathology departments, which in turn need to be UKAS-accredited centres. All histopathologists involved in reporting screening samples are required to participate in an appropriate EQA scheme. Cervical screening uses cytology, incorporating HPV testing, for initial investigation, which in turn leads to further histological investigation/treatment by cervical biopsy, cervical excision specimens or hysterectomy.

Screening has a high economic cost, not just in pathology, and therefore any screening test needs to fulfil a number of stringent criteria before it can be introduced UK-wide. In summary, the test must be for an important health problem, be simple, safe, validated and precise, and with existing policies in place for further investigation and treatment. Importantly, any benefits of screening tests must outweigh the potential harm resulting from having the test. Prostate-specific antigen (PSA) testing for prostate cancer is an example of one that does not fully meet the required criteria and for which introduction of national screening has not been approved. This is primarily because there is concern that it would lead to over-investigation and over-treatment of men who have no cancer or a low-risk cancer that does not require radical treatment.

1.15 Cancer registration

The National Cancer Intelligence Network (NCIN), operated by Public Health England, aims to improve cancer care and outcomes by promoting the national collection of high-quality data on patients diagnosed with cancer, and the subsequent availability of this data for audit and research. It does this through a network of UK organizations and the data collected cover many aspects of cancer care, including pathological diagnosis provided by the National Cancer Registration Service (NCRS). Reports generated in histopathology provide important pathological data that are submitted regularly via local cancer registries to the NCRS. These cancer statistics data are important for informing epidemiology, public health provision, and research. There are strict policies for collection, storage and access to the data. In January 2013 the Cancer Outcomes and Service Dataset (COSD) was established (replacing the National Cancer Database) and sets the standards for the histological information to be submitted regularly electronically to the cancer registries.

In many departments, a form of proforma reporting is used instead of free-text reporting, so that information required by COSD for the cancer registries is recorded consistently and is available in an easily transferable electronic format. Certain diagnostic category SNOMED codes (the standardized coding system for medical terms) that are added routinely to histopathology reports will automatically generate transfer of those reports to the cancer registry for analysis. Similar systems exist in other countries.

1.16 Laboratory information management systems

Record keeping is an essential component of the histopathology service (e.g. patient details, specimen details, macroscopic descriptions, numbers of blocks taken, block descriptors, stains, date of report, etc.) and a range of data has to be collected and placed on the departmental laboratory information management system (LIMS). A number of systems are available commercially and they play a pivotal role in the effectiveness of any department. A good system will help to streamline processes, reduce duplication of tasks, and reduce the risk of errors. It should also provide management information to aid decision-making, costing, and financial planning. It should also provide information to assist in audit, teaching, and training.

To reduce errors and streamline processes, barcode labels and readers are now in widespread use throughout the discipline. In addition, ancillary software systems have recently been developed to enhance departmental effectiveness (e.g. cancer reporting software, document control systems, incident reporting systems, interfaces with automated immunocytochemistry equipment, image capture systems, order-communications, etc.). A successful histopathology service must ensure that it has staff members who are computer literate in order to use this new technology to good effect. In the near future, interlaboratory links should help to develop histopathology networks.

1.17 Report production and distribution

Hard-copy reports are still commonly printed from the LIMS and submitted to the clinician by internal or external mail systems. Many establishments now allow access to the LIMS via the hospital network, thus allowing clinicians to access reports remotely. Results reporting systems, allied to order-communication systems, in time may do away with the need for hard-copy reports, and all reports could be viewed online.

1.18 Communication with clinicians

The main line of communication between the clinician caring for the patient and the histopathologist is the written report. This is filed in the patient's notes and is available through the hospital IT system. In some instances it may be necessary for the clinician to contact the histopathologist for advice on the content of the report and to discuss the implications for patient management. In addition, multidisciplinary team (MDT) meetings bring together all the clinical information, including any available imaging and the results of other laboratory tests (e.g. cytopathology, microbiology, haematology, biochemistry), and are particularly helpful in challenging cases where the definitive diagnosis is not clear and discussion can help to refine the diagnosis and guide patient management. Such meetings also review those patients who have recently completed treatment or patients who have recurrent disease. The histopathologist has a key role in communicating the diagnosis, along with any prognostic information obtained from the diagnostic biopsy material. If the treatment has involved surgery, the histopathologist accurately describes the extent of the cancer and whether or not the tumour has been adequately removed. In the case of certain surgical specimens it is necessary to correlate the pathological findings with intraoperative observations in order to establish the likelihood that the cancer has been completely removed.

1.19 Archiving

Key Point

Histopathology laboratories need a robust method to archive their specimen blocks and slides as material ideally should be retained for 30 years.

Laboratories must develop a policy for the retention and disposal of residual tissue following reporting. This is normally expressed in terms of the number of weeks a specimen is to be kept following reporting before disposal as clinical waste.

In the UK, histopathology blocks, slides, reports and request forms must be archived in accordance with the guidance issued by The Royal College of Pathologists and the Institute of Biomedical Science. In effect, histopathological material (i.e. blocks, slides and reports) must be retained for the lifetime of the patient for various reasons, including medicolegal purposes, effective patient treatment, research and teaching. Where possible, this means that blocks are retained for 30 years and slides are retained for 10 years.

1.20 Quality assurance

Ensuring the quality of a histopathology report is a key focus for the department and falls under the general heading of quality assurance. This can be defined as a planned and systematic series of actions which ensures confidence that the product or service fulfils the customer's expectations. In histopathology, this will incorporate internal quality control (IQC) and external quality assessment (EQA). The IQC measures employed aim to ensure that procedures are performed to expected standards. An example would be the use of known positive controls in histochemistry or with special stains. For example, a control slide known to contain tubercle bacilli should be included with every batch of slides stained with a Ziehl–Neelsen (ZN) stain. Only if the control slide is positive should the slides be submitted to the histopathologist for interpretation and reporting. It is imperative that the test sections be treated in exactly the same way as the control section.

Key Point

Control slides (both positive and negative) are essential for certain histological stains and histochemical reactions.

External quality assessment schemes are widespread throughout the field of pathology. Over 140 schemes operate from 24 centres based at major hospitals, research institutions, and universities throughout the UK. The services cover qualitative and interpretive investigations in andrology, clinical chemistry, genetics, haematology, histopathology, immunology, and microbiology. Specimens are distributed regularly to scheme participants and aim to cover the range likely to be encountered in clinical practice. Participants receive independent, objective, and impartial reports on their performance, enabling them to identify weaknesses and take appropriate action.

Education is the primary aim of EQA. United Kingdom participants who have persistent problems are offered advice and assistance by the scheme organizer/director and/or the relevant national quality assurance advisory panel. Schemes have close links with the professions, ensuring that their services are determined by clinical need.

In histopathology, schemes cover the diagnostic aspects of the service (e.g. UK NEQAS Breast Screening Pathology) and technical aspects (e.g. UK NEQAS Cellular Pathology Technique and UK NEQAS Immunocytochemistry and *In Situ* Hybridization). Further information is available at the UK NEQAS website. Other international schemes exist and remain popular (e.g. the Nordic scheme for immunohistochemistry).

It should be understood that quality assurance fulfils part of a wider context of quality management and clinical governance, which incorporates risk management, incident reporting, audit, staff training, staff competence, and accreditation.

Key Point

Knowledge of the microscopic appearance of the tissue structures a stain should and should not demonstrate is the key to providing good-quality slides for reporting.

Control slides (both positive and negative) are essential for certain histological stains and histochemical reactions.

Owing to the consequences of mislabelling specimens and loss or damage to irreplaceable samples, measures (IQC) to ensure the quality of the final result should be effective and robust.

High levels of quality assurance, incorporating both IQC measures and EQA, are essential if a clinician is to have the necessary confidence to take action (e.g. removal of a limb or the commencement of a programme of chemotherapy) on the strength of a histopathology report.

Accreditation provides assurance to clinical staff that the laboratory adheres to safe and effective practices.

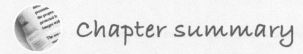

Chapter summary

After reading this chapter, you should know and understand:

■ the role of histopathology in the diagnosis of disease

■ the specimen journey through the laboratory

■ the principles of the Human Tissue Act 2004

■ the laboratory management systems that support an effective histopathology service

■ the role of UKAS (ISO 15189 Standards) in defining laboratory standards.

Further reading

● **Buesa RJ. Adapting lean to histology laboratories.** *Ann Diagn Pathol* 2009; **13** (5): 322–33.

● **Cross S ed.** *Underwood's pathology; a clinical approach* 6th edn. Edinburgh: Churchill Livingstone, 2013.

● **Health and Care Professions Council.** *Standards of conduct, performance and ethics.* London: HCPC, 2016.

● **Suvarna SK, Layton C, Bancroft JD eds.** *Bancroft's theory and practice of histological techniques* 7th edn. Edinburgh: Churchill Livingstone, 2012.

● **The Royal College of Pathologists.** *The retention and storage of pathological records and specimens* 5th edn. London: RCPath/IBMS, 2015.

Useful websites

■ Human Tissue Authority (**www.hta.gov.uk**)

■ Institute of Biomedical Science (**www.ibms.org**)

■ The Royal College of Pathologists (**www.rcpath.org**)

■ NHS Improvement (**https://improvement.nhs.uk**)

■ Nordic Immunohistochemical Quality Control (**www.nordiqc.org**)

■ Pathological Society (**www.pathsoc.org**)

■ UK Clinical Ethics Network (**www.ukcen.net**)

■ UK NEQAS (**www.ukneqas.org.uk**)

Discussion questions

1.1 What information is included on the histopathology request form and why is it important for the clinician to complete the form accurately?

1.2 Why are the majority of samples sent to the histopathology laboratory as 'fixed' specimens?

1.3 Why was it necessary to introduce the Human Tissue Act in 2004?

Acknowledgements

The authors are grateful to David Evans and Max Robinson, authors of this chapter in the first edition.

Answers to the self-check questions and tips for responding to the discussion questions are provided on the book's accompanying website:

 Visit www.oup.com/uk/orchard2e

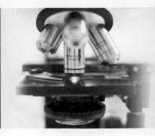

2

Fixation and specimen handling

David Muskett

Learning objectives

By the end of this chapter you should be able to discuss:

■ The need for timely specimen transfer to the laboratory.

■ The need for accurate specimen reception.

■ The principles of specimen fixation.

■ The need for specimen decalcification and the means by which this can be achieved.

■ The need for accurate patient details supplied with samples.

2.1 Introduction

> ### Key Point
> Good pre-analytical histopathology is the bedrock of a well-run laboratory.

In Chapter 1, the basic principles and steps of histopathology have been established. We will now look at what happens to specimens on their journey through the laboratory in more detail. In this chapter we will investigate the way in which biopsies and resections are first handled in the laboratory. Once specimens arrive in the laboratory they follow a process to the point of diagnosis. The process for most specimens remains the same until the first slide has been viewed for diagnosis. This differs from specimens received in blood science laboratories, which are often prepared and handled differently depending on the blood tube used and the tests requested.

The initial haematoxylin and eosin (H&E)-stained slide provides much valuable information about the state of the tissue, leading to the appropriate selection of supplementary tests.

2.1.1 In the clinical environment

Key Point

It is key for the laboratory to understand the needs of clinical users and to work effectively with them; likewise it is important for users to understand what the laboratory needs.

Proliferation rate

A measure of the number of cells within a tumour that are in an active process of cell division. Often called the Ki-67 index, it is defined as the percentage of tumour cells showing nuclear staining with KI-67 antibody. As a general rule of thumb, the higher the proliferation rate of a tumour the worse the prognosis.

Mitotic count

An investigation to see the number of cells that are dividing within the tissue. Mitotic counts are usually measured as a percentage, or a number, per high-power field.

Oestrogen receptor

A nuclear-bound protein transcription factor, which acts to up- or down-regulate transcription. Oestrogen receptors are particularly significant in breast cancer patients. Oestrogen receptor (ER) status is positive in about 80% of breast cancer patients. When positive, patients are suitable for specific drug therapies, which limit the response to oestrogen and thus limit disease progression.

Breslow thickness

A measurement of the thickness of a malignant melanoma lesion through the skin surface. Usually measured in millimetres, the Breslow thickness has a prognostic value; as a rule of thumb, the larger the measurement the worse the prognosis.

Cross reference

You can read more about public health considerations in Chapter 1.

The information required from each specimen taken differs depending on what sample is taken and the clinical picture. Some specimens have a known diagnosis and just need histological confirmation; some specimens are taken because a differential diagnosis has been reached and histological examination is required to distinguish which of the options is correct; some specimens are taken following an incidental finding and there was no suspicion of any significant pathology prior to the procedure.

What does a clinician need to know?

The key expectations from the histopathology report can be summarized as follows:

- Diagnosis of the disease or condition
- Margin clearance in tumour pathology
- Specific prognostic indicators
    a) **Proliferation rates** of tumours (e.g. lymphoma)
    b) **Mitotic count** per high-power field
    c) Ratios of specific protein expressions on or within cells (e.g. breast tumours and **oestrogen receptor** and progesterone receptor [ER/PR])
    d) Direct measurements of tumour invasion, such as **Breslow thickness** in malignant melanoma.

What does society need to know?

Although cellular pathology samples are reported in (usually) the local hospital, the information about the diagnosis forms part of a larger **public health** picture for the nation. Cancer statistics are taken in most countries and forwarded to a central office where statistical and demographic data is collected and analysed. This helps countries understand the changing face of health. It helps governments plan and focus health policy and resources.

2.2 Specimen collection

Key Point

Specimens should be tracked and transported quickly and safely to the laboratory.

Specimens need to be transported from the operating theatres and clinical areas to the laboratory. Sometimes this is from one part of a hospital to another and sometimes between hospital sites. In certain circumstances differing hospital organizations provide laboratory services for another hospital. Where specimens are transferred this should be done safely, in appropriate environmental conditions and in a timely manner. There needs to be an appropriate chain of custody from source to the receiving laboratory that allows locations of specimens to be noted. This is particularly important in the rare event of a lost specimen. The investigator should be able to locate the specimen down to a narrow field of areas.

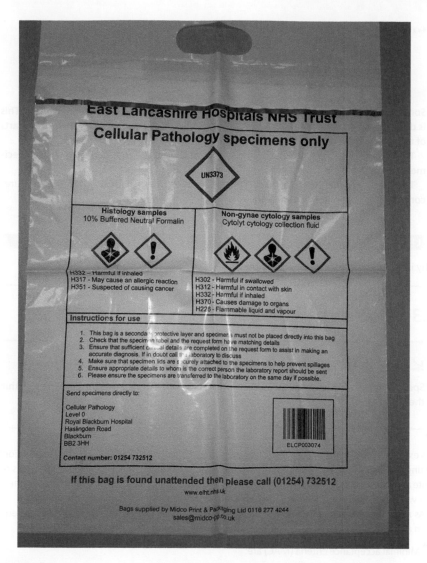

FIGURE 2.1
A specimen transport bag. Note the bag is barcoded to allow tracking through the stages of transport until it reaches the laboratory. The bag also contains some instructions for users and the contact details of the laboratory.

Specimens need to be transferred to the laboratory in a secondary protective layer either in a specimen box or transport bag (Figure 2.1).

2.2.1 Tracking specimens to the laboratory

The transport of specimens may be tracked to the laboratory in a number of ways.

1. When specimens are taken within the same site they are often walked up to the laboratory with a book in which specimens are signed for.

2. Fax sheets where the laboratory confirms receipt back to the clinic.

3. Specimens tracked to transport bags which are tracked between collection stations.

4. Electronic specimen ordering with an electronic receipting module.

BOX 2.1 Specimen resection transportation to the laboratory

Some laboratories prefer resection specimens to be transferred fresh to the department. This is done so that specimens can be inked and sliced to allow fixative to access the deep parts of the specimen.

This approach requires laboratory dissectors to be available on demand to slice specimens, and a free dissection bench.

There are also methods for vacuum-packing specimens in theatre for temperature-controlled transport to the laboratory.

SELF-CHECK 2.1

Why is it important to keep track of samples?

2.3 Specimen reception

Key Point

Specimen reception ensures the accurate matching of the specimen to the patient within the laboratory.

It is essential that the material for investigation is received in the laboratory in a suitable condition for testing (e.g. Box 2.1 and Box 2.2). For the laboratory to handle specimens correctly laboratories need quite a lot of information about what the sample is, which patient it is from, who is requesting the test, and who wants the report. Figure 2.2 shows a laboratory request form and specimen pot.

As an absolute minimum the following patient information should be provided on both request form and samples:

- Minimal acceptance criteria (MAC) are:
- Full surname
- Full forename
- One other identifier (e.g. date of birth, NHS number, hospital number).
- Details of the sample (e.g. skin, bone, etc.).

FIGURE 2.2

A specimen request form and specimen pot. The specimen and the request form must have matching patient details on the pot and form. Real patient and specimen details are not used in this image to maintain patient confidentiality. If specimen details on the pot and request form do not match then the sample should be rejected and either be returned to the clinic or the clinical staff asked to correct/amend the details.

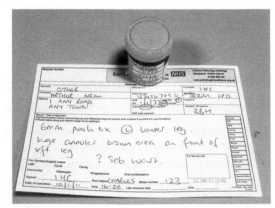

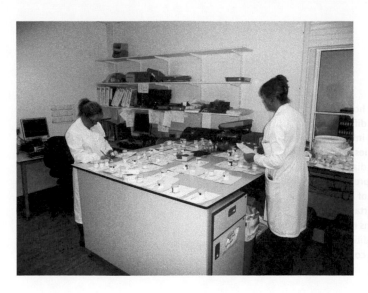

FIGURE 2.3
A busy specimen reception area. The specimens in the picture are biopsy samples and are sent in yellow-topped pots. The samples are being sorted and matched on the bench.

The request form may also ask for all of these items (if appropriate) in addition to the minimum data. The laboratory will provide instructions to users on how the specimen should be taken and transferred to the laboratory. Figure 2.3 shows a typical specimen reception area in a busy histology laboratory.

BOX 2.2 Specimen reception

When specimens are received into the laboratory it is important to check the details on the request form and the specimen pot. If there are any discrepancies, for example in the name and date of birth of the patient on the pot and on the request form, then the specimen should be returned for correction to the person requesting the specimen. A record of this error should be logged so that any patterns of mistake can be followed up with the service users.

SELF-CHECK 2.2

What are the implications of specimens not being linked correctly to the right patient?

Cross reference
See Chapter 17 where audit trails and quality issues are discussed in greater detail.

2.3.1 Clinical information

Key Point
Accurate and complete clinical information assists in creating a rounded clinical picture for the pathologist reporting the case.

When samples arrive in the laboratory, the type of specimen and the clinical history dictate the way samples are handled. If some vital clinical information is not supplied then it is possible that diagnosis can be compromised, incomplete, or incorrect (Box 2.3).

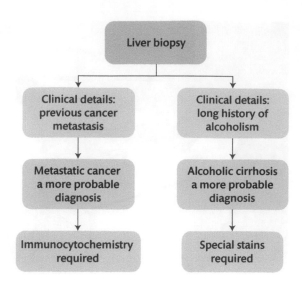

FIGURE 2.4
A flow chart showing how liver biopsies are handled differently as a result of the clinical information provided. Liver biopsies are usually only 2 mm in diameter and so the sample is precious, and therefore careful use of available material is very important. Wasting tissue sections may result in the need for an additional biopsy to be taken to confirm a diagnosis.

Cross reference
Read more about the identification of tumours in the immunocytochemistry and reporting chapters (Chapters 8 and 13, respectively).

For example, liver biopsies can be handled completely differently based on the clinical information provided. If patient 'A' has had a previous colonic cancer and had lymph node involvement with tumour, **immunocytochemistry** will be required to investigate the presence of metastatic cancer, as this is the most likely differential diagnosis. Patient 'B', who had a history of alcoholism and presents with decreasing liver function tests, will require special stains to investigate primary liver function. This is summarized in Figure 2.4.

CLINICAL CORRELATION: LIVER BIOPSY

The liver has many differing functions and a liver biopsy is a very valuable diagnostic tool for assessing a range of disease states. In the histopathology laboratory about six extra stains are routinely performed on medical liver biopsies. This gives lots of extra information. The amount of clinical material available is limited and must be used wisely.

Cross reference
Read more on special stains in Chapter 5.

BOX 2.3 *Full clinical information helps the laboratory to make a full diagnosis*

A single patient may have many biopsies taken. Therefore, it is important for the reporting pathologist to be aware of the previous clinical history. Often a small diagnostic biopsy—sometimes an endoscopic sample 2 mm in diameter, or a needle core of tissue 2 mm wide by 10 mm long—will be taken to assess the nature of the patient's cancer. This sample will lead to a diagnosis and the planning of treatment. The plan itself may result in further surgical procedures, known as a therapeutic biopsy or resection.

The storing of patient results enables any new pathology to be correlated with that identified in previous samples. This is of particular importance when monitoring patients with recurrent cancers.

Timeliness

The processing of samples, and return of results, can be affected by a number of time factors. For example, some laboratories can serve multiple hospitals, such that the sheer workload may place a limit on how quickly a sample can be processed. Also, while most laboratories provide a collection service for samples from GP surgeries within their service provider areas, the size of collection areas may mean that collections may only happen daily at best.

Most histopathology samples will not be available for reporting until the next working day from receipt at the earliest. Any specimen requiring more urgent handling will need to be highlighted and discussed with the laboratory (see also Box 2.4).

CLINICAL CORRELATION: TURNAROUND TIME

Patients with suspected cancer in the UK can expect to receive their results back within 14 days of the first GP appointment. Included in this time are the hospital appointment and the laboratory diagnosis. Rapid results mean the patients can be treated quickly, which helps with their clinical management. The laboratory will be monitoring turnaround data for all samples including key data on biopsy turnaround, collection to receipt times from clinics, and time taken on laboratory and reporting functions.

SELF-CHECK 2.3

Why is clinical information important?

2.3.2 Urgent samples

Urgent samples are received when the patient needs urgent clinical intervention based on the histopathology report. Samples may be urgent because the patient is on the operating table, as in the case of patients requiring rapid frozen sections, or they may have a rapidly deteriorating medical condition which needs clinical intervention. Patients who present with suspected cancer require their reports within two weeks so treatment can be planned.

Urgent samples fall into two groups:

- Frozen sections
- Urgent fixed specimens.

Frozen sections

Frozen sections offer a means to report histopathology specimens rapidly. The patients are often sedated, or under general anaesthetic, and in the operating theatre waiting for the diagnosis before the operation can proceed. The specimens are frozen using either liquid nitrogen, freezing sprays, a **Peltier plate**, or carbon dioxide.

Urgent fixed samples

Hospitals deal with many patients. Some can be treated in a measured manner with planned surgery and treatment. Other patients present with symptoms only when they are very ill. Patients who present with late symptoms are often difficult to diagnose and therefore urgent histopathology samples are removed from the patient. They may be **endoscopic biopsies** or **needle core specimens**. Urgent fixed samples include lesions or nodules which can be excised as a discrete entity but where clinicians are anxious to plan future surgery or treatment.

Peltier plate
A bimetallic strip through which an electric current is passed. The electric current causes one side of the bimetallic strip to cool; this is known as the Peltier effect.

Cross reference
You will read more about frozen sections later in this chapter and in Chapter 7.

Endoscopic biopsies
Tissue obtained using a flexible tube (endoscope) with a grip function on the end. The endoscope is inserted into the mouth or anus and allows samples to be taken from within the GI tract without the need for invasive surgery.

Cross reference
See also Case Studies 5.13, 9.15, 13.3 and 15.1 in Chapters 5, 9, 13 and 15, respectively, on malignant melanoma.

CASE STUDY 2.1 Urgent skin sample for suspected melanoma

A 63-year-old male patient presents at his GP with a slightly itchy, darkly pigmented lesion with an irregular border. In recent months the lesion has grown significantly. The GP suspects a malignant melanoma. A rapid appointment is made at the local hospital dermatology department and the patient is biopsied three days later. The excised skin lesion is placed in formalin and sent to the laboratory for urgent reporting. After processing, three levels are cut on the three blocks and the reporting pathologist suspects malignant melanoma, and immunocytochemistry is performed to confirm this. The case is reported and the results sent back to the consultant dermatologist and the GP. The whole process, from biopsy to report, took eight days, hence the process is urgent.

BOX 2.4 Working hours in histopathology

Historically, histopathology laboratories have offered a week-day office-hours service; however, in the push for reports to be returned more quickly, and the extended working hours seen in clinics and theatres, laboratories are considering Saturday and Sunday working patterns.

2.4 Cell and tissue preservation

Fixatives
Preservatives for cells and tissues.

Michel's transport medium
An isotonic salt solution which does not degrade or fix specimens.

Autolysis
The process of cellular degradation by the release of intracellular enzymes.

Eosinophilia
Enhanced staining with eosin where sections will look much more pink than usual.

Putrefaction
Decomposition of cells by bacterial or fungal action.

Fixation
The process of chemically preserving or stabilizing cells to prevent autolysis.

> ### Key Point
> High-quality tissue preservation is key in the majority of histopathology tests.

A majority of routine specimens received in the laboratory are suitable for formalin fixation, but not all of the subsequent tests required are compatible with fixation. Therefore, before the sample is taken, it is important to know which tests will be required and arrangements made to receive the samples either fresh or in **Michel's transport medium** in the case of skin samples for **immunofluorescence**. When tissue is removed from the body it dies due to the absence of oxygen and food, and the build up of waste material. The DNA, proteins, sugars, and fats start to deteriorate, initially through the build up of waste products and the uncontrolled release of proteases. This process is known as **autolysis**. Autolysed cells stained with haematoxylin and eosin (H&E) show enhanced cytoplasmic staining or **eosinophilia** (i.e. more pink) and reduced nuclear staining (less purple) due to the breakdown of RNA molecules in the cytoplasm and the breakdown of DNA molecules in the nuclei. Later, bacterial or fungal contamination can cause further destruction of cells and tissues, which is a process known as **putrefaction**. If the shape and structure of the cells deteriorate then diagnostic analysis becomes impossible. Therefore, the first part of the histopathology process involves making sure the cells do not deteriorate. Prevention of cellular deterioration is achieved by **fixation** or freezing. The nature of preservation in histopathology is to keep cells in as life-like a state as possible. For example, onions are pickled in vinegar to preserve them and keep them edible. At a cellular level, the process

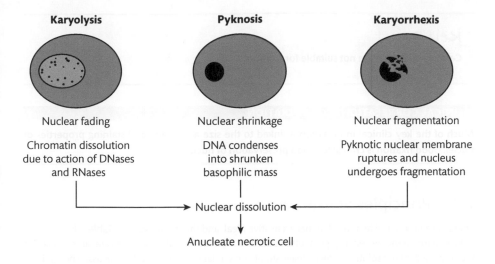

Karyolysis	Pyknosis	Karyorrhexis
Nuclear fading	Nuclear shrinkage	Nuclear fragmentation
Chromatin dissolution due to action of DNases and RNases	DNA condenses into shrunken basophilic mass	Pyknotic nuclear membrane ruptures and nucleus undergoes fragmentation

→ Nuclear dissolution ←

Anucleate necrotic cell

FIGURE 2.5

Diagram to show cellular changes that occur post-mortem (apoptosis and pyknosis). The aim of good fixation is to preserve material and prevent negative cellular changes such as these.

of autolysis is seen as **karyorrhexis** and **apoptosis** (Figure 2.5) and also **pyknosis**. The freezing of histopathology samples occurs only in a minority of cases where the tests required are incompatible with the chemicals used in fixation. Examples of tissues that should be frozen on receipt are muscle biopsies, specimens for immunofluorescence and suspected rare tumours where molecular studies may be of interest.

BOX 2.5 unusual fixatives

Admiral Nelson was placed in a barrel of rum to preserve his body until he returned to port after being killed on HMS Victory. He was later buried in St. Paul's Cathedral.

Fixation aims to preserve cells and tissue constituents in as close to a life-like state as possible. Essentially, it is concerned with the stabilization of proteins within the tissue and arresting the effects of autolysis and bacterial decomposition (Box 2.5). However, cell preservation is only part of the fixation effect. Fixatives impart additional benefits for the histologist as they allow the tissues to undergo further preparative procedures without change and make the cellular components more easily stained by dyes. It is important to realize that the appearance of the tissue after fixation is artefactual. The stabilization of proteins is necessary to prevent their diffusion during subsequent processing, but this also changes the structure and appearance of these proteins.

Information is available when the nucleus is examined. The size, shape, texture, and staining properties of the nucleus alter in differing pathological conditions.

Not all specimens received in the laboratory are suitable for fixation. This is because the subsequent tests required on some specimens are not compatible with fixation. It is important to know what tests will be required before the sample is taken. However, the majority of specimens received in the laboratory are received in fixative, which is ideal for the majority of routine samples. The others are most probably received either fresh or in **Michel's transport medium**. Michel's transport medium is not a fixative but a solution of salts plus an antibacterial agent, which acts to sustain biopsies in an osmotically balanced solution during transportation to the laboratory. It is used mainly with skin and mucosal samples for investigation of inflammatory disorders.

Specimens unsuitable for fixation are:

- Muscle biopsies for enzyme histochemistry.
- Skin/mucosal biopsies for investigation of inflammatory skin conditions.

Karyorrhexis

The destructive fragmentation of the nucleus of a dying cell whereby its chromatin is distributed irregularly throughout the cytoplasm.

Apoptosis

The process of programmed cell death. The nuclei are seen to reduce in size, stain much more intensely and show nuclear fragmentation, chromatin condensation, and chromosomal DNA fragmentation.

Pyknosis

The irreversible thickening of nuclear DNA within a cell during death.

Cross reference

As you will read in Chapters 11 and 12, the nucleus is the controlling part of the cell; it is the home of DNA.

Cross reference

You can read more about inflammatory skin disorders in Chapter 8.

> ## Key Point
>
> Certain specimens are not suitable for fixation.

CLINICAL CORRELATION: GOOD FIXATION

Much of the key clinical information is linked to the size and shape and staining properties of nuclei. Good fixation is critical for good preservation of nuclei.

2.4.1 Principles of fixation

There are a number of features that make a fixative ideal, and these are shown in Table 2.1.

In addition to the preserving agent, often salts or buffers are included. The salts are added to adjust the osmolality of the solution, which ideally should be similar to the fluid within the tissue being fixed. This ensures that cells do not shrink or swell. Figure 2.6 shows how red blood cells alter in solutions of differing strengths.

2.4.2 Mechanisms of fixation

Fixation is a chemical process by which the constituent molecules within cells can be manipulated in several ways (Table 2.2).

Cross-linking (or additive) fixatives act by binding amino acids within proteins to adjust their three-dimensional (3D) structure, preventing autolysis and putrefaction. Formalin fixation is not

TABLE 2.1   Features of an ideal fixative.

Factor	Reason
Kill cells quickly and evenly	This stops the build-up of harmful metabolites that disrupt the cellular appearance.
Penetrates tissues quickly and evenly	The solution diffuses through the tissue quickly.
Prevents autolysis and putrefaction	Stops cellular functions immediately, preventing self-destruction and microbial damage.
Does not shrink or swell the cell	Maintains the normal shape and size of the cell in relation to the size *in situ*. This allows for meaningful diagnostic and prognostic measurements.
Prepares the tissue for later treatment	Permits use of the tissue in a wide range of further tests. This includes making the tissue harder.
Prevents desiccation and drying of tissue	Keeps the cells hydrated.
Safe to use	Does not cause harm to the operator when using the fixative. Does not require expensive disposal regimes.
Reasonably priced	As large quantities of fixative are used in the routine laboratory, the cost should not be prohibitive.
Tolerant in use	Specimens are likely to be placed into fixative by non-histopathology staff in many different ways. A tolerant fixative allows subsequent testing of the sample, whether the specimen has been in the fixative 12 hours or 120 hours.

Hypertonic	Isotonic	Hypotonic

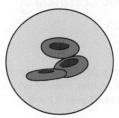 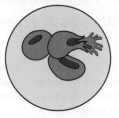

Cells lose fluid and shrink	Normal shape and size maintained	Cells swell and can rupture

FIGURE 2.6
Diagram showing how RBCs behave in solutions of differing concentration. The aim of an ideal fixative is to preserve cells without shrinking or swelling because the measurements of cells and tissues can be important in assessing prognosis (e.g. measurement of the Breslow thickness in malignant melanoma).

suitable when handling specimens for enzyme histochemistry as the cross-linking acts to denature many enzymes.

Precipitating or (non-additive) fixatives act by removing water from the cellular matrix, which acts to disrupt the 3D (tertiary) protein structure, thereby precipitating the protein.

The use of fixation results in significant changes to the tissue structure and components. These changes are beneficial in terms of tissue preservation; however, it is important to recognize that some tissue components are extremely **labile** and so would be readily inactivated by the use of these chemicals. As such, it is important to know what investigations may be required on individual samples so that the appropriate processing regimes can be employed. Fixation is a reversible process and much effort is undertaken to undo its effects (e.g. in **immunocytochemistry**) during antigen retrieval, which you will read more about in Chapter 8.

Well-fixed cells show good nuclear detail, being neither swollen nor shrunken, the integrity of the general architecture is not disturbed, and cellular proteins are well preserved for future tests.

Poorly fixed cells have poor nuclear detail and may be swollen or shrunken. The general architecture of the piece of tissue may be distorted, and cellular proteins may be lost. Fatty tissue is susceptible to poor fixation as the aqueous reagents do not penetrate fat well.

Labile
Able to undergo change easily (i.e. unstable).

Key Point

Poorly fixed specimens may not yield all the appropriate information. Poorly fixed specimens can seriously compromise diagnosis.

Tissue fixation is usually achieved by means of chemicals, but the same or similar effects can be achieved using heat. Heat is used to precipitate proteins and to prevent degradation; however, care must be taken not to overheat or damage the tissue. Microwave ovens can be used to heat at a steady temperature. Heating also allows fixation to take place at a much faster rate, reducing the fixation time from hours to minutes. Heat can also be used in combination with chemical fixatives, and this is covered later in the chapter, in Section 2.5.3, in relation to automated processors.

TABLE 2.2 Various types of fixative in common use and their modes of action.

Cross-linking	Precipitating	Compound
Glutaraldehyde	Alcohol	Picric acid
Formaldehyde	Acetone	

CASE STUDY 2.2 *Poor fixation can seriously impede cellular pathology reporting*

Fixation is essential to the steps undertaken in the histopathology laboratory. The four images below are from the same case. The two images on the left are of poorly fixed tissue and the two on the right are of well-fixed tissue. There is considerable difference in the staining intensity seen in the lower two images, both of which show staining for CD20, a B-cell marker (Figure 2.7 a–d).

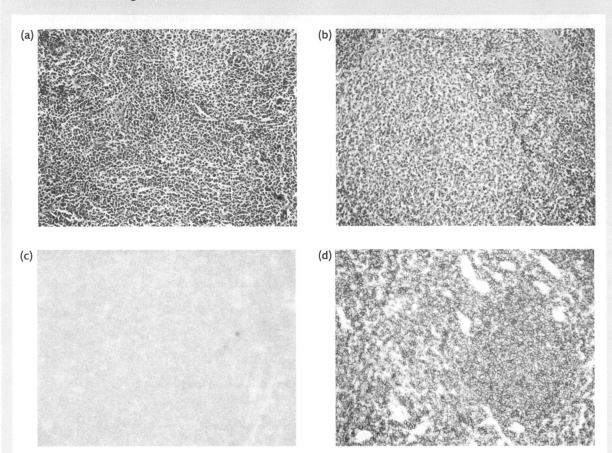

FIGURE 2.7

Four images from the same diagnostic case. Images **a** and **c** are from a poorly fixed piece of tissue; images **b** and **d** are from tissue that has been fixed for a longer period of time. **a.** A poorly fixed lymph node. Note that the nuclear detail and architecture are poorly preserved. **b.** A better fixed piece of the same lymph node. **c.** A CD20 marker for B cells on the poorly fixed tissue. Note the weak and erratic expression of the CD20 marker. **d.** A CD20 marker for B cells on well-fixed tissue from the same case. Note how it differs from that seen in Figure 2.7c. The localization of the marker is crisp and membrane-bound (see also Box 2.6).

BOX 2.6 CD20

CD20 is a membrane-bound protein found on most B cells, which are a subtype of lymphocytes present in the bloodstream and in secondary lymphoid organs such as the tonsil and spleen. They are also found at sites of inflammation. The CD20 protein can be demonstrated using targeted monoclonal antibodies, a good example of which is the clone L26 raised against a portion of the protein.

CLINICAL CORRELATION: LYMPHOMA

Lymphoma is a solid malignant tumour of white blood cells or lymphocytes. It is a common type of cancer that presents a number of diagnostic challenges to the laboratory. Many malignant lymphocytes look the same unless immunocytochemical methods are applied, making accurate diagnosis by H&E staining alone impossible.

Cross reference

You will find further information about the value of histopathology in the diagnosis of lymphoma later in this book.

SELF-CHECK 2.4

Why do laboratories use fixatives?

2.4.3 Factors affecting fixation

Fixation is a chemical process that is affected by a range of environmental factors (Table 2.3). The manipulation of these factors can accelerate the speed of fixation.

TABLE 2.3 Factors affecting the rate of fixation.

Temperature	The hotter the fixative, the quicker the fixation. Microwave processors utilize the heating of fixatives to allow quick processing schedules.
Size of specimens and penetration of fixative	Large specimens take longer to fix than small specimens. The penetration rate is the rate at which the chemicals permeate the tissue. This may be only four or five millimetres a day; consequently, large resections need slicing open before the processes of autolysis destroys the detail within the tissue.
Changes of volume	The larger the volume of the fluid to specimen ratio the more rapidly fixation will take place. It is recommended that there is 20 times as much fixative as specimen, although this is not always possible.
pH and buffers	The addition of buffer does slow the fixation process slightly, but it does ensure that the chemicals are at the correct pH. Acidic formalin fixatives react with tissues and can create pigments.
Osmolarity	Fixatives should be the same osmolarity as the cells they are fixing. This will help to prevent shrinking or swelling.
Concentration of fixatives	The stronger the fixative the more rapidly fixation takes place.
Duration of fixation	The longer tissues are in fixative the more complete the fixation will be.

2.5 Key fixatives

No single fixative is suitable for all preparations. Many different fixatives exist, although the number in routine use is now relatively small.

The most commonly used fixative in the UK routine laboratory is neutral buffered formalin solution.

It is important that laboratories use similar fixation regimes as this allows laboratories to review one another's cases more easily and to compare methodologies. Bouin's solution is occasionally used for testicular biopsies and for intestinal biopsies in cases of suspected Hirschsprung's disease, due to the enhanced nuclear detail achieved following fixation in this fixative.

2.5.1 Formalin solutions

Key Point

A formalin solution, such as neutral buffered formalin, is the main fixative used in routine histopathology.

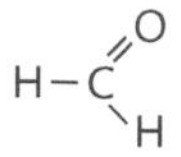

FIGURE 2.8

A molecule of formaldehyde, which is the active ingredient of formalin saline fixative. Note the double bond between the carbon and the oxygen, which gives the highly reactive aldehyde functional group.

Formalin is cheap, easy to make, keeps well on the shelf, and is easily transported. Formalin is an aqueous acidic solution that contains a concentration of dissolved formaldehyde gas (Figure 2.8). Acid formalin causes formalin pigment, which is a brown residue seen in red blood cells. Pigment is not seen when the pH of the solution is neutralized, so buffering agents are added in most circumstances. When purchased commercially in the UK it is usually supplied at a concentration of 37–40% formaldehyde. Traditionally, this solution has been considered to be 100% formalin. This solution is usually diluted (1 in 10) to give a formaldehyde concentration of 4%. This 10% formalin solution is the most commonly used fixative in routine laboratories (Boxes 2.7–2.12).

Use of formalin introduces a number of health and safety issues which impinge on the running of the laboratory.

Methylene bridges

$-CH_2-$ groups that link proteins.

Cross reference

You will read more about antigen retrieval in Chapter 8.

BOX 2.7 Formalin fixation: mode of action

Formalin in aqueous solution forms methylene glycol in a reversible reaction (Figure 2.9a).

Methylene glycol reacts with cellular protein moieties such as amine, guanidine, sulphydryl, and amide groups, and with lipids. The reaction with amine groups to form methylene bridges is seen in Figure 2.9b.

The fixation reaction is reversible and this feature is exploited in immunocytochemistry by the use of antigen retrieval.

$$H_2O + CH_2O \rightleftharpoons CH_2 (OH)_2$$

FIGURE 2.9A

The reversible reaction of formaldehyde with water to form methylene glycol.

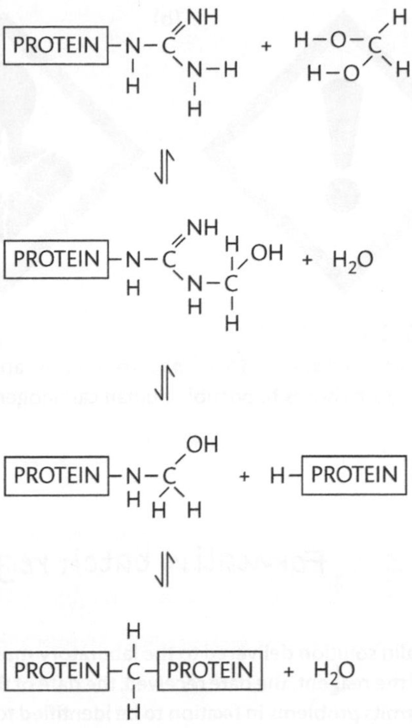

FIGURE 2.9B
The reaction of methylene glycol with proteins at the molecular level. The amine group of the protein (in this case the guanidine group of an arginine side-chain) is reacting with methylene glycol to form methylene bridges.

BOX 2.8 Health and safety: formalin

Colourless liquid
Causes burns (see Figure 2.10)
Very toxic by inhalation, ingestion, and through skin absorption
Readily absorbed through the skin
Possible human carcinogen (see Figure 2.10)
May cause allergic reactions
Causes watery eyes at levels over 20 ppm
First aid measures
Inhalation: remove to fresh air seek medical assistance if necessary.
Eye contact: rinse well with running water, seek medical advice if necessary.
Skin contact: rinse affected area, seek medical advice if necessary.

FIGURE 2.10
Global harmonized system (GHS) hazard symbols appropriate to formalin **a.** causes burns **b.** possible human carcinogen.

Global harmonized system (GHS) hazard symbols
An internationally agreed and recognized way of identifying hazardous chemicals.

BOX 2.9 *Formalin batch registration*

Each new batch of formalin solution delivered to the laboratory must be logged. The record should contain details of the reagent, the date received, the date of first use, and the date it is taken out of use. This permits problems in fixation to be identified to a specific batch.

2.5.2 How long does the fixation reaction take?

Key Point

Fixation rate

Fixation is divided up in to two parts: the penetration rate (the time it takes the fixative to reach the innermost part of the tissue), and the reaction time for the tissue to be fully fixed.

On average, the penetration rate for formalin in normal tissues is approximately 0.75 mm/hour at room temperature; therefore, the thicker the tissue the longer the fixation process will take. Once the formalin solution has penetrated the tissue fully, complete reaction takes approximately eight hours.

BOX 2.10 *Formalin fixation and the fixation of proteins*

Formalin is a protein fixative, but fixation of DNA is not ideal with this agent. Microscopically, the fixation process can be seen as cytoplasmic streaming on a periodic acid Schiff stain. As the formalin enters the cell the proteins are fixed first and any carbohydrate present is 'pushed' to the unfixed part of the cell, giving rise to the characteristic flow pattern that is seen microscopically (Figure 2.11).

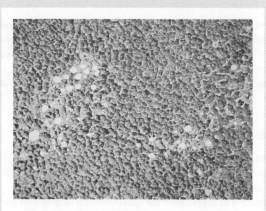

FIGURE 2.11

A PAS stain on a section of liver. Note that the glycogen positivity within each cell is uneven. This is known as cytoplasmic streaming. The fixative (formalin) fixes the protein but displaces the glycogen within the cell, which accumulates at the furthest point from the advancing fixative.

BOX 2.11 Formalin fixation: common errors and pitfalls

Inadequate length of fixation
Tissue not sliced before fixation
Faulty batches of solution
Incorrect pH of solution

SELF-CHECK 2.5

Why is formalin the fixative of choice in most histopathology laboratories?

2.5.3 Non-formalin fixatives (practical aspects)

Despite its tolerance and general all-round suitability, formalin is not the best fixative in all situations. Exceptions to the use of formalin as the initial choice of fixative include specimens requiring electron microscopy, where the use of glutaraldehyde (despite its inherent health and safety issues) remains the agent of choice.

Glutaraldehyde

Glutaraldehyde is an aldehyde fixative. It is a larger molecule (Figure 2.12) than formaldehyde and provides excellent **ultrastructural** preservation. It fixes tissue rapidly but does not penetrate tissue deeply, making it unsuitable for large samples. Specimens for electron microscopy are often cut into small (2 mm) cubes, which permits complete fixation of the tissue. Glutaraldehyde is a **respiratory sensitizer** and therefore must be handled with care.

Ultrastructural preservation

Preservation of the organelles (e.g. mitochondria, Golgi complex, etc.) within the cell.

Respiratory sensitizer

A chemical that irritates the lungs and may cause asthma.

Cross reference

You will read more about electron microscopy in Chapter 15.

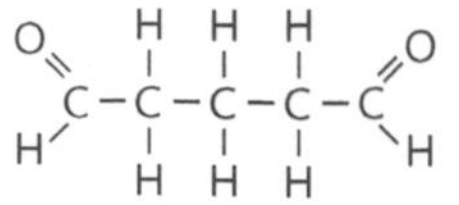

FIGURE 2.12

A molecule of glutaraldehyde. The structure is larger than that of formaldehyde and it has two aldehyde functional groups.

Bouin's fluid

Bouin's solution is a mixture of picric acid, alcohol, and formaldehyde. This yellow compound fixative is popular for the fixation of testicular biopsies, due to the improved appearance of the nuclear chromatin achieved in spermatogenic cells. It is also used for intestinal biopsies in the assessment of Hirschsprung's disease.

Others fixatives used even more rarely include Zenker's fixative, industrial methylated spirits, methanol, acetone, formaldehyde vapour, and commercial preparations.

Microwave fixation

The stabilization of proteins can also be achieved using microwave irradiation. This has the advantages of significantly improving the speed at which fixation can be completed and the absence of any noxious fixing chemicals.

An alternative approach is to supplement the usual chemical fixative with microwaves to speed up the fixation process. There is currently great interest in developing microwave-based automated tissue fixation and processing machines.

2.5.4 Specimens not for fixation

Key Point

Most specimens in the histopathology laboratory are received fixed or are for fixation; however, there are a few specimen types which must not be fixed.

Not all specimens to be investigated require fixation. Some specimens need to be handled more quickly than fixation can take place (i.e. in urgent cases). Some tissue elements react with the fixatives in a way that is unsuitable for diagnosis, such as samples for immunofluorescence studies, and where cells are required to be kept alive (i.e. cytogenetics samples).

Cytogenetics

Key Point

Cytogenetics can be a useful adjunct to routine histopathology in complex tumour cases.

Cytogenetics is the study of the structure of chromosomal abnormalities by the analysis of chromosome numbers. Tissue samples for cytogenetics analysis must be transferred in cytogenetic culture media, and sent directly to the cytogenetics laboratory.

CLINICAL CORRELATION: THE VALUE OF CYTOGENETICS

Cytogenetics is a branch of laboratory science that looks at chromosome abnormality and numbers. Cytogenetics is of particular interest in fetal and perinatal samples. Study of chromosomes can aid in diagnosis and explain the clinical presentation. In the cytogenetics laboratory, tissue samples are separated into cells and cultured to propagate them, from which DNA is extracted.

BOX 2.12 How do I know my tissue is well fixed?

The quality of tissue fixation is judged on morphology (the shape of the cells, their constituents, and tissues) and staining quality (the specificity of the staining reaction). Red blood cells should look bi-concave, and nuclear chromatin should be crisp and show aggregation into clumps towards the nuclear membrane. See Chapter 6 for further details about fixation artefacts.

Specimens for enzyme studies

Enzymes as proteins are fixed when a specimen is placed into fixative. Once in the fixative the cross-reaction adjusts the 3D structure of the molecule, rendering it unsuitable for further investigations, hence muscle biopsies are generally handled fresh.

2.6 Decalcification

> ### Key Point
>
> Bony specimens for routine processing need the calcium removing from the samples. This is a process known as decalcification.

After tissues have been fixed they are then ready for the next stage of laboratory investigation. Some tissues cut easily with a knife and require no further pretreatment. Some tissue structures (e.g. bone and teeth) are extremely hard due to the presence of a calcium phosphate salt (hydroxyapatite). This mineral is essential in life for these structures to perform their role, but unless this mineral is removed then the production of thin sections for microscopy will be problematic. The method of achieving this is termed decalcification as it is primarily calcium salts that are removed. However, during the process, materials other than calcium will also be removed, so a more accurate term to apply would be demineralization.

Calcium crystals may also be present in other tissues as part of a pathological process. Tissue such as breast may be X-rayed prior to being processed. The identification of this calcium has diagnostic significance and therefore it is important that it remains in the tissue.

> ### Key Point
>
> Specimens for investigation of metabolic bone disease are not suitable for decalcification.

Bone samples are not suitable for decalcification when they are to be studied for suspected disturbances to calcium metabolism (e.g. osteomalacia in adults or rickets in children). In these conditions, the amount of mineralized to non-mineralized bone is reduced. In order to be able to diagnose these conditions it is necessary to visualize the extent of both, and if the specimen is decalcified then it will be impossible to make this estimation. In these cases, the sample must be treated by embedding the **mineralized bone** into a hard embedding medium such as a plastic resin. This will permit suitable quality sections to be produced and stained.

Maceration

Loss of nuclear and cytoplasmic detail through degradation of connective tissue proteins.

Whichever decalcification method is employed there is a balance to be struck between speed of decalcification and preservation of cellular morphology. Generally, the speedier the rate of decalcification the greater the rate of destruction (**maceration**) of cellular morphology. This effect is exaggerated if tissue fixation has not been completed satisfactorily prior to commencing decalcification. The choice of decalcifying method and chemical will be influenced by the type of specimen investigated (i.e. a sample investigated for possible malignancy will be required much more rapidly than one for training and education purposes only). The strength of the acid affects the speed of decalcification.

Factors affecting the rate of decalcification are:

- Concentration of the acid used in the decalcifying agent
- Agitation of the tissue
- Saturation of calcium ions in the decalcifying solution.

Specimens must not be decalcified before fixation is complete as the decalcifying agent will cause excessive tissue maceration.

BOX 2.13 *Quality assurance*

Decalcifying agents are not suitable for work on specimens that require certain supplementary tests. Cellular iron detected using the Perls' method is removed when specimens are decalcified, leading to false-negative staining. Take care when interpreting decalcified sections.

2.6.1 Decalcifying agents

Key Point

Specimens may be decalcified by acid solutions or chelating agents.

Decalcifying agents fall into two main categories: acid decalcifiers and chelating agents.

Acids: Acid decalcifying agents act by reacting with the calcium in the tissue to form soluble salts.

Nitric acid: Very fast acting but produces the most tissue damage (see also Box 2.13). It is suitable for the controlled decalcification of very hard bones (e.g. skull).

Hydrochloric acid: This can be used alone or frequently as an ingredient of commercially available decalcifying solutions. Fast acting but produces less tissue damage than nitric acid.

Formic acid: This is much slower than nitric or hydrochloric acids and so its effect is more gentle. It is probably the most popular choice of decalcification fluid for most diagnostic histopathology applications.

Commercial solutions: A number are available on the UK and international markets. Most use hydrochloric acid but some use formic acid. Recently, formulations containing formic acid and formalin have been promoted that claim to permit 'concurrent fixation and decalcification', which contradicts the traditional edict of completing fixation before decalcification.

Chelating agents: These offer alternatives to the use of acids. They act as 'calcium sponges' continuously mopping up the free ionic calcium that is always present around mineralized bone. Chelating agents offer a gentler approach and may be the decalcifying agent of choice for tissue likely to require immunocytochemistry.

Ethylenediaminetetraacetic acid (EDTA): This is the main chelating agent used. Calcium removal is very slow and as a consequence there is minimal tissue damage. Probably the best option if there is no pressing demand for a speedy result. EDTA is the decalcifying agent of choice if immunocytochemistry is likely on the specimen (Box 2.14).

Trisodium citrate: This has a similar rate of demineralization as achieved with EDTA.

CLINICAL CORRELATION

Excessive decalcification can cause tissue damage or maceration. It is important to remove the tissue from this destructive solution as soon as possible.

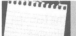

BOX 2.14 Bone marrow trephines

Bone marrow trephines are thin (3 mm) cores of bone usually taken from the iliac crest or sternum. Bone marrow is sampled to investigate the cellularity of the marrow, as in the case of suspected haematological malignancy or the investigation of anaemia of unknown cause. The core biopsy is fixed for 24 hours in formalin saline and then transferred to EDTA solution for 48 hours. The specimen is then processed along with other routine samples.

2.6.2 Testing the end point of decalcification

There are three key methods of checking whether the end point of decalcification has been reached:

- X-ray
- Chemical end-point testing
- Manual manipulation.

The 'end point' of decalcification occurs when all calcium ions have been removed from the specimen. A means of determining this point accurately is needed so that the tissue does not remain in acid solution longer than absolutely necessary. Use of X-rays provides the most complete assessment of decalcification, but is expensive. Chemical end-point testing makes use of the fact that insoluble calcium ammonium oxalate is produced from free calcium ions in the decalcifying fluid, with a cloudy solution indicating that decalcification is incomplete. Manual manipulation is the least specific method of assessing decalcification.

CLINICAL CORRELATION

Figure 2.13 shows a femoral head being sliced using a specially designed frame. The metal frame allows the slippery rounded femoral head to be held still before being sliced with a double-bladed hacksaw. The double blades of the hacksaw cut slices of 4 mm in thickness. This makes the specimen ideal for further fixation or decalcification.

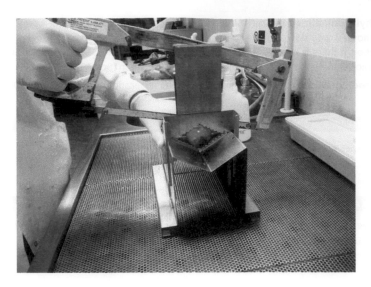

FIGURE 2.13
A femoral head in a specimen vice. The specimen is secured between metal teeth. The femoral head seen in the picture is being sliced by a special saw which has a double blade, allowing 4-mm-thick sections to be cut with 'relative' ease. The 4-mm slices can then be decalcified prior to processing. The decalcification process should take a few days.

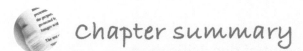

Chapter summary

In this chapter you have read about these important features:

- Speedy specimen transport from clinical areas such as theatres and clinics to the laboratory.

- Specimens need to be appropriately packaged to be transferred to the laboratory.

- Specimen details need to be accurately recorded on request cards and forms to ensure the correct diagnosis on the right patient.

- Clinical details are needed to help accurate diagnosis—failure to include appropriate clinical details may involve a waste of precious tissue to find out information not disclosed by clinicians.

- Fixation is essential for most specimens handled in the laboratory.

- Fixation involves preservation of tissue and prevention of autolysis and putrefaction.

- The most common fixative used in routine histopathology is formalin saline. It is a harmful solution and needs careful handling in the laboratory.

- Bony specimens are too hard for routine processing and need to be decalcified before processing starts.

Further reading

- Carson FL, Cappellano CH. *Histotechnology. A self-instructional text* 4th edn. EDS Publications, 2014.

- Kiernan JA. Formaldehyde, formalin, paraformaldehyde and glutaraldehyde: what they are and what they do. *Microscopy Today* 2000; **00-1**: 8–12.

- Open University. Introduction to histology (www.open.edu/openlearn/science-maths-technology/science/biology/introduction-histology/content-section-0).

- Orchard GE, Nation BR eds. *Cell structure and function*. Oxford: Oxford University Press, 2014.

- Suvarna SK, Layton C, Bancroft JD eds. *Bancroft's theory and practice of histological techniques*. Edinburgh: Churchill Livingstone, 2012.

 Discussion questions

2.1   Why do you think there are specimen acceptance criteria?

2.2   What are the changes cells and tissue undergo when they are removed from the body?

2.3   What are the principles of fixation?

2.4   What might be the implications of a poorly fixed specimen for accurate diagnosis?

2.5   What does formalin actually fix?

2.6   What are the key hazards associated with handling formalin?

2.7   What factors affect the speed of fixation?

2.8   What methods are used for decalcification?

2.9   How might the decalcification of tissues be speeded up? What automation could be used?

2.10 How is the end point of decalcification tested? What alternative methods are available? Which is the best and why?

Answers to the self-check questions and tips for responding to the discussion questions are provided on the book's accompanying website:

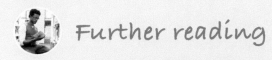 Visit www.oup.com/uk/orchard2e

3

Data recording and histopathological dissection

Vanda McTaggert, Sue Pritchard and Anne Warren

Learning objectives

After studying this chapter you should confidently be able to:

■ Accept specimens for histopathological examination.

■ Work safely in the dissecting room.

■ Gather clinical data relevant to specimen dissection.

■ Understand the basics of dissection and the macroscopic report.

■ Select appropriate tissue to ensure complete and accurate diagnosis.

Before considering the analytical aspects of histopathology it is vital to understand the need for appropriate data recording and dissection procedures. It is essential that identification checks are performed, to an agreed standard, throughout the analytic stage, so that the right report is generated for the right patient. The biomedical scientist (BMS) is key in ensuring this is completed. In addition, dissection techniques must be of the highest standard to ensure that the tissue sampled allows all the histological questions being asked by the requesting clinician to be answered. BMSs are increasingly advancing their skills to include dissection from simple cases to complex cancer resections. This is encouraged and supported by the additional qualifications (Diploma of Expert Practice and Advanced Specialist Diploma), available from The Royal College of Pathologists (RCPath; www.rcpath. org/) and Institute of Biomedical Science (IBMS; www.ibms.org). In addition, the College of American Pathologists (CAP; www.cap.org) has guidelines regarding experience required by non-medical staff prior to commencing dissection and the Royal College of Pathologists of Australasia (www.rcpa.edu.au/) has numerous dissection guidelines available for both medical and non-medical trained dissectors.

3.1 Pre-analysis

3.1.1 Specimen submission

As discussed in Chapter 2 we must first establish that the specimen has been submitted in the appropriate state for histological examination and that patient details on both specimen pot and request form fulfil the agreed criteria set by the laboratory. The biomedical scientist must ensure the integrity of the specimen is not compromised by inappropriate handling (e.g. wrong or insufficient fixative; see Chapter 2). Fresh tissue may be submitted for specialist techniques, clinical trials or research prior to light microscopy.

HEALTH & SAFETY 3.1

Known infected specimens should be identified to the laboratory with Danger of Infection labels and handled appropriately, but all tissue submitted is potentially hazardous. Hepatitis viruses, mycobacteria and HIV are some of the infective agents that you may be required to deal with. Adequate formalin fixation (24 hrs) will render most tissues safe to handle, but Category III cabinets are required to deal with pathogen 4 specimens, therefore most laboratories will not accept fresh tissue from known infected patients.

Attention to clinical history will ensure the specimen is for histopathological examination only and not for further specialist examination, as wrongly submitted samples lead to delay in diagnosis or inability to provide a detailed report. Each specimen must be given a unique laboratory number and then entered into the laboratory information management system (LIMS). Electronic tracking systems are now in use in many departments to minimize data entry and transcription error, but this does not negate manual checking. These details must be confirmed at every subsequent step throughout the laboratory process.

Good working practice advises that, where possible, similar types of samples are not given sequential numbers and therefore will not be handled in succession at the dissection bench, in case of cross-contamination.

SELF-CHECK 3.1

What are the minimum criteria for specimen reception and why are they essential?

3.1.2 Dissection room

Requirements of dissection room:

- clean
- well organized
- ventilated area
- adjustable dissecting tables with inbuilt downdraught extraction to draw formalin fumes away from the face (see Health & Safety 3.2), running water, macerator, and sluice drainage
- spillage kit.

Large resection specimens will need to be sliced/opened at time of receipt to ensure maximum fixative penetration. Gastrointestinal (GI) resections can present with a mixture of faecal material and haemorrhage (melena), which will make you appreciate good ventilation and sluice. More details on opening are given in Section 3.3.2.

HEALTH & SAFETY 3.2

Formalin is harmful through inhalation and ingestion, skin irritant, possible dermatitis, possible carcinogen. Maximum exposure 2 ppm.

Each table should be equipped with:

- a cutting board
- ruler
- scalpels/disposable blades
- forceps
- blunt-end scissors
- long-handled knife
- probe.

All instruments must be clean and if not disposable kept well maintained. Between use they should be wiped or washed in running water, and between sessions stored in an ortho-phthalahyde disinfecting solution (see Health & Safety 3.3). At all times be aware that fragments of tissue can be transferred from one specimen to another with possible serious consequences.

HEALTH & SAFETY 3.3

Avoid chlorine-based disinfectants where there is possible formalin interaction as this can react to release chlorine and other toxic gases.

In addition to dissection instruments you will require access to:

- a balance to record weights
- digital photography
- digital recording (for macro-descriptions)
- a standalone X-ray cabinet (can detect microcalcification in breast cases, calcium in bone samples being decalcified).

Key Point

All photographic/radiological images of specimens must be stored in accordance to Data Protection and Caldicott guidelines.

All laboratory equipment requires maintenance records and calibration logs to ensure safety, quality and accuracy.

Key Point

All specimens are potentially hazardous and should be treated accordingly.

Personal safety is paramount within the laboratory—every person working within the cellular pathology environment should be immunized against possible pathogens (e.g. hepatitis B).

Personal protective equipment (PPE):

- well-fitting gloves
- eye protectors
- aprons

is essential to all personnel working within the dissection room and must be worn at all times when handling specimens. While double gloving provides a better barrier it does not prevent puncture or cuts. It is good practice to change your gloves frequently. Laboratory coats must be worn in the laboratory; in the dissection room disposable aprons prevent splashing and contamination of the coat. You are advised to wear covered shoes to protect from formalin or contaminated fluid spillage and injury from falling instruments. Safety glasses or face masks will protect from aerosols and splashes: unsuspected cystic specimens can squirt fluid contents into the face of the unwary dissector. Remove and dispose of PPE before leaving the area and wash hands.

Keep the dissecting area clean:

- Wash the cutting board and instruments between cases.
- Beware of carry-over from instruments and gloves.
- Check for stray pieces of tissue or cassettes.
- Scrub down dissection area at end of working day.
- Discard disposable knives, scalpels, etc. into sharps containers.
- It is good practice to handle any Danger of Infection specimens at the end of the day then clean the area with suitable disinfectant immediately afterwards.

SELF-CHECK 3.2

What personal and environmental safety precautions should be taken in the dissection area?

Key Point

Due to the concentration level required during dissection, disturbances and distractions within the area should be kept to a minimum.

3.1.3 Preparation for dissection (pre-dissection)

For the BMS preparation will include:

- review of the cases to be dissected
- assignment of priority—urgent cases need to be flagged and treated appropriately
- assessment of complexity, to ensure cases are within the expertise of the dissector
- assessing if specimens require opening
- ensuring adequate formalin levels.

This will allow you to divide the workload according to complexity and urgency.

Tissue cassettes can be pre-printed with laboratory number/patient demographics/barcodes or cutting instructions depending upon laboratory protocol (Figure 3.1). At least two patient identifiers are advisable if the laboratory number is not yet assigned. This may be the case when carrying out a frozen section. Here patient name plus at least one other unique identifier should be used.

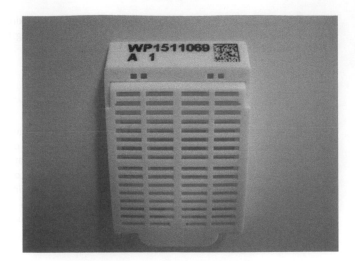

FIGURE 3.1
Cassette with 2D
Barcode and laboratory
identification.

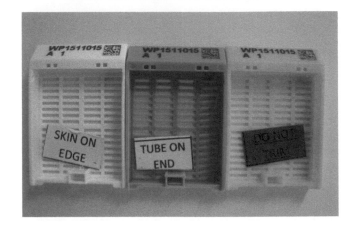

FIGURE 3.2
Tissue cassettes with
embedding and cutting
instructions.

Take care checking the cassette number against the case number before adding the selected tissue and ensure that the block key is an accurate record of the tissue taken.

Tissue cassettes are given incremental suffixes which allow you to record in a 'block key' which specific area of the specimen is represented. Each laboratory will have a standardized numbering system, for instance a specimen case with multiple pots (e.g. A, B and C) can be further divided into block A1 = resection margin, A2 = ulcerated area taken from pot A, B1 to B3 could represent central area from specimen in pot B and so on. The dissector can add cutting or embedding instructions to the block key and/or cassette. Coloured cassettes are often used to identify tissue type and thereby indicate specific embedding or cutting instructions (Figure 3.2).

3.2 Specimen types

The RCPath and IBMS have assigned tissues for dissection into specific categories, A, B, C, D and E, according to the level of complexity, knowledge and experience required to dissect. The definition of these categories is:

- A—Specimens requiring transfer from container to tissue cassette.
- B—Specimens requiring transfer but with standard sampling, counting, weighing or slicing.
- C—Simple dissection required with sampling needing a low level of diagnostic assessment and/or preparation.

- D—Dissection and sampling required needing a moderate level of assessment.
- E—Specimens requiring complex dissection and sampling methods (Tables 3.1 & 3.2).

The IBMS Diploma of Expert Practice assesses biomedical scientists on B and C type cases.

D and E type specimens are complex, requiring greater skill in dissection and much more in-depth knowledge of clinical disease processes and management of such. The IBMS Advanced Specialist Diploma assesses BMS on a selection of D and E cases.

The aim of the remaining part of this chapter is to examine the principles of dissection for a selection of specimens, to aid understanding of basic principles and to gain insight into the level of knowledge and skill required to dissect such specimen types.

TABLE 3.1 Specimens listed from Category A to C. Reproduced by kind permission of RCPath and IBMS.

A	B	C
1. Aural Polyp	1. Abscess or Sinus Tract (incl. Pilonidal Sinus)	1. Anus
2. Bladder Curettings	2. Appendix	2. Aorta
3. Bone Cores/Trephines	3. Benign Ovarian Cyst	3. Bone
4. Cell Blocks	4. Benign Skins	4. Branchial Cysts
5. Cervical Biopsies	5. Bullous Skins	5. Breast Duct Excision
6. Cervical Polyp	6. Cervix (Amputated)	6. Breast Reduction
7. Conjunctival Biopsies	7. Colonic Polyps (large)	7. Cervical Cone Biopsies
8. Endoscopic Biopsies	8. Cysts (all cysts—not solid)	8. Coronary Arteries
9. Incisional Skin Biopsies	9. Dental Cysts	9. Diverticular Disease Bowels
10. Myocardial Biopsies	10. Ectopic Pregnancy	10. Duodenum
11. Needle Core Biopsies	11. Endometrial Polyps	11. Femoral Head
12. Prostate TURPs	12. Epididymal Cysts	12. Fibroids
13. Skin Tags	13. Fallopian Tubes	13. Fresh Lymph Nodes
14. Small Colonic Polyps	14. Foreskin	14. Gastrectomy (benign ulcer)
15. Synovial Biopsies	15. Gall Bladder	15. Gastrointestinal Resections (non-neoplastic, non-inflammatory bowel disease)
16. Temporal Arteries	16. Ganglion	16. Jejunal Biopsies (capsule)
17. Testicular Biopsies	17. Gingiva	17. Lung—wedge
18. Uterine Curettings	18. Heart Valves	18. Muscle Biopsies
19. Vocal Cord Biopsies	19. Hydatid of Morgani	19. Myomectomy
	20. Lipomata	20. Nerves
	21. Lymph Nodes	21. Complex Ovarian Cysts
	22. Malignant Skin Biopsies (excluding MOHs)	22. Parathyroid Glands
	23. Meckel's Diverticulum	23. Placentas
	24. Molar Pregnancy	24. Salivary Glands—benign
	25. Nasal Polyps	25. Small Breast Lumpectomies (removed to confirm previously diagnosed benign disease)
	26. Nipple Biopsies	26. Soft Tissue Tumours (small)
	27. Perianal Warts	27. Solid Skin Lump
	28. Products of Conception	28. Thyroids
	29. Small Ovaries	29. Skin—wedge ear/eyelid
	30. Temporal Arteries	30. Spleen (benign)
	31. Tonsils	31. Stoma
	32. Uterus +/- Cervix (Negative History)	32. Suprapubic Prostatectomies
	33. Vas Deferens	33. Testes—simple
	34. Veins	34. Thyroglossal Duct Cyst
	35. Vertebral Discs	35. Ureter
		36. Urethra
		37. Uterus and Cervix (Positive History—CIN)

TABLE 3.2 Specimens listed for Category D & E. Reproduced by kind permission of RCPath and IBMS.

D & E	
1. Adrenal Glands	23. Mastectomy
2. Bladder—Cystectomy	24. Mediastinum MOHs skin biopsies
3. Bone Tumour Resections	25. Oesophagectomy
4. Breast Localization	26. Ovarian Tumours—mucinous
5. Breast Tumours—wide excision, large lumpectomies	27. Pancreatic Resections
	28. Neck Dissection
6. Brain	29. Penile Carcinoma
7. Bronchus—resection	30. Pleurectomy
8. Caecum (malignant or inflammatory bowel disease)	31. Pituitary
	32. Radical Prostatectomy
9. Cervix for Malignancy	33. Rectum (malignant or inflammatory bowel disease)
10. Colonic Resections (malignant or inflammatory bowel disease)	
	34. Renal Tumours
11. Eye	35. Salivary Gland Tumours
12. Gastrectomy (Carcinoma)	36. Small Bowel Tumour
13. Head and Neck Resection	37. Soft Tissue Tumours
14. Heart	38. Spinal Chord
15. Hirschsprung's Disease	39. Spleen (malignant)
16. Kidney	40. Testes—neoplastic
17. Laryngectomy	41. Thymus
18. Limb/Digital Amputation	42. Tongue
19. Liver	43. Uterine Carcinoma
20. Lung—Lobectomy	44. Vulvectomy
21. Lung—Pneumonectomy	45. Whipple's Resection
22. Malignant Breast Lump Resection	

3.3 Fundamentals of dissection

3.3.1 First steps

The majority of pathology laboratories deal with a large variety of histology specimens each week which require to be treated individually and with care. When first starting out in dissection, the BMS may not know where to begin. Starting with a clear understanding of what questions need to be answered on the histology report to guide the clinician regarding further patient management is the first fundamental step. This produces an understanding of which blocks need to be taken to allow production of a relevant, high quality histopathology report. Each laboratory will have Standard Operating Procedures (SOPs) in place outlining the dissection method for each specimen type based on RCPath/ CAP/RCPA guidelines. The RCPath/CAP/RCPA websites and specialized dissections books are available for guidance (see beginning of this chapter; also Rosai [1981]). Having read through and understood the guidelines it will start to become clear that regardless of specimen complexity the questions that need answering are often similar—*What is the pathology of the lesion? Is it completely excised?*

Key Point

Good Medical Practice: Have a clear understanding what questions need to be answered on the histology report before commencing dissection.

Regardless of specimen type it is essential you understand what needs to go in the final histopathology report. A lack of understanding in relation to this will lead to missed opportunities to manage the patient correctly. For example, not knowing that the closest excision margins are important in skin resections for basal cell carcinoma may lead a dissector to just sample the lesion randomly, without looking carefully for the closest margin (whether it be deep or peripheral), and sampling that specifically. The report may then state the lesion was fully excised when it was not. The patient will then not be managed correctly and will have an increased risk of recurrence.

Key Point

If unsure STOP and consult an experienced dissector.

For the dissector, preparation includes all points discussed in Section 3.1.3 above plus:

- Review of cases to be dissected, including the clinical histories given, making sure they are adequate; return of forms for relevant clinical history at this point and reassignment of cases can be planned into the, often very busy, day and can reduce delays later on.
- Ensuring they understand the information on the request form and what questions need answering in the histology report.
- Checking relevant clinical history from previous biopsies, radiological reports.
- Adherence to standard protocol set for each specimen type.

Key Point

Never handle more than one specimen at a time on the cutting board.

3.3.2 Opening

Many specimens require opening to aid fixation (see Chapter 2); for example intestinal resections, uteri and mastectomy specimens. Care should be taken when opening specimens and each case assessed individually (see www.rcpath.org/resource-library-homepage/publications/cancer-datasets.html). When opening one should consider the questions that need answering in the histology report and whether opening will affect the ability to do this adequately. Consider if the specimen needs inking or photographing prior to opening. Some macroscopic description and recording of measurements may be required before opening.

3.3.3 Marking specimens

Surgical margins are critical to assessment of the disease process and the true margin may only be microscopically visible if marked in some way at time of dissection. There are many dyes and inks that we can use which will mark the tissue without compromising the uptake of subsequent histological stains (e.g. Indian ink or commercially available Davidson Ink). These marking solutions are required to be robust enough to withstand the chemicals used in tissue processing. Surgical suture tags or staples applied to specimens enable you to orientate the specimen, making it possible to mark differentially the tissue margins using specified coloured inks (Figure 3.3). Some inks may contain elements that are picked up on X-ray and can mimic calcification, causing issues with assessment of specimen calcification in breast cases.

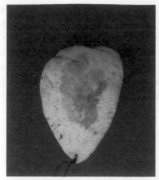 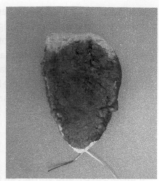

FIGURE 3.3
Differential marking of annotated skin.

■ 12 o' clock   ■ 3 o' clock   ■ 6 o' clock   ■ 6 o' clock
● Deep margin

Take care when inking specimens as the ink can run into areas you don't want it to. To reduce risk of this, ensure specimen is dry before inking and try to ink before cutting. Choose the area to be inked. Take care not to use excess ink on the brush—use of cotton buds can result in a more controlled inking technique. Allowing ink to dry before sectioning prevents ink being dragged onto the cut surface. Commercial solutions are available to aid the drying process. Always document the inking protocol used, as this should form part of the permanent record.

Key Point

Margins can be misinterpreted if ink is allowed to track through a specimen.

SELF-CHECK 3.3

What is the purpose of applying ink to specimens?

3.3.4 Gross descriptions

When first dictating gross specimen descriptions, it can be difficult to produce a succinct report that flows. Templates can help, but one needs to be mindful not to just go through the motions and fill in templates, but to think about every step taken. It is helpful to make rough notes and then dictate the report at the end, until practice and experience improve. One should ensure that important information is not lost in unnecessary description. For example, technical aspects of dissection are not needed, as there will be departmental SOPs describing these. Ensure you read through the final gross description to ensure all necessary information is present. It is helpful if you try and draw an image of the specimen based only on the gross description, or ask an assisting colleague to, when first starting dissection. It is important to audit and reflect on your practice.

SELF-CHECK 3.4

Do you understand common descriptive terms such as trabeculated, pedunculated, telangiectatic? Build a glossary of universal terms used to describe commonly seen features.

Gross descriptions of specimens must be transcribed either manually or by electronic dictation. It is essential that this is accurate as this will be the only record of the uncut specimen available to the reporting pathologist/clinician. If electronic description is used it is good practice to also write down key points/measurements, in case there is a problem with the electronic file and information is lost.

> ## Key Point
>
> Ensure you are familiar with the dictation system and speak clearly enough for the transcriber to understand. Gross descriptions should not be lengthy or flowery, but easily understood anatomical descriptions which convey an accurate portrayal of the specimen before you.

Generally the most important information to include is:

- Type of specimen and structures present
- Size (in 3 dimensions and in mm)
- Weight
- Colour
- Shape
- Consistency
- Presence of a specific lesion
  - If yes give size (in 3 dimensions, shape, colour, consistency, location in relation to specimen and distance to closest margins)
- Consider drawing diagrams, photography, use of digital photographic stations with annotation availability
- Block key.

Millimetres should be used at all times in the macroscopic and microscopic descriptions. Using the same unit of measurement in all areas of the report reduces errors.

Size and weight can be essential for further patient management and audit:

- The maximum dimension of a tumour is important in staging to guide patient management.
- Weight on its own can help differentiate between a normal and abnormal parathyroid gland.
- In the UK a surgeon should take no more than 20 g of tissue when performing an open diagnostic breast biopsy.

When dissecting try to leave the specimen so that it can be reconstructed afterwards, particularly in larger cases such as mastectomy. This allows review of the case and is also beneficial where extra sampling is necessary, as previous sites of block selection will be apparent to the reviewer who may not be the original dissector.

As you train in dissection it is essential to review and audit your workload. Ask yourself:

- Did you mention all required features/measurements?
- Are your gross descriptions clear and understandable?
- Did you sample the/an appropriate area?
- Are you oversampling?
- Have you followed the protocol?

It is important that you also review cases at the microscope so you can:

- correlate macroscopic features with microscopic findings
- appreciate the significance of the clinical history
- relate the pathological process with the patient pathway
- ensure appropriate block selection
- assess and reflect on your working practice.

3.4 Organ systems

The following is a review of common organ systems with a selection of case studies, highlighting the importance of correlation with pathological disease and clinical management.

3.4.1 Skin

Skin cases account for a large percentage of routine histopathological laboratory samples. Each component or structure within the skin (epidermis, dermis, glands, fat, etc.) gives rise to a vast array of pathologies from simple benign lesions to inflammatory conditions, autoimmune conditions, and premalignant to malignant tumours (see www.rcpath.org/resourceLibrary/g123-data-set-basal-may-2014.html; www.rcpath.org/resourceLibrary/dataset-for-the-histological-reporting-of-primary-cutaneous-malignant-melanoma-and-regional-lymph-nodes.html; and www.rcpath.org/resourceLibrary/g124_datasetsquamous_may14-pdf.html). Different anatomical areas of skin vary in their composition and are susceptible to particular dermal lesions. Table 3.3 gives examples of frequently seen conditions with which you should be familiar when dissecting skin specimens.

Skin specimens fall into two main categories: Diagnostic/Incisional and Excisional. It is important that you determine from the clinical history and the surgical procedure which category the specimen is in prior to dissection. Knowledge of surgical procedures and understanding their use in dermatology will help (Table 3.4).

Clinicians have been known to use **excision** as a general term for any excised piece of tissue and as dissector you must be on your guard. You may also see request forms reading 'lesion of skin' where you will interpret the clinical history, check for any procedural reference and assess the specimen to work out whether you are dealing with a diagnostic or excisional biopsy.

A diagnostic skin makes no attempt to remove the entire lesion: the aim is to confirm the clinical suspicion of a benign tumour, or to sample either a large lesion or a widespread pathology such as inflammatory diseases. Reporting of diagnostic skins will determine the best practice for patient management. Here the margins are of no relevance and your aim is to provide maximum quantity of tissue for the microscopic assessment.

The entire diagnostic sample is processed to give maximum yield on tissue sections (Figures 3.4 and 3.5). These samples can be scrappy and difficult to orientate, and, while ink marking is helpful to orientate skin biopsies at embedding, it can obscure these difficult biopsies even further. Multiple friable fragments should be wrapped or processed within specimen bags to prevent loss of diagnostic material or contamination of other tissue blocks.

TABLE 3.3 Commonly presented skin pathologies.

Benign	Skin polyps, basal cell papillomas/warts/seborrhoeic keratoses, cysts (pilar/epidermal), naevi, lipomas, dermatofibromas, neurofibromas, pyogenic granulomas, haemangiomas.
Inflammatory	Psoriasis, lichen planus, eczema, acne, rosacea, impetigo.
Autoimmune	Alopecia, dermatitis herpetiformis (DH), discoid lupus erythematosus (DLE), bullous pemphigus, systemic lupus erythematosus (SLE).
Premalignant	Actinic keratoses, Bowen's disease, lentigo maligna, melanoma *in situ*, dysplastic naevi.
Malignant (Non-melanoma)	Basal cell carcinoma (BCC), squamous cell carcinoma (SCC), keratoacanthoma.
Malignant (Melanocytic)	Malignant melanoma including: superficial spreading malignant melanoma (SSMM), lentigo maligna melanoma, nodular melanoma.

TABLE 3.4 Surgical procedures for skin specimens.

Surgical technique	Process	Removal of	Dissection procedure
Shave biopsy	Removal of surface layers using sharp blade.	All or part of lesion.	Count fragments, measure if single piece and process intact < 5 mm, bisect > 5 mm.
Curette & cautery	Skin scraping with heat applied to cauterize wound.	All or part of lesion.	Count/measure fragments and process all tissue.
Punch biopsy	Removal of circular disc of skin and underlying tissue 2–8 mm diameter. NB. Lesion may be curetted first to expose dermis.	All or part of lesion prior to carrying out excision.	Record number of pieces, measure diameter, > 5 mm bisect, < 5 mm process intact and bisect before embedding if appropriate.
Incisional/diagnostic	Elongated skin ellipses which include the lesion and some normal tissue.	Part of lesion prior to carrying out excision.	Measure, describe surface, bisect longitudinally where appropriate.
Excisional	Frequently elliptical but depends on size of lesion, site, closure technique.	Entire lesion with margin of normal skin.	Measure, describe any lesions, assess and sample through closest resection margins. Refer to Case study 3.1.
Mohs micrographic surgery shave excision (MMS)	Specialist technique (also Slow Mohs).	Tissue is removed in stages and examined microscopically until margins are clear.	See Chapter 7.

Key Point

Generally diagnostic biopsies are cut through the longitudinal axis while excisional biopsies are cut transversely demonstrating closest margin.

Excisional skins come in all shapes and sizes and you will find each must be assessed and dissected according to the shape and size of the specimen, the lesion, and the relationship of the two. The intention of excision is to remove the entire lesion with a margin of normal tissue. The representative tissue blocks must allow assessment of excision margins thereby providing a full report on which the clinician can base patient follow-up. Wedge excisions can be extremely complex to dissect and these cases are better discussed with or left to an experienced BMS/reporting histopathologist to handle.

As mentioned, the size and shape of skin, nature and position of abnormality, and importance of surgical margins will govern the selection of blocks in accordance with relevant SOPs. For a benign

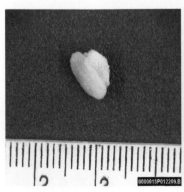
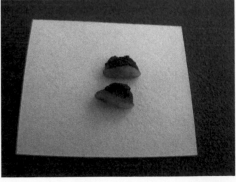

FIGURE 3.4
Punch biopsy >5 mm marked and bisected.

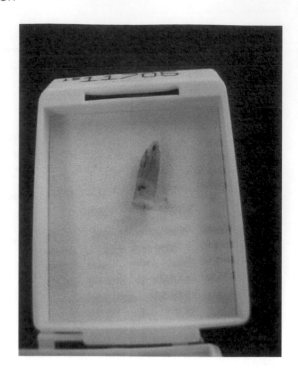

FIGURE 3.5
Punch biopsy < 5 mm processed
intact.

condition such as an epidermal cyst one block through the closest margin can confirm diagnosis and clearance (Figure 3.6).

Larger tumours or ill-defined lesions will need more extensive sampling with representative blocks showing the extent of tumour and surgical margins (Figure 3.7). Shaves from peripheral margins may be taken to more fully assess their status, but a Mohs procedure is the gold standard for full margin assessment (see Chapter 7).

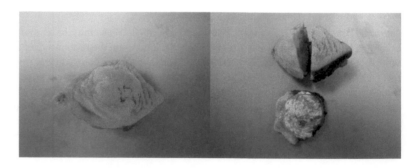

FIGURE 3.6
Clinically diagnosed cyst: a single block is taken across the central narrowest margin to show intact cyst.

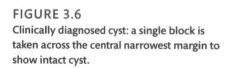

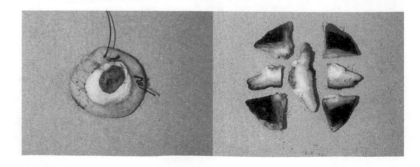

FIGURE 3.7
Central block with tumour and two margins plus cruciate of two other margins. Central block demonstrates the full face of tumour plus clearance at 12 o'clock and 6 o'clock margins, while cruciates demonstrate clearance at 3 o'clock and 9 o'clock.

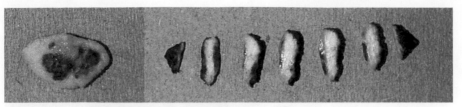

FIGURE 3.8
Transverse slicing where risk of tumour extending beyond macroscopic evidence.

Where an atypical or dysplastic naevus on clinical history or pigmented features is noted, at dissection you would block the entire lesion. If there is suspicion of malignant melanoma then block the entire specimen ≤10 mm and entire pigmented area if > 10 mm (Figure 3.8).

Key Point

Each skin must be assessed individually to note which margins are relevant to the final report.

Skin specimens are embedded on edge so that all layers from epidermis down to subcutaneous tissue can be assessed under the microscope. Sections through the tissue at different levels are routinely requested on diagnostic skins at time of dissection. It is important that the dissector identifies and cuts perpendicular to the skin surface and is careful when marking to ensure the skin surface is not obscured and the cut face is evident to the embedder.

Key Point

Failure to orientate skin correctly could destroy essential reporting features.

 CASE STUDY 3.1 *Basal cell carcinoma*

Request form clinical information: 58-year-old man presented to GP with 6-month history of typical rodent ulcer. Excision of proven basal cell carcinoma (BCC) right side nose. Suture marks superior.

BCCs are the most commonly occurring of malignant skin tumours and submitted in such numbers that they are frequently dissected by a BMS. The vast majority are accredited to sun exposure and predominantly arise on exposed areas of the head, neck and face as is the case here. Immunosuppression can predispose to BCC formation as can chemical or physical skin damage. Although BCCs are unlikely to metastasize, they are locally invasive and cause extensive damage making surgical removal the preferred option. A perimeter margin of healthy skin is removed along with the tumour cells to ensure complete eradication. There is the possibility of recurrence should excision be incomplete: an advisable surgical margin of 2–10 mm, and a 3-mm peripheral surgical margin will clear the tumour in 85% of cases (see Telfer *et al.*, 2008; www.cap.org/web/home/resources/cancer-reporting-tools/cancer-protocol-templates?_afrLoop=300658012556352#%40%3F_afrLoop%3D300658012556352%26_adf.ctrl-state%3Dmvxbk1597_4).

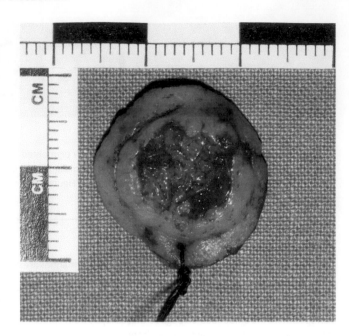

FIGURE 3.9
Annotated skin showing
ulcerated BCC.

At the bench first check patient demographics on the pot, form and cassette match before proceeding as follows:

Assess the clinical information:

- A clinical history of 'suspected BCC' denotes a clinical diagnosis, whereas 'proven BCC' indicates a previous incisional/diagnostic or punch biopsy has been carried out to confirm clinical suspicion. You may note scarring on the surface of a previously biopsied specimen on examination; the lesion may have been fully removed by the diagnostic biopsy, but the pathologist would be unable to comment on margin involvement.

- Check previous history especially if scar present. Previously incomplete excisions may be resubmitted as wider excisions as follow up or because of possible recurrence.

Examine the specimen (Figure 3.9):

- Inspect the specimen fully, dissect, LOOK, THINK and produce a macroscopic report.

- Note the shape of the skin – elliptical excisions are most common due to good cosmetic results but other shapes (e.g. rhomboid, rounded or oval) may be taken depending on the nature of the lesion and site of lesion. These can be difficult to orientate unless marked by surgeon.

- Note the colour of the skin surface—pigmentation could indicate a melanocytic lesion and tanned skin suggests frequent sun exposure.

- All skin specimens are measured (mm) in three dimensions.

- Note the presence and site of any suture. Here the suture is annotating the superior aspect allowing differential inking. In the absence of an orientation suture the entire surgical margin can be marked with a single colour identifying the surgical margin microscopically. A key of the inking protocol must be provided.

Surgical margins (peripheral and deep margins) must be assessed: inking greatly enhances the process, aiding the embedder to orientate correctly, and delineates the true margin on the tissue section allowing comment on adequacy of excision. Where the specimen is orientated using suture tags you can further differentiate the anatomical margins using coloured inks, allowing comment on specific margins. Depending on the size and position, the lesion can be sampled as seen in Figure 3.10.

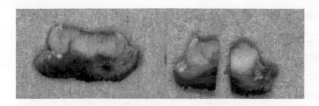

FIGURE 3.10
Transverse slice across narrowest margin plus cruciate blocks.

SELF-CHECK 3.5

Consider the orientation of the specimen: can you identify the medial and lateral margins given the details on the request form above?

- Photograph where appropriate (e.g. complex wedge biopsies and orientated skins) as this will corroborate the macroscopic description.

- Measure and describe any lesion in precise terms (e.g. macular, papular, warty, etc.). Here we have a centrally ulcerated lesion with rolled edges, the features which gave rise to their common name 'rodent ulcers'. Non-ulcerated BCCs may appear as pearly nodules.

- Comment on its relation/position on the specimen.

- Describe any other lesion present in relation to the main lesion, stating the distance between each.

- Note closest resection margin.

- Comment on cut surface (e.g. colour/cystic/solid/mucoid).

Macroscopic description given was: Rounded piece of skin measuring 21 mm × 19 mm, underlying tissue 5 mm. Suture tag marks the superior margin. Surface bears a central partly ulcerated nodule with rolled edges 16 × 15 × 6 mm. The closest resection margin is 2 mm at the medial margin. The nearest macroscopically noted margin is included in the tissue selection, but the microscopically measured distance to margin will be given in the report.

- The dissector should select tissue blocks to give the best representation of tumour relative to margins, taking into account the size of the lesion. A block containing the closest resection margin should be taken and any other margins which could be involved (Figure 3.10). Any other areas of abnormality must be sampled and included in the block key.

- Figure 3.10 shows the nodule had a homogenous pale cut surface characteristic of a BCC although they can also exhibit a cystic appearance. Block 1 was a transverse slice showing the full extent of the tumour and clearance at both the medial and lateral borders; block 2 contained the two cruciate margins demonstrating relationship of superior and inferior margins to the tumour.

CLINICAL CORRELATION

BCCs are classified as nodular, micronodular, cystic, superficial, infiltrative or morphoeic; the latter types have higher risk of recurrence. The extent of these lesions and margin clearance can only be truly seen and measured microscopically.

This was reported as a nodular BCC with infiltrative component, the excision margins were clear and the patient was put on 6 month follow-up to review the scar for possible recurrence. The microscopically measured margin clearance < 2 mm also infers higher risk of recurrence.

If excision had been incomplete the clinician would reassess the site and where appropriate remove further tissue—identification of a specific involved margin means the focus of the surgery at that margin, reducing the need to remove excessive tissue. Wider excision biopsies are submitted as a result of previously incomplete excision biopsy, suspected residual or recurrent clinical features around scars or where malignant melanoma has been diagnosed; skin with lesion including scarred area is submitted and extensively sampled usually by transversely slicing the entire specimen.

TABLE 3.5 Commonly occurring breast conditions/pathologies.

Benign	Fibrocystic change, fibroadenoma, hamartoma, papilloma, radial scar, complex sclerosing lesion, benign phyllodes tumour, gynaecomastia (in men).
Inflammatory	Granulomatous mastitis, fat necrosis, abscess, duct ectasia.
Calcification	Benign associated (columnar cell change, fibrocystic change, scarring, fat necrosis), malignant associated (DCIS, pleomorphic LCIS, invasive carcinoma).
Premalignant	DCIS, LCIS.
Malignant	Invasive ductal carcinoma not otherwise specified is the most common, followed by invasive lobular carcinoma; rarer types exist (metaplastic, micropapillary, apocrine, secretary, malignant phyllodes, angiosarcoma).

The characteristic features of basaloid tumour cells and peripheral palisading seen microscopically on H&E stain was sufficient to confirm the diagnosis, but in some cases immunocytochemistry may be required to differentiate tumours with similar morphology such as a trichoepithelioma (adnexal tumour). BCC is negative for CD34, EMA, P63 and CK20 while the trichoepithelioma is positive for all four markers.

3.4.2 Breast pathology

Breast lesions are common specimens received in the majority of pathology departments. Table 3.5 gives common breast conditions.

Breast lesions can be aspirated, biopsied or excised. Lesions are not normally excised unless there is a pre-excision diagnosis. Surgical procedures for breast specimens are given in Table 3.6, together with the basic dissection procedure. Please refer to RCPath guidelines for more details (www.rcpath.org/resource-library-homepage/publications/cancer-datasets.html; www.rcpath.org/resourceLibrary/pathologyreportingofbreastdisease-oct05-pdf.html).

TABLE 3.6 Surgical procedures and basic dissection procedure for breast specimens.

Surgical/radiological technique	Process	Removal of	Dissection procedure
Cyst aspiration	Drainage of cyst fluid.	All or part of cyst fluid. May or may not be sent for analysis depending on appearance and clinical/radiological impression.	Cytology specimen.
Fine needle aspiration	Sample lesional breast cells.	Part of lesion for diagnosis.	Cytology specimen.
Core biopsy	Needle biopsy (free hand, ultrasound or stereo-guided), normally 3–5 cores.	Part of lesion for diagnosis.	Count/measure cores and process all tissue, cut levels × 3.
Vacuum assisted biopsy	Needle biopsy under vacuum, more tissue removed than in core biopsy, so greater sampling achieved.	Breast tissue up to 2–3 cm, can be diagnostic or therapeutic (excision, for example, of a fibroadenoma).	Weigh tissue, count/measure cores and process all tissue, cut levels × 3 for diagnostic cases.
Punch biopsy skin/nipple	Removal of circular disc of skin and underlying tissue (2–8 mm diameter).	All or part of lesion for diagnosis.	Record number of pieces, measure diameter, > 5 mm bisect, < 5 mm process intact and bisect before embedding if appropriate.
Breast reduction	Can be unilateral or bilateral; surgical removal of breast tissue, often received in multiple pieces, some with overlying skin.	Breast tissue for cosmetic appearance/symmetry.	Weigh in total, count/measure pieces and describe +/− skin.

TABLE 3.6 Surgical procedures and basic dissection procedure for breast specimens. (*Continued*)

Surgical/radiological technique	Process	Removal of	Dissection procedure
Excision for benign pathology	Surgical removal of breast tissue.	All of lesion with narrow margin.	Weigh, measure in 3 dimensions (mm), ink, slice at 3–4 mm, describe external & internal surface, sample (see Case study 3.2).
Excision biopsy	Surgical removal of breast tissue < 20 g for diagnosis when pre-operative diagnosis not possible.	All or part of lesion for diagnosis.	Weigh, measure in 3 dimensions (mm), ink, slice at 3–4mm, describe external & internal surface, block in entirety.
Wide local excision	Surgical removal of breast malignancy with aim of clear margins (> 1 mm).	All of lesion with > 1 mm margin.	Orientate, weigh, measure in 3 dimensions (mm), ink, slice at 3–4 mm, describe external & internal surface, +/– X-ray/photograph, sample.
Mastectomy	Removal of all breast tissue +/– skin/nipple; can be prophylactic/risk reducing or therapeutic.	All breast tissue +/– malignancy (*in situ* or invasive disease).	Orientate, weigh, measure in 3 dimensions (mm), +/– skin, ink, slice at 10 mm, describe internal surface, +/– X-ray/photograph, sample.
Sentinel lymph node	Detection of sentinel lymph node by radioactive isotope +/– dye, surgical excision.	Sentinel lymph node.	Palpate node, measure in 3 dimensions (mm), slice at 2 mm perpendicular to long axis, block in entirety.
Axillary lymph node sample	Surgical identification of 4–6 low axillary lymph nodes, with excision.	4–6 low axillary lymph nodes.	Palpate nodes, count, measure largest in 3 dimensions (mm), slice, block in entirety (unless obviously involved by tumour).
Axillary lymph node clearance (ANC)	Surgical excision of all axillary lymph nodes in levels 1–3.	All axillary lymph nodes in levels 1–3.	Palpate nodes, count, measure largest in 3 dimensions (mm), slice, block in entirety (unless obviously involved by tumour).

SELF-CHECK 3.6

Can you list the common benign and malignant lesions that occur in the breast? Do you know what surgical procedures are used to treat these conditions?

CASE STUDY 3.2 *Benign breast lump*

Request form clinical information: Excision of a probable fibroadenoma from a 48-year-old female.

Standard patient/specimen identifications check should be made.

Assess the clinical information:

- Fibroadenomas are benign lesions of the breast. These are usually an oval/round, encapsulated mass consisting of white to grey homogeneous rubbery tissue that does not infiltrate into surrounding fat. They are more common in younger women (under the age of 30), and vary in size, but most are under 30 mm.

- Phyllodes tumours can mimic fibroadenomas. These are often more infiltrative with a leaf-like architecture. They are more common in older women (note the age of the patient in this case), and can be of variable size at presentation (10 mm to > 60 mm).

Previous histology reports and radiology reports may be searched for:

- There may be a previous core biopsy that showed features of a fibroadenoma.

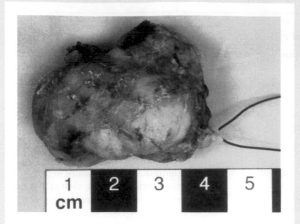

FIGURE 3.11
A moderately well circumscribed mass that has been 'shelled out' by the surgeon. It is approximately 40 mm in maximum diameter (it should be measured accurately, in three dimensions, in mm). Note the suture, which may be orientating the specimen.

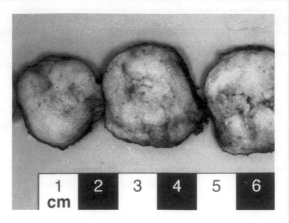

FIGURE 3.12
Slices of tumour with the specimen resection margin inked black and slight fragmentation centrally in two slices. This case was reported as a benign phyllodes tumour. The friable areas seen macroscopically showed increased cellularity, mitoses and a leaf-like architecture. The patient underwent a further excision to ensure complete removal of the lesion.

- The imaging (mammogram or ultrasound) reports may show a well circumscribed lesion, consistent with a fibroadenoma.

Examine the specimen (Figure 3.11), dissect, LOOK, FEEL and THINK and produce a macroscopic report:

- All breast specimens are weighed (g) and measured (mm), in three dimensions.

- The specimen is checked for orientation (clips or sutures). If orientated, then the specimen should be inked to allow specific margin assessment when reporting. A block key of the inking protocol is provided. If not orientated (which is normally the case in fibroadenomas), then the specimen can be inked in one colour.

- The specimen is serially sliced at 3–5 mm (Figure 3.12). If orientated, it is good practice to state in which direction slicing is (e.g. medial to lateral or superior to inferior), and how many slices there are. The cut surface should then be described. It is now that the dissector's knowledge of such specimens is called upon.

- If on slicing you see a well circumscribed, white to pale yellow, rubbery homogeneous mass, you can conclude this is in keeping macroscopically with a fibroadenoma

and sample accordingly. There are no evidence-based guidelines on how many blocks of a presumed fibro-adenoma should be taken. The dissector should comply with local standard operating procedures, taking into account the size of the lesion. A block containing the closest resection margin should be taken.

- However, if on sectioning the specimen contains a lesion that falls apart in places and looks friable with irregular outlines, the dissector should call on their knowledge and worry about the possibility of a phyllodes tumour, despite all pre-operative investigations favouring a fibroadenoma. If the dissector is not the reporting pathologist, they may want to call the reporting pathologist for their opinion, or they may wish to photograph the sliced specimen. What is certain is that more blocks will be taken of the lesion and specimen margin, to allow accurate classification, and excision status, of the lesion.

Learning points: It is essential to understand the pathology of the cases you are dissecting. Without the knowledge of fibroadenomas and phyllodes tumours one may not sample this case correctly. You may not have sampled the friable areas or taken enough blocks and the case may have been misdiagnosed as a cellular fibroadenoma.

3.4.3 Gastrointestinal

Gastrointestinal specimens are commonly received in the majority of pathology departments. Table 3.7 gives common gastrointestinal specimen types and associated pathologies, with Table 3.8 listing common surgical specimens and brief details on dissection methodology (www.rcpath.org/resourceLibrary/-giandp-tissue-pathway-nov09.html; www.rcpath.org/resourceLibrary/dataset-for-colorectal-cancer-histopathology-reports--3rd-edition-.html).

TABLE 3.7 Common gastrointestinal specimen types and associated pathologies.

Specimen site	Conditions/pathologies
Oesophagus	Benign—reflux oesophagitis, eosinophilic oesophagitis, Barrett's oesophagus, candida, herpes simplex, leiomyoma, schwannoma. Premalignant/indeterminate—squamous cell carcinoma *in situ*/dysplasia, glandular dysplasia, gastrointestinal stromal tumour. Malignant—squamous cell carcinoma, adenocarcinoma, metastatic disease.
Stomach	Benign—gastritis/ulcer, *Helicobacter pylori*, fundic gland polyp, hyperplastic polyp, inflammatory fibroid polyp, intestinal metaplasia, leiomyoma, schwannoma. Premalignant/indeterminate—glandular dysplasia, gastrointestinal stromal tumour, neuroendocrine neoplasm. Malignant—adenocarcinoma, neuroendocrine carcinoma, lymphoma, metastatic disease.
Duodenum	Benign—duodenitis/ulcer, coeliac disease, giardia, gastric/pancreatic metaplasia/heterotopia. Premalignant/indeterminate—glandular dysplasia, gastrointestinal stromal tumour, neuroendocrine neoplasm. Malignant—adenocarcinoma, neuroendocrine carcinoma, metastatic disease.
Small intestine (distal to duodenum)	Benign—ischaemia, Crohn's disease, tuberculosis. Premalignant/indeterminate—glandular dysplasia, gastrointestinal stromal tumour, neuroendocrine neoplasm. Malignant—adenocarcinoma, lymphoma, neuroendocrine carcinoma, metastatic disease.
Large intestine	Benign—benign polyps, ischaemia, diverticular disease, inflammatory bowel disease (Crohn's disease/ulcerative colitis), infective cause (*Clostridium difficile*, tuberculosis), NSAID-related disease. Premalignant/indeterminate—dysplastic polyps, gastrointestinal stromal tumour, neuroendocrine neoplasm. Malignant—adenocarcinoma, neuroendocrine carcinoma, lymphoma, metastatic disease.
Rectum	Benign—solitary rectal ulcer/mucosal prolapse syndrome, benign polyps, inflammatory bowel disease (Crohn's disease/ulcerative colitis), infective causes (lymphogranuloma venereum). Premalignant/indeterminate—dysplastic polyps, gastrointestinal stromal tumour, neuroendocrine neoplasm. Malignant—adenocarcinoma, neuroendocrine carcinoma, metastatic disease.
Appendix	Benign—acute appendicitis, mucocoele, benign polyps, lymphadenopathy, worms/parasites, inflammatory bowel disease. Premalignant/indeterminate—dysplastic polyps, neuroendocrine neoplasm, low grade appendiceal neoplasm. Malignant—neuroendocrine carcinoma, adenocarcinoma.
Anal region	Benign—benign polyps, haemorrhoids, fibroepithelial polyp, pilonidal sinus, fistulae. Premalignant/indeterminate—squamous cell carcinoma *in-situ*/dysplasia, glandular dysplasia. Malignant—squamous cell carcinoma, adenocarcinoma, basal cell carcinoma, anal gland carcinoma, melanoma, metastatic disease.
Gallbladder	Benign—cholecystitis, cholelithiasis, benign polyps. Premalignant/indeterminate—glandular dysplasia. Malignant—adenocarcinoma, metastatic disease.

TABLE 3.8 Common surgical specimens and brief details on dissection methodology.

Surgical/radiological technique	Process/removal of	Dissection procedure
Mucosal biopsy	Endoscopic cold or hot (diathermy) to remove part of lesion/normal appearing tissue.	Number of fragments, measure range of sizes, if attached to cellulose acetate or other, any other material present. Process all tissue, cut levels × 3.
Polypectomy	Endoscopic cold or hot (diathermy) to remove all or part of polyp.	Number of pieces, appearance (sessile or polypoid, colour, ulcerated), measure in 3 dimensions; stalk length +/– diameter of base. Ink base if seen, if > 5 mm bisect or serially slice (preserve stalk). Process all tissue.
Endoscopic mucosal resection (EMR)	Endoscopic procedure to remove all or part of lesion with more/deeper tissue than biopsy or polypectomy.	State if pinned, number of pieces, appearance, measure in 3 dimensions, ink base, serially slice. Process all tissue.
Appendicectomy	Surgical removal of appendix (laparoscopic or open) for management of appendicitis or removal of neoplasm.	Measure length and maximum diameter +/– attached fat, describe serosa, serially slice transversely and bisect tip longitudinally, describe wall, lumen, any lesions (appearance, size, location distance to margin). Block half of tip, transverse section (at least 1), margin, any lesions.
Oesophagectomy/ gastrectomy	Surgical removal of part of oesophagus +/– all or part of stomach, or removal of all or part of stomach only, can be laparoscopic or open. For excision of benign (ulcer, gastric sleeve for obesity, abscess, fistula, diverticulum, polyp), or malignant (with > 1 mm margin), pathology.	Benign & malignant—describe specimen type, measure length of oesophagus and stomach, measure length of lesser and greater curve, describe serosa, wall, mucosa, luminal contents, lymph nodes and any lesions (location, appearance, size, distance to margins), photograph. For more details and sampling see www.rcpath.org/resourceLibrary/g006oesophagealdatasetfinalfeb07-pdf.html; www.rcpath.org/resourceLibrary/dataset-for-the-histopathological-reporting-of-gastric-carcinoma.html.
Intestinal resections (small bowel resection, right/left hemicolectomy, sigmoidectomy, anterior resection, anterior peritoneal resection)	Surgical removal of part or all of segment of small/large bowel, can be laparoscopic or open. For benign (ischaemic segment, perforation, inflammatory bowel disease, diverticula, polyp, volvulus, intussusception), or malignant (total excision of malignant lesion with > 1 mm margin), pathology.	Benign & malignant—describe specimen type, measure length and maximum diameter, describe attached fat, serosa, wall, mucosa, luminal contents, lymph nodes and any lesions (location, appearance, size, distance to margins), photograph. For more detail and sampling see www.rcpath.org/resourceLibrary/-giandp-tissue-pathway-nov09.html; www.rcpath.org/resourceLibrary/dataset-for-colorectal-cancer-histopathology-reports--3rd-edition-.html; and Case study 3.3.
Trans-anal mucosal resection (TAMIS)	Trans-anal surgical removal—all of lesion with more/deeper tissue than biopsy or polypectomy (to muscularis propria).	Should be pinned, number of pieces, appearance, measure in 3 dimensions, ink base, serially slice. Process all tissue.
Cholecystectomy	Surgical removal of gall bladder +/– stones, can be laparoscopic or open. To manage symptoms, or to characterize lesion/s seen on imaging.	State if received opened, measure length and maximum diameter +/– any attached organs, describe surface, wall, mucosa, luminal contents and any lesions, lymph nodes Block cystic duct margin, section of neck, body, any lesions or lymph node.
Pancreatectomy (pylorus-preserving pancreatoduodenectomy, Whipple's resection, distal pancreatectomy)	Surgical removal of part or all of the pancreas to control symptoms/duct obstruction, assess radiological suspected tumour, remove neoplasm. Can be laparoscopic or open.	State specimen type, measure in 3 dimensions, extrapancreatic bile duct length +/– any attached organs, describe external appearance, ink margins, describe cut surface (location, size, appearance, margin distance of any lesions). For more detail and sampling see www.rcpath.org/resourceLibrary/dataset-for-the-histopathological-reporting-of-carcinomas-of-the-pancreas--ampulla-of-vater-and-common-bile-duct.html.

CASE STUDY 3.3 *Diverticular disease*

Request form and clinical information: 68-year-old male, sigmoidectomy for severe diverticular disease.

Standard patient/specimen identifications checks are made. Assess the clinical information:

Diverticulae can be congenital or acquired. The most common form is acquired diverticular disease. Increased intraluminal pressure leads to diverticula formation, which typically form where arteries pierce the muscularis propria, as this is where the colonic wall is weakest. Most people with diverticular disease remain asymptomatic, with only up to a quarter becoming symptomatic. Complications include diverticular inflammation (diverticulitis), bleeding, abscess formation, fistula formation, stenosis, adhesions, and rupture with associated peritonitis. The request form gives little information, only 'severe diverticular disease'. Checking of previous pathology reports, imaging, patient notes (electronic or paper), or discussion with the surgeon would aid the dissection process and ensure it is of high quality. If no further information is available at dissection look for all possible complications in the specimen.

Examine the specimen, dissect, LOOK, FEEL & THINK and produce a macroscopic report:

- All colorectal resections are examined on receipt in the laboratory to see if opening is required to aid fixation. Intestine is opened along the antimesenteric border longitudinally, unless a lesion is present. Lesions are best left intact if possible to allow for accurate macroscopic description. However, if the pathology present has caused the lumen to become narrow, it may be necessary to slice into the bowel transversely to ensure fixation is adequate, but do not slice all the way through, to retain integrity while fixing. The luminal contents should be washed out gently with water. A note of the luminal contents is made (blood, faeces). Care should be taken so as to not damage the mucosa. Photographs may need to be taken before opening, and this should always be considered. If on examination there is concern of unexpected neoplasia, the histopathologist responsible for the specimen should be informed. It may be necessary to ink relevant resection margins at this time. The opened specimen will require further fixation in an adequate volume of formalin (see Chapter 2). Fixation time will vary depending on the specimen type and may be up to 48 hours.

- The type of resection is stated, in this case sigmoidectomy.

- The maximum length and diameter of the bowel is measured in millimetres. If the diameter is variable this is described and the range of diameters given.

- The maximum dimensions of any attached fat/mesentery are given.

- It is best to then describe the specimen from outside to inside so as to not miss any important features (see Table 3.9).

- This case shows a sigmoidectomy measuring 150 mm in length and up to 45 mm in diameter, with attached fat measuring 150 mm × 135 mm × 25 mm (see Figure 3.13). The serosal surface is haemorrhagic with a purulent exudate, in keeping with peritonitis and perforation. A perforation was carefully looked for. This was identified 70 mm from one resection margin (see Figure 3.14). The wall was thickened throughout due to fibrosis, measuring up to 15 mm in thickness (range 10 mm to 15 mm). The mucosa

TABLE 3.9 Description of the specimen from outside to inside.

Serosa	Colour and focal changes of colour, purulent exudate (pus on surface). Perforations (if present state location, measurements, shape, number). Adhesions. Strictures or puckering (if present state location, measurement and number).
Wall	Thickness, if variable state and describe giving range of thicknesses. Fibrotic. Fistulae. Sinus tracts. Abscess.
Mucosa	Colour. Nature—normal, atrophic, haemorrhagic. Look for diverticular disease, but also pseudomembranes, cobblestone, pseudopolyps, polyps, tumour mass, ulceration, and if present describe the extent and relationship with margins. For diverticula describe the approximate number, presence of associated abscess, fibrosis or perforation.

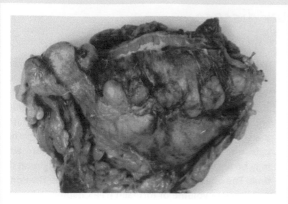

FIGURE 3.13
External appearance of colectomy specimen.

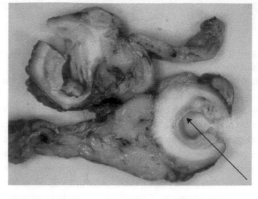

FIGURE 3.15
Slices across colon showing flattened firm area (arrow)
and diverticula.

showed approximately 10 diverticula, in the form of 'holes'
within the mucosa. The mucosa showed a focal firm, flattened area, but no polyps (see Figure 3.15). The worry here
was that this firm, flattened area could be a 'hidden' carcinoma within the diverticular segment. This was described
as a 'firm, fibrotic area of the mucosa measuring 9 mm ×
8 mm, present 57 mm from the closest resection margin
and 140 mm from the mesenteric cut margin'. The specimen was sliced transversely at 10 mm intervals, ensuring
the firm, flattened area was sliced through and thoroughly
examined. The sections showed out-pouches of mucosa
consistent with diverticula, with an area associated with

abscess formation and perforation. This was separate from
the firm fibrotic area. This showed slightly firmer white
tissue involving the mucosa, but the submucosa and muscularis propria looked normal and intact. This was slightly
worrying for carcinoma and the reporting histopathologist
was called.

- The histopathologist agreed carcinoma needed excluding and instructed the dissector to sample the flattened,
  firmer area in its entirety and to also look for all lymph
  nodes within the specimen, to identify and block separately the apical lymph node (lymph node closest to the
  mesenteric margin) and to sample the resection margins.

- Block selection included resection margins, apical lymph
  node, all other identifiable lymph nodes, all of the flattened fibrotic area and representative blocks from the
  diverticular disease including the abscess and area of perforation. Block key produced.

- Microscopically, diverticular disease was confirmed with
  associated abscess formation, perforation and acute peritonitis. In addition, separate from the diverticular disease
  and area of perforation there was an 'early' adenocarcinoma. The flattened firm area was a 'hidden' adenocarcinoma which infiltrated very focally and superficially into
  the submucosa. There were no lymph node metastases or
  vascular invasion. The patient was discussed at the multidisciplinary team meeting and underwent thoracic and
  abdominal CT scans and full colonoscopy, which showed
  no other abnormality. No further treatment apart from
  follow-up for bowel cancer was required. Three years on
  the patient remains fit and well.

Learning points: It is essential to understand the pathology of the cases you are dissecting. Diverticular disease and

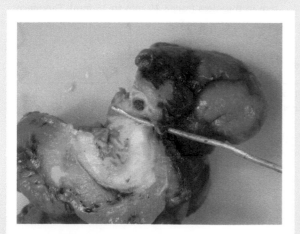

FIGURE 3.14
Area of perforation associated with diverticula indicated
by a probe.

colon cancer are both common diseases in patients of this age group and can co-exist. Diverticular disease can make it difficult to identify cancers by endoscopy or radiological imaging (CT/MRI scan). The dissector needs to be aware of this and carefully look for features suggestive of carcinoma in these specimens. The dissector here ensured the patient was given the correct and full diagnosis, enabling further management. The patient may not have done so well if the carcinoma was missed due to poor quality dissection, especially if lymph nodes were involved or if the cancer had already spread.

3.4.4 Endocrine

Endocrine specimens include cytology, biopsies and resections from the thyroid, parathyroid and adrenal glands. In addition there are neuroendocrine neoplasms of the gastrointestinal tract. Not all specimen types are seen in all departments. More common specimens within this specialized area include thyroid specimens for benign disease. Table 3.10 gives common endocrine specimen types and associated pathologies, with Table 3.11 listing common surgical specimens and brief details on dissection methodology. Please also refer to the Royal College of Pathologist Cancer datasets for endocrine neoplasms (www.rcpath.org/resourceLibrary/tissue-pathways-for-endocrine-pathology--january-2012-.html; www.rcpath.org/resourceLibrary/thyroid_dataset_feb14.html; www.rcpath.org/resourceLibrary/g081_datasetgiendocrine_sep12-pdf.html).

TABLE 3.10 Common endocrine specimen types and associated pathologies.

Specimen site	Conditions/pathologies
Adrenalectomy	Benign—treatment for Cushing's or ectopic adrenocorticotrophic hormone syndrome (usually bilateral excision), adrenal mass on imaging (diagnosis uncertain), infective lesion, congenital conditions. Premalignant/indeterminate—adrenal medullary hyperplasia in multiple endocrine neoplasia type 2. Malignant—carcinoma, metastatic disease.
Parathyroid gland	Benign—primary, secondary or tertiary hyperparathyroidism, adenoma, hyperplasia, cysts. Malignant—carcinoma.
Thyroidectomy/thyroid lobectomy	Benign—multinodular goitre, follicular adenoma, hyperplastic nodule, Graves' disease, autoimmune thyroiditis, Hurthle cell neoplasm. Malignant—papillary carcinoma, follicular carcinoma, medullary carcinoma, anaplastic carcinoma, lymphoma.

TABLE 3.11 Common surgical specimens and brief details on dissection methodology.

Surgical/radiological technique	Process/removal of	Dissection procedure
Adrenal gland	Surgical removal of unilateral or bilateral adrenal gland. If laparoscopic removal may be slightly more disrupted.	Measure in 3 dimensions, weigh and ink. The head, body and tail of the gland should be identified, and the gland sliced from head to tail. Describe appearance of the cortex, the presence or absence of nodules (give the maximum dimension of any nodules). Note the distribution of the medulla. One block taken from the head, body and tail. Consider additional blocks if there are focal abnormalities.
Parathyroid gland	Surgical removal of one or more parathyroid glands. May receive with request for frozen section.	Weigh with suitable high quality scales, measure in 3 dimensions, state colour and consistency. Bisect small glands, cut larger glands into parallel slices, through the vascular pole where possible. Glands should have margins inked prior to dissection if a diagnosis of carcinoma is being considered (large glands, thick capsule or surgical/radiological suspicion).

continued

TABLE 3.11 Common surgical specimens and brief details on dissection methodology. (*Continued*)

Surgical/radiological technique	Process/removal of	Dissection procedure
Thyroid gland	Fine needle aspiration (FNA) specimens for diagnosis. Surgical removal of thyroid gland/lobe for symptom relief, cosmetic reasons, or removal of mass lesion/Thy3+ FNA lesions.	FNA—cytology specimen. Lobectomy/total thyroidectomy—state nature of specimen and laterality if applicable. Orientate the specimen and measure each lobe and isthmus in 3 dimensions & weigh. Describe the capsule (intact or not) & external surface of specimen. Look for any attached parathyroid glands or lymph nodes. Ink resection margins. Cut into 5-mm slices in the horizontal plane and describe the cut surface. Measure and describe colour/consistency of any nodules. Process any parathyroid glands or lymph nodes. For inflammatory and diffuse lesions sample at least two blocks from each lobe. For multinodular goitres sample one block from representative nodules, up to five from each lobe. Any encapsulated nodule should be treated as a potential neoplasm and sampled accordingly (www.rcpath. org/resourceLibrary/thyroid_dataset_feb14.html). Block any unusual areas.

CASE STUDY 3.4 Thyroid adenoma

Request card clinical information: 55-year-old woman with a thyroid nodule rapidly increasing in size. Left thyroid lobectomy performed.

Standard patient/specimen identification checks are made prior to dissection.

As is good practice, previous histology results were reviewed and revealed that an earlier core biopsy from the nodule had been diagnosed as a 'follicular neoplasm'. It was not possible to ascertain whether the lesion was benign or malignant, as the growing edge of the lesion is not seen on the biopsy, hence a lobectomy was performed.

Next examine the specimen, dissect, LOOK, FEEL & THINK and produce a macroscopic report. Thyroid lobectomy specimen dissection is detailed in Table 3.11.

In this case the lobectomy specimen weighed 11 g and was 45 × 27 × 24 mm max. It had a smooth outer surface. The tracheal aspect was inked red and the remaining surgical margins blue. Transverse slicing revealed a 25 mm solid lesion (see Figure 3.16). This was cream in colour with small areas of haemorrhage and had an apparent surrounding capsule. No other nodules were noted. The lesion was sampled in its entirety, with additional blocks from the background macroscopically normal thyroid tissue. No parathyroid glands or lymph nodes were found.

Microscopic examination revealed an encapsulated lesion composed of a solid proliferation of colloid-poor microtubules, differing in appearance from the surrounding thyroid gland which also showed pressure effects due to the presence of the expanding lesion. There were no nuclear features of a papillary carcinoma. There was no necrosis. The capsule was not invaded or breached. No lymphovascular invasion was seen. The lesion was clear of the surgical margins, the closest

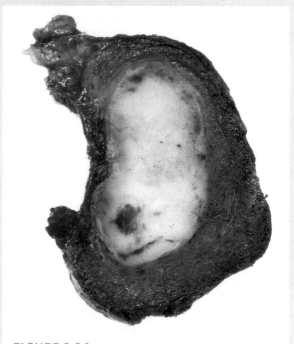

FIGURE 3.16

Section through thyroid lobe and tumour showing fibrous capsule and relationship of tumour to the inked surgical margins.

being the tracheal aspect, with a minimum distance from the margin of 1 mm.

Diagnosis: Follicular adenoma.

Encapsulated thyroid nodules ideally need to be sampled in their entirety, as capsular invasion and vascular invasion are the key features for distinguishing between a follicular adenoma and a carcinoma. It is important to note whether the background thyroid gland contains multiple nodules, as this may indicate a hyperplastic process with a dominant nodule, rather than a solitary neoplastic lesion.

Key Point

Knowledge of the different types of lesions that occur within an organ enables correct sampling of the specimen.

SELF-CHECK 3.7

Why is it helpful to have a methodical approach to specimen dissection?

3.4.5 Genitourinary

Genitourinary specimens are received from a number of different organs, i.e. the bladder, prostate, testis, penis and kidney, as part of the investigation of a variety of conditions. A list of the more common pathological findings at the various organ sites is given in Table 3.12.

TABLE 3.12 Common pathological findings at various organ sites.

Specimen site	Conditions/pathologies
Bladder	Benign—cystitis (acute/chronic/granulomatous), follicular cystitis, cystitis cystica, cystitis glandularis, malakoplakia, interstitial cystitis, amyloidosis, papilloma (urothelial, papilloma), nephrogenic adenoma, keratinizing squamous metaplasia, diverticulae, fistulae. Pre-malignant/indeterminate—urothelial carcinoma *in situ* (CIS). Malignant—urothelial carcinoma (commonest), rarer adenocarcinoma, squamous cell carcinoma, neuroendocrine carcinoma, metastases.
Prostate	Benign—benign prostatic (nodular) hyperplasia. Pre-malignant/indeterminate—high grade prostatic intra-epithelial neoplasia (HGPIN). Malignant—prostatic adenocarcinoma (commonest), neuroendocrine carcinoma, metastases, urothelial carcinomas arising in the prostatic urethra.
Kidney	Benign—chronic/acute pyelonephritis, xanthogranulomatous pyelonephritis, hydronephrosis, renal calculi, benign tumours (oncocytoma, angiomyolipoma, metanephric adenoma, papillary adenoma), polycystic kidney disease, non-functioning kidney. Pre-malignant/indeterminate—urothelial carcinoma *in situ* (CIS) in the renal pelvis. Malignant—renal cell carcinoma (clear cell commonest, but many types), urothelial carcinoma arising in the pelvi-calyceal system, metastases.
Ureter	Benign—stricture (congenital or acquired), pelvi-ureteric junction obstruction, calculi, duplex ureter (congenital). Pre-malignant/indeterminate—urothelial carcinoma *in situ* (CIS). Malignant—urothelial carcinoma, metastases.
Testis and epididymis and related structures	Benign—torsion/infarction, epididymal cyst, appendix testis and epididymis, epididymo-orchitis, adenomatoid tumour, lipoma of spermatic cord, hernia sac, hydrocele. Pre-malignant/indeterminate—testicular intra-tubular germ cell neoplasia/germ cell neoplasia *in situ*. Malignant—germ cell tumours (seminoma/non-seminomatous/mixed), lymphoma, metastases.
Penis	Benign—balanitis xerotica obliterans (lichen sclerosis), various skin lesions. Pre-malignant/indeterminate—urothelial carcinoma *in-situ* of penile urethra, penile skin intraepithelial neoplasia (PeIN). Malignant—squamous cell carcinoma, urothelial carcinoma, metastases.

As with other organ systems, genitourinary specimens submitted for histopathology range from small biopsies to major resections and will require particular handling during dissection. Typical small biopsy specimens, such as those from the bladder, prostatic urethra or ureter, usually only require a documented gross description and simple transfer into cassettes for routine processing and cutting of standard levels. Other biopsies may need to undergo set protocols for laboratory handling, such as spare intervening unstained sections to be retained for immunohistochemistry, as are frequently required on prostate core biopsies to enable the diagnosis of tiny cancerous lesions. Such specific requirements need to be conveyed to the laboratory from dissection by means of different cassette colours or labelling as detailed in local protocols; otherwise precious biopsy tissue may be lost at section cutting. Testicular biopsies submitted as part of the clinical investigation of infertility are best received in a different fixative from buffered formalin (e.g. Bouin's) that gives optimum preservation of the nuclei of the germ cells for the assessment of spermatogenesis. A summary of typical genitourinary specimen types is given in Table 3.13, with a brief overview of the dissection procedure.

TABLE 3.13 Typical genitourinary specimen types, with a brief overview of the dissection procedure.

Surgical/radiological technique	Process/removal of	Dissection procedure
Mucosal biopsy (any site)	Cystoscopic cold or hot sampling of abnormal/normal areas.	Number of fragments, measure range of sizes. Process all tissue. Cut levels × 3.
Bladder tumour resection or 'curettings'	Cystoscopic transurethral resection of bladder tumour (TURBT), with removal of tumour and sampling of underlying deep tissue to assess invasion.	Weigh and measure in aggregate. Process all tissue (unless very large). Cut levels × 3 for small tumour specimens.
Cystectomy	Removal of bladder, partial (for diverticulae, fistulae, tumour localized to the bladder dome) and radical (total) for treatment of malignancy.	Radical cystectomy usually includes the prostate (with or without the penile urethra) or the uterus and adnexae. Dissection involves examination and sampling of the tumour to determine the grade and stage, plus surgical margins (www.rcpath.org/resourceLibrary/dataset-for-tumours-of-the-urinary-collecting-system--renal-pelvis--ureter--urinary-bladder-and-urethra.html).
Prostate needle core biopsy	Core biopsy sampling via transrectal or transperineal route. Extended protocols for wider and systematic sampling of the prostate and 'targeted' biopsies from lesions visible via ultrasound or MRI scanning.	Number of fragments, measure range of sizes. Process all tissue, ensuring cores are kept flat. Minimal number of cores per cassette advised, to ensure full face section of all cores obtained. Cut levels or serial sections, with spare unstained retained for immunohistochemistry.
Prostate chippings resection	Transurethral resection to relieve bladder outlet obstruction.	Sampled according to local protocols. Discussed further in text.
Prostatectomy	Removal of the entire prostate by open, laparoscopic or robotic technique as a treatment for prostate cancer. Includes the seminal vesicles.	Prostatic carcinoma is often not visible by naked eye, therefore the gland is weighed, orientated, inked, measured and entirely processed, most frequently with the central portion in transverse slices processed in mega blocks and the apex and base in small blocks so that all margins can be assessed (www.rcpath.org/resourceLibrary/dataset-for-histopathology-reports-for-prostatic-carcinoma.html).
Kidney biopsy	Percutaneous approach, with needle cores taken from mass lesions visible on radiological images.	Number of fragments, measure range of sizes. Process all tissue. Cut levels/serials to allow spares for immunohistochemistry.

TABLE 3.13 Typical genitourinary specimen types, with a brief overview of the dissection procedure. (*Continued*)

Surgical/radiological technique	Process/removal of	Dissection procedure
Kidney	Partial nephrectomy, for complete removal of lesions but allowing maximum conservation of renal tissue. Simple nephrectomy, to remove non-functioning kidneys, benign lesions (that are large or at risk of haemorrhage) or failed transplant kidneys. Radical nephrectomy, to remove renal tumours known or suspected to be malignant. May also include the adrenal gland. For ureteric tumours arising in the renal pelvis or ureter, a nephro-ureterectomy is performed, with removal of the kidney and the entire ureter, including the distal portion embedded in the bladder wall.	Partial nephrectomy: Measure in 3 dimensions; weigh; ink to denote intra-renal and capsular margins; cut into parallel slices; describe and measure lesion and its relationship to the margins. Blocks should include most/all of lesion depending on size, with the margins included, plus a block of the background normal tissue. Simple nephrectomy: see Case study 3.5. Radical nephrectomy (renal tumours): weigh; measure kidney with fat and kidney without fat. Describe and measure attached ureter and the adrenal gland or hilar lymph nodes if present. Ink the outer aspect where tumour might involve the margin. Inspect the hilar vessels, i.e. renal vein, for the presence of tumour thrombi. Slice kidney from the lateral border. Describe and measure any tumours, stating the location and relationship to margins. Select blocks to sample different areas of the tumour and those where it is adjacent to normal kidney, the renal sinus fat, the renal pelvis and the perinephric fat. For ureteric tumours, the tumour will be in the pelvis and/or ureter and should be sampled appropriately for typing grading and staging and margin assessment (www.rcpath.org/resourceLibrary/dataset-adult-renal-parenchymal-cancer-histopathology-reports.html).
Ureter	Partial removal for strictures.	Measure length and diameter, describe and sample abnormal areas and the surgical margins.
Orchidectomy	Removal of testis for benign conditions, such as torsion or during a hernia repair, or to remove a tumour.	See Case study 3.6 for benign testicular pathology. For tumours, the dissection procedure is similar, but with additional special attention to describing the tumour location, size, appearance and consistency. Blocks need to include generous sampling of the tumour for tumour typing and blocks to show its relationship with the tunica albuginea/vaginalis, the rete testis and the spermatic cord in order to determine the tumour stage (www.rcpath.org/resourceLibrary/dataset-for-the-histological-reporting-of-testicular-neoplasms.html).

Some specimens, although not requiring detailed dissection, may need careful handling for subsequent optimal orientation at embedding. For example, in order to confirm that a vasectomy has been successful, histological examination needs to be able to confirm that the resected tissue is a vas deferens and also that a full transverse section has been achieved (Figures 3.17 & 3.18). Similarly, resected sections of ureters, taken at cystectomy (bladder removal) for bladder cancer, need appropriate inking, slicing and correct orientation to confirm that the appropriate ureteric surgical margin is free of pre-malignant disease (urothelial carcinoma *in situ*) or tumour. Failure to do this means that it may not be possible to confirm to the urologist that the ends of the ureters implanted into ileal conduits (small intestine segments fashioned to collect urine as a bladder substitute) are likely to be disease free.

This 12-mm segment of vas deferens (Figure 3.17) needs to be cut into pieces of appropriate length so that it can be identified as a tubal structure at embedding. Failure to cut the specimen appropriately or to alert the embedder that the pieces need to be upright may mean that the specimen

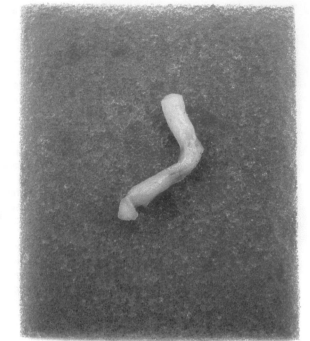

FIGURE 3.17
A 12-mm segment of vas deferens; slices of appropriate length must be cut so that it can be identified as a tubal structure at embedding. Failure to cut the specimen appropriately or to alert the embedder that the pieces need to be upright may mean that the specimen is incorrectly embedded, making confirmation of successful vasectomy impossible.

is incorrectly embedded flat and after initial sectioning a full cross-section (Figure 3.18) cannot then be obtained, even after re-embedding. This is potentially problematic for the patient, as successful vasectomy cannot be confirmed histologically.

Key Point
Poor handling of specimens at dissection and embedding may have significant clinical consequences.

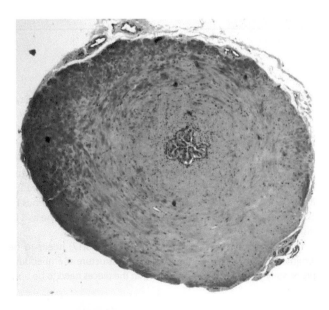

FIGURE 3.18
Complete cross-section of a vas deferens.

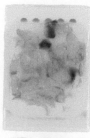
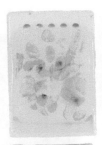
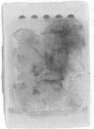
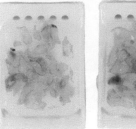
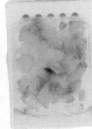
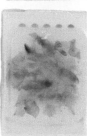

FIGURE 3.19

Blocks of sampled prostatic chippings removed for presumed benign prostatic hyperplasia (BPH; i.e. nodular enlargement of the prostate). They are weighed and a proportion sampled, including any 'yellow' areas of potential cancerous tissue identified macroscopically.

Selection of tissue for processing from transurethral resection specimens ('chippings') obtained at cystoscopy from the bladder or prostate is determined by the clinical scenario. Bladder tumour resections are ideally processed in their entirety, so that the tumour can be examined fully and diagnosed and graded correctly histologically. This also means that all deeper tissue (lamina propria and detrusor muscle) present can be examined for the presence or absence of invasion by urothelial carcinoma. Prostate chippings, however, removed most often for relief of symptoms of difficulty in passing urine (bladder outflow obstruction), may be too numerous to process. The main purpose of histological examination of these specimens is to detect incidental prostatic cancer that is clinically significant, i.e. requires treatment, so reference is needed to local protocols to determine the proportion of tissue that should be processed in order to best achieve this. Extra blocks may be required if areas suspicious, but not diagnostic, of cancer are seen on the sections from the initially selected tissue sample (see Figure 3.19).

Penile biopsies and lesions identified on circumcision specimens are often processed according to skin protocols and may be reported by dermatopathologists, because of the nature of the lesions arising in penile skin.

Penile resections, however, are uncommon and are only performed at a limited number of surgical centres.

Large urological resection specimens for cancer of the bladder, kidney, prostate and testis require advanced dissection skills. However, large resections for presumed benign disease are also frequently encountered. It is therefore advisable to examine these carefully for unsuspected neoplasms and to routinely take some additional blocks that might otherwise be necessary should this incidental finding occur.

> **ORC**
> See Section 3.4.1.

CASE STUDY 3.5 Renal calculus

Request form clinical information: A 60-year-old man has a nephrectomy for a non-functioning kidney.

The approach to handling of simple nephrectomy specimens for benign disease is similar for a variety of different diagnoses. Attention to the clinical history is important so that specific areas of the specimen may be examined in more detail, if required. For example, if a history of a ureteric stricture (narrowing) is given as a cause of hydronephrosis (dilated fluid-filled kidney), it is important to locate and examine the stricture site for a possible cause and to sample that area.

Once the necessary identification checks have been made, it is important to examine the specimen, dissect, LOOK, FEEL & THINK and produce a macroscopic report:

- Weigh the specimen.
- Measure the kidney with perinephric fat and the kidney alone.
- Describe the external appearance of the capsule, noting scars, adherence to fat.
- Measure and describe appearance of the ureter, noting any strictures or dilated areas.
- Identify and inspect the renal vessels (artery and vein) at the hilum for unsuspected tumour or abnormalities.
- On opening (slicing from the lateral aspect) describe the appearance of the cortex and medulla, noting the thickness and the presence of any scarring or abscesses.
- Describe the appearance of the pelvi-calyceal system—is it dilated, distorted, or expanded (hydronephrosis), and are there calculi present? See Figures 3.20 and 3.21.
- Check for lymph nodes at the hilum—although not often present, they should be processed if identified.
- The adrenal gland is not normally present in simple nephrectomy specimens.

Blocks need to include the ureteric margin, the renal cortex and medulla (in particular any visible lesions) and the renal pelvis. The hilar blood vessel margins are sampled in case of an incidental tumour and can be included with the ureteric margin section to keep block numbers to a minimum.

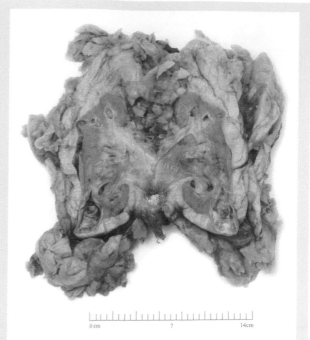

FIGURE 3.20
The kidney pictured is mildly hydronephrotic (dilated), the cortex and medulla are atrophic (shrunken) and scarred. Small cortical cysts are also present.

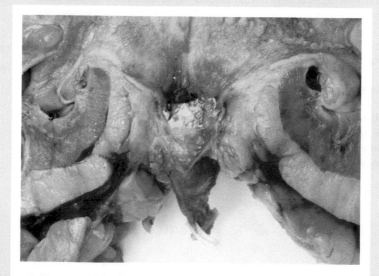

FIGURE 3.21
Careful inspection of the kidney in Figure 3.20 reveals a calculus (renal stone) obstructing the pelvi-ureteric junction, which has led to the changes in the kidney.

CLINICAL CORRELATION

Hydronephrosis may be due to obstruction to urine outflow and subsequent back pressure on the kidney, due to nodular enlargement of the prostate, a bladder tumour obstructing the ureteric orifice, or tumours, strictures or calculi obstructing the ureter.

Key Point

Use the clinical details to guide you to areas of the specimen that may need detailed inspection.

CASE STUDY 3.6 Testicular infarction

Request form clinical information: A 23-year-old man has an orchidectomy due to torsion.

Torsion of the testis occurs when the spermatic cord (from which the testis is suspended) twists and compresses the blood vessels within it. If prolonged for several hours without surgical intervention or spontaneous resolution, there will be haemorrhage and infarction of the testis due to the consequent obstruction to its vascular supply.

Examine the specimen, dissect, LOOK, FEEL & THINK and produce a macroscopic report:

- Measure the specimen, which usually includes both the epididymis and testis.

- Measure the length of spermatic cord present (may be short, unlike orchidectomy specimens excised because of the presence of a tumour).

- Describe the external appearance, usually dark purple/black and dusky with torsion.

- Slice the specimen transversely along its length, describe the appearance and consistency of the cut surface (Figure 3.22) and carefully inspect for any unexpected lesions, which should be described and sampled.

- Sample the spermatic cord margin (in case of an incidental tumour), the testis and epididymis.

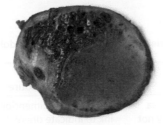

FIGURE 3.22
Transverse section of testis showing haemorrhage and dilated blood vessels in the fat and in the adjacent epididymis. Although apparently normal in colour, on microscopic examination the testis was infarcted.

> **Key Point**
>
> Some tissue may be processed in case an unexpected malignancy is found at microscopic examination. This is because dissection of the specimen may make it difficult to find key areas/structures on revisiting the specimen for extra blocks.

3.5 Head and neck pathology

Head and neck specimens are rarer specimens, not seen in all departments. However, more common specimens within this specialized area include nasal polyps and tonsils. Specimens may consist of hard tissue (bone/teeth), which will need decalcification. Please refer to Chapter 2 for information on decalcification of hard tissues. Table 3.14 gives common head and neck specimen types and associated pathologies, with Table 3.15 listing common surgical specimens and brief details on dissection methodology (www.rcpath.org/resourceLibrary/head-and-neck-pathology--may-2014-.html; Dahlstrom *et al.*, 2012; Slootweg, 2005).

TABLE 3.14 Common head and neck specimen types.

Specimen site	Conditions/pathologies
Oral cavity	Benign—benign keratosis, polyps, odontogenic cysts, mucocoele. Premalignant/indeterminate—squamous cell carcinoma *in situ*/dysplasia. Malignant—squamous cell carcinoma.
Nasal cavity	Benign—inflammatory polyp. Premalignant/indeterminate—dysplasia. Malignant—carcinoma, lymphoma, metastatic disease.
Salivary glands	Benign—sialadenitis, sialithiasis, pleomorphic adenoma, Warthin's tumour, Sjögren's syndrome. Premalignant/indeterminate—dysplasia. Malignant—carcinoma, lymphoma, metastatic disease.
Larynx, pharynx and tonsil	Benign—chronic tonsillitis, keratosis, leucoplakia. Premalignant/indeterminate—dysplasia. Malignant—squamous cell carcinoma, lymphoma, metastatic disease.
Neck	Benign—reactive lymphadenopathy, thyroglossal cyst, branchial cyst. Malignant –metastatic disease, lymphoma.

TABLE 3.15 Common head and neck surgical specimens and brief details on dissection methodology.

Surgical/radiological technique	Process/removal of	Dissection procedure
Mucosal biopsy/excision (any area)	Surgical removal of ellipse of mucosa with underlying tissue, may or may not be orientated, may be sent fresh for immunofluorescence. Removal of: part or all of lesion.	Measure in 3 dimensions, describe mucosal surface, ink to indicate orientation, for excision specimens sample closest margin (often by transverse section across short axis). Process all tissue.
Incisional biopsy (any area)	Elongated mucosal ellipses which include the lesion and some normal tissue. Removal of: part or all of lesion.	Measure in 3 dimensions, describe surface, ink to indicate orientation, bisect longitudinally where appropriate. Process all tissue.

TABLE 3.15 Common head and neck surgical specimens and brief details on dissection methodology. *(Continued)*

Surgical/radiological technique	Process/removal of	Dissection procedure
Teeth	Surgical removal often with attached cyst or resection specimen, rarely for tooth disorder. Removal of: all of tooth +/− attached tissue.	Notation, site, morphology, caries, fillings, colour, root number & morphology, resorption. Decalcification or ground section for enamel defects. Incisors, canines & premolars section in bucco-lingual plane, molar teeth meso-distally. At least one block of cross-section.
Cysts (odontogenic and non-odontogenic)	Surgical removal of cyst and usually small amount of surrounding tissue.	Normally multiple fragments, record number and 3 dimensions of largest, bone present, relation to tooth, wall thickness, nodules, keratin. Process all of fragmented lesions, representative slices of larger cysts.
Salivary glands	Surgical removal of minor or major salivary gland tissue for symptom relief or removal of mass lesion.	Measure in 3 dimensions, weigh and ink, describe external and cut surface (lesion seen, dimension, appearance, capsulated, closest margin). One block per 10 mm of lesion at least, margins, adjacent tissue, lymph nodes, other attached organs.
Jaw lesions	Surgical removal of benign and malignant lesions by enucleation as multiple fragments or as one excision specimen.	Multiple fragments—number of pieces, dimensions of largest and in entirety, appearance, process all if small sample or representative pieces. Resections—orientate, photograph, measure in 3 dimensions, attached mucosa, teeth, lesion (dimensions and margins), ink, +/− section with bone saw and decalcify. Process all if small sample or representative sections.
Nasal cavity	Surgical removal of benign and rarely malignant lesions, often as small fragments/polyp or excision specimen (rare).	Number of fragments, largest in 3 dimensions, appearance (colour, texture, polyp, ulcerated), if any hard tissue may need decalcification. Process all if small sample or representative sections.
Tonsil	Surgical removal of both or one tonsil for symptom relief or neoplasia.	Orientate if possible & ink deep margin, measure in 3 dimensions, weigh, section 4–5 mm transverse slices, describe surfaces. Process 2 blocks if normal (unless excised for unknown primary when all tissue is blocked), more representative blocks if lesion.
Larynx	Partial or total laryngectomy specimens usually for malignancy, rarely for benign disease.	Orientate, measure in 3 dimensions, ink margins, decalcify, section longitudinally or transversely, describe mucosa, lesion (dimensions, closest margin, invasion of cartilage), attached organs, lymph nodes. At least 4 representative blocks: lesion, margins, attached organs, lymph nodes (www.rcpath.org/resourceLibrary/head-and-neck-pathology--may-2014-.html).
Neck lesions	Fine needle aspiration (FNA) & core biopsy specimens for diagnosis, cyst excision, lymph node excision for diagnosis, neck dissection for treatment of malignancy/staging.	FNA—cytology specimen, core biopsy measure number and length & process all. Cysts—measure in 3 dimensions, attached tissues, thickness of wall, external and internal surfaces, contents, serial slices, take representative sections. Lymph node—<5 mm embedded whole, 5–10 mm bisected through hilum, >10-mm section at 4 mm, take representative samples. For neck dissections orientate, measure in 3 dimensions, describe attached structures, palpate/visualize and process all nodes (www.rcpath.org/resourceLibrary/head-and-neck-pathology--may-2014-.html).

CASE STUDY 3.7 *Benign parotid tumour*

Request card and clinical information: 42-year-old male, partial parotidectomy for 2-cm nodule, FNAC?? Warthin's tumour, but not certain. Heavy smoker and drinker.

Standard patient/specimen identifications checks are made.

Assess the clinical information:

The most common mass lesion within the parotid gland is a pleomorphic adenoma, closely followed by a Warthin's tumour. Both are benign lesions. However, malignant salivary gland tumours can occur and in some cases intraparotid lymph nodes may be involved by metastatic disease (especially metastatic squamous cell carcinoma), all of which should be considered in a patient of this age with a history of heavy smoking, drinking and a mass lesion in the parotid. It would be worthwhile looking at the fine needle aspirate (FNAC) report. In this case it showed some cellular debris and a small number of lymphocytes, but no epithelial or malignant cells. Overall classification was non-diagnostic. This is not too helpful at dissection, apart from informing the dissector there is at present no definite diagnosis of the lesion.

Examine the specimen (Figure 3.23), dissect, LOOK, FEEL & THINK and produce a macroscopic report:

- All salivary gland tissue specimens are weighed (g) and measured (mm), in 3 dimensions.

- The specimen is checked for orientation by the surgeon (clips or sutures). If orientated the specimen is inked to allow orientation at the time of reporting. A key of the inking protocol is provided. If there is no orientation (normally the case for presumed benign disease), then the specimen is inked in one colour.

- The specimen is serially sliced at 3–5 mm, usually along the transverse axis. If orientated it is good practice to state which direction slicing is (e.g. medial to lateral), and how many slices there are. The cut surface should then be described.

  - Colour and consistency.
  - Look for a mass lesion (present or absent). If present:
  - Number; if more than one tumour, designate and describe each tumour separately.
  - Size in millimetres (at least the maximum diameter should be given, but it is good practice to give in 3 dimensions).
  - Appearance—circumscription, colour and consistency (solid, rubbery, soft, hard, cystic, gelatinous, necrotic).
  - Distance to margin (mm).

- Are any other abnormalities present? For example, separate cysts or stones.

- Look for lymph nodes—if present describe and measure range of lymph node size.

Submit representative sections:

- Surgical resection margins.
- Mass lesion.
  - If < 30 mm, it may be appropriate to submit all the tumour.
  - If > 30 mm, at least one section per 10 mm of tumour.
- All macroscopically different areas particularly at the edge of the tumour.
- Tumour interface with non-lesional tissue.
- Surgical resection margins.
- Submit all lymph nodes & identify the site of each.

Block allocation key should be provided.

This was a mass of grey tissue measuring 70 mm × 62 mm × 30 mm and weighing 45 g. It had not been orientated by the surgeon, so the margin of the whole specimen was inked black. The external surface showed no abnormality. On sectioning there was a well circumscribed solid lesion measuring 37 mm × 34 mm × 24 mm, which was rubbery in consistency, with a homogeneous white cut surface. There were no cystic or necrotic areas seen. The lesion was 2 mm from the closest resection margin. No other abnormalities were seen and no lymph nodes identified. Four blocks from the lesion were taken, including the closest resection margin, together with a block of background normal appearing salivary gland tissue. A block key was provided.

This case was reported as a benign Warthin's tumour, completely excised.

Learning points: This was a benign Warthin's tumour, which was completely excised, with a margin of 2 mm. Dissection, description and block selection allowed this diagnosis to be made confidently. It also allowed the resection status to be given. The surgeon can now inform the patient this was a benign lesion which was completely excised with a very low risk of recurrence.

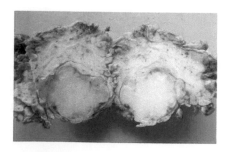

FIGURE 3.23
Bisected parotid gland containing a well-circumscribed solid lesion.

3.6 Gynaecological cases

Gynaecological cases include the uterus, cervix, Fallopian tubes (FT), ovaries, vagina and vulva, any of which can be submitted individually or as part of a larger resection specimen, depending on the clinical presentation (www.rcpath.org/resourceLibrary/tissue-pathways-for-gynaecological-pathology--january-2015-.html). Common pathologies of each component are given in Table 3.16. The dissector should be aware of the various surgical techniques used to obtain gynaecological specimens depending on investigation (see Table 3.17).

TABLE 3.16 Common pathologies in gynaecological tissue.

Specimen site	Conditions/pathologies
Cervix	Cervicitis, cervical polyp, hyperplasia, HPV infection, leiomyoma (uncommon), cervical intraepithelial neoplasia (CIN) also known as high grade squamous intraepithelial neoplasia (HSIL), cervical glandular intraepithelial neoplasia (CGIN), invasive carcinoma of the cervix.
Fallopian tube	Salpingitis (hydrosalpinx, pyosalpinx), ectopic pregnancy, paratubal cyst, endometriosis.
Ovary	Non-neoplastic cysts (e.g. follicular, inclusion, fibromas, teratomas [dermoid], etc.), hyperplasia, polycystic ovary syndrome, malignant cysts and tumours of epithelial, stromal and germ cell derivation.
Uterus	Endometritis, endometrial polyp, adenomyosis, endometriosis, leiomyoma, hyperplasia, endometrial carcinoma (usually adeno), stromal tumours, adenomatoid tumours (rare), leiomyosarcomas (uncommon).
Vagina	Vaginitis (e.g. *Trichomonas vaginalis*—commonly sexual transmitted disease [STD], *Gardnerella vaginalis*, herpes simplex, *Candida albicans*).
Vulva	Any skin disorders, commonly lichen planus, lichen sclerosis, lichen simplex chronicus, herpes, STD, vulval intraepithelial neoplasia (VIN).

TABLE 3.17 Surgical techniques.

Surgical technique	Removal of	Reason
Fine needle aspiration (FNA)	Cystic fluid from ovary.	Cytological investigations.
Peritoneal aspiration/washings	Ascitic fluid.	Investigation of neoplasia.
Pipelle biopsy	Endometrial curettings.	Investigation of endometrial abnormality.
Cervical dilation and curettage (D&C)	Larger sampling of endometrium.	Investigation of endometrial abnormality (requires general anaesthetic).
Hysteroscopy	Endometrial biopsy, sampling or removal of polyps.	Endometrial investigations, identification and removal of polyps per vagina.
Endocervical biopsy	Small piece cervical tissue.	Investigation of CIN or CGIN.
Colposcopic biopsy	Punch biopsy of cervical tissue.	Investigation of CIN or CGIN.
Cone biopsy, LLETZ, knife biopsy	Affected area of cervix.	Treatment of CIN or CGIN.
Amputation of cervix	Entire cervix.	Pelvic floor repair/prolapse.
Laparoscopy	Biopsy sample if appropriate.	Investigation endometriosis.
Polypectomy	Endometrial or cervical polyp.	Removal of cervical or endometrial polyps.
Oophorectomy	Ovary.	Elective with hysterectomy, torsion, genetic predisposition to ovarian cancer (BRCA 1 & 2 carriers), endometriosis, polycystic ovarian disease, malignancy.
Cystectomy	Benign cyst only.	To preserve function of tube or ovary where benign cyst.

continued

TABLE 3.17 Surgical techniques. (*Continued*)

Surgical technique	Removal of	Reason
Salpingectomy	Fallopian tube.	Sterilization, treatment ectopic pregnancy, salpingitis, as part of hysterectomy.
Salpingo-oophorectomy	Fallopian tube and ovary.	See above.
Laser ablation		Therapeutic treatment menorrhagia.
Myomectomy (Fibroidectomy)	Leiomyoma.	Removal of subserosal or submucosal leiomyoma without hysterectomy.
Hysterectomy simple/subtotal • Abdominal—preferred method for large uterine bodies • Laparotomy—where no endometrial abnormality (may be morcellated) • Vaginal—usually post-menopausal small uterus and for prolapse repair	Uterus +/− cervix.	Uterovaginal prolapse, abnormal menorrhagia, failed laser ablation, presence of leiomyoma. To confirm or establish diagnosis, to type and grade tumours and to stage by assessing depth of spread and serosal involvement.
Radical/total abdominal hysterectomy	Uterus, both FTs and ovaries, cervix and upper third of vagina.	Treatment endometrial cancer and to type, grade and stage tumour.

When faced with multiple components as part of one surgical procedure (e.g. total abdominal hysterectomy), you should develop a methodical system, dealing with each element as an individual specimen while demonstrating the connection where pertinent (e.g. cut through hilum of ovary in continuity with Fallopian tube creating one block showing morphology and relationship of both the ovary and the tube).

Key Point

Where request card states uterus, cervix, both tubes and ovaries included, ensure you identify, describe and sample all components.

CASE STUDY 3.8 *Fibroid uterus*

Request form reads: 47-year-old female, history of dysmenorrhoea over 6 to 8 months; prolonged heavy painful periods, fibroid uterus. Sterilized 20 years ago.

Heavy, painful or prolonged menstruation (menorrhagia, dysmenorrhoea) and abnormal bleeding (post-coital or intermenstrual bleeding), uterovaginal prolapse, adenomyosis, endometriosis and leiomyomas are the most common clinical reasons for carrying out hysterectomies for benign conditions. Examples of common findings when dissecting the uterus are given in Table 3.18.

TABLE 3.18 Common uterine presentations.

Condition	Findings
Adenomyosis	Ranging from quite subtle striated pattern in the myometrium to extensive proliferative pattern indicating the presence of endometrial gland and stroma within the myometrium, often accompanied by hyperplasia of the myometrium giving thick bulky corpus. The glands can be cystic with haemorrhage giving brown speckling.
Leiomyoma (common term: fibroid)	Circumscribed pale whorled appearance, can be multiple, larger may show red/brown degenerative areas with 'beefy' consistency indicating ischaemic change, mucinous myxoid degeneration, haemorrhage, and necrosis or calcified areas. Benign smooth muscle tumours arising from myometrium. Can also arise from cervix, fallopian tubes, or uterine ligaments. A subserosal leiomyoma can become detached and implant on another part of the pelvic serosa and would be submitted separately from the uterus specimen. Submucosal leiomyomas may present as a polypoid lesion protruding into cavity. Leiomyosarcomas are rare malignant forms of leiomyomas, whiter and generally softer than benign leiomyomas usually with areas of necrosis/haemorrhage and indistinct edge.
Endometrial polyp	Broad based or pedunculated, can protrude into cervical canal. Generally firmer texture than endometrium with darker colour and possible cystic cut surface. Hyperplasia can appear as one or more small polyps while adenocarcinoma and adenosarcoma may also present in the form of a polyp.
Endometriosis	May not be apparent macroscopically; usually diagnosed histologically; endometrial glands and stroma on outer surface of the uterus. More obvious around fallopian tubes, ovaries, broad ligaments if present often in association with adhesions. Cyclical bleeding causes haemorrhage, pain and scarring, tubes and ovaries may appear welded together, and possible formation of 'chocolate cyst' in the ovaries due to altered blood.

CLINICAL CORRELATION

This patient had been prescribed drugs to ease the bleeding, but after discussing the options available decided to have a hysterectomy. Due to the uterine size leiomyomas were suspected. On examination cervix was healthy.

Prior to dissection:

- Check previous history/radiological findings—here we have recent pipelle sampling which showed secretory phase endometrium, no endometriosis, hyperplasia or malignancy, but very scanty sample. Ultrasound scan (USS) confirms bulky enlarged uterus with possible multiple leiomyomas, anteverted uterus enlarged to 12/14 weeks' size. Cervical smear history normal. From this information you can proceed to dissection of this as a benign therapeutic hysterectomy.

Any suspected malignant endometrial tumour would be dissected by histopathologist or well trained, experienced BMS.

At the bench:

- Check patient demographics on pot, request card and cassettes match, then follow dissection procedure below.

Correlate all the clinical information:

- Read clinical history on form noting which components have been included.
- Note patient's age or menopausal status if given.
- Confirm specimen includes all parts mentioned on request card—in this case the

uterus and cervix only have been submitted. Conservation of the ovaries is desirable in premeno-pausal women to avoid hormonal imbalance and early menopause but only where the ovaries are healthy, otherwise they would be removed. Patient was sterilized, no FTs mentioned on request form or seen, but in other cases stumps of discontinuous FT may be visible at cornu, with or without sterilization clips *in situ*.

Key Point

Always check pot/bucket for any separate tissue pieces. Ovaries or FTs may be detached during difficult procedures and sent loose in container.

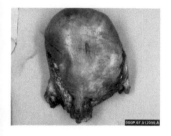

FIGURE 3.24
Posterior view of distorted uterine body.

- Orientate the specimen using peritoneum, round ligaments, FTs and ovaries where present as guides; the posterior peritoneal reflection (Pouch of Douglas, lying between uterus and rectum) extends further inferiorly than anterior peritoneal reflection (bladder side), round ligaments are anterior to fallopian tubes and ovaries posterior. Depending on distortion and presence of adnexae this can be difficult. In this case the posterior peritoneal/anterior peritoneal reflections were the only landmarks with the posterior extending almost to cervical margin (see Figure 3.24).

Key Point

Marking one aspect of uterine body with ink can help maintain orientation during dissection and block selection particularly of the more grotesquely misshaped specimens.

Examine the specimen, dissect, LOOK, FEEL & THINK and produce a macroscopic report:

- Describe and measure specimen in three dimensions (mm): fundus to external os (fundus to stump/neck where cervix conserved), transversely (cornu to cornu), and anterior to posteriorly; a weight can also be included.
- Note presence and site of any attached vaginal tissue (none noted here).
- Comment on serosal aspect, note presence of pedunculated nodules, sub-serosal nodules or any disruption (possible site of leiomyomectomy or uterine perforation). Comment on any grey/brown adhesions or haemorrhagic areas on serosal surface as this would suggest possible endometriosis (pipelle sample was scanty; cannot rule out endometriosis).
- According to clinical history patient was sterilized but there may be stubs of fallopian tubes at cornu.
- Bisect uterine body in either sagittal or coronal plane—although a matter of preference this gives you optional approach for grossly distorted specimen while maximizing examination of uterine cavity. Gentle probing through the endocervical canal will allow you to gauge the direction of the uterine cavity for best cutting plane.
- The uterine body is cut at intervals 90° to sagittal bisection for full examination; macroscopic findings not noted at initial examination could go undiagnosed. Subtle histological findings may necessitate review of specimen and selection of further blocks.
- The uterus is a dense muscular organ and early bisection is recommended to allow penetration by formalin and reduce autolysis, of particularly relevance for leiomyoma (this case) and endometrial cancer cases. Majority of cases must be left for extended fixation before selecting blocks. This specimen was moved into larger appropriately labelled container and left for a further 24 hours to allow adequate fixation.

- Comment on the appearance of endometrium (e.g. thickened, cystic) and myometrium which can display features of adenomyosis (thickened with striated woven pattern and scattered narrow brown slit-like spaces). In this case wall grossly distended and no obvious features seen.

Key Point

If on opening you see any malignant feature (e.g. friable endometrium), you would stop immediately and refer to experienced dissector.

Where there are multiple nodules they should be counted, largest measured, and further defined by their position in the uterine body as subserosal, intramural or submucosal. Describe the cut surfaces. These nodules are firm with typical appearance of a leiomyoma—firm, pale whorled, circumscribed mass (Figure 3.25).

- Record presence of intra-uterine device (IUD can be associated with uterine perforation). Threads may be visible at cervical os and alert you to their presence. Two were noted in this specimen, which due to distortion would be difficult to remove.

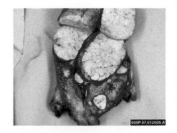

FIGURE 3.25
Firm, pale, whorled, circumscribed masses showing the typical appearance of a leiomyoma.

CLINICAL CORRELATION

Intrauterine device (IUD/IUCD) or coils are routinely used as a contraceptive device and are often prescribed for prevention and treatment of menorrhagia, dysmenorrhoea, pelvic pain, endometriosis and adenomyosis. These release hormones which can affect the morphology of the uterine body, including leiomyomas.

Key Point

While it is important to give macroscopic description and examine fibroids fully, if there are no abnormal features it is unnecessary to sample and examine every one microscopically.

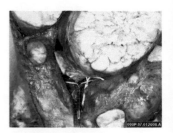

FIGURE 3.26
Sagittal section with ×2 IUD *in situ*.

This case described as 'markedly enlarged uterus and cervix 220 mm × 150 mm × 120 mm, unremarkable parous cervix 13 mm diameter. No FTs or ovaries. On opening, several large well circumscribed intramural nodules, largest 95 mm maximum dimension. Two plastic IUCD devices present within endometrial cavity.'

Further dissection and block selection following extended fixation:

- Check patient demographics, request form and cassettes.

- Re-check clinical history and read through/listen to gross description already given.

- Follow protocol for non-malignant hysterectomy minus adnexae.

- Sample any areas described on serosal aspect of specimen.

- Amputate cervix and take one block from anterior cervix and one from posterior cervix, to evaluate transformation zone. If scarred or incomplete cervix noted then would be concerned that there had been previous surgery for abnormality and would require further investigation. This patient had no previous cervical abnormality, but if suggestion of CIN noted on selected blocks case would be revisited and rest of cervix blocked.

> ### Key Point
>
> If abnormal cervical history of cervical intraepithelial neoplasia (CIN II & III/HSIL), you would treat cervix in same manner as cone biopsy; orientate, transversely slice and lay each tissue block in order on sequential cut face. Process entire cervix. If the cervix is conserved then the patient will continue with cervical screening programme.

- Sample any cervical polyps (none noted here).
- If you see no gross abnormality of the endometrium or myometrium the standard practice is to select one block from anterior wall and one from posterior wall to incorporate endometrium, myometrium and serosa. Composite blocks can be taken where walls are beyond capacity of tissue cassettes.

CLINICAL CORRELATION

It is important to have full clinical history to prevent misinterpretation of findings on examination. If patient had undergone endometrial ablation as therapeutic treatment for menorrhagia, then the cut surface will exhibit scarring; hormonal treatment and Tamoxifen can also alter the architecture of leiomyomas.

- This case presented with multiple leiomyomata which were described. There were no areas of soft brown necrosis, calcification or myxoid change. Select representative blocks from leiomyomata which demonstrate their relationship to serosa, myometrium or endometrium. Any variation from typical white whorled/nodular appearance as described should be sampled more extensively.
- Block any other incidental findings, suspected adenomyosis, endometrial polyps noting the site; include the base of the polyp in continuity with the endometrium. Note presence of caesarean section scars, important to sample when the history indicates obstetric complications.

Final report issued: Cervix unremarkable. Endometrium largely inactive with areas of breakdown and mild chronic endometritis. The myometrium contains numerous benign leiomyomata. No malignancy seen.

CLINICAL CORRELATION

Patient recovered well, although required transfusion for post-op anaemia, although bleeding not excessive at op. Reviewed at gynaecology clinic: vault well healed, Hb normal, scar healing well, no tenderness. Abdominal and pelvic examination at review unremarkable. Discharged to GP care.

3.7 Storage and retention

Any residual tissue remaining after selection of tissue blocks for diagnosis must be retained for a minimum of four weeks as per RCPath guidelines, CAP and CLIA retention is two weeks after final report (http://home.ccr.cancer.gov/LOP/intranet/PolicyManual/GeneralPolicy/CAPCLIA.asp), while Australian regulations stipulate one month after final report (www.commcarelink.health.gov.au/internet/publications/publishing.nsf/Content/npaac-retention-lab-records-toc~npaac-retention-lab-records-app-1) before disposal.

Stored specimens must be traceable and retrievable should further re-examination or sampling be necessary; storage period should be from date of last sampling. Disposal of human tissue is carried out in accordance with clinical and related waste management procedures. The laboratory will use an accredited company to uplift and destroy by incineration all specimens deemed suitable for disposal.

An important exclusion from this is tissue related to a pregnancy (with exception of placenta), which must be handled in a sensitive and respectful manner and not included with routine cellular pathology samples. Best practice advises parent(s) or guardian must sign a consent form indicating their wishes regarding examination and indicating their choice of private arrangement or shared cremation (www.rcn.org.uk/professional-development/publications/pub-001248). If requested, tissue may be returned to patient and must be double bagged and sealed to prevent leakage.

Where there is no residual tissue, the empty pots should be stored until the report is with clinician; this allows the pathologist to check any discrepancy between microscopic findings and sample details on the pot or clinical history and also provides evidence if a clinician queries the report (e.g. if wrong patient details were put on pot and request card at time of biopsy).

Key Point

Any pregnancy-related tissue must be handled sympathetically and follow a sensitive pathway. Parent/guardian wishes must be evidenced prior to examination.

Tissue retained for clinical trials, research, or tissue banking must have ethical approval and patient consent, and be recorded and stored in accordance with national guidelines.

Guidelines can be found via:

- Human Tissue Act 2004 UK, RCPath guidelines

- Human Tissue Act (Scotland) 2006, RCPath guidelines

- US Food and Drug Administration (FDA)

- Human Tissue Act/ALRC, National Pathology Accreditation Advisory Council (NPAAC) Guidelines for the Retention of Laboratory and Diagnostic Material.

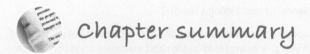

Chapter summary

After reading this chapter you should now know how to:

■ Accept specimens for histopathological examination.

■ Work safely in the dissecting room.

■ Gather clinical data relevant to specimen dissection.

■ Understand the basics of dissection and the macroscopic report.

■ Select appropriate tissue to ensure complete and accurate diagnosis.

You should have a clear understanding of the importance of cross-checking patients' details and laboratory numbers at all stages of the process, and have knowledge regarding appropriate PPE and safe working in the dissection room. This should include working with high-risk category cases. Regarding dissection you should have knowledge of the role of the BMS in dissection, from assisting medical personnel to performing dissection independently. The main take home messages relating to dissection are always to work only in your field of expertise, always to ask if you are unsure of any aspect of dissection (from terminology on the request form to unusual findings during dissection), and to audit and reflect on your own practice regularly. One must always remember these are precious, often 'once only' specimens that need to be dissected at a high level of quality so that the patient's histopathology report is of high quality to guide future treatment.

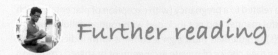

Further reading

- Allen DC, Cameron RI. *Histopathology specimens. Clinical, pathological and laboratory aspects*. London: Springer, 2004: 235–67.

- Calonje E, Brenn T, Lazar A, McKee PH. *McKee's pathology of the skin* 4th edn. Elsevier, 2012.

- Cotran RS, Kumar V, Collins T, Robbins SR. *Pathological basis of disease* 6th edn. Philadelphia: Saunders, 1999: 1047–65.

- Dahlstrom J, Coleman H, Johnson N, Salisbury E, Veness M, Morgan G. *Oral structured reporting protocol*. Surry Hills, NSW: The Royal College of Pathologists of Australasia, 2012.

- Patterson JW. *Weeden's skin pathology* 4th edn. London: Elsevier, 2015.

- Rosai J. *Ackerman's surgical pathology* 6th edn. St Louis, MO: Mosby, 1981: 937–55.

- Slootweg PJ. Complex head and neck specimens and neck dissections. How to handle them. *J Clin Pathol* 2005; 58 (3): 243–8.

- Telfer NR, Clover GB, Morton CA. Guidelines for the management of basal cell carcinoma. *Br J Dermatopathol* 2008; 158 (7): 35–48.

Discussion questions

3.1   The process of specimen dissection involves many steps. How would you minimize the risks involved at each of the following levels?
I.   Specimen reception
II.   Staff protection
III.   Waste disposal

3.2   What are the possible consequences of mislabelling a sample?

3.3   Macule, papule and keratotic horn are macroscopic terms used to describe skin lesions. Do you understand the terms and can you give examples of benign and malignant conditions which may show these features?

3.4   A 25-year-old male is referred by GP with pilonidal sinus. What is the most common site and how does it arise? Which surgical procedure would you expect to be performed? Do you know the laboratory procedure for dissection and block selection of the specimen? Outline the possible macroscopic and microscopic features.

3.5   Request card gives a clinical history of alopecia. Where does the handling of this specimen vary from punch biopsy for diagnosis of actinic keratosis, and explain why?

3.6   Describe the techniques available to reach a pre-operative diagnosis in a 64-year-old female with a palpable lump in her breast.

3.7   A sigmoid colectomy specimen is sent to the laboratory with the clinical details 'perforated diverticular disease'. What is diverticular disease and what are its complications?

Answers to the self-check questions and tips for responding to the discussion questions are provided on the book's accompanying website:

 Visit www.oup.com/uk/orchard2e

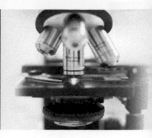

4

Routine processing, embedding and staining

David Muskett

Learning objectives

By the end of this chapter you should be able to:

- Discuss the principles and practices of tissue processing.

- Discuss the reagents used in tissue processing.

- Discuss reagent management for tissue processing.

- Discuss the role and principles of cryotomy.

- Discuss the principles and pitfalls of embedding.

- Discuss the role and principles of routine staining.

- Discuss systems to maintain the quality of work within the laboratory.

4.1 Introduction

In the previous chapters we have looked at specimen collection, reception, handling and dissection. In this chapter we will look in more detail at the laboratory processes which follow specimen dissection. As described in the earlier chapters most histopathology specimens follow a similar path of collection, fixation and dissection. The processes described in this chapter follow on in this chain. Once the specimen has been handled as described in Chapters 2 and 3, it is then available for reporting, which is described in Chapter 13.

4.2 **Tissue processing**

Key Point

Supporting media

Tissue processing involves preparing tissues so that they are infiltrated with a supporting medium. The supporting medium is usually paraffin wax but can be resin.

Cross reference

For more information about section cutting, see Section 4.5.

Cross reference

For more information about resin processing of tissue see Chapter 15.

The aim of tissue processing is to prepare tissue in a supporting medium ready to be cut into thin sections, in order to observe individual cells under the microscope (see Table 4.1). This means being able to produce slices (sections) at a thickness of 2–6 microns, about the thickness of a single cell or 1/10th the thickness of a human hair. The most commonly used embedding medium is paraffin wax. When solid, paraffin wax has a consistency very similar to that of the tissue itself and this assists with the subsequent sectioning process. Wax, however, is immiscible with water so the tissue cannot simply be transferred from water to wax. Instead, the tissue must transfer through a number of intermediary steps until it is able to be impregnated with wax. This is termed paraffin processing.

The tissue blocks prepared during specimen dissection are immersed in a number of different chemical solutions. These solutions act to prepare the tissue for mixing with an embedding medium, in most cases paraffin wax, although resin is sometimes used for hard tissue (e.g. bone or teeth) and material which needs to be cut into sections thinner than about 2 microns (about half the normal thickness; e.g. specimens required for electron microscopy). Paraffin wax is the embedding medium of choice for the vast majority of routine specimens, because it is cheap, easily handled when both molten and solid, is non-toxic, and is hard enough to support the cutting of thin sections.

Processing is not always straightforward. Different types of tissue require slightly different processing regimes. In most laboratories this is not always possible as there will be a range of different tissue types appearing on any one day, a limited amount of tissue processors and limited time. Generally, processing is a compromise of a number of different factors to give the best overall balance of quality of processing, timeliness and cost. Tissues are generally processed together in an overnight batch, but this may result in poor processing of fatty tissue and particularly hard tissue.

TABLE 4.1   **Four stages of tissue processing.**

Fixation	Fixation is the first part of most processing schedules. If specimens are well fixed this can be a very short part of the programme. Specimens may be processed unfixed or in a part fixed state and before the next stage is started they must be completely fixed.
Dehydration	Removes water from the section.
Clearing	To act as a link between the dehydrator and wax. The solution must be miscible with both the dehydrating agent and the wax. Clearing is the term that was applied due to the observed effect that some of these chemicals had upon the tissues. Many have a similar refractive index to the tissues and this caused a resultant transparency or 'clearing' of the tissues after immersion for a suitable time. Not all of the reagents used for this purpose actually clear the tissue so other terms have been suggested, e.g. ante-media, but the use of clearing agents has remained steadfastly popular. Most of these chemicals are organic solvents and all are toxic to a greater or lesser degree. The purpose of clearing agents is to act as a reagent which is miscible with both alcohol and wax. Xylene is probably the most widely used agent but it suffers from rendering the tissue more brittle and harder than many of its alternatives, particularly if incubation is protracted.
Impregnation	To infuse all parts of the tissue structure with the embedding medium (most commonly wax but can be resin) in preparation for subsequent embedding into a solid block.

In the processing schedule a number of reagents are used of each type. The changing of the reagents ensures the increasing purity of the reagent as the samples pass through. This ensures that as the samples migrate to the next type of reagent all traces of the previous reagent are removed. For example, tissues are dehydrated using alcohol solutions. All the water needs to be removed before the samples enter the clearing agent. If this does not happen then processing will not be successful. Having said this, tissue processing is a reversible process and placing wax blocks in the processing reagents in reverse order allows tissue to be taken back to an aqueous state; this can be important when the first attempt at complete processing has been unsuccessful.

Key Point

Reagent quality

Poor quality, contaminated or 'dirty' reagents can have a negative effect on tissue processing.

4.2.1 Fixation

This has been covered in Chapter 2.

Cross reference

You can read more about fixation in Chapter 2.

4.2.2 Dehydration

A number of dehydrating solutions are available but the most popular are industrial methylated spirit (IMS), which is primarily ethanol and isopropyl alcohol (synonyms—isopropanol, propan-2-ol and 2-propanol). Isopropyl alcohol can act as both dehydrating and clearing agent.

Whichever option is chosen, it is preferable to start with a more dilute alcohol and gradually increase the concentration rather than to immediately introduce a higher alcohol concentration as the tissue is more adversely affected by the latter option by displaying increased shrinkage artefacts.

Cross reference

See xylene-free processing in Section 4.3.4.

HEALTH & SAFETY: INDUSTRIAL METHYLATED SPIRIT

- Highly flammable.
- Harmful by inhalation and if swallowed.
- Requires specialist disposal.
- If industrial methylated spirit (also known as industrial denatured alcohol [IDA]) comes into contact with eyes or skin it needs to be washed well in running water.

4.2.3 Clearing

Clearing agents are chemicals which are miscible with the dehydrating agent and the tissue infiltrating agent; in routine practice this tends to be industrial denatured alcohol as the dehydrating agent and xylene as the clearing agent. (Xylene is more correctly known as di-methylbenzene). The name clearing agent comes from the fact that dehydrated samples placed in these agents tend to become 'more transparent' to the naked eye, hence the term cleared. Chlorinated hydrocarbons such as trichloroethanol have been popular as clearing agents in the past due to the efficient removal of lipids, but have fallen out of use due to safety and environmental concerns.

■ **Flammable.**

■ **Harmful by inhalation and in contact with skin, is irritating to eyes and skin.**

■ **Xylene waste must be disposed of as specialist disposal.**

■ **If skin becomes splashed with xylene it must be washed well away under running water. If xylene is splashed in eyes, following rinsing under running water, medical advice should be sought.**

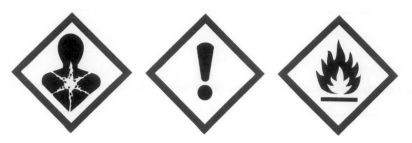

4.2.4 Impregnation—properties of wax

Paraffin wax is a crystalline hydrocarbon, which is quite brittle, derived from the petrochemical industry. Pure paraffin wax is not ideal for routine histopathology and the optimal preparation is created by adjusting the additives to the wax mixture. The optimal wax preparation should have:

- Good penetration of tissue so that processing is even—dimethyl sulphoxide (DMSO) is added to assist with this.
- Good ribboning properties—microcrystalline wax is added to assist with this.
- Good adhesion between the tissue and the supporting medium—a variety of additives may be included to assist with this, for example ceresin, beeswax, rubber or asphalt.

4.3 Tissue processing in practice

It is important to establish the correct processing schedules before you start processing the tissue blocks (see Box 4.1). This is done by a process of testing various timings and processing environmental pressures to find the best protocols for each set of circumstances. This is the process of tissue processing validation. The key criteria you are looking to optimize are:

- overall morphology
- chromatin detail
- tissue integrity.

4.3.1 Reagents used in tissue processing

One of the main reagents used in tissue processing is industrial denatured alcohol as the dehydrating agent. Commonly the alcohols are graded in strength from 70% industrial denatured alcohol aqueous, to 90% industrial denatured alcohol, to 100% alcohol. A few changes in the strength of the alcohol are usually performed. This is to ensure that the tissue is completely and effectively dehydrated.

Tissue which has not processed well may be impossible to cut. Poor processing is due to the retention of water within the tissue and can be redeemed by dehydrating the tissue properly. The tissue

BOX 4.1 Processing schedule validation

Tissue processing schedules are validated by using surplus clinical material not required for diagnosis. The size of the tissue pieces used in the validation is dependent upon how quick the processing schedule is and what guidance the manufacturers offer.

blocks will need to have the wax removed before this can happen and are usually soaked in xylene before being placed back in alcohol solutions. The forward processing scheme is then followed (see Chapter 6 on Artefacts).

METHOD 4.1 Routine processing

Samples are routinely processed overnight, using the typical schedule of reagents and times outlined below.

Tissue processors should be linked to an alarm system or a member of staff may be contacted to attend to the samples if the machine fails.

Formalin (1 hour)
70% Alcohol (1 hour)
90% Alcohol (1 hour)
100% Alcohol (1 hour)
100% Alcohol (1 hour)
100% Alcohol (1 hour 30 minutes)
Xylene (1 hour)
Xylene (1 hour)
Xylene (1 hour)
Wax (2 hours)
Wax (2 hours)
Wax (2 hours)

Key Point

Reagent management

Tissue processing reagents need close management. It is important that reagents do not become too contaminated by use and are refreshed regularly. Often this is controlled by the processing reagent management system, which indicates when defined threshold levels of solvent usage have been reached (see Figure 4.1).

The reagents which are loaded into the tissue processor are by and large hazardous and volatile. The reagents, when in the tissue processors, are pumped in and out of the reaction chamber and warmed up. This leads to gaseous build-up. The gaseous reagents are captured by being exhausted through **activated charcoal filters**. Activated charcoal filters are a constituent part of all enclosed tissue processors. The purpose of the filters is to remove solvent and formalin vapours that are by-products of the pumping of reagents in and out of the reaction chamber. The activated charcoal filters act to react with the solvent vapours released by the chemicals. The vapours are 'locked' into the filter and are rendered safe.

Weekly tissue processor change log

Processor name   Asset code   Date sheet started   Sheet number

Date	1	2	3	4	5	6	7	8	9	10	11	12	13	1	2	3	Initials
	NBF	70% IMS	96% IMS	99% IMS	99% IMS	99% IMS	99% IMS	Xyl	Xyl	Xyl	Flush Xyl	Flush IMS	Water	Wax	Wax	Wax	

Batches

NBF		96% IMS		99% IMS		Xylene		Wax	

FIGURE 4.1

A processing record change sheet. Note the space to log the reagent details and batch number. It is also important to keep a record of who has made the reagent change and when.

4.3.2 Equipment

How does tissue processing take place? Tissue processing may be performed manually, with the histologist moving the material by hand, or may be automated. There are a number of different types of processor—carousel, enclosed process flow and microwave—all of which work on the same principle, i.e. bringing tissues into contact with processing solutions for a fixed period of time then transfer to the next solutions. We will look at each processing type in turn.

Hand processing requires the tissues to be moved by hand between the reagents (see Box 4.2). All subsequent methods of processing have developed from this.

Factors affecting processing:

- heat
- mixing
- vacuum.

BOX 4.2 Hand processing

Hand processing requires the tissues to be moved by hand between the reagents. This is a very time-consuming process and in practice this does not happen often. Generally, it is only used for small urgent diagnostic biopsies. The reagents can be warmed to enhance processing speed.

A typical hand processing schedule for an urgent renal biopsy would be as follows; reagents should be warmed to 45°C and the paraffin wax to 60°C:

1. Formalin (15 minutes)
2. 70% alcohol (15 minutes)
3. 90% alcohol (15 minutes)
4. 100% alcohol (15 minutes)
5. 100% alcohol (15 minutes)
6. Xylene (15 minutes)
7. Xylene (15 minutes)
8. Paraffin wax (15 minutes)
9. Paraffin wax (15 minutes)

Practically it is best to handle reagents in a fume cupboard or hood to help contain fumes.

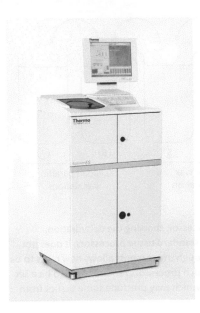

FIGURE 4.2
An enclosed tissue processor. The touch screen allows the programme to be selected and monitored. The reagents are stored in bottles within the doors on the front of the machine. (Image courtesy of Thermo)

Automated processing schedules are either carousel, enclosed, process-flow or microwave. Most laboratories operate routine processing with enclosed processors but process flow machines are becoming of increasing interest in large laboratories. The major drawback with any automated processor is that the flexibility to adapt regimes for different tissue types is lost as all specimens undergoing a particular protocol will all be treated identically.

Carousel tissue processors originated in the 1950s and represented the first attempts to automate tissue processing. In essence they copied the manual processing regime and automated the transit from one processing reagent to the next using timer clocks. Their use meant that many more samples could be processed at any one time, and in particular this automated transfer facility meant that processing schedules could be run overnight and timer delays incorporated into processing cycles so that schedules could be operated over weekends and public holidays. A major drawback with carousel processors is that the tissue samples are extremely vulnerable whilst being transferred from one processing reagent to the next.

Enclosed processors contain all the reagents within the machine. The tissue blocks are contained within a chamber and the reagents are pumped in. The tissue blocks are processed in batches and most tissue processors hold in excess of 200 blocks on each cycle. The length of time each reagent is in contact with the specimens is computer controlled. Enclosed processors have developed increasingly complex safety systems to ensure the integrity of samples and to monitor reagents. If a blockage prevents the entry of a solution the processor may skip to the next reagent or incubate further with the previous reagent (Figure 4.2).

The **continuous processing machine** is a type of tissue processor that allows material to be added to the processor at varying points during the day (see Figure 4.3). This way of handling tissues offers a 'Lean' way of processing material when it is needed, usually in more frequent, smaller batches. The principle of the machine is very similar to the carousel processor where the specimen moves through a series of reagents. The end point is that wax-impregnated blocks come out at various points within the day. This allows work to flow out of the machines on to the next stage of embedding.

Microwave processing is a way of increasing the speed of tissue processing by using the microwave process (see Figure 4.4). Standard processing reagents of industrial methylated spirit and xylene cannot be used. Bespoke proprietorial reagents are used that are better able to respond to the effects of the microwaves. Microwave tissue processing schedules are able to process biopsy samples in a few hours.

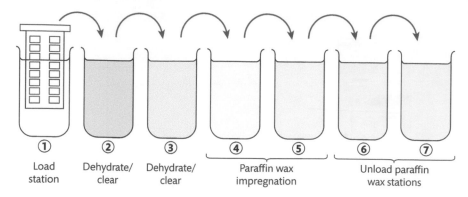

① Load station
② Dehydrate/ clear
③ Dehydrate/ clear
④ ⑤ Paraffin wax impregnation
⑥ ⑦ Unload paraffin wax stations

FIGURE 4.3

Diagrammatic representation of a continuous tissue processor, showing the dehydration, clearing and paraffin wax infiltration steps. Unlike most standard tissue processors, it does not include an initial fixation station. Moving the tissues through the reagents allows new racks to be loaded once the first reagent station is clear; however, such processors require tissue to be a set thickness to allow appropriate penetration of reagents, which may preclude some tissues from being processed in this way.

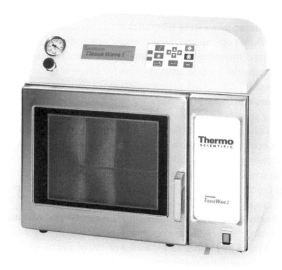

FIGURE 4.4

A microwave tissue processor. The instrument is programmed with the times in each reagent. (Image courtesy of Thermo)

Lean technology

Lean technology is a concept derived from manufacturing industry. It is the process of analysing the steps of the process to ensure the most efficient work patterns. Within tissue processing this is the concept of reducing batch size to the smallest number possible with the aim of ensuring work moves progressively through the laboratory without any waiting steps.

QUALITY 4.1 INSTRUMENT ALARMS

Tissue processing equipment does not always work perfectly and as such may break down while a processing run is in progress. This can often be in the night! Tissue processors are fitted with alarms which highlight when a processing run fails.

Laboratories should test the alarms as part of their routine maintenance cycle for the processors.

Histopathology specimens are generally run in batches overnight although continuous throughput or **Lean technology** is now being applied so that smaller batches can be processed, so that peaks and troughs of workload can be eliminated. This results in the service being more efficient and reduces turnaround time for the results of some samples. Additional processing schedules exist for small urgent pieces of tissue or for larger pieces which require longer time in the reagents.

4.3.3 Further considerations about tissue processing

In more recent years, tissue processing has become more tailored to the specimens under investigation (e.g. fatty specimens processed alone or biopsies processed together on rapid schedules). This, in combination with a push towards improving laboratory safety, has led to a range of developments.

4.3.4 Xylene-free processing

Interest in the use of processing regimes which do not require the use of xylene or similar clearing agents is largely due to the health and safety concerns associated with the use of these chemicals and a desire to eliminate their use in laboratory practice. Advances in processor technology have reduced the effect of problems that were encountered with this concept in previous years.

Isopropyl alcohol (IPA) can be used either in combination with ethanol, where the IPA is used in place of xylene, or as both dehydrating and clearing agent. In either situation the ability to use high temperatures within the modern tissue processor retort improves the rate at which IPA is driven from the tissue as molten wax is introduced.

4.3.5 Processing fatty tissue

Because of their high lipid content these types of specimens may need extended times in processing reagents, particularly dehydrating and clearing agents, in order to achieve the required effect. This commonly includes samples from breast tissue or skin and soft tissue samples. This may mean that these types of specimen are segregated from others and processed by a separate regime created specifically for this purpose. In addition, if xylene-free processing is being considered, then additional time may be required to ensure complete removal of IPA prior to wax impregnation.

4.3.6 Large blocks

As processing equipment has improved and reporting demands have altered there has been a return to a need for larger blocks. The larger blocks allow more tissue to be seen on a slide; this is important as it allows specimen margins to be seen in the context of where the pathology (often cancer) is seen. This helps with tumour staging and with patient treatment.

4.3.7 Tissue reprocessing

The process of tissue processing is reversible and where processing has been unsuccessful, i.e. all the water has not been removed from the tissue, then the material can be rehydrated and the process recommenced (see Box 4.3).

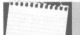

BOX 4.3 Tissue reprocessing

Laboratories should keep a log of what material has been reprocessed, from what tissue processor, and on what schedule.

Collecting these data allows laboratories to understand if material is processed on the correct schedule with appropriate reagents.

4.3.8 Hard tissues

Hard tissues such as tendon, nail, and decalcified bony structures may benefit from pre-treatment with tissue softening agents, either phenolic-based solutions or surfactants, before final processing. This helps to soften the tissues for easier sectioning.

HEALTH & SAFETY: PHENOLIC-BASED SOLUTIONS

Phenolic-based solutions are highly carcinogenic and flammable. They need to be handled with care and stored in flameproof containers.

Chlorocarbons

Chlorocarbons are organic compounds consisting of carbon-based molecules with chlorine and hydrogen. Once they were commonly used but this is declining due to environmental and health considerations.

4.3.9 Neuropathology samples

Neuropathology samples are generally much softer than routine histology samples. They have a higher fat content on average than routine histology specimens. Samples of brain and nerve are quite fragile and can become easily damaged, and require a slightly different output, e.g. sections need to be thicker so that you can follow nerves through the tissue. Processing reagents are often richer in **chlorocarbons**, such as carbon tetrachloride or chloroform, which remove the lipid from the tissue more easily than some other reagents.

4.3.10 Resin processing

> ### Key Point
>
> **Resin processing**
>
> Resin processing is used when particularly hard tissue requires sectioning and when very thin sections are required.

Cross reference

See Chapter 15 for more on resin processing and electron microscopy.

Resin processing is an alternative to paraffin wax processing. Tissue is fixed and dehydrated in the same way, but instead of xylene a dilute resin mix is used and progressively the amount of the resin is increased until the tissue is immersed in pure resin. At this point the resin is cured and a hard supportive medium surrounds the tissue.

SELF-CHECK 4.1

What are the four steps of tissue processing?

4.4 Embedding

> ### Key Point
>
> **Correct orientation**
>
> Embedding is the orientation of tissue within a supportive matrix. Correct orientation of tissue enables a full diagnosis of the pathology of the specimen.

Once tissue has been processed it needs embedding in a manner to allow sectioning. The aim of embedding is to orientate tissue to allow for the maximum amount of diagnostic information to be retrieved. This involves ensuring the macroscopic cut surfaces are flat on the base of the embedding mould and the tissue is correctly orientated. Most material is embedded into a mould that has the plastic cassette in which the tissue is placed attached to the back. This allows the material to be held in a manner which allows the tissue to be gripped firmly in a clamp and thin sections to be made (see Box 4.4). Figure 4.5 illustrates use of an embedding centre. The way in which tissue is placed for embedding is very important. Correctly orientated tissue allows viewing and interpretation to happen easily. Incorrectly orientated tissue prevents this. Large square samples from resections must be placed flat within the tissue mould to allow for an even cross-section of tissue to be prepared.

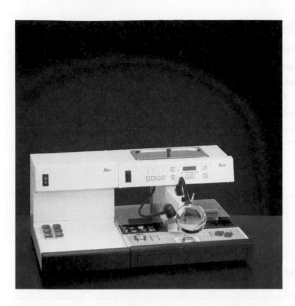

FIGURE 4.5
An embedding centre with attached cold plate. (Image courtesy of Leica Microsystems)

What is the purpose of embedding?

4.4.1 Embedding equipment

For most laboratories, the volume of work requires the use of a designated embedding centre. Most histology equipment suppliers produce embedding centres which all have the same basic features:

- A heated wax tank which keeps wax molten. This tank is thermostatically controlled to keep the wax just above its melting point.
- A heated wax tap or dispenser which allows molten wax to be dispensed on demand.
- A chilled plate which sits under the wax dispenser tap. This is used to make the molten wax solid and is especially useful to secure the correct orientation of the processed tissue.

 BOX 4.4 *Aids to embedding*

Embedding is a labour-intensive process which needs knowledge of the tissue, an understanding of the pathology under investigation and some consideration of the practical implications of section cutting.

Cassettes are now available that allow tissues to have a fixed orientation established at the time of specimen dissection. This means if a specimen is required to be embedded on edge then the sample is orientated and fixed either within a series of soft spikes, which hold the tissue, or within a sponge.

4.4.2 Tissue orientation

The correct orientation of tissue is essential for good histopathology. Some larger pieces of tissue are cut as slabs of tissue and can be embedded flat within a mould. Others, for example, a piece of skin, need to show all the epithelial strata to allow a routine diagnosis. Failure to get this step performed correctly can have significant implications for appropriate subsequent microscopic evaluations.

During the embedding process tissue is exposed to the work surfaces of the embedder. Some tissues are prone to break up when handled and are known as friable.

The friable fragments need to be cleared up after each case so that tissue from one patient does not enter the block of another patient. This could have very serious effects as cross-contamination of one patient's material to another could lead to misdiagnosis and inappropriate treatment.

Tumours such as bladder and some colon cancers can be particularly friable.

4.5 Microtomy

> ## Key Point
>
> **Microtomy**
>
> Microtomy is the process of producing a thin tissue section.

4.5.1 Equipment

Microtomy is a repetitive task and as such staff undertaking long periods of microtomy may be subject to musculoskeletal repetitive strain conditions. Within each laboratory, risk assessments should be in place to ensure the safety of staff.

Microtome

Tissue sections are prepared on a machine called a microtome. This word comes from the Greek micro—small, and tome—cut.

Tissue sectioning is the part of the histology process in which microscope slide preparations are made from the embedded tissue pieces. The instrument used to cut tissue sections is known as a **microtome**. There are many different manufacturers of microtome, all with slightly different designs, yet fundamentally all microtomes operate in the same way. A piece of tissue is held in a clamp and moves over the blade. A thin sliver of tissue is taken from the top of the block and at the end of the block flow the machine increments the block forward for the next section. Alternative styles of microtome hold the knife firm and move the block in a similar fashion.

The produced slide preparations are translucent and can vary in thickness from 0.1 μm to 50 μm. The thinnest sections are required for electron microscopy and the thickest sections are required for neuropathology techniques.

Good section cutting is facilitated by tissue blocks being cut from a medium which is about the same hardness as the tissue. Wax embedding is not really suitable for tissue which is very hard. Tissues which are very hard either need to be softened or embedded in a harder medium such as resin. The microtome is an essential piece of equipment in the histology laboratory. Microtomes are available in a number of different forms. The rotary microtome is by far the most popular, and can be semi-automated. The sledge and sliding microtome are popular in some laboratories for the simplicity of use and quality of sections. Whatever the type of microtome, the basic function is the same, to prepare tissue sections of a known thickness in a consistent manner (see Figure 4.6 and also Box 4.5).

For routine diagnostic specimens embedded in paraffin wax the objective is to cut a slice from the tissue that is approximately one cell in thickness. In practice this means that samples are routinely sliced (*sectioned*) at approximately 4 μm. Multiple sections are often required from the same block and the microtome must be able to provide ribbons of sections.

Each block contains many sections' worth of material and it is important to go sufficiently deeply into the block to obtain an appropriate cross section of material; also, it is equally important not to waste material. It is quite possible that numerous additional tests will be required. The way each block is sectioned depends on a number of factors; the type of tissue, the size of the tissue or the clinical history. Some blocks will require a single section for H&E, some require a number of sequential sections,

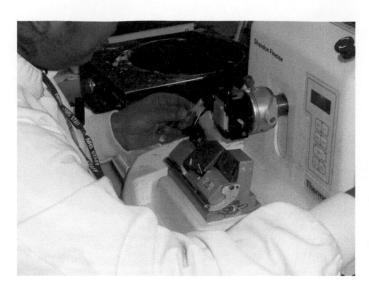

FIGURE 4.6
A microtomy station showing sections being cut. Note in this case the microtomist sits face on to the microtome and controls the block with their right hand and picks sections of from the blade with their left hand.

to follow a lesion or tissue element through the tissue, and this is known as 'serials'. Some require a number of sections distant to each other through the block to look at random parts sequentially; this is known as 'levels'. Looking at various sections through the material allows you to see the clinical picture in three dimensions. Often an H&E slide alone is required but there are specimens which need multiple different types of stain to obtain a diagnosis, e.g. liver biopsy, renal biopsy.

QUALITY 4.2 SECTION DEPTH

When tissue blocks are cut it is essential that the microtomist goes deep enough into the block. Sections should be complete and show a representative portion of tissue within the block. If the section is incomplete then it is possible that the key pathology within the tissue may be missed and a patient not treated appropriately.

The cut sections are floated out on a water bath (Figure 4.7) which is heated to about 50°C, just below the temperature that the wax melts. The warm waterbath allows creases that occur in the section preparation to be eased out.

Modern microtomy stations are now available linked to a PC, barcode scanner and slide label printer, allowing information about the block to be stored and subsequently transferred to the slide. Use of such systems minimizes transcription error and saves time.

QUALITY 4.3 TISSUE SECTION QUALITY

The floating out is an important part of the process. Sections need to be floated out for the appropriate length of time: if they are floated out for too short a length of time then sections may be creased, if they are floated out for too long then sections may disaggregate or disintegrate.

HEALTH & SAFETY: MICROTOME BLADES

Microtome blades are extremely sharp and it is easy to injure yourself, particularly if concentration wanes. If you feel your concentration flagging, take a short break and return later. This can be managed by varying tasks around the laboratory or taking prepared slides for staining.

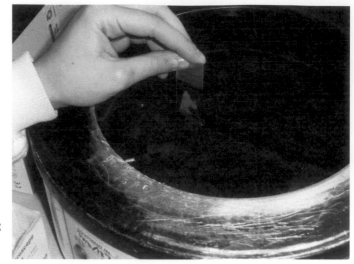

FIGURE 4.7
A section taken from the surface of a waterbath. The microtomist's fingers are held away from the water to prevent squamous cells being transferred to the tissue section.

Cross reference
The use of special stains and immunocytochemistry will be explored in later chapters (Chapter 5 and Chapters 8 & 9, respectively).

Some cases will require the examination of deeper levels within blocks. This may be when a lesion is described clinically and not seen, or histology elements are not seen completely. About 80–90% of diagnoses may be made by the H&E stain slides alone, but in the remaining 10–20% of cases further sections and stains are required to elucidate the diagnosis. These stains may be either tinctorial methods (special stains) or immunocytochemistry. The pathologist will report these additional slides in conjunction with the original H&E slide, and not instead of it.

SELF-CHECK 4.3

What are the key health and safety risks associated with microtomy?

4.5.2 Factors affecting section cutting

There are a number of factors which affect the quality of cut sections. These factors include:

- Sharpness of the cutting blade.
- Rigidity of the knife and specimen holder.
- Hardness of the tissue and focal calcification.
- Blood within the tissue.
- The coldness of the blocks.
- Rigidity of the knife in the specimen holder.

The cutting blade needs to be sharp and free from defects. Most laboratories use disposable blades which are clamped within a knife holder. As more tissue is progressively cut the knife becomes blunt. Any pieces of calcium can nick the knife causing sections to score.

4.5.3 Coldness of blocks

Blocks need to be cool in most circumstances. The colder the block the harder the wax will be, the harder the supporting matrix, the easier it is to cut thin sections. There is a point at which, if blocks are too cold, the tissue itself becomes too brittle to section and ribbon easily. This means that the integrity of the overall section is spoiled, and the sections may appear chattered (see Chapter 6 on artefacts).

BOX 4.5 *Automated microtomy*

Microtomy is a very labour-intensive process and an experienced microtomist may only cut 150 blocks in a day. As yet no working automated microtomy system is available to match the skill and dexterity required to produce high-quality tissue sections.

SELF-CHECK 4.4

What factors affect tissue section quality when cutting a block?

4.5.4 Rotary microtome

In this design the tissue block and knife are held in the vertical plane. Turning the handle (flywheel) one complete revolution advances the tissue towards the blade at whatever thickness has been set. As the two make contact a sliver of wax, containing the tissue, is shaved from the surface of the block (see Figure 4.6).

4.5.5 Sledge microtome

This version works similarly to the rotary microtome with the exception that both block and knife are positioned horizontally and the block is slid backwards and forwards in this plane making contact with the knife. As the block is slid back towards the operator on runners (or a sledge) an advance mechanism is operated which raises the block towards the knife by the required section thickness.

4.5.6 Freezing microtome

The sample is frozen onto the cassette holder. The blade is then drawn over the tissue sample to produce the section.

4.5.6 Cambridge rocking microtome

Although not used in many establishments, the Cambridge 'rocker' has had an important role in the development of microtomy. The tissue block rocks on a stand against a blade. The resultant sections are cut in an arc from the block. The simple design of the Cambridge rocker has made them long-lasting and easy to repair.

4.5.7 Microscope slides

Microscope slides are made of glass, which is transparent but suffers from being very brittle, shattering easily, and is very heavy in great numbers. In routine histopathology, slides are generally 75 mm × 25 mm, which correlates well with the width of the common processing cassette. The end of the slide is usually frosted so that pencil labelling can be easily applied. Once the section is mounted upon the slide it is drained and heat fixed to the slide once water has cleared from between the section and the glass.

It is important when you prepare good quality sections that you don't spoil all your effort by the use of inappropriate microscope slides. It is important slides should be clean and free from specks of dust so that the tissue section is not disrupted or torn. Commonly slides are either uncoated or coated to aid adhesion of sections on to the slide. The coating of slides can be from a number of sources, such as albumin (egg white), 3-aminopropyltriethoxysilane (APES), and positive charged coating.

4.5.8 Special considerations

Hard material

Hard material such as bone may need a different approach to softer tissues. Brittle material such as heavily keratinized skin or thyroid colloid may need softening prior to sectioning; this can be done with water, phenolic-based reagents or surfactant-containing softening agents. Recent comparative studies suggest that softening agents containing surfactants perform better on a cross-section of hardened tissue types, with the additional benefit of fewer health and safety issues.

Blood within the tissue

Blood does not process well and dries out. When dry the blood cracks on cutting. Blocks containing blood cut much better when they are soaked or cut from wet ice.

Lymph nodes

These are very cellular specimens and so tend to look very crowded under the microscope when sectioned at 4 µm. Far better cellular resolution is achieved if these are sectioned routinely at 2 µm.

Renal biopsies

As with lymph nodes, the resolution of the glomerular basement membrane is much improved if sectioned routinely at 2 µm.

Amyloid

The demonstration of amyloid variants with Congo red solutions is improved if thicker sections than usual are obtained. Ideally these should be sectioned at a thickness of around 8 µm.

Neuropathology sections

Thicker sections are most suited to many of the tinctorial and metallic impregnation methods used. Thicknesses of 15–50 µm are frequently encountered to be able to view and follow nerves through the section.

4.6 Cryotechniques and cryotomy

Key Point

Cryotomy

Cryotomy allows the rapid sectioning of unfixed material by freezing fresh tissue. The ice formed within the tissue acts as the supporting matrix.

Cryotechniques are laboratory methods using tissues that have been frozen solid. Freezing techniques may be used for a variety of reasons, including speed, and preservation of cell enzymes or avoidance of chemical fixatives due to interference with the method under investigation. Tissues may be frozen by liquid nitrogen, card-ice (solid CO_2), electrical plates or fluorocarbon spray. It is important to freeze tissue quickly and evenly to prevent ice crystal artefact.

Key Point

Ice crystal artefact

Ice crystal artefact is avoidable. Blocks must be cooled quickly and evenly.

Ice crystal artefact occurs when tissue is damaged by ice crystal formation that occurs as the tissue is frozen. If water within the tissue freezes slowly it forms large crystals, which disrupt and damage the cell (see Chapter 6).

When a tissue block is frozen the ice forms the supportive medium for the tissue, in the same way that paraffin wax does in routinely fixed specimens. Once the tissue is frozen it may be cut into sections using an instrument known as a cryostat.

4.6.1 Equipment

HEALTH & SAFETY: FROZEN SECTIONS

Tissue handled in cryostats may contain high-risk microorganisms such as TB, HIV or hepatitis B. It is therefore essential that a cryostat can be decontaminated and fumigated to disinfect the microtome and cooling chamber.

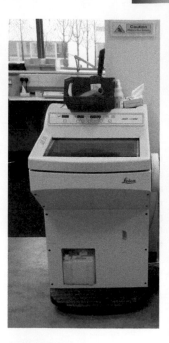

FIGURE 4.8
Cryostat.

A cryostat is a microtome housed in a freezer unit (Figure 4.8). The chamber around the microtome is cooled and temperatures are usually between –15 °C and –25 °C. The front housing has a glass panel which closes off the unit from the warm air of the room.

Frozen sections are more difficult to cut thinly, i.e. <5 μm, and do not allow for the examination of material in as much detail as paraffin-processed tissue. In other words, the morphological features are not as well preserved in frozen sections compared to paraffin-processed tissue. However, for the microscopic investigation of muscle enzyme activity cryostat prepared frozen sections are essential.

Frozen sections are a way of reporting histology samples rapidly—for example, when a patient is in theatre and the results may inform the action the surgeon takes next. Sectioning of these samples is made possible by freezing the tissue to provide a firm supportive matrix from the water within the tissue frozen as ice. Sections are usually a few microns thicker than usual at about 5 μm. Frozen sections are received when the patient is operated on and the course of the surgical intervention is dictated by the histology. The surgeon often wants to know whether a mass is malignant or not, if it needs removing or if the patient requires surgical palliation. Patient results from frozen section specimens should be phoned back to the operating theatre within 20 minutes of receipt. Common frozen sections are taken from abdominal cavity nodules or lymph nodes looking for the presence of cancer (see Chapter 7).

Cross reference

See the muscle biopsy case study in Chapter 5.

CASE STUDY 4.1 *Frozen section*

A surgeon is about to remove a skin lesion (suspected BCC) from close to the patient's eye. The aim of the operation is to remove the lesion but not too much surrounding skin so that the cosmetic change to the patient's face is minimal.

A frozen section is selected by the surgeon as it allows for the margins of the skin to be examined quickly to assess for the cancer. This allows the surgeon the opportunity to leave the skin wound open until the report for the frozen section is available. If the margins of the lesion are clear, then the tumour is completely clear and the patients wound can be stitched up. If the margins are not clear, then a further sample will be required to ensure clear margins.

METHOD 4.2 Urgent frozen sections

- On arrival, the time is noted, the tissue is described and a small representative piece is placed on a labelled chuck. The specimen is frozen down.
- Frozen sections are cut at 5 μm, usually two per slide.
- The slide is labelled with patient details.
- The slide is fixed in formalin or another fixative such as **Clarke's** for a minute.
- Rinse in water.
- Stain in Gill's III haematoxylin for 2 minutes.
- Rinse.
- Acid alcohol—2 dips.
- Rinse.
- Blue.
- Eosin—30 seconds.
- Rinse.
- Dehydrate, clear and mount.
- Pass to pathologist for reporting with request form.

Clarke's fixative

An alcohol and glacial acetic acid solution that provides rapid fixation but poor tissue penetration. This fixative is ideal for fixing fresh sections adhered to a slide.

Key Point

Frozen sections

Formalin fixation and paraffin wax processing takes several hours to complete even for very small diagnostic samples. The use of frozen sections achieves a thin section suitable for staining and microscopic examination within usually 20 minutes.

SELF-CHECK 4.5

What are the key infection risks associated with frozen sections?

Some enzymes are labile to the chemicals used in conventional paraffin wax processing. Frozen section processing removes the need for these chemicals so that these enzyme sites can be demonstrated. Many **enzyme histochemical** methods demonstrate enzymes which are damaged by formalin fixation, therefore frozen sections must be used with these samples.

4.6.2 Investigation of inflammatory skin disorders

Patients may develop rashes and bullae that require investigation. Small skin samples should include lesional (i.e. the blistered area) and perilesional (i.e. adjacent, visibly uninvolved) skin. These samples are taken and sent to the laboratory fresh, or in a non-fixative solution (Michel's transport medium is often used). The differential diagnosis includes pemphigoid, which has linear immunoglobulin deposited at the dermo-epidermal junction. Investigation of these immunoglobulins is best done with immunofluorescence techniques. These methods use antibodies labelled with fluorescent dyes to mark antigens deposited in the tissue. The dark background of the immunofluorescence test provides excellent contrast with the brightly staining antigens.

The number of antibodies used in immunofluorescence techniques is limited often to IgG, IgA, IgM, C3c and fibrinogen.

Certain laboratory tests are prohibited by the use of formalin; this is so with immunofluorescence as formalin fixation causes autofluorescence under UV light.

4.7 Haematoxylin and eosin staining

Key Point

Haematoxylin
Haematoxylin is the main stain used for routine diagnosis in histopathology.

QUALITY 4.4 ASSURING THE QUALITY OF STAINING REAGENTS

When sections are mounted and heat fixed on to slides they are available for staining. Staining follows one of a number of strands:

- General morphology stains such as H&E.
- Special stains looking for specific tissue elements identified by chemical interaction between dyes and the tissue (e.g. elastin stains; see Chapter 5 for more details).
- Immunocytochemistry. The interaction of antibodies and tissue elements.
- Molecular techniques. Investigations into the DNA and RNA of the cell.

4.7.1 The haematoxylin and eosin stain

The prepared sections mounted on the microscope slides are translucent and require staining. The H&E stain is the first stain performed on most material when it enters the laboratory. It has the advantage over other stains that it provides a good staining of the majority of tissue components and is cheap. Most importantly, it gives lots of information about the cell nucleus (see Box 4.6). The eosin stain gives a good demonstration of connective tissue and cytoplasmic elements. H&E-stained slides provide sufficient diagnostic information to be able to report 80–90% of all cases; in the remaining 10–20% of cases further tinctorial, immunocytochemistry or molecular tests are required.

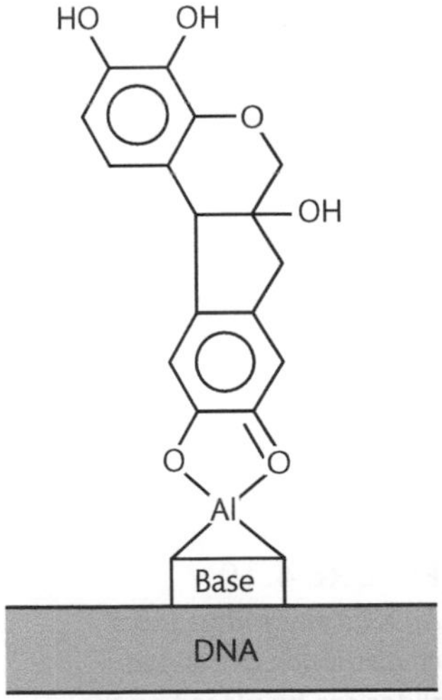

4.7.2 Haematoxylin

Haematoxylin is a dye originally derived from the logwood tree, a tropical hardwood tree found in Central America. Haematoxylin itself stains tissue poorly and for effective staining to take place it needs to be **oxidized** and linked to a **mordant** (Figure 4.9).

Staining may be either **progressive** or **regressive**. Progressive staining is where the tissue is stained until the point that all tissue elements are stained correctly. This requires fine control of the reagents. Regressive staining is where the sections are over-stained and excess stain is removed using a dilute acid.

Common haematoxylin solutions used in the laboratory are:

- Carazzi's haematoxylin
- Ehrlich's haematoxylin
- Gill's haematoxylin
- Harris haematoxylin
- Mayer's haematoxylin.

FIGURE 4.9
Interaction of a haematoxylin molecule with a mordant and the tissue.

BOX 4.6 *Reagent testing*

Before haematoxylin and eosin reagents are brought into routine use they should be tested to see that they are fit for purpose. The easiest way to do this is to stain a control slide with the solutions and check the results for quality. Once the staining is viewed as satisfactory then the batches are authorized for use and this is documented and signed off.

4.7.3 Eosin

Originally eosin was derived from crushed beetles; now it is manufactured synthetically. The eosin molecule is negatively charged and binds to the positively charged components within the cytoplasm. Eosin solutions are either prepared in alcoholic or aqueous solutions. The synthetic form is often combined with acetic acid and/or calcium chloride to enhance the staining. There are two main types: eosin Y and eosin B.

4.8 Staining equipment

The staining of routine sections in most laboratories is no longer carried out by hand and automated staining machines are used. The purpose of an automated staining machine is to hold the slides in a series of reagents in order for a set period of time. Automated staining machines save a lot of laboratory time but do require some regular routine maintenance. Many of the reagents used by the staining machines are harmful and vapours from these machines need to be controlled. Fans and activated charcoal filters are used to do this.

Most staining machines available on the market allow the storing and use of multiple programmes. This allows for slides of different material to be stained for different lengths of time.

Types of automated histology stainers:

Linistainers consist of a basic chain (very similar to a bicycle chain) which is attached to an electric motor which runs at a constant speed. The length of time in each reagent is determined by the width of the staining pot used i.e. wider staining pots have the slides immersed in them for a longer period of time. Although linistainers are very simple they provide possibly the ultimate in lean staining. A single slide can be added to the machine at any time and there is no batching.

There is an end trough containing xylene where the stained sections are stored prior to coverslipping.

XY stainers are histology stainers with a robotic arm which places the slide racks in each staining pot for a fixed length of time. The staining time is programmed and is not dependent on the width of the staining pots as with linistainers. Multiple racks of slides can be stained at any one time. XY stainers provide a flexible approach to staining together with a rapid throughput of slides (Figure 4.10).

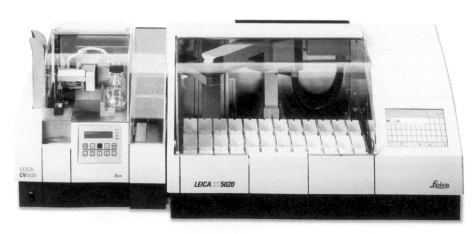

FIGURE 4.10
An XY stainer linked to a coverslipper. Unstained slides can be placed on the machine and a coverslipped end-product is then available. (Image courtesy of Leica Microsystems)

Tape coverslippers: The principle of the tape coverslipper is that the tape is unrolled over the section then cut. This is a quick process but some laboratories have had problems when archive sections have had their tape coverslips fall off with time.

BOX 4.7 Integrated stainers and coverslippers

Modern equipment now encompasses stainers linked to coverslippers so that the process of staining and coverslipping can be automated. This has the clear benefit of speed and efficiency and will allow greater numbers of slides to be stained and mounted. These machines can also cope with staining numerous racks of slides at the same time during the staining programmes. The computerized software on these machines will enable the programming of numerous staining procedures, and the machines are programmed to calculate the most efficient and quickest sequence of rack movement to achieve the optimum slide turnaround time.

4.9 Coverslips

Once the slides are stained, the preparations need to be made permanent by putting a protective covering over the tissue section, usually either glass or a plastic film. Coverslips are thin pieces of glass used to cover tissue sections and protect them from damage. This protective layer sits on top of a mountant, which must have the same refractive index as the glass slide and the coverslip. This helps to prevent refraction artefacts.

Coverslipping can be done by hand or automatically. There are a number of basic aims for coverslipping:

- To place a coverslip over the section.
- To ensure that sufficient mountant is present to prevent retraction.
- That there is not too much mountant that the top of the coverslip becomes encrusted with mountant.
- That there are no air bubbles trapped under the coverslip.

4.9.1 Automated coverslippers

Automated coverslippers have been developed to speed up the coverslipping process in the laboratory. They use either glass coverslips or plastic strips on tissue sections (see Box 4.7).

4.9.2 Automated glass coverslippers

Glass coverslippers place individual glass coverslips over the tissue section. The mountant is usually added to the slide and the coverslip is flexed by the machine in order to remove any trapped air bubbles. Coverslips need to be sufficiently robust to withstand a small amount of flexing.

SELF-CHECK 4.6

Why are automated staining machines used routinely?

4.10 Quality assurance

> **Key Point**
>
> **Quality**
> The assurance of the quality of work produced by the laboratory is an ongoing challenge.

Quality assurance (QA) is the activity of providing evidence needed to validate the quality of work carried out within the laboratory, and that activities that require good quality are being performed effectively. Appropriate quality assurance is a core component of every laboratory's function. Quality control gives evidence that the tests being carried out are accurate and specific. This evidence may be provided internally within the organization by internal quality control (IQC) or by reference to an external body providing external quality assessment (EQA). IQC is paramount to ensure that processes are functioning effectively, but this must be supplemented by EQA so that the possibility of site-specific bias is reduced.

4.10.1 Internal quality control

Internal quality control is the system followed in the laboratory to maintain the quality of the work. This will involve ensuring that the stains carried out are checked for their specificity and accuracy of staining. As a minimum the routine haematoxylin and eosin stain should be checked at the start of each day (see Box 4.6). In most laboratories this process is automated so this involves the checking of the first section stained using the staining machine. The IQC slides produced are stored for review and audit.

Block checking

After sections are cut and stained the blocks are checked against the slides cut so that the shape of the sections is checked and the patient name and case number are checked.

Microscope checking

Each slide, or a selection of slides from a case, is/are checked under the microscope for staining quality and for quality of microtomy. Sections that are of poor quality are rejected and a replacement section is cut.

The key items investigated when microscope checking slides are:

- Is the fixation OK?
- Is the section suitable?
  - Deep enough?
  - Representative?
  - Are there any cutting defects? Creases? Folds? Scores?
- Is the staining of good quality?
- Is the coverslipping OK? Are there any air bubbles?
- Is the presentation OK? Is the section central?
- Are the correct patient details on the slide?

SELF-CHECK 4.7

What is internal quality control?

4.10.2 External quality assessment

External quality assessment is a process whereby the slides produced in different laboratories are checked against each other. This permits maintenance of inter-laboratory standards. It also allows laboratories to be informed of staining methods which need to be reviewed and improved. Separate schemes exist for diagnostic aspects of histopathology work. There are two main EQA schemes relevant in the UK—UKNEQAS for Cellular Pathology Technique (CPT) and UKNEQAS for ICC and ISH. Similar schemes exist in other countries.

UKNEQAS CPT assesses the quality of H&E-stained material selected from scheme participant files and also assesses a range of special stains used on material distributed by the scheme organizers.

Cross reference

See Chapter 6 for commonly seen IQC failures.

Cross reference

For more details about EQA in immunocytochemistry, see the immunocytochemistry chapters (Chapters 8 & 9) later in this book.

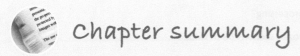

Chapter summary

Tissue processing

Tissue processing is the chemical treatment of tissues to produce tissue within a supportive medium which allows the thin sectioning of tissue.

Embedding

Once tissue is processed it needs to be orientated within a mould and mounted to a cassette. Orientation needs to be correct to the tissue type.

Sectioning

Tissues are sectioned at about the thickness of a single cell so a 'monolayer' of cells is present on the slide. The sections are transparent so need to be stained.

Routine staining

Haematoxylin and eosin is the routine stain. The positively charged haematoxylin binds to the negatively charged DNA within the nucleus. The net positive charge on the cytoplasm reacts well with the eosin molecule.

Cryotomy

Where rapid sections are needed within 10 minutes of the specimen arriving in the laboratory then the specimen is frozen and the ice within the specimens forms a supportive matrix.

Quality assurance

Why quality assurance steps are important.

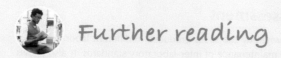

Further reading

- Cross S. *Underwood's pathology: a clinical approach* 6th edn. Edinburgh: Churchill Livingstone, 2013.

- Farne H, Norris-Cervetto E, Warbreck-Smith J. *Oxford cases in medicine and surgery* 2nd edn. Oxford: Oxford University Press, 2015.

- Kumar P, Clark M. *Kumar & Clark clinical medicine* 9th edn. Edinburgh: Churchill Livingstone, 2016.

- Orchard GE, Nation BR eds. *Cell structure and function*. Oxford: Oxford University Press, 2014.

- Suvarna KS, Layton C, Bancroft JD eds. *Bancroft's theory and practice of histological techniques* 7th edn. Edinburgh: Churchill Livingstone, 2012.

Discussion questions

4.1   What is the purpose of tissue processing?

4.2   In what circumstances might frozen sections be of value?

4.3   What thicknesses of section are used in microtomy? Why?

4.4   Why are internal quality control steps of value?

Answers to the self-check questions and tips for responding to the discussion questions are provided on the book's accompanying website:

 Visit www.oup.com/uk/orchard2e

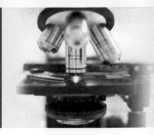

5

Stains in action

David Muskett and Guy Orchard

Learning objectives

After studying this chapter, you should be able to:

- Describe the key principles of tissue staining.

- Describe the scope and clinical significance of special stains in diagnosis.

- Describe the practicalities of ensuring the quality of control material for special stains.

- Describe how material is prepared for examination of stained sections under the light microscope.

- Describe various types of staining, and how they are used.

- Be conversant with the reasons for using some of the routine and specialized staining methods in the diagnostic process.

- Be aware of health and safety aspects associated with staining of tissues in a laboratory environment.

5.1 Introduction

Fixed and processed tissue lacks contrast, and appears largely colourless despite containing numerous individual entities. In Chapter 4 we learned about routine staining, which is most commonly carried out using the haematoxylin and eosin (H&E) method. There are circumstances where the initial stain will not reveal sufficient information and subsequent demonstration methods are required. Various coloured dyes and stains can be used to emphasize the different structures present. These stains have evolved over many years, and in the modern diagnostic histopathology laboratory there are dozens of methods available to colour many entities to give contrasting appearances.

Most of these methods rely on chemical principles whereby structures of a specific chemical nature can be stained selectively with the appropriate dyes. Often, two or more dyes can be used to provide vivid contrast of the various structures within the tissue.

Many of the dyes used today in histological demonstration were first introduced over one hundred years ago, not for histological use but in the colouring of fabrics such as cotton. Many natural dyes from plants were used until the late 1800s when synthetic dyes were introduced. Dyes such as madder date back thousands of years. Other dyes such as cochineal, indigo, and logwood (haematoxylin) are still used today.

5.2 Underlying principles of staining

Key Point

Special stains form part of a raft of supplementary tests available to selectively demonstrate tissue components and other entities.

When tissue sections have been prepared they are almost transparent (see Chapter 4). To obtain useful clinical information tissue sections need to be stained and various tissue elements need to be selectively demonstrated. There are many methods for selectively demonstrating tissue elements within tissue sections. The various methods can be divided as:

- routine morphological staining
- special stains
- vital stains
- immunocytochemistry
- *in situ* molecular methods.

Many special stains have been in use for many decades yet a number of methods have retained a very significant role in diagnostic histopathology. Most of the methods rely on chemical interactions between the tissue and chemicals/dyes applied.

There are many different types of 'staining', whereby specific structures can be shown in a variety of colours. Simple staining is often based on the attraction of opposites.

Once tissue sections are prepared (usually but not always at about 4 microns thick) they can be rehydrated (in histological terms, taken to water; see Box 5.1).

BOX 5.1 Taking sections to water

Wax is removed in xylene.
The xylene is rinsed out with 100% industrial denatured alcohol, then 90%, then 70%, then the sections are transferred to water (Figure 5.1).
This is the first part of many demonstration methods.

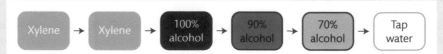

FIGURE 5.1
The process of taking sections to water. Slides (usually in racks) should be immersed in each solution for 15–20 seconds, then drained and moved to the next reagent.

SELF-CHECK 5.1

How do special stains supplement routine staining?

5.2.1 Histochemical

This utilizes a true chemical reaction in the tissue and matches what would happen if the reaction was performed in a test tube. The tissue will be fixed, as many histochemical reactions would 'disintegrate' the living cell. The periodic acid Schiff (PAS) reaction to demonstrate carbohydrates and the Perls' Prussian blue method to identify haemosiderin are examples of histochemical methods.

5.2.2 Lysochrome

> **Key Point**
>
> Lysochromatic staining utilizes the property of preferential solubility as a mode of action.

This is the 'staining' of neutral lipids/fats whereby elective solubility allows the dye molecules to leave the solvent in which they are dissolved (usually weak alcohol) and enter the lipid. This occurs as a result of the hydrophobic nature of the lipid. Effectively, the dye is more soluble in the lipid than in the solvent in which it is initially dissolved. Examples are seen in the use of Sudan dyes (I, II, III, IV) and Oil red O.

5.2.3 Impregnation

> **Key Point**
>
> Impregnation is the characteristic staining method for silver stains.

Impregnation is the deposition of silver within a specified area on a tissue section and can be described as either:

- Argyrophil, where a reducing agent (e.g. formalin) is required to produce a black deposit on, for example, reticulin fibres.
- Argentaffin, where no reducing agent is needed, as in the case of the demonstration of enterochromaffin cells.
- Ion exchange, as seen in von Kossa's method to detect bone mineralization—here, the phosphates and carbonates form insoluble salts in conjunction with the silver solution which is blackened following treatment with ultraviolet (UV) light or hydroquinone.

Classically, impregnation is seen in the demonstration of reticulin fibres using silver salts which will be reduced to form a black coating/deposit around the individual fibres, making them look slightly thicker than they are in reality. The dense black coloration provides good contrast, making the result excellent for photography, as well as being effectively permanent, with no fading over a long period of time (in excess of one hundred years). Dyed sections often fade after much shorter periods (10 years). Metal impregnation is also used in neurological methods to demonstrate, for example, glial cells and nerve fibres.

5.2.4 Injection

Loosely described as staining, injection involves the introduction of a coloured compound into the tissue to highlight various structures (e.g. red and blue latex dyes injected into arteries and veins to show the blood system of organs, or air spaces filled with coloured latex in the lung). Both would then have the tissue macerated, leaving a cast of the coloured entities.

5.2.5 Fluorochrome

Staining is effected by combining a fluorochrome with a tissue entity, which is then visualized under fluorescent light. Examples are seen in the demonstration of amyloid with thioflavine T, and acid alcohol-fast bacilli using auramine/rhodamine. In each case, small quantities of substance or numbers of microorganisms can be seen to fluoresce brightly, while they may be overlooked in conventional staining.

5.2.6 Trapping agents

As the name suggests, a trapping agent prevents the escape of dye that has entered the tissue entity. A classic example is seen with Gram's stain, where iodine is used as a trapping agent to form large aggregates with the dye (crystal violet). This prevents or slows the loss of colour in Gram-positive organisms during treatment with acetone or alcohol, but allows Gram-negative organisms to lose the crystal violet colour (blue) and be stained in a contrasting colour (red) with a counterstain such as neutral red.

Differentiation

The removal of excess dye from tissue to provide a good balance/contrast of stained and unstained elements to aid identification.

5.3 Differential action of dyes

Optimizing special stains is a fine art and tissue sections are either stained up to the correct level (progressive staining) or overstained then cleaned up or differentiated (regressively stained). In progressive staining the dye is left on the section long enough for the desired depth of coloration to be achieved. In practice, this means that we need to remove excess dye from tissues.

The differentiating agents used are:

- mordants
- acids
- oxidizing agents (see Figure 5.2).

(a)

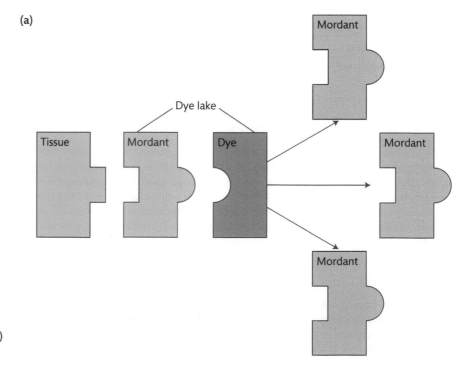

FIGURE 5.2
Differentiation with a) mordants, b) acid alcohol and c) oxidizing agents.

(b)

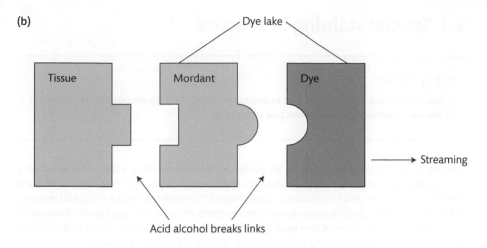

(c)

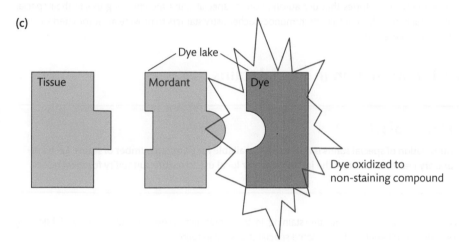

FIGURE 5.2
(*Continued*)

While it has been shown that chemical affinity (attraction of opposites) plays a major role in the staining process, it must be appreciated that this is not the sole consideration.

The depth of colour is affected by:

1. Chemical affinity
2. Density
3. Permeability and diffusion of dye.

On the other hand, red blood cells (RBCs) are chemically reactive (acidophilic), dense and relatively impermeable. Therefore, they are not easily dyed, except by a rapidly diffusing dye.

SELF-CHECK 5.2

What are mordants?

SELF-CHECK 5.3

What is the meaning of the terms progressive and regressive staining?

5.4 Special staining in practice

Key Point

Special stains have retained their role in diagnostic histopathology despite the development of immunocytochemistry and molecular techniques.

Each histopathology laboratory will have an area set aside for special stains, either together with any automation or separately with a down draft bench and/or a fume cupboard. There needs to be ready access to running water and ready access to distilled water. There also needs to be a fridge for reagents. The fridge needs to be divided up into areas for new reagents, those ready to use but which have been tested, and those in use. Solvent bins need to be close at hand. A microscope should be available to check stains as they are progressing and to review the quality of the finished product.

Increasingly, laboratories that use automation for special stains are choosing to site their special staining machines adjacent to their immunocytochemistry stainers to provide an automated staining section (see Figure 5.3).

5.4.1 Automation in special stains

Key Point

Automation of special stains is now readily available for a limited number of stains. Each laboratory needs to evaluate the instruments for local use to ensure suitability for local needs.

As well as the automation of routine staining, instrumentation now exists to automate special staining procedures. The benefits of automated special stains are as follows:

- Standardized staining times for protocols.
- Standardized repeatable conditions applied to slides.
- Specific controls of temperature applied to slides.

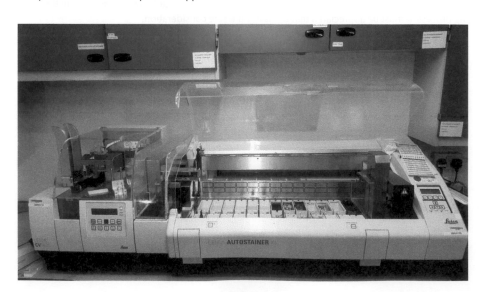

FIGURE 5.3
Automated staining machine with coverslipper to the left. Inside the machine is a robotic arm which is programmed to immerse slides in each reagent for the correct time.

- Multiple slides handled the same way easily.
- Frees up time for staff to carry out other activities.
- Audit trails of reagents linked to slides.

There are a few disadvantages:

- Inability to adapt the stain to the specific needs of each slide based on specific internal control assessment.
- The preservatives used within the staining reagents limit the sensitivity of reagents.
- Limited number of special stains available—it is unlikely that any staining machine will cover a full repertoire of tests in any laboratory, but this is an expanding area of development.
- Limited shelf life of kits, usually in the range of 12–18 months.
- Kits generally quite large (50–75 tests) with a shelf life of about 12 months so the laboratory needs to process sufficient tests for the acquisition of the machine to be viable for the tests.
- Staff training on the equipment/de-skilling of competency for manual special stains skills.
- Cost—for the capital purchase of the machine versus lease rental cost versus cost of staff time carrying out tests.

Most instruments currently available operate on the same principle, using fixed-volume dispensers (like spirit optics in a pub) adding a known volume of reagent on to a slide. This sits on a programmable pad where the temperature is adjusted according to the needs of the section and stain (Figure 5.4). The instrument will also have a mechanism to prevent the slide from drying due to evaporation or through use of slide-covering technology (e.g. an oil-based liquid medium or a rigid cover/tile).

(a)
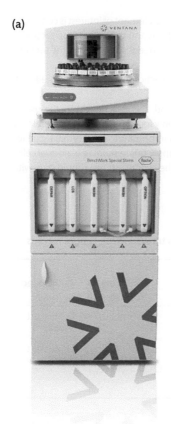

(b)
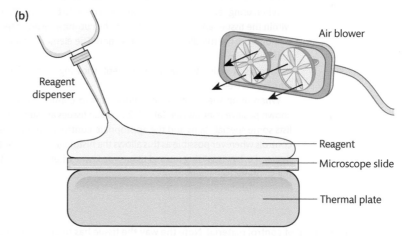

FIGURE 5.4
a) A commercial automated special stains machine. Up to 20 slides can be placed in the carousel, which sits beneath the tray of barcoded reagents. Bulk washing buffers sit below the main reaction area and are dispensed onto the slides as per the programme employed. The instruments are compact and permit tight audit of the reagents used on each slide via the computer interface. b) Mechanism of slide staining (hot plate, slide and reagent).

Note the top layer acts to prevent the slide drying out and allow the staining reaction to be carried out under applied heat.

SELF-CHECK 5.4

What are the key advantages of automating special stain procedures?

5.4.2 Quality control processes for special stains

> **Key Point**
>
> The appropriate control of special stains is the key way the quality of the tests is controlled within the laboratory. Control material needs to be carefully selected and evaluated.

Using appropriate control material is the key to assessing whether a test has been performed well. It is important to use normal elements wherever possible, but for some special stains this is not possible. Most infective agents (fungi, viruses and mycobacteria) are non-commensal and therefore pathological tissue sources are required. Expression levels of the element of interest ideally should be seen as different concentrations so that a proper assessment of the accuracy of the stain can be made. Records of the control material should include details of who, when, and what tests have been performed (see Table 5.1). There also should be a link to what reagents are used. This is generally documented automatically by automated staining methods but with manual methods a system of reagent linkage needs to be adopted. This is the general principle of traceability.

When using sections to control stains you need to be aware that the element of interest is contained within the tissue sample. This is achieved by cutting a series of sections and staining the top section, a section from the middle and the last section. The element of interest needs to be in all of the sections to be suitable.

Records of which test sections are kept, showing what control section has been performed with which tests (see Box 5.2).

When using special stains, it is important to control the method; this is achieved by the use of known positive controls (see Table 5.2). Certain tissues are suitable only for some special stains. Table 5.1 lists some special stains and the appropriate control material. It is important to use normal tissue for controls wherever possible as this allows the histologist to ensure appropriate staining of normal cells/tissues, i.e. by visualizing normal tissue you know whether or not the cells of interest should stain with the solutions (see Figure 5.5).

TABLE 5.1 Example of a record of control material. Note the way the tissue has been handled is tracked in the control records.

Control block number	Case number	Significant pathology	Days in formalin	Processing schedule type	Date taken	Taken by	Authorized for use with	Authorized by/date
A23	H,17.123	Carcinoid tumour	2	Routine overnight	23/1/17	DM	Grimelius	D Muskett 25/1/17
B24	H,17.269	TB–infected lymph node	3 (fixed for 48 hours before slicing)	Routine overnight	25/1/17	JC	ZN	D Muskett 7/2/17

BOX 5.2 Quality management with staining solutions

Accurate records of date received, date acceptance tested and date first used should be recorded for reagents in use in the laboratory. Expiry dates should be noted and reagents removed from service before the expiry date is reached.

For in-house solutions the lifespan of the solutions will need to be established by experimentation. Orcein solution, for example, has a limited lifespan and will not work well after about 3 months. What will be seen with solutions used outside of their working life is that the staining will be less (and increasingly non-specific) and background staining will increase.

TABLE 5.2 Appropriate control material for special stains.

Method	Tissues	Notes
Alcian blue	Colon	Stains acid glycoproteins, glycoproteins found in the colonic crypts
Alcian blue/periodic acid Schiff (AB/PAS)	Salivary gland	Salivary gland has both acidic and neutral mucins
PAS	Liver	Glycogen is stored in normal hepatocytes
DPAS	Stomach	Neutral mucins
Reticulin	Liver	To show connective tissue architecture
Martius scarlet blue	Mature placenta	To demonstrate fibrin
Perls'	Liver with haemosiderin	Haemochromatosis-positive case
Elastin	Lung or young skin	To show fine and coarse elastin fibres in the connective tissue and blood vessels
Orcein	Liver infected with hepatitis B	Shikata's stain for hepatitis B surface antigen
Amyloid	Tissue with amyloid deposits	Often taken from previous positive tissue
Gram stain	Tissue infected with bacteria	
Ziehl–Neelsen	Tissue infected with *Mycobacterium*	
Wade–Fite	Tissue infected with *Mycobacterium leprae*	

SELF-CHECK 5.5

What are the reasons for using positive controls in special staining procedures?

(a)

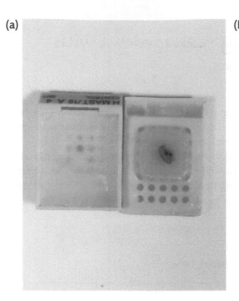

(b)

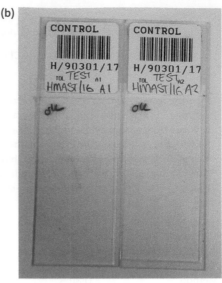

FIGURE 5.5
Use of control blocks is an important part of maintaining staining quality, and confirming that a stain has worked: a) Two control blocks of skin containing mast cells. Each block is uniquely identified and traceable to the case of origin; b) Two control slides stained with toluidine blue. Control slides and test slides are treated identically, and therefore absence of positive staining in the test is due to absence of heparin, rather than the stain not working.

5.5 Carbohydrates, mucins and glycoprotein demonstration

Key Point

Carbohydrates and glycoproteins are of major interest within histopathology, as they are present within normal tissue, e.g. liver and pathological tissue (e.g. liver and pathological tissue).

Mucin and glycoprotein stains are some of the most commonly performed special stains because of the key role glycoproteins and carbohydrates play within the body (see Table 5.3 and Box 5.3).

TABLE 5.3 Sources of mucins and their demonstration.

Glycoprotein family	Subtype	Location	Demonstrated by (method)
Acid	Weakly sulphated	Colon	AB pH 1.0, colloidal iron, mucicarmine
		Oesophagus	AB pH 2.5
Neutral		Stomach	DPAS
		Cervix	DPAS
		Bronchus	DPAS
		Vagina	DPAS
		Prostate	DPAS
Mixed		Salivary	AB/DPAS

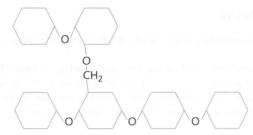

FIGURE 5.6
Glycogen macromolecule.
Note the hexose sugars joined
together.

Carbohydrates in tissue sections are usually present as either glycogen or a type of mucin, a term used to describe glycoproteins, which are proteins with attached sugar molecules (Figure 5.6).

Glycoproteins are secreted by epithelial cells (Figure 5.7).

The main normal functions of glycoproteins are as follows:

- cell to cell interactions

- hormones

- structural proteins

- lubrication of epithelial surfaces

- protection of the body from proteolytic enzymes (i.e. those produced in the stomach).

They are of particular interest to histologists because in pathological conditions the location and quantity of glycoprotein expressed changes.

SELF-CHECK 5.6

What are the key functions of glycoproteins in the body?

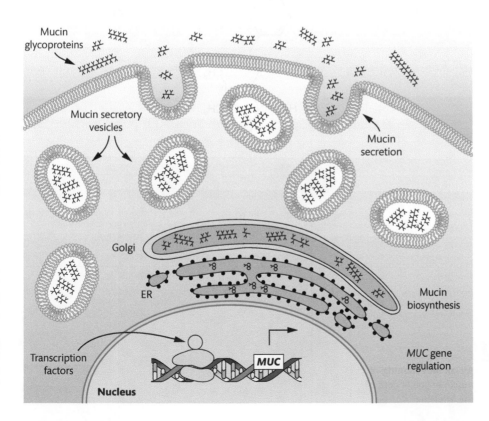

FIGURE 5.7
Glycoproteins are formed
by transcription of the *MUC*
gene. The protein structure is
synthesized in the endoplasmic
reticulum and Golgi complex
and secreted as vesicles.

5.5.1 Acidic glycoproteins

Acid mucins contain sulphated and carboxyl ester groups. The composition of each type of glycoprotein has a different chemical formula.

The most common demonstration method is by the Alcian blue stain (see Figures 5.8 and 5.9).

The selective demonstration of acid glycoproteins can be achieved by adjusting the acidity (pH) of the staining solution by the use of different types of aqueous acids at pH 1 (using hydrochloric acid), at pH 2.5 (using 3% acetic acid) or pH 3.1 (using 0.5% acetic acid). Hyaluronidase can also be selectively removed using **hyaluronic acid**.

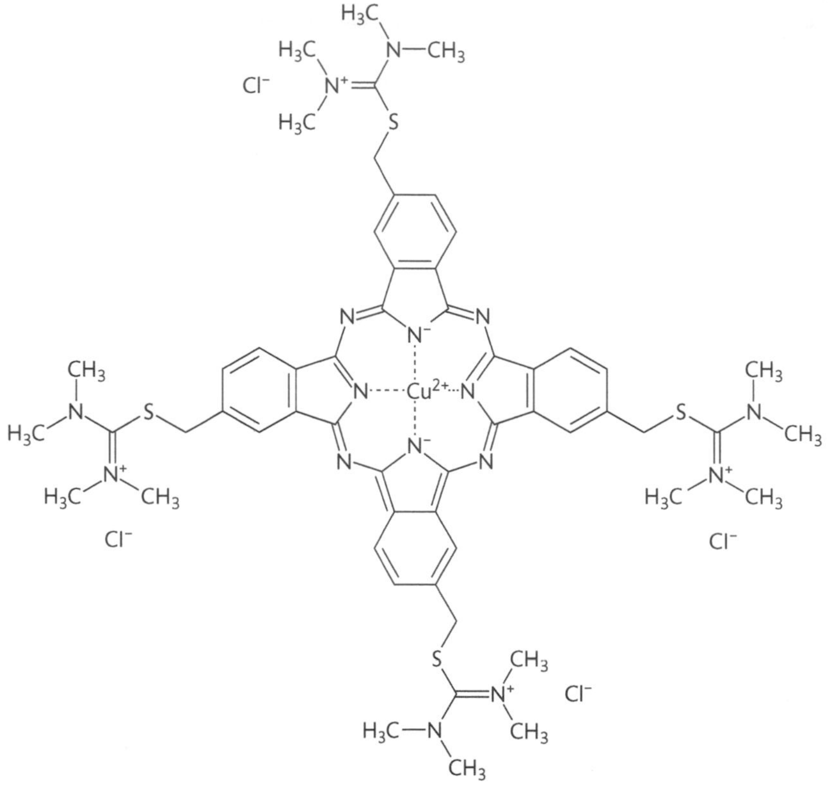

Hyaluronic acid

Hyaluronic acid is an ionic, non-sulphated glycosaminoglycan distributed widely throughout connective, epithelial and neural tissues (e.g. synovium and synovial fluid, skin, aorta, umbilical cord, cartilage and bone).

FIGURE 5.8

Alcian blue molecule. Note the copper (Cu) ion at the centre of the molecule, which gives the stain its distinctive colour.

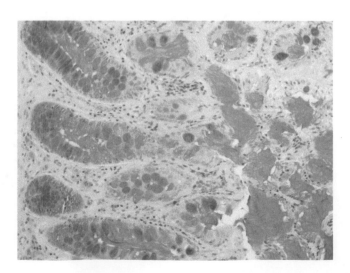

FIGURE 5.9

Alcian blue staining of mucin in goblet cells of the intestine.

5.5.2 Neutral glycoproteins

Neutral glycoproteins are found at various sites around the body including stomach, bronchus, prostate, cervix and vagina.

CLINICAL CORRELATION

Gargoylism (also known as Hurler syndrome)

A congenital syndrome in which mucopolysaccharides (glycosoaminoglycans) are accumulated within the tissue due to a lack of an enzyme, alpha-L-iduronidase. The symptoms of Hurler's syndrome include:

- mental retardation
- coarse facial features
- skeletal deformities
- joint deformities.

BOX 5.3 Periodic acid Schiff (PAS) method

The periodic acid Schiff reaction is a versatile method commonly used in histopathology. It is easy to perform and reliable, giving crisp, easy to interpret results over a wide range of tissues (Figure 5.10).

The method was first established in the 1940s by McManus and is used to demonstrate neutral glycoproteins, as well as glycogen. The presence of glycoproteins in the basement membrane allows the method to be of value in renal pathology (Figure 5.11; see also Box 5.4).

The presence of glycogen in the cell wall of fungi allows the method to be of use in infective agent pathology (see Section 5.6).

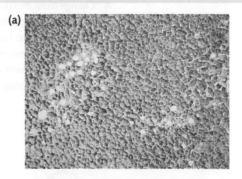
(a)

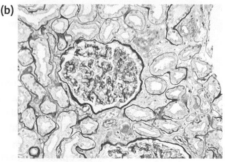
(b)

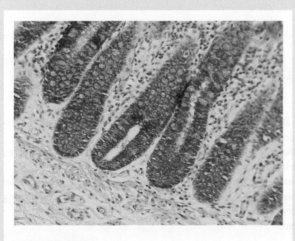

FIGURE 5.10
Periodic acid Schiff staining of intestinal mucin.

FIGURE 5.11
Periodic acid Schiff staining of a) glycogen in liver, and b) basement membranes in the kidney.

CLINICAL CORRELATION

Metaplasia

Metaplasia is a common pathological condition for which glycoprotein stains can be of use.

Metaplasia is described as a reversible change (meta-change) in shape (plasia) from one cell type to another in the presence of a stimulus (Figure 5.12). Metaplasia often represents an adaptive response to environmental stress. Metaplasia can be the result of normal physiological processes or the result of pathological changes.

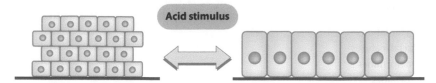

FIGURE 5.12

The process of metaplastic change. Metaplasia is the reversible process of a change of histological cell type due to the presence of an external stimulus. The diagram shows a change from stratified squamous epithelium to columnar epithelium in the presence of an acid stimulus. In the early stages of metaplasia the process is reversible. In certain circumstances metaplasia may develop into cancer and thus diagnosis is key to helping to prevent this development.

Examples of metaplasia include:

■ Change from mucus-secreting epithelium to stratified squamous epithelium in the bronchi as a result of cigarette smoking.
■ Change in cervical epithelium from stratified squamous epithelium in the presence of the female sex hormones oestrogen and progesterone.
■ Change from stratified squamous epithelium of the oesophagus to glandular columnar epithelium in the presence of acidic conditions.

CASE STUDY 5.1 *Barrett's oesophagus*

A 47-year-old male presents at his GP with chronic gastro-oesophageal reflux and heartburn. He is referred to the endoscopy unit at the local hospital.

On endoscopy, changes to the oesophageal mucosa were noted (see Figure 5.13). The area was biopsied and sent to the histopathology laboratory for examination.

The normal stratified squamous epithelium of the oesophagus was seen to be replaced with glandular epithelium. This metaplastic change was caused by a change in pH, causing the epithelium to adapt to the stimulus.

Treatment is by antacid agents.

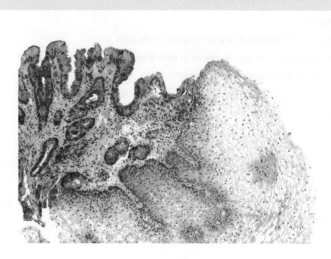

FIGURE 5.13

Histological appearance of normal oesophageal squamous epithelium (right) and the glandular epithelium of Barrett's oesophagus (left). (Credit: CC BY-SA 3.0)

CLINICAL CORRELATION

Barrett's oesophagus

Barrett's oesophagus is a common disease characterized by **acid reflux** into the oesophagus from the stomach (Figure 5.14). It occurs in about 2% of the adult population and is more common in men than women, and increases with age.

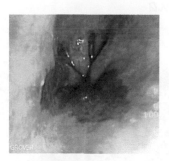

FIGURE 5.14

Macroscopic appearance of Barrett's oesophagus, as viewed towards the stomach.

Reflux occurs as a result of the cardiac sphincter becoming weakened.

Symptoms include heartburn, a sour taste in the mouth, and feeling bloated.

Diagnosis is often by endoscopy and a biopsy sent for histopathology. Treatment is by a number of means including losing weight, giving up smoking, and relaxing, as well as by medication such as antacids and **proton pump inhibitors**.

Acid reflux

The clinical condition in which gastric acid is released into the oesophagus.

Antacids

A type of medication that helps to control the acidity of your stomach.

Proton pump inhibitors

Drugs which reduce the amount of acid the stomach produces.

Key clinical uses of carbohydrate and glycoprotein methods:

- fungal demonstration
- changes in the location and level of glycoprotein expression
- changes to glycogen levels or glycoproteins in liver biopsy
- changes in glycogen levels in muscle biopsy
- demonstration of changes to the basement membrane in kidney and skin biopsies
- investigation of glycogen storage disorders.

CLINICAL CORRELATION

Mucin production and malignancy

Increased mucin production occurs in many adenocarcinomas (malignancies of glandular epithelium) including cancers of the:

- **pancreas**
- **bronchus**
- **breast**
- **stomach**
- **ovary**
- **colon.**

Identification of the glycoprotein type (acidic, neutral or mixed, or via specific immunocyto-chemistry antigen) can assist in the identification of metastatic tumour deposits. In well-differentiated epithelial tumours (i.e. tumours which closely resemble the tissue from which they are derived), staining can assist in the identification of the primary source.

CASE STUDY 5.2 *Gastric carcinoma*

A 63-year-old man presents at hospital with haemoptysis. After admission and stabilization, a gastric biopsy is taken under endoscopic investigation. The clinicians suspect a gastric carcinoma.

On microscopic investigation, gastric goblet cells are seen as large distended cells with large, central, mucus-containing vacuoles. The nucleus is seen to be pressed against the cell membrane to produce so-called signet ring cells (Figure 5.15).

The content of the vacuole was investigated with a DPAS stain and was seen to be positive, confirming the presence of neutral glycoprotein.

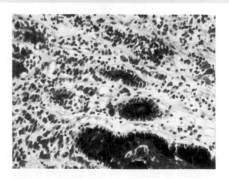

FIGURE 5.15
Diastase periodic acid Schiff (DPAS) staining showing the presence of so-called signet ring cells scattered throughout the tissue.

CLINICAL CORRELATION

Gastric cancer

Gastric cancer is the fourth most common cancer worldwide. It is a tumour of stomach epithelium and amounts to nearly 2% of all cancers diagnosed. Nearly half of all the people affected are over 75 years of age. Incidence is highest in white men and lower in females and other ethnicities.

CASE STUDY 5.3 *Alpha-1-antitrypsin*

A 61-year-old man presented to his GP with jaundice of un-known origin, and was referred to the local hospital for further investigations. Following initial biochemical tests, a liver core biopsy was taken and the sample sent to the laboratory. An initial H&E and a standard panel of liver stains was performed (H&E, PAS, DPAS, reticulin, HVG and Perls') was applied. Microscopic examination of the slides revealed the following:

H&E staining showed eosinophilic cytoplasm (i.e. brighter pink than would normally be expected)—see Figure 5.16a.

Most of the special stains were unremarkable yet staining with DPAS (Figure 5.16b) demonstrated the presence of mucin granules within the cytoplasm of the cells, an abnormal finding. The presence of DPAS-positive globules in the cytoplasm confirms α-1-antitrypsin deficiency.

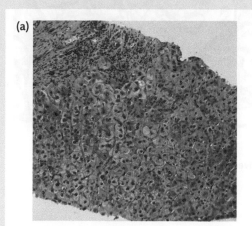

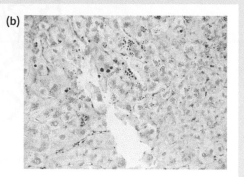

FIGURE 5.16
Liver showing alpha-1-antitrypsin deficiency: a) H&E b) DPAS.

CLINICAL CORRELATION

α-1-antitrypsin deficiency

Alpha-1-antitrypsin deficiency is an inherited genetic disorder found in a gene on chromosome 14. The incidence is about one in 1600 for Caucasians from north-west Europe but less for other racial groups. The abnormal protein results in the lack of a protein α-1-antitrypsin which is normally produced in the liver.

Disease severity varies from patient to patient, as over 70 variants of the disease have been identified. Age at diagnosis varies (from childhood to adulthood) but it is not uncommon for patients to be over 50 years of age at diagnosis.

Treatment of α-1-antitrypsin is complicated as the major aim is the maintenance of lung function. There is no direct 'cure' but enzyme therapy may be offered, known as augmentation therapy, where α-1-antitrypsin enzyme is given by intravenous therapy.

BOX 5.4 Glycogen stains for basement membrane

Glycoproteins are a constituent of basement membranes, which are mainly composed of type IV collagen, a structural protein. The presence of glycoproteins within basement membranes can be utilized when using special stains for glycogens (e.g. PAS and Jones methenamine silver (Figure 5.17) techniques for the interpretation of renal histopathology).

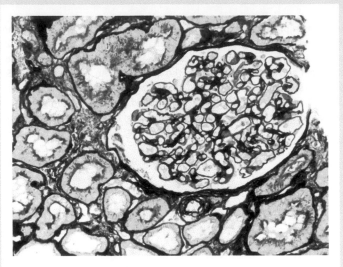

FIGURE 5.17
Methenamine silver staining of a needle core biopsy of kidney.

5.5.3 Heparin

Heparin is a sulphated glycoprotein secreted by mast cells. Mast cells are a myeloid-derived granulocyte, present in the tissue. The role of mast cells is in allergy and host defence against helminth parasites. They are involved in responses against other pathogenic infections, wound healing and inflammatory disease (Figure 5.18).

CLINICAL CORRELATION

Mast cell disease (mastocytosis)

The presence of too many mast cells, or mastocytosis, can occur in two forms—cutaneous and systemic. The most common cutaneous (skin) form is also called urticaria pigmentosa, which occurs when mast cells infiltrate the skin. Systemic mastocytosis is caused by mast cells accumulating in the tissues and can affect organs such as the liver, spleen, bone marrow and small intestine.

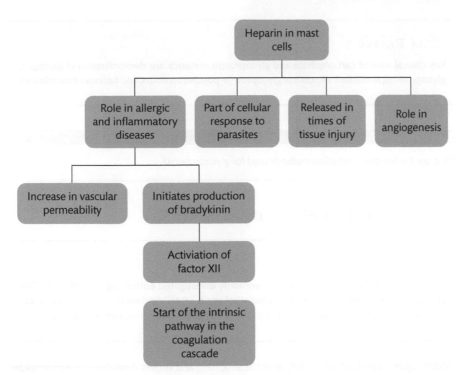

FIGURE 5.18
Heparin is stored exclusively in mast cells within the body and has a role within the immune response to parasites. Mast cells are also indicated in a number of pathological conditions including mastocytosis, asthma and eczema.

CASE STUDY 5.4 Mast cells in section

A man aged 30 with dark skin presented with pigmented plaques on his buttocks and hips. The clinically suggested diagnosis was eczema. A biopsy was taken for histopathological investigation. The H&E revealed a heavy infiltrate of mast cells within the dermis mainly occupying the papillary and reticular dermal compartments. Toluidine blue stain demonstrated the metachromatic nature of the stain and the histamine granules within the mast cells (Figure 5.19). These findings confirm that the gentleman had urticaria pigmentosa, exhibiting extensive mastocytosis. Treatment is by **topical** antihistamines.

Topical treatment
Treatment applied directly to the lesion.

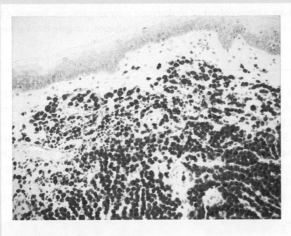

FIGURE 5.19
Metachromatic staining of mast cells (toluidine blue).

Key Point

Key clinical uses of carbohydrate and glycoprotein methods are demonstration of glycogen, glycoproteins, metastatic deposits of glycoprotein-positive tumours, and basement membrane.

What are the key demonstration methods used for glycoproteins?

5.6 Infective agent demonstration

Key Point

Infective agents are some of the most commonly investigated entities by special stains. The investigation of infective agents by histopathology is often incidental and microbiological typing and sensitivity are obviously the primary investigations where infection is suspected.

Infective agent is a term which encompasses bacteria, fungi and viruses. Amoebae are seen occasionally, as are larger parasites such as worms.

In haematoxylin and eosin-stained sections, the presence of microorganisms can be indicated by an inflammatory response. This can be a characteristic as in caseating granulomatous inflammation, which is indicative of tuberculosis infection (see Chapter 13).

There are many special stain methods available and more recently many immunocytochemistry, cell homogenate and *in situ* methods to supplement these tests. The accurate subtyping of specific species requires immunocytochemistry and molecular methods.

5.6.1 Bacteria

Key Point

Bacteria constitute a large cohort of prokaryotic microorganisms. Typically, these are a few micrometres in length. Bacteria have a number of shapes, ranging from spheres to rods and spirals.

Bacteria constitute a large group of prokaryotic organisms. Bacteria are primarily subtyped on the chemical properties of their cell wall. The thick cell wall retains Gram stain components and is termed Gram-positive and the thinner wall of the Gram-negative organisms does not retain Gram stain reagents (see Boxes 5.5 and 5.6). Alongside these two groups there is a smaller yet still significant group called mycobacteria. Mycobacteria form a distinct subgroup of organisms sufficiently significant in histology to demand a specific entry. Mycobacteria differ from other bacteria by the presence of a thick lipid-rich coat. The mycobacteria are differentially stained by the retention of a phenol-derived stain in the presence of an acid solution. Figure 5.20 shows examples of these two types of staining.

How are bacteria classified?

(a)

(b)

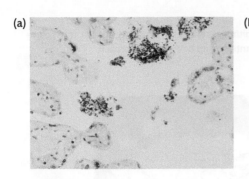
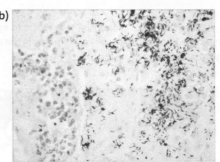

FIGURE 5.20
Microorganisms: a) Gram-negative bacteria, b) Mycobacteria demonstrated by the Ziehl–Neelsen method.

BOX 5.5 The Gram stain

The Gram stain was designed by Hans Christian Gram, a Danish microbiologist who first published his findings in 1884. This method is still in use today 130 years later!

The stain divides bacteria into two main groups based upon their staining properties, Gram stain positive and Gram stain negative.

The procedure has 3 steps (see also Figure 5.21):

1. Staining with crystal violet. This imparts colour to everything.
2. Treatment with an aqueous solution of iodine and potassium iodide. This reagent contains triiodide ions, which form a water-insoluble complex with the dye.

$$[Crystal.violet]^+ + I_3^- \rightarrow [Crystal.violet - I_3]$$

3. Extraction of the dye–iodine complex with an organic solvent such as ethanol or acetone. The solvent extracts dye from some types of bacteria (Gram negative) but leaves other types (Gram positive) fully stained unless the extraction is greatly prolonged. The second dye of contracting colour is then applied.

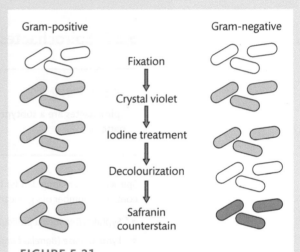

FIGURE 5.21
Diagrammatic representation of Gram staining.

BOX 5.6 Helicobacter pylori

Helicobacter pylori previously known as *Campylobacter pylori* is a Gram-negative microaerophilic bacterium found in the stomach (Figure 5.22). Two Australian scientists, Barry Marshall and Robin Warren, in 1982 found that it was present in a person with acute then chronic gastritis and gastric ulcers, thereby indicating the link between these conditions and the organism. Acute gastritis is characterized by neutrophil infiltration, while chronic gastritis is characterized by the presence of lymphocytes, plasma cells and macrophages. It is associated with peptic ulceration (which can be treated) and, less commonly, gastric cancer. Histopathological diagnosis depends on demonstration of typically curved bacilli in the biopsy specimen. *Helicobacter pylori* occur primarily in mucus adjacent to epithelial cells at the mucosal surface, most commonly in the antrum and body of the stomach.

(a) 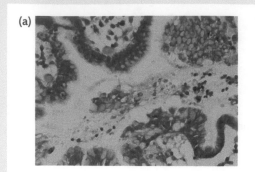   (b)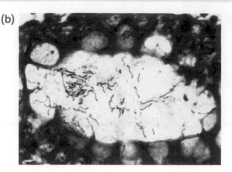

FIGURE 5.22
Helicobacter pylori: a) Giemsa b) Warthin and Starry.

5.6.2 Spirochaetes

> ### Key Point
>
> Spirochaetes are a subtype of bacteria, spiral in shape, with a distinct histological staining pattern.

Spirochaetes are long slender bacteria which twist and coil upon themselves. The spirochaete group contains a number of significant organisms, including:

- Syphilis (*Treponema pallidum*)
- Lyme disease (*Borrelia burgdorferi*).

These can now be identified by immunocytochemical means. Employing antibodies directed against epitopes associated with the spirochaete structure, it is now possible to demonstrate them within histological paraffin-embedded sections. There are also serological assays which can be used to check for these infections.

CLINICAL CORRELATION

Syphilis

Syphilis, if untreated, can cause progressive systemic damage. It affected a number of composers over the last few centuries and its effects are seen in a number of their musical compositions.

The Czech composer Beidrich Smetana was affected by tinnitus caused by his syphilis, and the effects of this is seen in his String Quartet Number 1—From My Life where a high-pitched line is heard mirroring his tinnitus.

The composer Frederick Delius is suspected to have become infected in the 1890s when he was sent to Florida as an orange farmer. By the 1920s he was completely paralysed and wheelchair-bound, but with the help of an amanuensis (Eric Fenby) to transcribe his dictation, was able to compose up until his death in 1934.

5.6.3 Mycobacteria

The two key mycobacterial organisms of interest histologically are:

- *Mycobacterium tuberculosis*—the cause of tuberculosis
- *Mycobacterium leprae*—the cause of leprosy.

Key point

Tuberculosis

Mycobacterium tuberculosis is the most clinically significant acid-fast bacillus. It is the causative agent of tuberculosis. Tuberculosis is the second most significant infectious cause of death, after HIV. Tuberculosis affects over 1.7 billion people and kills 1.7 million people each year. Over 50 million people worldwide are co-infected with HIV and TB.

CASE STUDY 5.5 Tuberculosis

A 55-year-old woman presented to her local hospital emergency department with a lesion which was thought to be a **haematoma**. The swelling was drained and did not appear to be a haematoma. An incisional biopsy of skin was performed.

Subsequently, she developed a right submandibular swelling with discharge. A 1.5 cm crater formed surrounded by a 2 cm halo of dusky skin. The provisional diagnosis was either infectious agents (necrotizing fasciitis or infected lymph node) or fat necrosis.

A further specimen was sent for frozen section, which showed an initial blister formation in the dermis (Figure 5.23a). A subsequent Ziehl–Neelsen (see Box 5.7 for mechanism) showed magenta staining rod-shaped organisms within a granulomatous inflammatory background, confirming a *Mycobacterium* infection (Figure 5.23b).

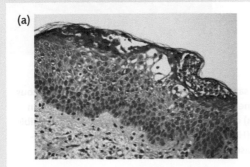
(a)

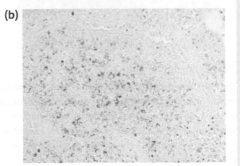
(b)

FIGURE 5.23
Tuberculosis of the skin: a) H&E stain, b) ZN stain.

CLINICAL CORRELATION

Mycobacterium infection

If left untreated, *Mycobacterium* infection can be fatal. Treatment is usually with two antibacterial agents for 6 months. It may be several weeks before the patient starts to feel better after starting a course of treatment.

Haematoma

A localized collection of blood outside a blood vessel. The breakage may be spontaneous in the case of an aneurysm or caused by trauma.

Key Point

Leprosy

The leprosy bacillus is less acid and alcohol fast than the tubercle bacillus and is frequently discoloured by the standard Ziehl–Neelsen technique. Therefore, a modified Ziehl–Neelsen (Wade–Fite) is necessary for the demonstration of *Mycobacterium leprae*. In this method the sections are dewaxed gently and are only minimally exposed to organic solvents, thus protecting the acid and alcohol fastness of the organism.

CASE STUDY 5.6 *Leprosy*

A 35-year-old gentleman from Delhi, India, arrived in an A&E department presenting with multiple open sores on his skin. Swabs were taken for microbiological investigations and a biopsy was performed and sent to the histopathology laboratory. Routine H&E revealed focal necrosis with oedema. There was a dense inflammatory infiltrate composed predominantly of histiocytes/macrophages with some eosinophils. (Figure 5.24a). A request for a Wade–Fite stain demonstrated large numbers of *M. leprae* bacilli within the macrophages (5.24b), confirming that the man had leprosy.

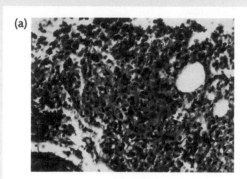

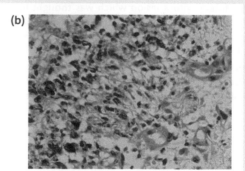

FIGURE 5.24

The infective agent *Mycobacterium leprae* is the causative agent of leprosy. Patients with lepromatous leprosy develop nodules in the dermal and subcutaneous compartments of the skin, which contain deposits of macrophages filled with mycobacteria: a) dermis showing features that indicate a possible infection, but the bacteria are not clearly identified (H&E, original magnification ×40); b) magenta-stained mycobacteria clearly seen within the cytoplasm of the macrophages (Wade–Fite, original magnification ×40).

CLINICAL CORRELATION

Leprosy

Leprosy is caused by a slow-growing bacillus, *Mycobacterium leprae*. It is transmitted via droplets from the nose and mouth of untreated patients with severe disease, but is not highly infectious. If left untreated, the disease can cause nerve damage, leading to muscle weakness and atrophy, and permanent disabilities.

Leprosy can be easily treated with a 6–12-month course of multidrug therapy. Each year over 150,000 new cases are reported.

HEALTH & SAFETY 5.1

Mycobacterium tuberculosis remains one of the key infective agent hazards to health in the cellular pathology laboratory. The TB organism is a potential danger in fresh specimens received into the laboratory from theatres or clinic.

One problem with warning the laboratory is that the clinical presentation of tuberculosis shares a number of symptoms with the clinical presentation of **lymphoma**.

The shared symptoms include:

- Weight loss
- Night sweats
- Pyrexia.

Lymphoma

Lymphoma is a lymphoid neoplasia which is distinguished from leukaemia by cellular proliferations involving discrete tissue masses in lymph nodes, secondary lymphoid organs such as the spleen, or extra-nodal such as the stomach. Leukaemia usually involves widespread involvement of circulating tumour cells in the bone marrow and circulating blood stream.

BOX 5.7 *Mechanism of mycobacterial staining*

In the Ziehl Neelsen (ZN) method for acid-fast tubercle bacilli the tissue section is over-stained with the Kinyouin's solution and differentiated with acid alcohol. The solution is then counterstained with a contrasting methylene blue solution. See Figure 5.25.

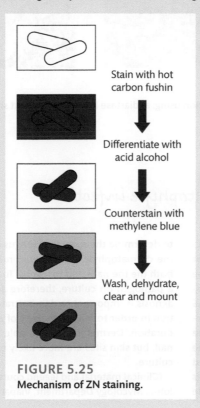

Stain with hot carbon fushin

Differentiate with acid alcohol

Counterstain with methylene blue

Wash, dehydrate, clear and mount

FIGURE 5.25
Mechanism of ZN staining.

Fungi

Key Point

Fungi are unicellular nucleated organisms seen as either yeasts, hyphae or spores. Fungi can be identified by diastase PAS and Grocott methods (see Figure 5.26).

Fungi are eukaryotic unicellular organisms which contain nuclei and cell walls. They may be organized as hyphae (chains of cells connected together) or yeasts (unicellular buds).

Key fungal organisms of interest histologically:

- *Candida*
- *Cryptococcus*
- *Aspergillus*
- Zygomycosis.

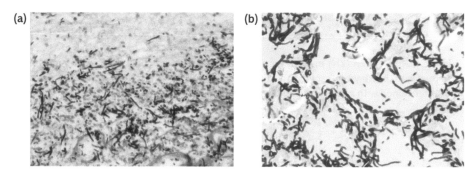

FIGURE 5.26
Fungal hyphae demonstration using: a) diastase PAS and b) Grocott silver staining.

CASE STUDY 5.7 *Dermatophyte infection*

A teenage boy presented with a suspected fungal foot infection. Toe nail clippings and toe web scrapings were taken for mycological assessment. Histological examination of the toe nail H&E (Figure 5.27a) revealed keratotic nail tissue. Special stains for fungal investigation were performed. The PAS (Figure 5.27b) revealed the presence of fungal hyphae (purple/magenta colour). On higher power (Figure 5.27c) the hyphae are seen to be regularly septate and there is some dichotomous branching. Similar features are demonstrated using a Grocott stain (black in Figure 5.27d). These findings were consistent with fungal infection, but it is not possible to determine the species of fungus on histology. On culture the dermatophyte *Trichophyton rubrum* was isolated from both the toe nails and toe webs. Toe nails often fail to grow a pathogen on culture, therefore accurate microscopic diagnosis is important to demonstrate the presence of infection in order to initiate therapy of an appropriate type and duration. Dermatophytes are able to infect both skin and nail, but skin sites are more likely to yield the pathogen on culture.

(Clinical material and legend courtesy of Dr Sue Howell, St. John's Mycology Department, Viapath, St. Thomas' Hospital)

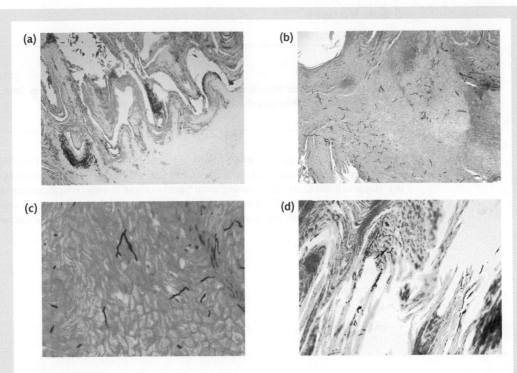

FIGURE 5.27
Keratotic nail tissue with fungal infection: a) H&E, b) PAS (original magnification ×20), c) PAS (original magnification ×40), and d) Grocott silver stain (original magnification ×20).

Pneumocystis carinii

Pneumocystis carinii is a fungal infection. It is an opportunistic pathogen often seen in immune compromised patients, who are either compromised by disease (e.g. patients with end stage HIV infection) or by the use of immunosuppressive therapy (e.g. patients who have undergone organ transplants). Samples of bronchial or lung biopsy or bronchoalveolar lavage specimens may be sent to the laboratory with the specific request to rule out *Pneumocystis* infection. The wall of the microorganism is rich in glycogen and is well demonstrated as bi-concave unicellular discs with the PAS and Grocott stains (Figure 5.28).

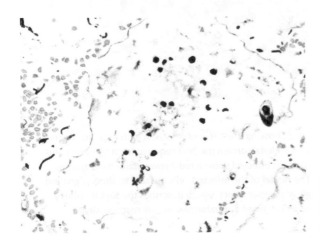

FIGURE 5.28
Bi-concave unicellular discs typical of *Pneumocystis* infection (Grocott silver stain).

5.6.4 Viruses

Key Point

Viruses are unicellular organisms which consist of genetic material either as DNA or RNA and a protein coat. They lack the ability to reproduce by themselves.

Viruses are unicellular organisms which consist of genetic material and a protein coat. They lack the ability to reproduce without a host cell. Viruses are the causative organism of some infectious diseases (e.g. Hepatitis B and C), as well as causing some types of cancer, namely cervical carcinoma and squamous carcinoma of the head and neck. Both cancers are caused by human papilloma virus infection. The common demonstration of viruses is done by special stains, as well as immunocytochemistry and molecular methods.

Key viral infections are:

- Hepatitis B
- Cytomegalovirus
- Herpes simplex virus
- Epstein–Barr virus.

CASE STUDY 5.8 Hepatitis infection

A 31-year-old intravenous drug user presented at his GP with the following symptoms:

    Abdominal pain.
    Dark urine.
    Fever.
    Joint pain.
    Loss of appetite.
    Nausea and vomiting.
    Weakness and fatigue.
    Yellowing of skin and the whites of the eyes (jaundice).

Blood tests were taken and sent to the local lab for investigation. When returned, the results showed abnormal liver function test results. Following referral to the hepatologist at the local hospital a liver biopsy was performed. Initial microscopic findings showed a ground glass appearance to the cytoplasm of the hepatocytes. A Shikata's orcein stain was performed which confirmed the presence of hepatitis B infected cells (Figure 5.29).

Note

If many hepatocytes are affected, the antigen appears as fine granules, either spread diffusely throughout the cytoplasm or concentrated in the cytoplasm peripheral to the sinusoidal space. This is responsible for the overall ground glass appearance. When single cells are involved, the hepatitis B surface antigen appears as oval, round or irregularly shaped aggregates in the cytoplasm, especially in the perinuclear region.

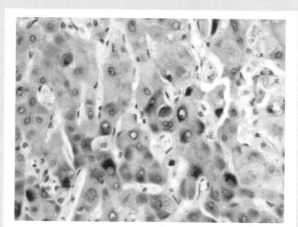

FIGURE 5.29

Liver showing the effect of infection with hepatitis B virus. This Shikata's orcein method requires fresh solutions and the cells infected show a red-brown stained cytoplasm. The nuclei of the infected cells are said to show a 'ground glass' stopper effect, which describes the slightly blurry and ill-defined appearance seen microscopically.

5.6.5 Protozoa

Protozoa are unicellular nucleated organisms. Protozoa may be detected by H&E stain and include *Giardia* and worms.

5.7 Extracellular proteins and connective tissues

Proteins are a normal constituent of tissue and therefore their presence in sections is never questioned (Table 5.4). The main reasons for staining are:

- Raised or depleted amounts of a specific protein (i.e. reticulin protein in bone marrow).
- Inappropriate deposition of normal proteins (e.g. collagen deposition in collagenous colitis).
- Deposition of pathological proteins (e.g. amyloid).

Extracellular proteins are often described as connective tissue. The main functions of connective tissue are:

- Structural.
- Mechanical and protective.
- Transport of nutrients and metabolites.
- Storage of energy-rich lipids, water and electrolytes.
- Defence against pathogenic organisms.
- Tissue repair.
- Thermogenesis.
- Insulation.

Trichrome staining figures prominently in the assessment of extracellular proteins and connective tissue, the principles of which are shown in Figure 5.30.

TABLE 5.4 The main extracellular proteins of interest and their key demonstration methods.

Protein	Stain	Results
Elastin	Miller's elastin/van Gieson	Elastin—Black Collagen—Red Fibrin—Yellow
Fibrin/Collagen	Martius scarlet blue (MSB)	Fibrin—Red Muscle—Red Collagen—Blue
	Masson trichrome	Muscle & Erythrocytes—Red Collagen—Blue
	Phosphotungstic acid Haematoxylin	Fibrin—Blue Collagen—Orange/Red Muscle—Blue
Collagen III (Reticulin)	Reticulin methods (there are many different methods often named after the scientists who devised them, e.g. James, Gordon and Sweet)	Reticulin—Black Other collagen types (if untoned)—Tan
Collagen IV	Periodic acid Schiff/ Haematoxylin	Basement membrane—Pink Nuclei—Blue
Amyloid	Congo red Sirius red Thioflavin T Crystal violet Immunocytochemistry methods	Congo red staining imparts apple green birefringence using cross-polarizers (refer to Chapter 14 for the definition of birefringence). Thioflavin T requires the use of the fluorescent microscope (Refer to Chapters 8 and 14 for information regarding immunofluorescence). There are several antibodies which can be employed for amyloid demonstration (e.g. Amyloid P).

(a)   **Effect of cell structure and dye molecule size**

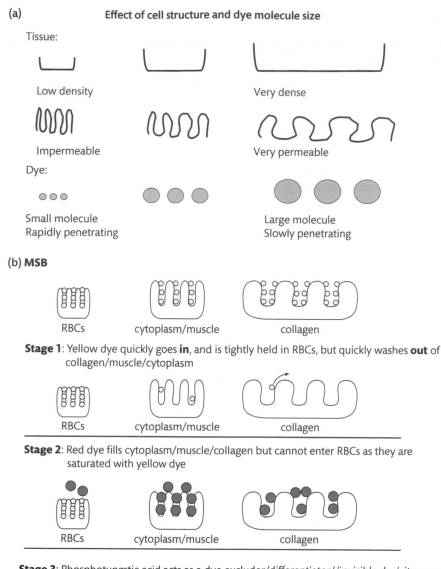

(b) MSB

Stage 1: Yellow dye quickly goes **in**, and is tightly held in RBCs, but quickly washes **out** of collagen/muscle/cytoplasm

Stage 2: Red dye fills cytoplasm/muscle/collagen but cannot enter RBCs as they are saturated with yellow dye

Stage 3: Phosphotungstic acid acts as a dye excluder/differentiator/ 'invisible dye', it competes with and turns red dye out of tissue in the order of collagen, muscle, cytoplasm. The reaction is stopped when collagen is only faintly stained.

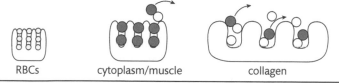

Stage 4: Collagen simply needs to be filled with blue dye, then rinse, dehydrate/clear/mount. (*NB: if aniline blue is left too long it will eventually compete with the other dyes. If this happens, the preparation is useless*).

FIGURE 5.30
Principles of trichrome staining; a) effect of cell structure and dye molecule size; b) Martius Scarlet Blue (MSB) as an example of trichrome staining.

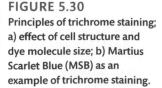

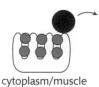
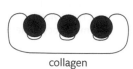

5.7.1 Elastin

> ### Key Point
>
> Elastin is a normal protein expressed in skin, blood vessels and the respiratory system. It can be demonstrated with Miller's elastin stain and orcein stain.

Elastin fibres are normal constituents of skin, the respiratory system and blood vessels. Histologically, the interest in elastin focuses on the levels found in different tissues; for example, is the level increased or decreased or the normal pattern disturbed? Elastin fibres are divided up into three types:

- Oxytalin (fibrillar).
- Elauni (amorphous).
- Elastic (mixed).

Elastic fibres are assembled into filaments and contain large amounts of the simple hydrophobic amino acids valine, glycine, alanine and proline. The hydrophobic property is exploited in elastin staining using non-polar alcoholic solutions; an example of this is Miller's elastin stain.

CASE STUDY 5.9 Temporal arteritis

A 68-year-old female presents at her GP with a chronic headache which has steadily worsened over the previous five days. The pain is on the left side of her head and has not moved. An examination of her cranial nerves reveals reduced visual acuity in the left eye and not the right. The left side of her scalp is tender to the touch.

She has blood tests taken for erythrocyte sedimentation rate (ESR) and C-reactive protein (CRP) and is referred to ophthalmology urgently. A temporal artery biopsy is taken and sent to the laboratory for investigation (Figure 5.31).

Artery biopsies for investigation of temporal arteritis need accurate embedding so that the lumen is in clear cross-section when examined microscopically.

(a)
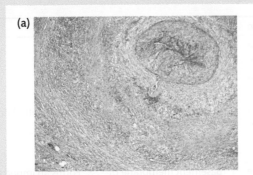

(b)
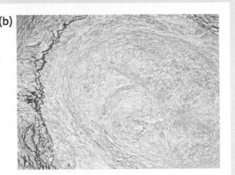

FIGURE 5.31
Temporal arteritis: a) The normal lumen of the temporal artery is blocked and large numbers of inflammatory cells are seen (H&E stain, medium power); b) The lumen of the artery is blocked and not evident, and the encircling elastin fibres have a frayed appearance (Miller's elastin stain, high power).

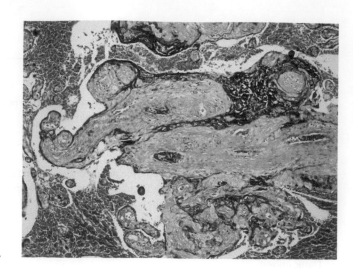

FIGURE 5.32
Fibrin deposition (red)
in the placenta (Martius
scarlet blue [MSB] stain).

5.7.2 Fibrin

Fibrin is an insoluble fibrillary protein formed by the polymerization of soluble fibrinogen into insoluble fibrin (see Figure 5.32) which is seen in damaged tissue. It is a transient protein in the repair process that follows injury and thus its staining properties change with age; however, early fibrin is difficult to stain.

Assessment of fibrin demonstration on H&E stain can be difficult as it has a non-specific eosinophilic appearance; hence special stains are used, the key methods being Masson trichrome, Martius scarlet blue and phosphotungstic acid/haematoxylin.

5.7.3 Collagen

Collagen is a connective tissue protein that provides tensile strength by virtue of molecules that form a triple helix thread. There are four key types of collagen (see Table 5.5).

TABLE 5.5   **Main types of collagen.**

Type of collagen	Structure	Location	Note
Collagen I	Rope-like structure	Skin, dermis, tendon, bone, ligaments and cartilage	
Collagen II	Rope-like structure	Hyaline and elastic cartilage	
Collagen III (also known as reticulin)	Rope-like structure	Blood vessels, parenchymal organs, bone marrow, lymphoid tissue, smooth muscle nerve and lungs	Stained with reticulin
Collagen IV	Sheet-like structure	Basement membrane of skin and kidney	Forms an important barrier between the body and the outside world; damage can result in serious medical conditions. Stained with Jones' methenamine silver and PAS.

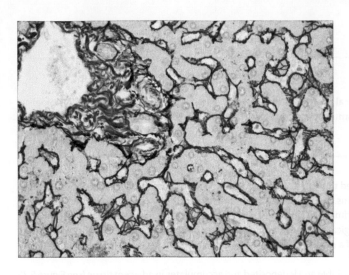

FIGURE 5.33
Reticulin network of
the normal liver (silver
staining).

5.7.4 Collagen III (Reticulin)

Reticulin is a normal protein produced by fibroblasts that provides a supporting matrix in cellular organisms such as the spleen, liver, bone marrow and lymph node (see Figure 5.33).

Reticulin staining is used to identify changes in the normal architecture and deposition and whether or not it is the cause of the patient's pathology. The reticulin stain comes in a number of variations based upon the names of the persons who described the method (e.g. James, Jones, Gordon and Sweet).

CASE STUDY 5.10 *Fibrosis of the bone marrow*

A 53-year-old man presents to his GP with general weakness, weight loss and breathlessness. The patient had also been suffering from more colds recently. Initial investigations included a blood test which showed depleted erythrocytes, leucocytes and thrombocytes. A referral to the haematologist at the local hospital was made. Following review of the initial laboratory test results, a bone marrow trephine biopsy of iliac crest was performed. The sample was sent to the laboratory for analysis. Following decalcification and processing the initial H&E was reviewed (see Figure 5.34a). The specimen was seen to be very cellular with no fatty spaces remaining as is normally seen. The silver stain for reticulin (see Figure 5.34b) showed a high density of reticulin fibres, much higher numbers than are normally seen, confirming fibrosis.

(a) 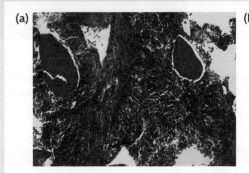   (b)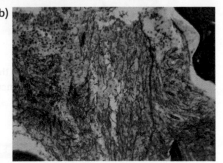

FIGURE 5.34
Bone marrow trephine specimen showing excess reticulin and the typical appearance of fibrosis: a) H&E staining; b) silver staining.

5.7.5 Amyloid

Key Point

Amyloid is a pathological protein; it does not exist within the body as a normal physiological protein. Once accumulation of amyloid has started it disrupts the normal functioning of tissues.

Amyloid is the term applied to a range of abnormal fibrillar proteins which are deposited as pathological extracellular proteins. It may be part of an inherited condition or sporadic in occurrence. Amyloid is regarded as a primary disease protein and also as a secondary by-product of other disease processes (e.g. haematological and chronic inflammatory disorders). Amyloid is deposited as part of the incorrect processing of a range of proteins (see Table 5.6 for the main types of amyloid and their source).

The residue formed is insoluble and is deposited and accumulates in adjacent tissue (see Figure 5.35 in Box 5.8). Once deposited amyloid is not easily removed. Protein fragments vary in size from 8000 to 30,000 Daltons (Da).

BOX 5.8 Demonstration of amyloid

Amyloid deposits stain with Congo red, a dye originally used in the cotton industry, and produces pathognomonic red-green birefringence under polarized light microscopy. The lozenge-shaped Congo red molecule reacts with the fibrillary beta pleated sheets.

Alternative amyloid stains are Sirius red, thioflavin T, crystal violet, and a range of antibodies for use with immunocytochemistry.

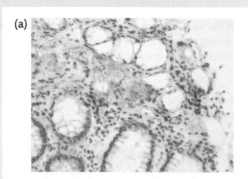
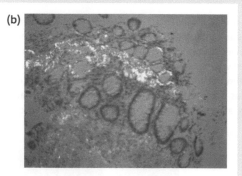

FIGURE 5.35
Amyloid a) stained with Congo red, and b) the same preparation viewed under polarizing microscopy to show the typical apple green birefringence due to the amyloid (beta-pleated sheet)-dye interaction.

CLINICAL CORRELATION

Key causes of sporadic amyloid deposition

- Chronic diseases.
- Chronic infection.
- Tuberculosis.

- Osteomyelitis (inflammation of the bone due to bacterial infection).
- Chronic inflammatory disease (a major cause of amyloidosis).
- Rheumatoid arthritis.
- Ankylosing spondylitis.
- Malignancy.
- Multiple myeloma.

There are over 20 types of amyloid but the main types of amyloid seen in histopathology are shown in Table 5.6.

TABLE 5.6 Types of amyloid.

Amyloid	Source
AL amyloid	Immunoglobulin light chains
AA Amyloid	Serum amyloid-associated protein
B2 amyloid	Beta-2-microglobulin amyloidosis
AB amyloid	AB amyloid is associated with Alzheimer's disease
AS amyloid	
AP amyloid	Amyloid serum P is a subtype seen in many deposits

SELF-CHECK 5.9

Is amyloid protein a normal physiological protein?

CASE STUDY 5.11 Amyloidosis

A 78-year-old female presented at her GP with weight loss and diarrhoea, with a clinical diagnosis of colitis. Endoscopic biopsies were taken and the initial H&E staining showed an amorphous pink band. To elucidate the source of the amorphous band, special stains using Congo red (? amyloid) or Masson trichrome (? collagen) were performed. The Congo red stain stained red under brightfield illumination, and when visualized under polarized light showed apple green birefringence (see Figure 5.35 in Box 5.8).

5.8 Lipids

Lipids are a varied group of fats, most of which contain long-chain fatty acids. Lipids are a normal constituent of tissues and cells, being present in all cell membranes. Some cells are specially adapted for the storage of lipids and are termed lipocytes. Lipids have a role as storage molecules, protection and insulation.

Lipid demonstration requires tissues to be handled differently from routine formalin-fixed, paraffin-embedded tissues. Routine processing removes lipids from tissue so therefore tissues must be frozen and cut as frozen sections to preserve the lipids within the tissue. Demonstration is with either Oil Red O or Sudan Black stains which act as **lypsochromatic dyes** (Figure 5.36).

Lypsochromatic dyes

Lypsochromatic dyes are dyes that are more soluble in the substance to be demonstrated than in the substance they are prepared in. For example, Oil Red O staining solution is worked up in 60% aqueous isopropyl alcohol, the solution of which is about at the point of saturation. However, the dye is much more soluble in cellular lipid. Lypsochromatic solutions should always be filtered before use.

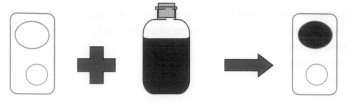

FIGURE 5.36
Lypsochromatic staining. The technique utilizes a dye product that is only partially soluble in the staining solution. When the staining solution is applied to tissue sections the dye product is more soluble in fat contained within cells. Care should be taken when using the solutions as they need filtering before use.

Examination of lipid within sections focuses on two areas:

- Pathological accumulation of lipids within cells (i.e. due to metabolic errors—lipid storage disorders).
- Lipid presence in the wrong place (i.e. lipid embolism following broken bones).

Cross reference

For further details about the role of the Coroner see Chapter 16.

Lipids accumulate in thecoma tumours and in atherosclerosis but these pathologies are of limited interest in routine histopathology.

 CASE STUDY 5.12 *Medium chain acyl CoA dehydrogenase (MCAD) deficiency*

A 6-month-old child died suddenly and unexpectedly in his cot. Due to the sudden nature of the death and the lack of any previous medical history a post-mortem examination is ordered by the Coroner. On macroscopic examination of the body no obvious cause of death could be established, so with the permission of the Coroner tissue was taken for histological assessment. Tissue was taken for paraffin processing. Heart, liver and kidney tissue was taken for frozen sections to investigate the possibility of lipid storage disorders.

Paraffin processing revealed vacuoles in the cytoplasm of the hepatocytes (see Figure 5.37a). Oil Red O staining of frozen sections revealed pathological depositions of cytoplasmic lipid (see Figure 5.37b).

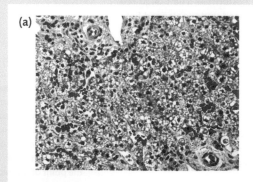
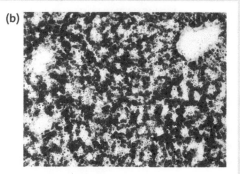

FIGURE 5.37
Intracellular lipid deposition in the liver: a) H&E stain; b) Oil Red O stain on frozen section.

> ## Key Point
>
> Lipid staining is not common in histopathology, but when it is performed it does have a valuable diagnostic role.

CLINICAL CORRELATION

Lipid storage disorders

Lipid storage disorders are a group of metabolic inherited disorders characterized by the accumulation of lipids within cells, due to the overproduction of lipid or decreased metabolism. Lipid storage disorders are rare (incidence in the region of 1-2 per 100,000 live births).

Clinical presentation is diverse storage in CNS can lead to a neurodegenerative course, with loss of skills or failure to attain developmental milestones. Storage in visceral cells can lead to organomegaly, skeletal abnormalities, bone marrow dysfunction, pulmonary infiltration, and other manifestations.

Examples of lipid storage disorders include, Fabry, Farber, Gaucher and Niemann–Pick diseases.

5.9 Pigments and minerals

Pigments are a group of coloured molecules that may be produced naturally by the body or introduced. Pigments are often categorized as:

- Endogenous
- Exogenous
- Artefactual.

5.9.1 Endogenous pigments

Endogenous pigments are those produced by the body and can be normal cellular constituents and also the result of pathological change.

Key endogenous pigments are:

- Melanin
- Iron
- Copper
- Lipofuscin.

There are a number of endogenous pigments which look very similar (often brown and granular) on routine H&E staining. As a result of this special stains are used to differentiate the pigments. This also explains why often pigment stains are asked for in pairs or groups to differentiate the pigments.

Melanin

Melanin (Figure 5.38) is a normal biological pigment found in skin, the retina of the eye and the substantia nigra of the brain. As a constituent of skin (see Figure 5.39), it acts to provide protection to cells from the harmful rays of the sun. Within the eye, the black colour of melanin absorbs stray light and prevents reflection of the sun's rays. Melanin is produced by cells known as melanocytes or naevocytes.

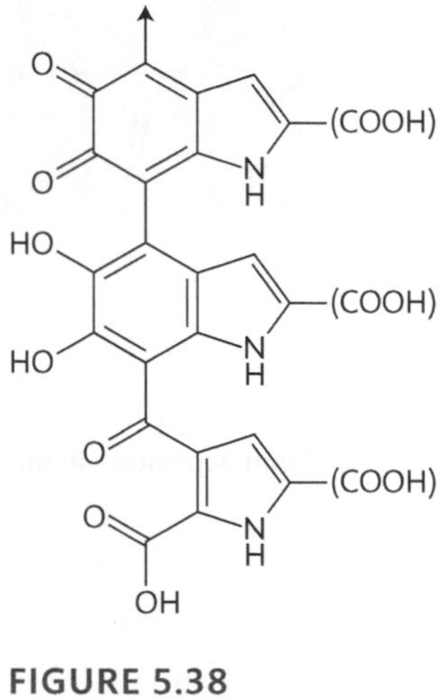

FIGURE 5.38
Melanin, a normal biological pigment found in the skin.

CASE STUDY 5.13 *Malignant melanoma*

A 32-year-old female who enjoyed holidaying in the Mediterranean recently returned with an irregularly pigmented, raised and inflamed, pigmented lesion on the back of the calf. On closer inspection the lesion had a variegated pigmentation, was raised, and had an irregular outline. There was also pronounced reddening and inflammation surrounding the lesion. The woman stated that she only had a small discrete mole at the site previously and the changes had appeared rapidly on her return from holiday. The lesion was excised with a clear margin. Under routine H&E staining the lesion appeared to have an asymmetric pigmented lesion with upward migration of melanocytes throughout the epidermis and invasion into the dermis. The melanocytic cells showed mitotic activity with pronounced nuclear atypia. The lesion was classified as a superficial spreading malignant melanoma. A secondary wider excision of the area was recommended.

The woman was informed of the risks of sunbathing and also the increased risks of developing skin cancer. The paler the skin type, the increased risk of developing skin cancer.

'The only good sun tan is the one that comes out of a bottle' Cancer Research UK.

Sun tan = sun damage

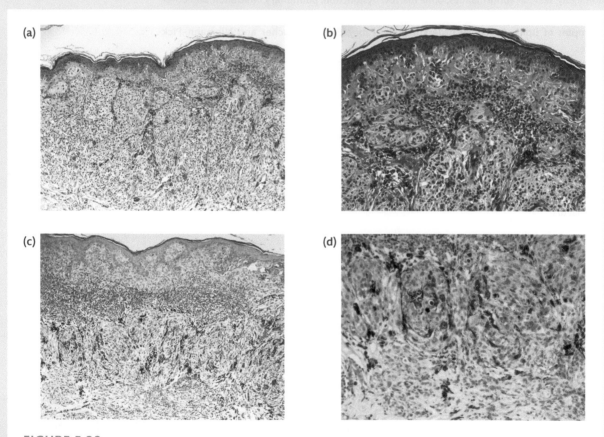

FIGURE 5.39
Melanin deposition in the skin: a/b) H&E staining; c/d) Masson–Fontana silver staining.

Key points

Melanin

- Polymerized macromolecule.
- Produced by melanocytes.
- Black in colour. Melanin is a major contributor to skin colour.
- Acts as a protective molecule in the skin, absorbing UV light (280–320 nm).

Iron

Iron is an essential mineral within the body. The body holds about 3–4 grams of iron, mainly within haemoglobin; most of the remainder is stored within iron storage proteins ferritin and haemosiderin. Iron is an essential component of haemoglobin and of **metalloprotease** enzymes. Low levels of iron within the body lead to low haemoglobin and to **anaemia**. Iron may be deposited in damaged tissues and is responsible for the dark coloration typical of a bruise.

It is important to note that histological investigation is not the best way of identifying increased iron levels in the body, which is best performed in biochemistry using a serum ferritin method.

Metalloprotease

A protease enzyme whose catalytic mechanism involves a metal.

Anaemia

A condition in which there are reduced numbers of red cells or a deficiency of haemoglobin in the blood.

CASE STUDY 5.14 Haemochromatosis in a liver biopsy

A 25-year-old woman presented at her GP with fatigue, weakness and a palpably enlarged liver. An initial number of haematological and biochemical blood tests were taken. Following review of the results, she was referred to the local hospital for further investigations. The hepatologist examined the patient and a tru-cut liver biopsy was performed and sent to the laboratory. In light of the clinical information provided a range of special stains was performed. The H&E showed some brown pigment in the cytoplasm of the hepatocytes. A Perls' stain was performed and the liver showed an increased deposition of iron (Figure 5.40; usually iron is not visible to the naked eye on a normal Perls' stain).

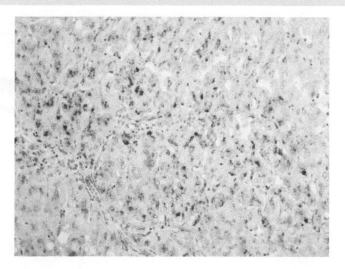

FIGURE 5.40
Increased deposition of iron in the liver due to haemochromatosis (Perls' stain).

Haemochromatosis

Haemochromatosis (or bronze diabetes) is a relatively common inherited disease characterized by increased iron absorption and iron deposition, which is commonly seen in the liver. Haemochromatosis can lead to fibrosis and organ failure. Treatment is primarily very simple by venesection (i.e. draining iron-rich blood). If diagnosis is early enough the outcome can be very good.

Copper

Copper is an essential trace metal which is present within a number of enzymes including cytochrome oxidase. Copper is difficult to identify histologically as levels at which it is found are too low for visualization. In routine practice copper levels are best measured in biochemistry via serum copper, serum caeruloplasmin and urinary copper assays. However, a liver biopsy can be helpful and rhodamine and stain may help identify copper deposits in copper overload disease states.

There are two inborn errors of copper metabolism:

- Menke's syndrome (see Box 5.9).
- Wilson's disease (see Box 5.10).

BOX 5.9 *Menke's disease*

Menke's disease is a fatal genetic disorder seen in male infants who often present with strikingly peculiar kinky hair (pilo torti; Figure 5.41). Clinical presentation is by growth failure, mental retardation, lesions of the major blood vessels and bone disease.

Where there is a clinical suspicion of Menke's disease, a few strands of hair are sent to the laboratory for examination under the dissecting microscope.

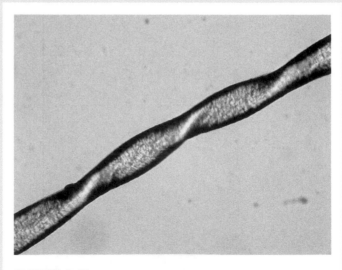

FIGURE 5.41
'Kinky' structure of hair seen in Menke's disease.

BOX 5.10 Wilson's disease

Wilson's disease is a rare genetic condition arising as a result of an anomaly on chromosome 13. Clinical presentation is often in adolescents and young adults, although the disease has been first noted in older patients.

Symptoms include unexplained neurological and/or hepatic disease.

Histologically, copper may be seen on rhodamine staining of the liver biopsy following negative staining of brown pigment in the liver by Perls' stain (Figure 5.42). Confirmation of Wilson's disease is by measurement of the amount of copper in a liver biopsy, which is usually greater than 250 µg/g dry weight in patients with the disease.

Wilson's disease is treatable and can be managed by the administration of chelating agents which promote copper excretion.

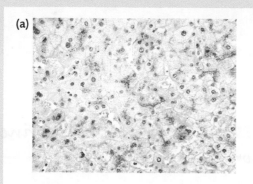
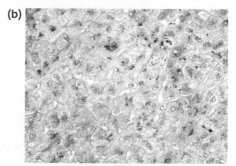

FIGURE 5.42
Wilson's disease and abnormal deposition of copper in the liver: a) rhodamine and b) orcein staining.

Lipofuscin

Lipofuscin is a yellow/brown 'wear and tear' pigment. It accumulates in cells with increasing age and is a product of the breakdown of red blood cells. Levels of lipofuscin increase with age and it is sometimes referred to as the aging pigment. It is commonly seen in cardiac myocytes and neurons.

Bile pigment

Bile pigment is a commonly observed feature of liver biopsies, often seen as green on tissue sections. There are a number of demonstration methods available to selectively demonstrate bile pigments, including Gmelin and Schmorl.

Neuroendocrine granules

Neuroendocrine granules are normally found in cells of the neuroendocrine system, which includes the α and β cells of the pancreatic islets of Langerhans, Paneth cells, adrenal cells, thyroid and pituitary cells (Figure 5.43). Their function is to control glandular activity. Neuroendocrine cells are found in ductless glands developed from the invaginations of epithelial surfaces. Typically, they secrete peptide and steroid hormones. Neuroendocrine tumours (or carcinoid tumours) are the most common malignancies of the neuroendocrine system.

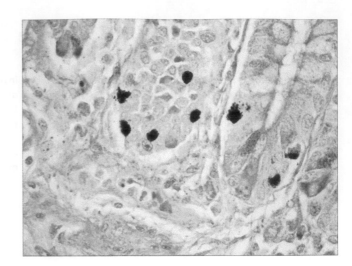

FIGURE 5.43
Neuroendocrine cells
stained black in the
intestinal mucosa
(Grimelius stain).

CASE STUDY 5.15 *Neuroendocrine carcinoma*

A 67-year-old man presented at his GP with flushing of the skin, diarrhoea, wheezing, a fast heart beat and bouts of sudden low blood pressure. Blood tests were sent to the biochemistry laboratory and a diagnosis of carcinoid was suggested. A scan followed in radiology and a gastrointestinal biopsy was taken.

Initial H&E staining showed cells with prominent clumping of nuclear chromatin, without the cells looking frankly malignant, and numerous cytoplasmic granules were seen. A Grimelius stain was performed and the cytoplasmic granules stained dark brown/black, confirming their neuroendocrine origin and a diagnosis of carcinoid tumour.

Surgery and removal of the tumour is often curative.

CLINICAL CORRELATION

Neuroendocrine tumours

Carcinoids are a rare type of tumour with approximately 1200 new cases diagnosed each year in the UK, with men and women affected equally. Such tumours are usually found in adults over 30 years of age.

Most tumours are found in the appendix and the small intestine. Less commonly, they may arise in the lung or pancreas, and rarely in other parts of the body.

Carcinoid tumours often grow slowly and it may be several years before symptoms appear and the tumour is diagnosed.

5.9.2 Exogenous pigments

Exogenous pigments are external elements introduced into the body, often from the environment. The key exogenous pigments seen in histopathology are carbon and asbestos.

Carbon

Carbon is present in the atmosphere and is inhaled as smoke and smog (i.e. everyday city air). Over time carbon breathed in gets trapped in the respiratory mucus and ends up in the macrophages in the lymph nodes draining the lung. It causes no wider pathology and is clinically insignificant.

Asbestos

Asbestos is not a pigment but a fibre. Asbestos fibres were used to lag pipes and as insulation material in the 1950s and 60s. When individual asbestos fibres are released and breathed in then they can lodge at the edge of the lung. The fibres are too big to be engulfed and remain. They rub against the pleural cavity causing initial inflammation. This develops into neoplasia and later malignancy.

CASE STUDY 5.16 Asbestosis and mesothelioma

A 71-year-old former shipyard worker presents to his GP with shortness of breath. Initial investigations show reduced lung capacity and reduced lung function. A lung biopsy showed a fibrous lesion. His clinical history and the histological picture suggested asbestos.

A Perls' stain was requested. On examination, the dumb-bell asbestos fibres (see Figure 5.44) appeared to be in close proximity to macrophages which stained positively with the Perls' stain. This supported the diagnosis of asbestosis.

Once asbestosis was identified, the man was able to approach a solicitor to make a claim against his former employer for compensation for his asbestosis.

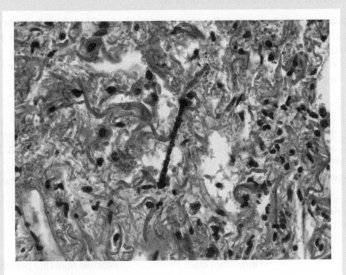

FIGURE 5.44
Asbestos fibre showing the typical dumb-bell appearance (H&E stain; original magnification ×400).

5.9.3 Artefactual pigments

Artefactual pigment is a term to describe pigments introduced into tissue sections as part of the processing regimes used on tissue.

Formalin pigment accumulates in tissue that has been fixed using acidic formalin. Formalin pigment is created by the action of an acid formaldehyde solution on haemoglobin. By using buffered formalin solutions, the occurrence of formalin pigment can be largely avoided.

Mercury pigment is seen in tissues fixed in a mercury-based solution. This is not an artefact commonly seen today as the use of mercury-based fixatives has declined. Evidence of mercury pigment is now increasingly confined to archived samples.

5.10 Liver biopsy

Liver biopsy assessment represents a defined area of special staining in histopathology. Clinical indicators for needle core biopsy of liver for medical conditions are listed as:

- Acute viral hepatitis.
- Chronic hepatitis.
- Alcoholic liver disease.
- Cholestatic liver disease.
- Cirrhosis.
- Immunodeficiency disorders (e.g. HIV and the viral hepatitis conditions hepatitis A, B and C).
- Fever of unknown origin.
- Metabolic disorders.
- Focal lesions.
- Monitoring therapy in patients undergoing hepatotoxic treatment.
- Hepatic allografts (biopsies pre- and post-liver transplantation).
- Vascular disorders.
- Hepatomegaly and abnormal liver function tests.

The initial biopsy is usually requested after an array of biochemical tests broadly termed liver function tests (e.g. prothrombin time, albumin, bilirubin, aspartate transaminase, alkaline phosphatase, transaminases, gamma-glutamyl transpeptidase).

A detailed clinical history is essential for a complete histopathological report, the substance of which relies on a panel of special stains (Table 5.7).

TABLE 5.7 Key stains used in the assessment of liver biopsies.

Stain	Result	Reason
Haematoxylin & eosin	General tissue architecture.	
Periodic acid Schiff (PAS)	Investigation of glycogen.	The liver is the main storage organ for glycogen.
Diastase periodic acid Schiff (DPAS)	Investigation of neutral carbohydrates.	
Perls'	Blue cytoplasmic granules.	
Reticulin	Fibres stain black.	Reticulin fibres are present normally between the cells in a number of tissues. The level of reticulin is what is being demonstrated rather than the presence or absence.
Haematoxylin & van Gieson	Fibrin red, collagen yellow, nuclei blue/black.	Investigation of fibrosis.
Orcein	Either cytoplasmic staining of protein or coarse granular ground glass appearance of hepatitis B infected cells.	Ground glass appearance due to presence of virus particles in the cytoplasm.

CASE STUDY 5.17 *Liver cirrhosis*

A 60-year-old male with a large alcohol intake (greater than 50 units per week) presents with increasing jaundice. Initial blood tests to investigate his liver function show abnormal results (raised alanine aminotransferase, raised aspartate aminotransferase, raised alkaline phosphatase and raised gamma glutamyl transferase). He is referred to his local hospital and after a clinical examination and review of his lab test results a tru-cut biopsy of liver is performed.

Initial tests include a liver set of special stains and an H&E. The H&E showed a changed liver architecture (see Figure 5.45a). There was fatty change and a nodular change to the liver seen on the HVG (see Figure 5.45b) and reticulin stain (see Figure 5.45c)

The results of the biopsy confirm alcoholic cirrhosis. Patients are managed by asking them to stop drinking: often this can be a very difficult process, but this can improve the prognosis of five-year survival to almost 90%.

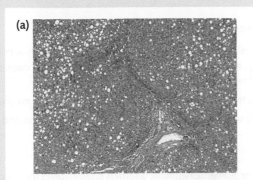

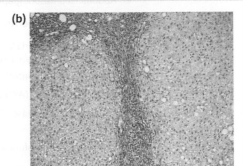

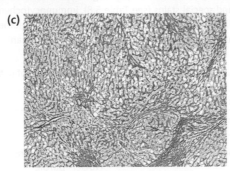

FIGURE 5.45
Alcoholic cirrhosis of the liver showing fatty and nodular changes as illustrated by a) haematoxylin and eosin; b) haematoxylin and van Gieson; and c) reticulin staining.

Key Point

In the investigation of liver disease, the use of biochemical and histological methods is often quite complementary.

5.11 Native renal biopsy

Renal disease is an increasingly specialist area of histopathological investigations. Correlation of clinical and laboratory features is a must for an accurate diagnosis and type of a kidney disease (renal disease) or glomerulonephritis.

The following investigations are considered important to ascertain the diagnosis and type of glomerulonephritis:

Investigations for likely diagnosis of glomerulonephritis:

- Clinical presentation.
- Urine analysis (proteinuria, haematuria and electrophoresis).
- Microscopy of urinary sediment.
- Intravenous pyelography (IVP: Radiological investigation).
- Abdominal ultrasonography.

There are four common indications for renal biopsy:

- Significant proteinuria/nephrotic syndrome (>1 g/L, or PCR > 100 mg/mmol) with two normal sized, non-obstructed, kidneys and no obvious cause (usually considering the diagnosis of a glomerulonephritis or interstitial nephritis).
- Acute kidney injury (AKI) with two normal sized, non-obstructed, kidneys and no obvious cause.
- Chronic kidney disease (CKD) with two normal sized, non-obstructed, kidneys and no obvious cause.
- Renal transplant dysfunction.

The assessment of a renal biopsy for glomerulonephrotic disorders often involves the use of traditional H&E and special stains (see Table 5.8), immunocytochemistry involving the detection of immunoglobulin deposits at the basement membrane of the glomeruli, and transmission electron microscopic evaluations of the architectural features of the Bowman's capsular areas.

TABLE 5.8   Key stains used for the assessment of native renal biopsies.

Stain	Result	Reason
Haematoxylin & eosin	Nuclei—purple Cytoplasm—pink	General tissue architecture
Periodic acid Schiff	Basement membrane—pink Nuclei—purple	
Picro Mallory trichrome		
Congo Red	Amyloid seen as extracellular amorphous red deposit	
Jones methenamine silver with haematoxylin & eosin	Basement membrane—black Deposited immunoglobulin	
Elastic van Gieson	Elastic fibres stain black	To monitor the health of blood vessels

5.12 Muscle biopsy

Muscle biopsy techniques are one of the key specialist areas of histopathology investigations. The tissues taken require pre-analytical attention to detail to ensure that the tissue is optimally preserved for evaluation. The subsequent investigations encompass staining procedures covering traditional tinctorial special stains, enzyme histochemical methods and immunocytochemistry assessments, as well as evaluations of electron micrographs. The tissue type presents with inherent difficulties compared to most other tissue types principally due to its contractile properties, its susceptibility to freezing artefacts, and its sometimes complex embedding requirements (transverse sectioning [TS] for patho-logical interpretations). Please refer to Orchard and Nation's *Cellular structure and function* textbook in this series for more detailed explanation of muscle structure. Nearly all examples of skeletal muscle biopsy removal from patients are 'open investigations, with invasive procedures, often on quite frail and vulnerable patients who often carry an increased risk due to the operative procedures'. The pro-cedures will quite often involve the removal of multiple samples to be assessed by numerous staining and electron microscopic procedures. In more recent times tissue is also removed for immunoblotting techniques, which are quite often required in cases of metabolic disorders, or similarly DNA extrac-tion for gene analysis or indeed in some cases biochemical assessments for respiratory chain enzymes or perhaps fibroblastic culture. Generally speaking muscle biopsies from the quadriceps in the thigh are preferred. These may be needle biopsies, which are generally rapid to perform and less invasive. However, they may be more challenging to orientate correctly. Similarly, more popular are the open biopsies which are performed under general anaesthetic. However, the site and yield of tissue re-moved is quite often governed by the clinical features of the individual patients under assessment. The majority of pathological assessments of muscle are made on frozen sections of muscle cut in TS. This underlines the critical need to ensure tissue is correctly orientated before cryotomy. The tissue is also susceptible to freezing artefacts and as such must be frozen down quickly. Any residual water remaining in the sarcoplasm will readily form ice crystals and form a peppered or holey appearance under the microscope. In addition, these small holes may also be confused with vacuole formation, which is commonly seen in some of the inherited metabolic myopathies. In order to prevent ice crystal artefacts, and to minimize the loss of antigenicity and optimize enzyme activity, muscle must be snap frozen in isopentane cooled in liquid nitrogen.

The preliminary investigations encompass a battery of histological and histochemical tests per-formed on cryostat sections orientated and embedded in OCT for transverse sectioning (TS) and cut at 10 microns. These preliminary investigations will rarely define an exact diagnosis but will enable the establishment of a particular category of muscular disease, for example myopathic or neurogenic disorders. See Table 5.9 for the main routine histological and histochemical methods. Needless to say

TABLE 5.9 Routine histological and histochemical methods used in muscle biopsy assessment (adapted from Costin-Kelly N, *The Biomedical Scientist*, December 2008).

Staining method	Demonstration features
H&E	Morphology, fibre basophilia, inflammatory cells.
Modified Gomori's trichrome (GT)	Morphology, ragged red fibres, nemaline rods, tubular aggregates, cylindrical bodies, cytoplasmic bodies, rimmed vacuoles, connective tissue.
Nicotinamide adenine dinucleotide-tetrazolium reductase (NADH-TR)	Cores, target/targetoid fibres, lobulated fibres, intermyofibrillar disruption, neurogenic atrophy. Fibre types I & II.
Succinic dehydrogenase (SDH)	Mitochondria.
Cytochrome oxidase (COX)	Mitochondria, COX deficiency.
COX-SDH	Cox-negative fibres.
Adenosine triphosphatase (ATPase at peri-incubation pH 10.4, 4.6, 4.3)	Fibre types I, IIA, IIB and IIC.
Acid phosphatase	Lysosomal activity, lipofuscin, phagocytosis, macrophages.
Oil Red O (ORO)	Neutral lipid—intrafibre lipid droplets, interstitial adipose tissue.
Periodic acid Schiff (PAS) with diastase digestion (DPAS)	Glycogen, necrotic fibres, denervated fibres. PAS-positive/diastase-resistant inclusions.
Additional stains	
Phosphorylase	Deficiency = type V glycogenosis (McArdle's disease).
Phosphofructokinase	Deficiency = type VII glycogenosis (Tarul's disease).

the H&E stain can be extremely helpful in defining broad morphological features when performed on well prepared and orientated cryostat sections.

In order to comprehend the importance of these stains and what they can reveal it is important to understand that, firstly, muscle is composed of several fibre types which will have differences in their metabolic pathways used to generate ATP. Secondly, each fibre functions as part of a motor unit.

There are three main fibre types. Type I contract slowly and are capable of sustained activity due to a slow but regular supply of ATP. They are described as 'slow twitch' fibres. Type II fibres can be subdivided into two sub-types: Type IIA and B. Type IIA are described as 'fast twitch, fatigue-resistant fibres'. Type IIB fibres are described as 'fast twitch, fatigue-sensitive fibres'.

The H&E stain can demonstrate changes in size and shape of fibres, internalization of nuclei, fibre splitting, vacuolated fibres, basophilic (regenerating) fibres, necrotic fibres and those undergoing phagocytosis. The modified Gomori trichrome stain (GT) has many benefits but is particularly useful to delineate 'ragged red fibres' which are seen in some mitochondrial disorders. The GT stain is also useful to demonstrate connective tissue components with clarity and delicacy.

The histochemical stains include the NADH-TR reaction which demonstrates mitochondria and the membranes of the sarcoplasmic reticulum, while SDH and COX demonstrate mitochondrial enzymes only. The NADH-TR reaction, SDH and COX stains are important for demonstrating the central cores, minicores, core-like areas or general unevenness of staining associated with congenital myopathies. The SDH and COX stains can confirm pathological changes seen in the NADH-TR reaction. Together with the GT stain they can define mitochondrial abnormalities.

Myosin ATPase also can be used to define fibre types. The techniques depend on the assurance of good pH control. It is a time-consuming technique that requires dedicated time to ensure that the procedure is carried out correctly. The ATPase technique is very useful in demonstrating the large group atrophy and fibre type grouping seen in the spinal muscular atrophies (SMA).

Acid phosphatase detects lysosomal activity and is useful in studies of some storage disorders and vacuolar myopathies.

PAS with and without diastase demonstrates fibre glycogen. Its main application is the demonstration of glycogen storage diseases (glycogenosis; Figure 5.46).

Oil Red O (ORO) stains neutral lipids red. Increased intrafibre lipid is seen in fatty acid oxidation disorders (FAOD) and also in some mitochondrial disorders.

Immunocytochemistry (ICC) has expanded its role in this area; focusing on identifying the presence or not of specific proteins implicated in selective muscular dystrophies, for example. In addition, there are also disorders involving abnormal protein surplus in some forms of structural myopathies.

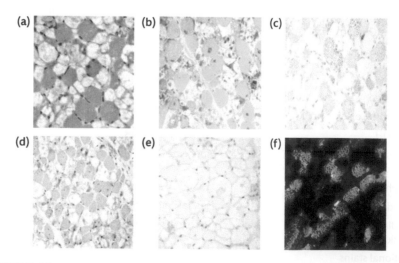

FIGURE 5.46

Severe infantile form (Pompe's disease) of type II glycogenosis: a) H&E; b) modified Gomori trichrome; c) oil Red O; d) acid phosphatase; e) PAS with prior digestion with diastase; and f) PAS (adapted from Costin-Kelly N, *The Biomedical Scientist*, December 2008).

Similarly, ICC can help in the diagnosis and differential diagnosis of inflammatory muscle disease. ICC can also help in defining muscle fibre development, maturation and regeneration.

Electron microscopy is useful to identify minicores in cases of irregular mitochondrial distribution. Of importance is the use of EM to define myelin inclusions in cases of Niemann–Pick C disease, granular osmiophilic inclusions (GRODs) of Batten disease, etc.

5.13 Nerve biopsy

Principally nerve biopsies can provide information on potentially treatable causes of neuropathy. Neuropathy may be caused by a host of conditions such as vasculitis, sarcoidosis, amyloidosis and leprosy. The nature of the biopsy is that it is an invasive procedure and so tends to be only employed in progressive neuropathy cases. In most cases of neuropathy it is the lower limbs that are affected. It is the superficial peroneal with the peroneus brevis muscle, or the sural nerve with the vastus lateralis or the gastrocnemius muscle that are usually assessed. In cases where the upper limbs are affected it is usually the superficial radial nerve, a branch of the ulnar nerve in the dorsum of the hand, that is biopsied. (Refer to the muscle and bone chapter of *Cell Structure and Function* in the OUP *Fundamentals of Biomedical Science* series.)

Pathologically nerve biopsies are obtained and prepared by three methods:

- One nerve piece (0.5 cm in length) is fixed in neutral buffered formalin and embedded in paraffin.
- One piece (0.5 cm in length) is placed in Michel's transport medium or frozen in liquid nitrogen.
- One piece (2.0–2.5 cm in length) is placed in glutaraldehyde for semithin plastic sectioning and also for 'teased' myelinated nerve fibre assessments.

Assessments of tissue embedded in paraffin will yield valuable information in defining the disease process, most notably in establishing the underlying condition in cases of amyloidosis, sarcoidosis, vasculitis and leprosy. The use of accompanying special stains, such as Congo red, thioflavin T or S for amyloid demonstration in amyloidosis, and elastic van Gieson (EVG) for elastic fibres, along with the use of Perls' stain for haemosiderin, can be useful in cases of vasculitis. In some cases, stains to demonstrate fibrinoid deposits may be useful, such as MSB. The use of immunohistochemistry techniques can be useful in selective cases. A good example would be the use of transthyretin or immunoglobulin light chains that can cause two types of amyloid neuropathy.

Generally, transverse sections of semithin plastic resin-embedded material will improve the morphological detail observed and are more useful in the analysis of myelinated fibres because they can demonstrate small myelinated fibres, onion bulbs and other structures with greater clarity than can be seen in paraffin-processed tissues. Generally, semithin sections are stained with toluidine blue as a post-embedding step, having been stained with osmium tetroxide in a pre-embedding step. This approach can help distinguish axonal disorders from primary demyelination disorders. Results can be quantified and can provide evidence to indicate a loss of myelinated fibres. The loss of myelinated fibres is generally an indication of axonal loss with secondary degeneration of myelin sheaths.

In the case of acute primary demyelination of nerve fibres, the axons effectively appear stripped of myelin sheaths. Additional information can be seen using electron microscopy as there are often wider myelin lamellar changes in certain entities.

Segmental remyelination occurs often without onion bulb formation but it cannot always be distinguished from fibres that have undergone axonal regeneration and remyelination in semithin sections (Figure 5.47). For this purpose, the method of 'teased' myelinated fibre analysis is employed. It is a helpful procedure for identifying demyelinating and axonal features. Analysis involves the quantification of abnormalities in a minimum of 50 teased myelinated fibres and comparison to the data of age-matched normal control subjects.

In practical terms nerve biopsy evaluation has limited diagnostic value, with some authors reporting that it helped confirm diagnosis in 14–45% of all biopsies examined, but yet could provide valuable supportive evidence for diagnostic purposes in up to 70% of cases.

There can be some complications from nerve biopsy procedures. These include neuroma or pain with paraesthesia or neuralgia. There can be loss of sensation in certain parts of the body affected (e.g. the foot).

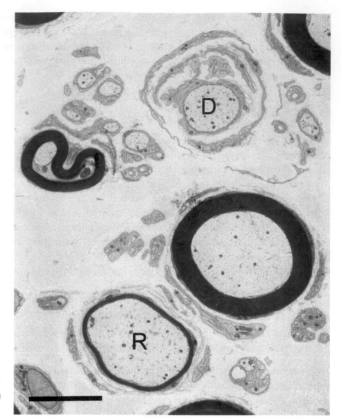

FIGURE 5.47
Recent demyelination (D)
and remyelination, where
the new myelin sheath (R)
is thinner than normal.

For what are the three samples of nerve tissue taken in routine investigations following an invasive
nerve biopsy procedure?

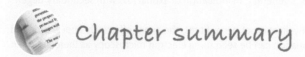

Chapter summary

Special stains provide a valuable adjunct to H&Es, ICC and molecular methods. Although the role of
special stains is limited they still have a place alongside the other methods. Increasingly, instrumentation is allowing the automation of special stains.

Glycoproteins and carbohydrates

■ Carbohydrates have a varied role in the body.

■ Staining of glycoproteins can be useful in the demonstration of adenocarcinoma and
metaplasia.

Infective agents

■ Histopathology can provide useful information about infectious agents.

■ Histopathology is not the method of choice to demonstrate infective agents—that is microbiology.

■ Infective agents are rarely well demonstrated upon H&E stain.

■ The presence of infective agents is often suspected by inflammatory processes within tissue.

Pigments and minerals

■ Melanin, iron and copper pigments are often seen as brown cytoplasmic pigments and are difficult to distinguish.

■ Melanin and iron stains are often requested together.

External proteins

■ Elastin stains can be used in the diagnosis of temporal arteritis.

■ Amyloidosis is a progressive disease characterized by abnormal protein processing, and may be demonstrated by Congo red.

Lipids

■ Lipid stains are used mainly to investigate lipid accumulation disorders, which represent a rare group of diseases.

■ Observation of lipid accumulation is not possible on paraffin-processed tissue and therefore frozen sections must be used.

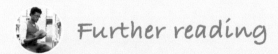 Further reading

● Collington SJ, Williams TJ, Weller CL. Mechanisms underlying the localisation of mast cells in tissues. *Trends Immunol* 2011; **32** (10): 478–85.

● Costin-Kelly N. Collecting and handling muscle biopsies. *The Biomedical Scientist* 2008; **52** (6): 491–5.

● Costin-Kelly N. Histological analysis of a muscle biopsy. *The Biomedical Scientist* 2008; **52** (12): 1063–70.

● Therapath Neuropathology. Nerve biopsy (www.therapath.com>tests.nerve).

● Suvarna KS, Layton C, Bancroft JD eds. *Bancroft's theory and practice of histological techniques* 7th edn. Edinburgh: Churchill Livingstone, 2012.

Useful websites

■ British Association of Dermatology (**www.bad.org.uk**).

■ Web MD treatment for α-1-anti-trypsin deficiency (**www.webmd.com/lung/copd/features/treatments**).

- α-1-antitrypsin deficiency support (**www.alpha1.org.uk**).
- Lyme disease network (**www.lymenet.org**)
- National Institute of Allergy and Infectious Diseases (**https://www.niaid.nih.gov/**)

 # Discussion questions

5.1 Discuss the complementary roles of special stains and immunocytochemistry.

5.2 Discuss the histological features seen on H&E staining that may indicate the need for stains to demonstrate infective agents.

5.3 Discuss the value of mucin stains in the diagnosis of metaplasia.

5.4 Discuss the role of special stains in the diagnosis of liver disease.

5.5 Describe the investigative tinctorial and histochemical stains and what they demonstrate in muscle biopsies.

Acknowledgement

The authors wish to acknowledge the work undertaken by Harry Elliot, who wrote 'Staining—principles and demonstration techniques' in the first edition.

Answers to the self-check questions and tips for responding to the discussion questions are provided on the book's accompanying website:

 Visit www.oup.com/uk/orchard2e

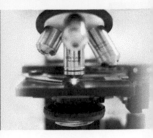

6

Artefacts

Guy Orchard, Chantell Hodgson and Brian Nation

Learning objectives

After studying this chapter, you should be able to:

- Appreciate the key artefacts in histological procedures.

- Identify the key causes of artefacts in this context.

- Understand what actions are required to attempt to rectify these artefacts.

- Develop a broad comprehension of the process of histopathological tissue analysis and to begin to appreciate the complex skills and understanding required to enable the identification of technical failures, and how to plan to reduce the risks of occurrence.

6.1 Introduction

Up to this point you will have read about the processes and procedures that enable us to fix, cut and stain tissue for histological assessment. In addition, there is an inherent need to appreciate the skills required to identify problems in the process of histopathological assessment. Put more simply, as a trained and competent biomedical scientist, you will be required to develop an appreciation of how to identify when processes or procedures go wrong, identifying the cause of any given problem within this multi-step procedure. In addition, you will be required to develop an understanding of what actions are required to rectify any of these problems.

Key Point

What is an artefact?

In the broadest sense, artefacts can be defined as:

1. An object made by a human being, which is typically cultural or historical. This explains the use of the word in historical studies of archaeological landmarks and cultural civilizations.

2. Something that is observed in a scientific investigation or experiment that is not normally present, but occurs as a result of the process of preparation or investigation.

3. An inaccurate observation, effect or result, often arising from the technology used in a scientific investigation or from experimental error.

Points 2 and 3 are scientifically related and together explain the use of the term artefact in histopathological processes and procedures.

6.2 Concepts and classification criteria

It is worth considering how the term artefact (derived from art and factum) has come into such widespread use. Ironically, artefacts are not facts at all, but rather a miscomprehension or misinterpretation of something observed and taken as a fact.

Artefacts in histopathological studies can be commonplace and have a profound impact on the outcome of any investigations, but how then do we classify them?

There are many classifications systems, all of which have merits and will focus on key techniques or procedures in which artefacts can occur (e.g. tissue fixation, section cutting or section staining). The problem with this approach is that you can be drawn into the detail of artefact production pertaining to very selective processes or procedures without an appreciation of the overall picture. It is important to remember that the presence of an initial artefact subsequently creates others later in the processes employed to analyse tissue for histological investigation. Therefore, it would seem sensible to adopt a classification system that provides a good overview rather than in-depth detail of the very specific events, processes or procedure that can cause artefacts.

Key Point

How do we classify artefacts?

Whichever classification method you adopt, it will be largely determined by the frequency of artefacts encountered. The specialized techniques and procedures employed will determine the length, breadth and depth of the classification system employed.

Adopting a classification that looks at artefacts in specific compartmentalized areas of histopathological techniques is a good approach. For example, starting at the beginning of the process we have surgical procedures, followed by fixation, tissue processing, embedding, microtomy, section mounting, staining and coverslipping.

Alternatively, a more rounded and simplistic approach is to look at a classification system based on just two steps: pre-analytical, essentially covering artefacts produced before the sample is received by the laboratory; and post-analytical, which covers all artefacts produced during the laboratory analysis pathway.

6.3 Pre-analytical artefacts

Pre-analytical artefacts are largely due to the processes and procedures undertaken prior to specimen receipt in the histopathology laboratory. They relate to the need to ensure that Good Clinical Practice (more precisely **Good Surgical Practice**) is followed while removing tissue samples from patients, to reduce their impact on viable tissue harvesting. The artefacts encountered can be split into two main groups:

1. Tissue dehydration prior to fixation issues (Figure 6.1).

2. Mechanical trauma or damage to the tissue due to surgical procedures which directly affects the tissue. These would include:

   i) Crushing/pinching of the tissue from the use of forceps (Figure 6.2).

   ii) Leaching of autolytic enzymes from ruptured cells, resulting in localized tissue damage.

   iii) Fragmentation of the tissue (Figure 6.3).

   iv) Haemorrhagic changes as a result of rupturing blood vessels. (Figure 6.4).

Key Point

Good Surgical Practice (GSP) requires a good understanding of the clinically suspected diagnosis of the patient's condition. It concentrates on the practice of safe, timely and competent surgical intervention. It ensures patients are prioritized and treated according to their clinical needs.

In terms of the removal of histological material, GSP would encompass consideration of the patient's condition and supportive surgical care requirements, the surgical procedure to be performed, the selection of the appropriate surgical instruments to be used, and attention to the time period between removal of the tissue and placing it in appropriate fixative or transporting medium.

It is well known that, once removed from the human body, tissue will begin to break down very quickly. The tissue will dehydrate and this will cause it to begin to break down, a process termed autolytic change. This involves the lysis of cell membranes and the release of enzymes that can cascade the autolytic process still further and affect other cells in the surrounding tissue environment. This breakdown of cells can be surprisingly swift and, if left unchecked, may result in a tissue sample being unsuitable for histological assessment in a diagnostic setting. These changes can be seen most commonly

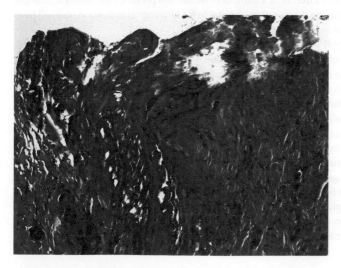

FIGURE 6.1
The effect of dehydration prior to fixation.

(a)
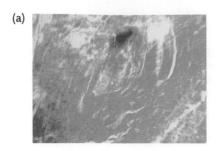

(b)
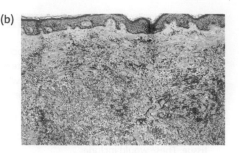

FIGURE 6.2
a) Crushing and b) pinching effects caused by the use of forceps.

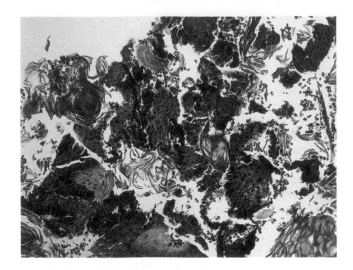

FIGURE 6.3
Fragmentation of tissue.

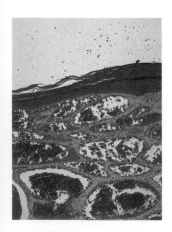

FIGURE 6.4
Haemorrhagic changes as a result of rupturing blood vessels.

in affected cells as nuclear pyknosis, karyolysis and vacuolization in the cytoplasm. These changes are more commonly seen in autopsy of post-mortem samples. These effects can be reduced, although not stopped, by storing tissue at 4°C. There is also an increased risk of the introduction and widespread distribution of common commensal and opportunistic microbiological organisms. In order to address the onset of autolysis, the use of a fixative or a transport medium will prevent these autolytic changes from taking place and stabilize the tissue, making it suitable for histological evaluation. You will have read about this in more detail in previous chapters.

These changes may not only start as a consequence of dehydration of the tissue but may result from the subsequent effects of the surgical process. A good example of this is the crushing or pinching artefacts seen due to the use of forceps. The more cellular the tissue the more likely the crushing or pinching effects will be seen on subsequent histopathological examination. These effects are non-reversible. The release of cellular enzymes (lysozymes) and their effects are generally seen around the edges of the tissue sample, where the forceps were in contact with the tissue. When handling delicate lymphoid tissue samples, this is a particular artefact that must be avoided as it may decrease the viable tumour cells and impact on tissue assessment.

Similarly, the use of cauterization during the surgical procedure can also damage the tissue sample and produce autolytic changes (Figure 6.5). In addition, vacuolization and coagulation of involved connective tissue fibres can be seen. The affected tissue is dehydrated and this can result in subsequent acidophilic staining, giving it a much darker blue/purple colour than one would see in unaffected tissue. Fragmentation can occur if the material is keratotic and the surgical procedure has removed only a very superficial sample; for example, in the case of a shave excision of a warty cutaneous lesion.

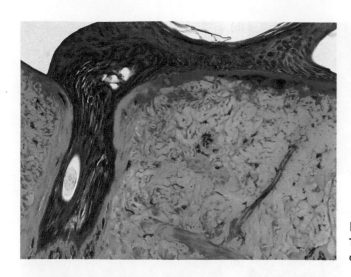

FIGURE 6.5
The effect of heat damage on skin.

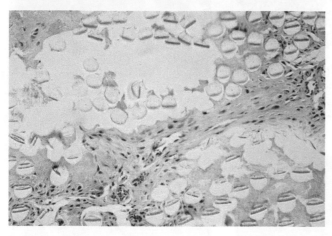

FIGURE 6.6
Dissolvable sutures seen in cross-section.

Surgery often involves the use of sutures (or metal staples) for closure or attachment, or to act as a marker for orientation of the sample. Sutures and staples are inert and extremely resistant to any fixative or solvent used in histopathology. Ideally, they should be removed at specimen dissection, but this is not always possible. They will not necessarily damage the tissue but they will cause damage to any knife used to dissect the sample, or the microtome blades used to section the paraffin block. If not removed, sutures may be seen in cross-section in tissue sections and they are also strongly birefringent (Figure 6.6).

During surgery, cotton fibres from cotton-based dressings or cellulose fibres from wooden instruments or appliances may get trapped on the tissue sample. Alternatively, epithelial samples from the gastrointestinal tract may include food debris of a cellulose nature. These items are generally resistant to fixation and subsequent histological processing, and may cause damage resulting in tears or scores in tissue sections. Similarly, starch grains from surgical gloves may become trapped on the tissue samples. These grains are strongly birefringent and exhibit a classical Maltese cross appearance under polarized light (Figure 6.7).

Occasionally, tissue may need to be assessed by frozen section (see Chapter 8). The process of freezing tissue commonly involves the use of cryosprays or liquid nitrogen, and will result in tissue damage due to the production of ice crystals. The tissue will appear shrunken with spaces between the frozen cells or tissue fibres. The nuclei of affected cells may appear shrunken and darker, and cytoplasmic detail is often pale and less discernible. These effects can be exacerbated if the freezing and subsequent thawing process is repeated (Figure 6.8).

Haemorrhagic artefacts can be seen in samples of tumours that have abundant blood vessels (e.g. pyogenic granuloma or angiosarcoma). Such tumours are delicate and the blood may act to maintain

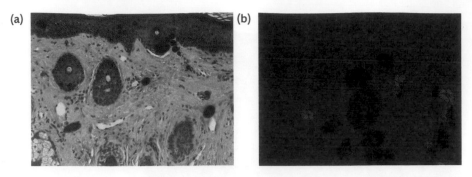

FIGURE 6.7
Starch grains on a) H&E-stained skin, and b) showing birefringence and characteristic Maltese cross appearance.

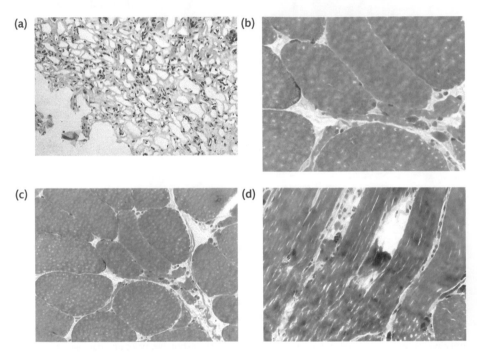

FIGURE 6.8
Freezing artefact in a) kidney and b–d) muscle tissue.

the integrity of the tissue. Once the blood supply is cut off, the structures can be damaged. Abundant blood deposits will also slow down the process of fixation and decrease the fixative's ability to penetrate deeply into larger specimens. (Figure 6.9).

The majority of these pre-analytical artefacts can be prevented as follows:

- Good clinical judgement in selecting the appropriate biopsy site.
- Adequate specimen depth to avoid fragmentation.
- Fast and efficient fixation immediately following tissue removal.
- Appropriate handling of the tissue sample, including careful use of forceps, or use of a suture as an alternative.
- Small incisional biopsies and delicate strips of tissue placed on card or sponges and then immersing in fixative, to reduce the curling and shrinking effect.

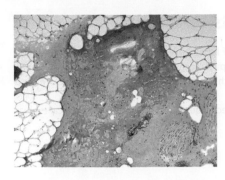

FIGURE 6.9
Pigmentation due to haemorrhage or dried blood.

- Avoid sources of foreign bodies during the surgical process. Examples include starch grains from some surgical gloves, or cotton wool deposits from swabs.

- Careful attention to the effects of heat and drying following use of cautery instruments or lasers. This can be reduced by use of cutting rather than coagulation electrodes, so that low current is produced, reducing the heating effect but allowing cutting and liberation of the tissue sample.

SELF-CHECK 6.1

What are the main artefacts seen in pre-analytical procedures, and how can they be prevented?

Table 6.1 shows the causes and effects of key artefacts that can occur in the pre-analytical stages of histological tissue sampling, and their appropriate remedies.

TABLE 6.1 The cause and effect of the key artefacts that can occur in the pre-analytical stages of histological tissue sampling, and the appropriate remedies.

Artefact	Appearance	Cause	Commonly associated with	Solution	Prevention
Tissue dehydration	Autolytic changes	Delay in fixation	Autopsy/post-mortem specimens		Immediate fixation following tissue removal/ use of transport medium
Mechanical trauma/damage	Crushing effects (often on outer edge of specimen)	Forceps or other surgical instruments	More common in incisional than punch biopsies		Delicate use of forceps/ suture as an alternative to forceps
Heat damage	Strong staining in affected areas/ loss of nuclear and cytoplasmic detail	Cauterization of tissue	Surgical procedures		Awareness of effects of heat and drying due to cautery instruments/lasers
Sutures/clips/ staples	Fragments or fibre bundles/metal	Suture material from surgical procedure	May or may not be of pathological significance	Removal if visible/ possible	Removal if visible/possible before processing to prevent damage to knife edge/tissue block
Starch granules	Maltese cross on birefringence	Powder from surgical gloves	Surgical procedure/ specimen dissection		
Ice crystals	Spaces within processed tissue	Ice crystals formed due to freezing/ distortion of tissue architecture	Freeze-drying methods	Use of isopentane with liquid nitrogen	Avoid freezing of tissue before processing

6.4 Post-analytical artefacts

Post-analytical artefacts are produced as a result of laboratory procedures and techniques, and there is greater emphasis on appreciating their impact because quality control procedures will need to define what they represent and facilitate the introduction of measures to reduce their incidence.

These artefacts can be aligned to specific steps or techniques in the process of histological evaluation (Tables 6.2–6.7), as follows:

- Fixation
- Specimen dissection (cut up)
- Tissue processing
- Embedding
- Microtomy
- Staining (tinctorial and immunocytochemical)
- Coverslipping and mounting
- Automated machine failures
- Molecular contamination
- Miscellaneous.

SELF-CHECK 6.2

Describe the two main groups of artefact that can occur when undertaking a surgical procedure and subsequently performing histological assessments. How do we group artefacts that occur in the laboratory?

6.4.1 Fixation

Various artefacts can occur as a result of fixation. These can be controlled effectively if the procedure is carried out correctly and under the correct conditions. There are a number of factors that will affect the process of fixation, and you will have read about these in the previous chapters. The key points to remember are:

- type of fixative and its component constituents
- pH of the fixative
- volume of fixative used
- temperature at which fixation occurs
- nature of the specimen being fixed
- duration of fixation.

Fixative type

The type of fixative and its constituents can cause artefacts. Formalin can produce a brown/black birefringent pigment, usually in association with red blood cells. This occurs if the sample is left in formalin for a long period of time and particularly if the formalin is not buffered (neutral pH). Often seen in tissue rich in blood (e.g. placenta or spleen) it occurs as a result of acid formalin reacting with haemoglobin to form acid formaldehyde haematin pigment. It can be removed from deparaffinized tissue sections by treating them with alcoholic picric acid solution prior to subsequent staining. Ensuring formalin is buffered and that tissue is not left in fixative for long periods of time will virtually eliminate occurrence of this artefact (Figure 6.10).

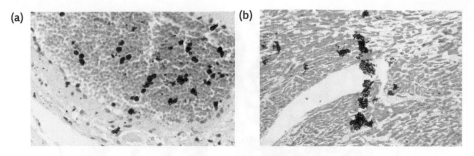

FIGURE 6.10
Presence of pigment due to fixation: a) formalin, b) mercury.

Traditional fixatives not popularly used today, such as Zenker and Helly, contain mercuric chloride, which can produce black pigmentation in the tissue. This can be removed by treating deparaffinized sections with Lugol's iodine solution, followed by bleaching in sodium thiosulphate solution. Owing to the highly toxic nature of mercury and its harmful effects, fixatives such as Zenker are no longer widely used.

Bouin's fixative contains picric acid and thus results in yellow coloration of the tissue. This fixative is useful when use of connective tissue stains is required, and is beneficial when dealing with testicular and gastrointestinal tract samples. Its main advantage over neutral buffered formalin is crisper nuclear staining, but it can cause extensive shrinkage of larger specimens. The coloration can be removed by placing sections in 70% ethanol, lithium carbonate or another acid dye applied separately during a subsequent staining procedure.

Key Point

As a general rule, the composition of different fixatives determines their effectiveness. It is important to appreciate that although 10% neutral buffered formalin is regarded as the 'gold standard' fixative, its popularity is due to the fact that it is suitable for most tissue types and subsequent histological investigations. Many other fixatives can offer improvements over formalin for specific areas of histological investigation, but cannot match the overall versatility and suitability for such a wide range of histological techniques, whether it be for conventional H&E staining, special stains, immunocytochemistry or indeed retrospective molecular techniques such as PCR.

Fixative pH

In routine formalin fixation, neutral pH is critical to ensure that appropriate cross-linking of methylene groups occurs, which is important for many immunocytochemically demonstrated antigenic epitopes. In addition, neutral pH ensures that formalin pigment does not form. The pigment generally forms at pH < 5.7, and production increases over the range pH 3.0–5.0. For these reasons, formalin is now often buffered using phosphate, cacodylate, bicarbonate, Tris or acetate. Osmolality is also important here, as hypertonic and hypotonic fixatives will cause increased shrinkage and swelling, respectively. Generally, the best morphological results are achieved when the fixative is very slightly hypertonic (400–450 mOsm). Most ideal fixative solutions should be as close to isotonic as possible.

Fixative volume

This is critical and as a general rule specimens should be fixed in volumes that are at least 20 times the volume of the specimen. Generally, neutral buffered formalin will penetrate and fix tissue at a rate of

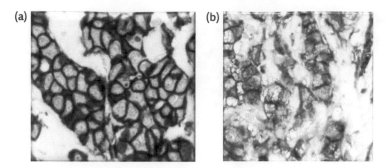

FIGURE 6.11
HER2 staining following a) good fixation, and b) poor fixation (original magnification ×40). (Courtesy UK NEQAS ICC and ISH Scheme.)

1 mm per hour, but this is highly variable and will depend on a host of factors including the density and porosity of the tissue specimen. If an inadequate volume of fixative is used, penetration rates will be affected—a situation compounded by short incubation or immersion times. In such cases, some antigenic epitopes will not be fixed adequately and so weak labelling of target antigens can give rise to false-positive or false-negative results. Evidence of this can be seen in studies of HER2 expression in breast tumour analysis (Figure 6.11).

Temperature of fixation

It is well known that temperature has a significant bearing on the speed at which tissue samples are fixed. Generally, the speed of diffusion of molecules increases with rising temperature, and this manifests itself as an increased rate of penetration of fixative through tissue—the higher the temperature the faster the penetration and the quicker the fixation process. This is the main reason why microwave ovens are used to assist in the fixation of samples. It is important, however, not to overheat samples as this can also cause artefacts, most notably tissue disintegration or drying of small tissue samples. There is also the complex issue of compromised antigenic epitopes, as fixation may not be optimal for the full range of antigens which need to be preserved.

There is a host of specimen-selective issues that can cause artefacts if due care and attention is not paid. Examples of tissue types that require selective attention with regard to fixation include lymphoid organs, eyes, breast, lung and brain tissue. These are either highly cellular, as in the case of lymphoid tissue, and are prone to autolytic change, or contain large amounts of lipid, which reduces the penetration of the fixative, as in brain tissue. It is well known that a whole brain commonly takes up to two weeks to fix appropriately. In the case of eyes, careful insertion of cuts into the globe (avoiding key structures such as the retina and iris) is required. Again, if these are not performed appropriately then artefacts will occur and morphology and tissue preservation will be compromised. Similarly, structures that have an outer capsule or are dense in nature may be difficult to penetrate and so the fixative may not gain sufficient access to central portions of the tissue. This can result in artefacts which demonstrate 'zonal' variation in fixation. This results in variations in staining both tinctorially and also immunocytochemically (Figure 6.12).

This artefact is not just unique to dense tissues or tissues with an outer capsule, but can be seen in cases where fixation exposure has been too short or the ratio of fixative to specimen mass is not adequate. We will talk more about this when we consider artefacts that can occur during specimen dissection. Another interesting and unusual fixation artefact is 'streaming'. This is most commonly seen in liver tissue. Hepatocytes contain relatively large amounts of glycogen within the cytoplasm of the cell and the streaming occurs as displacement. Precipitation occurs as a direct result of the predominant directional flow of the formalin into the cell, effectively pushing the glycogen to one side of the cell. This effect can be demonstrated with a PAS or carmine stain for glycogen demonstration (Figure 6.13).

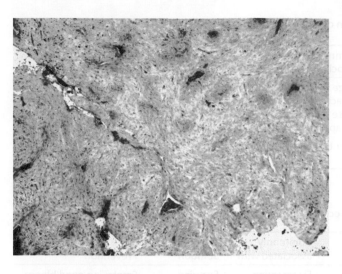

FIGURE 6.12
Weak and patchy
haematoxylin and eosin
(H&E) staining (original
magnification ×10).

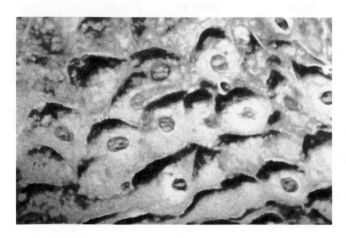

FIGURE 6.13
Effect of streaming artefact
on glycogen in liver
cells (PAS stain, original
magnification ×40).

TABLE 6.2 The cause and effect of the key artefacts that can occur due to fixation, and the appropriate remedies.

Artefact	Appearance	Cause	Commonly associated with	Solution	Prevention
Formalin	Brown/black birefringent pigment	Acid formalin reaction with haemoglobin/red blood cells forming acid formaldehyde haematin pigment	Red blood cells/ blood-rich tissue	Treating cut tissue sections with alcoholic picric acid solution following deparaffinization	Ensuring formalin is buffered and tissue is not left in fixative for long periods of time
Zenker/ Helly	Black pigmentation	Mercuric chloride fixatives		Treating cut tissue sections with Lugol's iodine solution followed by bleaching in sodium thiosulphate solution	Use of zinc salts instead of mercuric chloride (these do not produce artefact pigment)/use of alternative fixative
Bouin	Yellow tissue coloration	Picric acid		Treating cut tissue sections with 70% ethanol/lithium carbonate/another acid dye	

(continued)

TABLE 6.2 The cause and effect of the key artefacts that can occur due to fixation, and the appropriate remedies. (*Continued*)

Artefact	Appearance	Cause	Commonly associated with	Solution	Prevention
Zonal fixation	Uneven staining/red blood cell lysis	Fixative penetrates at different rates/levels within the tissue	Large specimens, especially those that are encapsulated	Ensuring sufficient fixation time/volume	Opening specimen where possible
Streaming effects	Displacement of glycogen	Directional flow of fixative into cells	Liver tissue		

TABLE 6.3 The cause and effect of the key artefacts that can occur as a result of specimen dissection, and the appropriate remedies.

Artefact	Appearance	Cause	Commonly associated with	Solution	Prevention
Cross-contamination	Transfer of residual tissue	Tissue left on dissecting blade or on dissecting board/transferred to next dissected specimen	Fragmenting tissue	Ensuring blades are cleaned between each tissue sample	Employing 'good biopsy practice'
Tissue inking	Displacement of dyes from original site of application	Application of marker dyes	Orientation of fresh or fixed surgical specimens		Small brushes/orange sticks to apply minimal amount of dye
Foam inset	Porous pattern	Foam biopsy pads			Use of alternatives/tissue wrap/mesh tissue safes
Tissue moulding	Triangular/star-shaped holes on outer surface of tissue	Tissue too large for biopsy cassette			Ensure 'thin' sections of tissue taken for processing

TABLE 6.4 The cause and effect of the key artefacts that can occur as a result of processing and embedding, and the appropriate remedies.

Artefact	Appearance	Cause	Commonly associated with	Solution	Prevention
Poor wax impregnation	Soft 'watery' tissue/unable to section adequately/contains holes where tissue not processed	Residual water in tissue	Incomplete dehydration	Reprocessing the tissue block	Processing schedules to accommodate dehydration depending on tissue type
	Excessive shrinkage		Excessive dehydration		Processing schedules to accommodate dehydration depending on tissue type
	Hard tissue		Excessive clearing		Schedules to accommodate clearing depending on tissue type
Crystal composition (e.g. cholesterol)	Needle-like crystal clefts	Crystals dissolve during processing leaving gaps in tissue			

TABLE 6.4 The cause and effect of the key artefacts that can occur as a result of processing and embedding, and the appropriate remedies. (*Continued*)

Artefact	Appearance	Cause	Commonly associated with	Solution	Prevention
Cross-contamination	Transfer of residual tissue	Forceps not thoroughly cleaned before opening next tissue cassette to embed	Fragmenting tissue	Ensuring embedding forceps cleaned between each tissue sample	Immersing embedding forceps in molten paraffin wax wells
Incorrect orientation	Suspected lack of all expected cell layers in tissue type	Incorrect orientation		Re-embedding	Attention to embedding protocols

TABLE 6.5 The cause and effect of the key artefacts that can occur as a result of microtomy, and the appropriate remedies.

Artefact	Appearance	Cause	Commonly associated with	Solution	Prevention
Knife marks and scores	Scores and scratches parallel to the direction of sectioning	Blunt blade/trauma to blade		Regularly changing blade/use fresh blade	Use one blade to trim down the blocks to full face/use new blade to take sections
Trimming artefact	Tears and rough-edged holes within section	Rough trimming pulling tissue fragments from face of block		Full-face polishing	Employing 'good microtomy practice'
Chatter/vibration	Variation in section thickness causing stripes of alternate staining intensity	Vibrations/movement of knife edge	Varying tissue densities/hard tissue	Use of softening agents/cut thinner sections	Ensuring adjustable microtome settings securely fastened and tight/employing 'good microtomy practice'
Tissue folds/creases	Creases and folds in tissue section giving double layers	Variable expansion of section when floating on water bath	Varying tissue density/hard tissue	Warm water bath/manual stretching of tissue sections from microtome blade	Careful microtomy and flotation of sections
Tissue displacement	Cells become detached and move over other areas of the section	Blunt knife/excessive rough trimming	Hard or friable tissue		Employing 'good microtomy practice'
Water bubbles (under tissue sections)	Circular areas of lifting/altered staining patterns	Bubbles arise from the water bath		Using trimmed curl of paraffin wax to act as a cone, placing under the surface of the water and directly under entrapped bubble	Attention when floating out sections to remove bubbles/knocking of water bath/skimming water surface with paper tissue sheet to remove freed bubbles
Squames	Contamination by material not in the block (usually above the section)	Scalp/hands of sectioner			Employing 'good microtomy practice'/use of surgical gloves/hand cream
Water contamination	Contamination by material not in the block (usually above the section)	Fragmented tissue/plant algae/commensal bacteria		Water bath topped up constantly during day/completely replaced at end of day	Using distilled water/wiping around water bath with clean tissue paper

TABLE 6.6 The cause and effect of the key artefacts that can occur as a result of section staining, and the appropriate remedies.

Artefact	Appearance	Cause	Commonly associated with	Solution	Prevention
Residual wax	Patchy/incomplete staining	Residual wax preventing penetration of dyes		Additional xylene treatment and re-staining	Attention to staining protocols
Incomplete staining	Tidal mark	Low stain level		Re-stain	Ensure adequately filled pots
OCT residue	Patchy/incomplete staining	Residual OCT preventing penetration of dyes	Frozen sections	Additional water treatment and re-staining	Attention to frozen section protocols
Stain deposit	Precipitate deposited on tissue section and/or slide	Undissolved/unfiltered stain	Alcoholic stains	Re-stain	Use sealed jars/filter stains to reduce surface evaporation

TABLE 6.7 The cause and effect of the key artefacts that can occur as a result of section mounting, and the appropriate remedies.

Artefact	Appearance	Cause	Commonly associated with	Solution	Prevention
Scratches/tears	Areas of section missing	Manual/automated cover slipping		Avoid direct contact of the mounting equipment with tissue surface	Attention to section mounting protocols
Air bubbles	Air bubbles under coverslip	Air bubbles within the mountant		Squeeze air bubbles out from under coverslip by applying gentle pressure	Attention to section mounting protocols
Mountant retraction	Opaque areas over tissue section	Areas of mountant have dried back from coverslip edges	Sections drying too quickly/insufficient mounting media	Clear and remount	Application of sufficient mounting media/not allowing slides to dry completely
Contaminant on slide	Squames/floaters/fibres/pencil or ink deposits	Contamination by non-biological or biological material, excluding dye/reagent deposits, usually above the section between section and coverslip		Remount/recut	Ensure clean working environment
Water present	Droplets of water under coverslip/opaque under microscope	Inadequate dehydration		Return sections to alcohol and re-dehydrate, clear and mount	Ensure alcohol baths changed regularly/dehydration stages are long enough
Residual wax	Refractile areas of undissolved wax are visible	Residual wax from sectioning		Additional xylene treatment and re-staining	Attention to staining/mounting protocols
Drying	Air bubbles over nuclei	Tissue section allowed to dry before coverslip applied		Clear and remount	Application of sufficient mounting medium/not allowing slides to dry completely

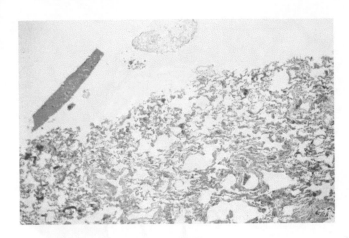

FIGURE 6.14
Cross-contamination
of one specimen with a
fragment of another.

6.4.2 Specimen dissection

Specimen dissection (cut up) represents another laboratory-based process that can produce a selective assortment of artefacts, some of which are highly significant and can cause difficulties with pathological interpretation. The most significant artefact is cross-contamination from one specimen to another. This involves the transfer of residual tissue, often left on the dissecting knife blade or on the dissecting board, being transferred to the next specimen. This may involve the transfer of tumour cells, which can have a significant impact in terms of the evaluation of the subsequent tissue sections stained from the processed blocks (Figure 6.14). This artefact can be avoided by ensuring that the dissecting blade is wiped clean between each tissue sample and ensuring the use of appropriate disposable towelling to wipe down the dissection board surface. The issue of cross-contamination is not unique to specimen dissection, and can occur at tissue processing, embedding, section floating out on waterbaths, and even during section staining.

CLINICAL CORRELATION

There have been well-documented cases of specimen cross-contamination reported in the media and also medical press. These cases have often resulted in an inappropriate treatment being given to the patients involved. The most serious cases often occur with cancer investigations and can result in some instances of extensive, inappropriate surgical procedures being applied on the wrong patients. Fortunately, these cases are extremely rare; however, they do raise awareness of the need to be diligent and ensure all routine checks are enforced rigorously.

As well as tissue cross-contamination, another artefact can occur as a result of inking tissue samples with marker dyes. These are used to identify true tissue margins on the subsequent tissue sections produced from the tissue blocks. On smaller tissue samples excessive application of marker dyes can result in displacement. The dye may also penetrate into the tissue or appear on the tissue surface, rather than simply appear around the outside edge of the tissue. The use of small brushes or orange sticks to apply the dyes and ensuring residual dye is blotted from the sample generally reduces the incidence of this artefact (Figure 6.15).

A less well known artefact produced as a result of specimen dissection relates to the use of foam pads to secure small samples into tissue processing cassettes. These pads also ensure the tissue is securely placed in the cassette. If the tissue is sandwiched between foam pads it will restrict the shrinkage and 'curling' of the tissue during processing. Once the cassette lid is placed on top of the foam–tissue sandwich and snapped shut, there can be pressure effects on the tissue sample. This effect is often termed 'tissue moulding' and reflects the porous pattern of the foam pads on the surface of the tissue sample. This can be avoided by using other methods to secure the tissue within the cassette (e.g. tissue wrap paper sheets) or by employing dedicated 'sieve-like' mesh tissue safes.

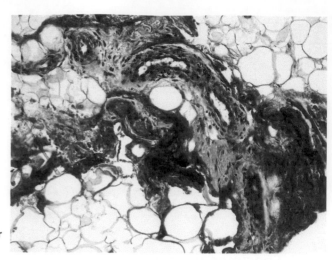

FIGURE 6.15
Penetration of blue marker
dye in a skin sample.

6.4.3 Tissue processing

This is probably the least understood area in which artefacts are produced, mainly because processing has become a fully automated process.

It is also fair to say that poor fixation will invariably lead to poor processing. As you will have read in earlier chapters, processing involves three principal steps:

1. Dehydration: using graded alcohols (70–99%), typically industrial methylated spirit (IMS), which will remove water from the tissues.

2. Clearing: using xylene, as alcohol and paraffin wax are not miscible. For this reason, xylene is used to remove all remnants of alcohol before the final step.

3. Impregnation: with molten paraffin wax.

These three steps will each take several hours and involve several changes of reagent. This is the main reason why most processing of histological tissue samples is performed overnight using an automated processing machine.

The main causes of artefacts from this process are either derived from 'under' or 'over' processing of tissue samples. This means running a processing schedule that is either too long or too short in terms of exposure to the reagents. This is invariably associated with mistakes made in selecting the right programme to run, or as a direct result of a machine failure during any run cycle. It can be related to mistakes made when changing reagents. This may entail placing the reagents in the wrong sequence on the machine or as a consequence of overuse of already exhausted reagents. Invariably, artefacts are created when errors occur during dehydration or wax impregnation.

If dehydration is not completed, residual water will remain in the tissue, which is not miscible with xylene. This will hamper the 'clearing' process and lead to poor wax impregnation. The end result is that the tissue will be soft, watery and will not section, containing holes where the tissue has not been processed. The best course of action is to reprocess the tissue block. In order to do this the wax will need to be removed and the tissue brought back through xylene and then alcohol, in a reverse rapid fashion, so that it can be reprocessed on a longer processing schedule. The greater the fat content, the more water the tissue contains and the longer the exposure to alcohol needed in the dehydration step to remove the water. Tissues such as breast and brain commonly require prolonged processing schedules to accommodate the longer dehydration and wax impregnation steps required (Figure 6.16). If dehydration is prolonged then there will be excessive shrinkage, which in turn leads to poor wax impregnation. Similarly, if clearing (step 2) is too long it will harden the tissue, again making wax impregnation difficult. The result will be hard tissue that is difficult to section for microscopic evaluation, a situation made worse if the tissue is already quite dense in nature (e.g. a highly keratotic piece of skin, or decalcified bone).

Some mention should also be made of labile substances which can be lost as a result of the processing schedule but which leave reminders of their presence prior to processing. The best example

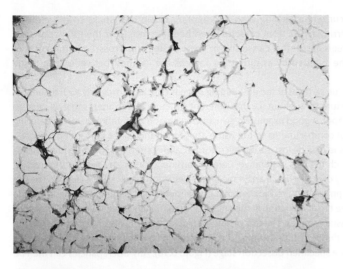

FIGURE 6.16
Poorly processed lipoma.

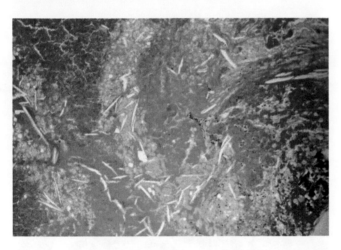

FIGURE 6.17
Cholesterol clefts.

here is crystal composites. These include cholesterol, which is dissolved by the alcohol used in the dehydration step, and leaves cut-like slits in the tissue. These are referred to as 'cholesterol clefts' (Figure 6.17).

A good example of crystal formation is seen in cases of gout and pseudogout. Gout is caused by monosodium urate monohydrate crystals and pseudogout is caused by calcium pyrophosphate crystals. Like cholesterol, these crystals will not survive tissue processing and so angulated spaces are left in the tissue. Patients with gout, particularly women, are at increased risk of vascular disease.

6.4.4 Tissue embedding

The artefacts that can occur in this process are:

- Tissue carry over.
- Incorrect tissue orientation.
- Heating or drying effects.
- Introduction of foreign structures.

Tissue carry over can occur when dealing with fragmenting tissue that sticks to the embedding forceps when transferring tissue from cassette to embedding mould. If the forceps are not thoroughly cleaned between cases, this can result in the transfer and cross-contamination of tissue samples. This can be avoided by ensuring the forceps are cleaned between each tissue sample.

Correct orientation of tissue samples at the embedding stage is critical, particularly with tissue that is not homogenous in structure throughout (i.e. has different structural components that all need to be seen under the microscope). A good example is skin, in which good orientation involves ensuring both epidermal and dermal compartments of the tissue are seen. If this is not performed correctly, then critical areas of the tissue may be lost during microtomy. Careful attention to embedding protocols when dealing which such tissue is imperative. Careful consideration of any specific embedding instructions provided for any complex tissue at the specimen dissection stage is also valuable. The use of all the appropriate equipment required for optimal embedding must be applied. These include anglepoise lamps to increase the illumination at the embedding centre, and magnifying equipment to aid visualization of small tissue samples. The use of embedding logs should also not be understated, as they help to indicate to the person performing the embedding how many pieces of tissue were placed in each cassette at the specimen dissection stage (Figure 6.18). Any discrepancies can then be identified immediately.

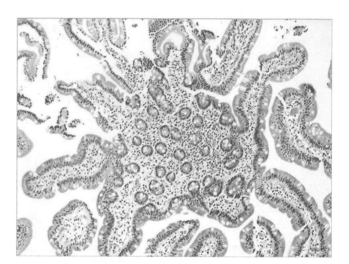

FIGURE 6.18
Poor orientation of an intestinal biopsy during embedding.

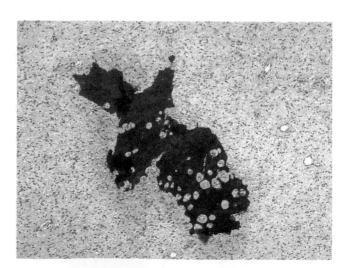

FIGURE 6.19
Carry over of tissue from the surface of the floating out water bath.

Heating or drying effect is an unusual artefact, but can occur with delicate, friable tissue samples. This manifests as drying or excessive shrinkage of the tissue, often around the edges, with the cellular detail damaged or destroyed. This may happen if the hot plate is too hot when placing tissue samples in the moulds, or if the process of tissue orientation is problematic, resulting in the tissue being exposed to heat for a long period of time.

6.4.5 Microtomy

There are a multitude of artefacts that can be produced as a result of the process of producing tissue sections from paraffin blocks. In this section we will also include artefacts produced from the section floating out step on waterbaths (Figure 6.19). The key artefacts are:

- Knife marks and scores.
- Trimming artefact.
- Chatter/vibration.
- Tissue folds/creases.
- Tissue displacement issues (including knife-back debris).
- Entrapped bubbles under tissue sections.
- Squames (floating on the waterbath and picked up with tissue sections).
- Water contamination (in the waterbath).

An video demonstrating how incorrect microtomy technique can produce knife marks and scores, and tissue folds/creases can be viewed on the book's accompanying website: www.oup.com/uk/orchard2e

Knife marks and scores are seen as lines which appear to be drawn through the tissue section, parallel to the direction of sectioning. They are produced as a result of the blade having been blunt at a specific point or multiple points along its length. This occurs either as a result of the blade losing its sharp edge due to continued usage, or as a direct result of damage to the blade (Figure 6.20). For example, this can occur when cutting heavily keratinized skin or tissue containing focal areas of calcification (e.g. prostate or uterine fibroids). They may also occur if there is foreign material in the tissue block (e.g. a metal staple or a suture), or pieces of hard debris (e.g. grit or dirt) that have penetrated the wax block prior to final sectioning. Brushing the knife edge with forceps when removing sections will also damage the blade. It

(a)
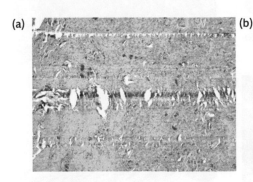
(b)
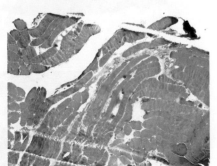

FIGURE 6.20
Scores in tissue caused by a) tissue constituents or b) a damaged blade.

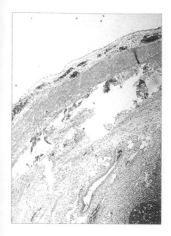

FIGURE 6.21
The effect of rough trimming.

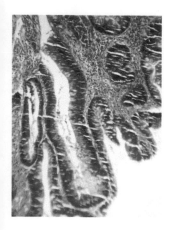

FIGURE 6.22
Appearance of chatter due to a poorly secured or blunt blade.

is very important to reduce these artefacts by changing the blade regularly and using a fresh blade as soon as any cutting artefacts are detected. A good approach is to use one blade to trim down the blocks to expose the full face of the tissue, and a fresh blade to take the final sections for staining. Sections produced with knife marks are generally not acceptable unless the tissue contains areas of focal calcification.

Trimming artefact appears as either rips or holes in the tissue section, often with the edges lifting. This indicates that the full face of the tissue has not been 'polished' and retains the effects of the rough trimming performed to expose the tissue (Figure 6.21).

Chatter/vibration can be either coarse or fine, the latter often being termed the 'venetian blind' effect. Coarse chatters tend to occur when cutting tissue blocks of varying tissue density (e.g. tissue containing cartilage and also soft tissue components). It is a physical effect resulting from sectioning both hard and soft tissue components, resulting in movement of the block in the holder, or slight movement of the blade. This causes a very slight 'step' effect. Fine chatters are caused by tiny vibrations in the knife edge as it passes through tissue which is either hard or brittle in composition (Figure 6.22). Essentially, this effect can be related to processing issues, as poorly processed tissue may be harder and more brittle than optimally processed material. Overheating of tissue during embedding will compound this problem, as will excessive rough trimming. The best approach to avoid these artefacts is to ensure that the microtome is properly serviced and that all adjustable settings are tightened securely. The use of softening agents is also advocated (e.g. Cellsoft). Finally, cutting sections on a thinner setting (e.g. 3 microns) is also a good approach.

Folds and creases are the direct result of compression artefact caused by two hard objects (i.e. knife and tissue block) coming together. The tissue will be cut but it is compressed. These effects are made worse if the tissue is dense, hard, or contains variable soft and hard tissue components. Creases and folds can also occur when cutting really soft tissue which is highly cellular (e.g. lymph node). Harder tissue generally will shrink less than the softer tissue during processing. Once cut, sections are floated on a waterbath at around 40°C, which takes advantage of the liquid's surface tension. Sections that are compressed and then floated on a warm waterbath will be stretched, and this will remove the majority of folds or creases created from the sectioning process. The folds and creases can be removed by ensuring good microtomy technique to ensure sections are lifted off the cutting edge of the blade and stretched manually before floating on water. In the case of difficult tissue blocks, floating out for longer than normal will help to reduce the effects of finer folds or creases (Figure 6.23a and b).

Tissue displacement is an artefact sometimes seen when cutting hard tissue such as bone. It is seen when softer tissue such as connective tissue surrounding the harder tissue is displaced during the cutting process, often causing it to be realigned along the direction of cutting, moving over other areas

(a)

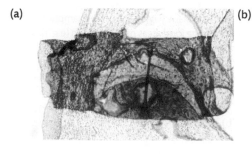

(b)

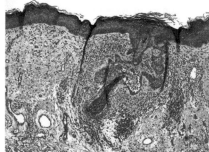

(c)

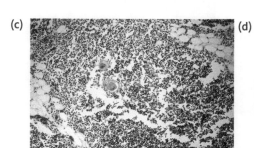

(d)

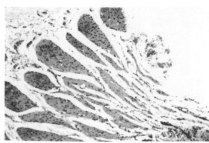

FIGURE 6.23
Examples of a) folds, b) creases, and c/d) tissue displacement.

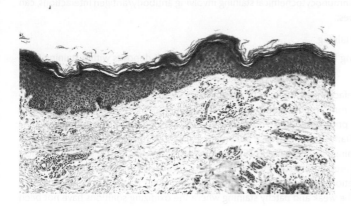

FIGURE 6.24
Squamous cells overlying the stain section.

of the section. This can be caused by the block being sectioned on a blunt portion of the knife, or as a result of rough trimming of the block (Figure 6.23c and d).

Entrapped bubbles are often the result of bubbles that rise to the surface of the waterbath either due to heating or if the bath is agitated or knocked. If not removed, the bubbles subsequently burst during the section drying process and create altered staining patterns or lifting in the area of the bubble entrapment. They can be removed from the water by knocking the bath and skimming the surface with a tissue paper sheet to remove the freed bubbles. Entrapped bubbles can be removed by using a trimmed curl of paraffin wax directly under the surface of the water beneath the bubble entrapped under the section.

Squames are another artefact related to floating out sections on a waterbath. Squamous cell contamination is relatively common and often arises from squames detaching from the skin surface and landing on the water. These are picked up with the section and will be stained and appear randomly on the slide. They appear as anucleate pink-stained cells on haematoxylin and eosin-stained slides (Figure 6.24).

Water contamination due to cross-contamination from one specimen to another is possible as a result of a section breaking up and transferring on to other slides while floating out. Similarly, contaminated water containing plant algae or commensal bacteria is another source of artefacts. This can be avoided by using distilled water, and by ensuring that the water is topped up constantly during the day and replaced at the end of the day. Wiping around the waterbath with clean tissue paper will also reduce contaminating debris that could transfer on to histological slides.

A final important point about microtomy and tissue section floating out is to ensure that appropriate slides are used. In cases of hardened tissue or where immunocytochemistry or *in situ* procedures are requested, it is imperative that adhesive slides are used to prevent tissue detachment.

Key Point

Surface tension is the elastic tendency of liquid, which makes it acquire the least surface area possible. It is a principle evident in most ecosystems. In the arthropod world, the water boatman is denser than water but is able to run along the water surface because it utilizes the principle of surface tension. Water has a high surface tension because of the attraction between water molecules (72.8 milliNewtons per metre at 20°C), which is much higher than most other liquids.

SELF-CHECK 6.4

Explain the various artefacts that can occur during tissue microtomy and how these can be avoided.

6.4.6 Tinctorial and immunocytochemical staining artefacts

Artefacts arising from the process of staining, whether it be conventional tinctorial methods involving H&E and special stains or immunocytochemical staining involving antibody/antigen interactions, can be divided in two main types:

- Incomplete or patchy staining.
- Contamination involving the staining solutions or precipitation of deposits within staining solutions.

In the case of staining artefacts resulting in incomplete or patchy staining, the causes are relatively easily defined. The most common cause is the presence of residual wax which has not been removed during the dewaxing step, prior to staining. This results in poor dye penetration, resulting in patchy staining of the tissue. Similarly, there may be a tidal mark across a stained slide due to a low level of stain in one of the staining vessels (Figure 6.25). Unstained areas of tissue may also be seen following inadequate use of preparatory staining solutions prior to use of a final staining solution, an example being tissue oxidation with potassium permanganate and oxalic acid in a melanin bleaching procedure. The result will be weak and patchy staining where the oxidizing solutions have not been removed.

Frozen section material is embedded for sectioning in a cryostat using an optimal cooling temperature (OCT) embedding medium. This provides support for cryotomy in much the same way as paraffin wax does in routine tissue sectioning. The OCT is removed by washing in running tap water once the sections are cut and attached to slides. If washing is inadequate then OCT will remain and prevent penetration of the reagents used subsequently, resulting in patchy staining.

Staining artefacts due to precipitation or deposits can arise as a result of undissolved stain remaining in the solution, or, more commonly, solid crystalline deposits remaining in the solution. This can be exacerbated in alcoholic staining solutions as the evaporation rate from the staining solution is considerably more rapid than with non-alcoholic solutions. Similarly, certain dyes are more prone to oxidation on contact with air and will precipitate more readily once applied to tissue sections; a good example is neutral red counterstain (Figure 6.26). To reduce these artefacts, it is important to ensure that measures are taken to minimize surface evaporation of dyes. In addition, dyes that are prone to oxidation should be filtered regularly to remove precipitation products.

Stain entrapment artefacts can be seen in immunocytochemistry when the final chromogen is trapped beneath the section (Figure 6.27), and gives the appearance of an amorphous stain precipitate. This occurs primarily because the section has lifted or detached in part from the slide, allowing the chromogen to gain access beneath the section. Hard or keratotic tissues are particularly prone to this artefact.

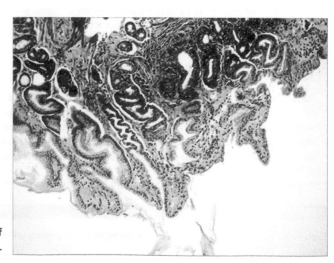

FIGURE 6.25
Incomplete eosin staining possibly due to position of section or level of reagent.

(a) 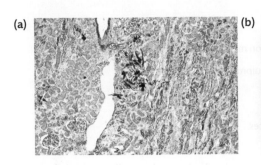 (b)

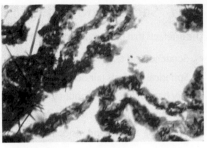

FIGURE 6.26
Two examples of stain deposit.

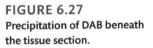

FIGURE 6.27
Precipitation of DAB beneath the tissue section.

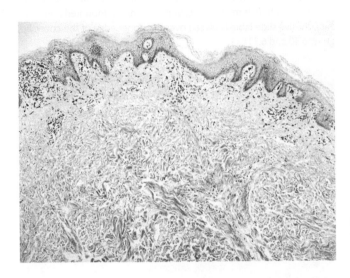

FIGURE 6.28
Background DAB staining of collagen fibres (original magnification ×10).

Staining artefacts due to contamination are generally related to the formation of microbial growth within the staining stock solutions. This can occur if solutions are not used regularly or if they are kept in warm environments. Filtering the solution will remove the microbial growths. Placing a minute amount of antimicrobial crystals (e.g. thymol) in the staining solution may also help. However, the best course of action is to ensure that the solution is dated and replaced regularly to reduce the risks of contamination. Also, use CE-marked commercial products where possible.

In immunocytochemistry procedures, artefacts may arise as a result of insufficient blocking steps, to reduce the incidence of non-specific staining for endogenous enzymes such as alkaline phosphatase and peroxidase, which are present in certain cell types. Plasma cells and eosinophils, for example, are known to be rich in endogenous peroxidase and will require longer blocking times to quench the enzymes present. If these are not adequately blocked they will be detected in the final reaction steps, as they rely on peroxidase or alkaline phosphatase chromogenic reactions to develop the final reaction colour. Similarly, non-specific staining of connective tissue components can occur if insufficient attention is paid to the pre-digestion or heat-induced epitope retrieval steps. In addition, antibody titres should be monitored carefully. In instances when background staining is seen, careful attention to the washing and antigen retrieval steps and antibody dilution factors in the standard operating procedure (SOP) should eliminate this undesirable staining (Figure 6.28).

6.4.7 Section mounting

The artefacts that can occur as a result of section mounting are mainly as follows:

- Scratches and tears from the mounting equipment.
- Spherical artefacts (air bubbles).
- Dry back of the tissue mountant.
- Contamination from a wide range of sources.
- Air-drying artefact and residual water/wax.

Scratches and/or tears can occur during both manual and automated coverslipping procedures, but are far more common following manual procedures. These usually arise as a result of damage by forceps or the edge of the coverslip catching the surface of the section, creating a 'score'.

Spherical artefacts or air bubbles are produced when lowering the coverslip onto the tissue mountant and applying pressure to remove entrapped air. Inadequate pressure may result in air bubbles remaining under the coverslip (Figure 6.29).

Dry back of tissue mountant is a phenomenon that can result when an inadequate volume of mountant is used to coverslip the tissue section. It may also occur if sections are mounted and dried too quickly, or alternatively if the adhesive slide label is placed over the upper edge of the coverslip, causing an extraction effect (Figures 6.30 and 6.31).

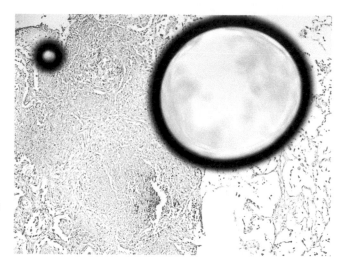

FIGURE 6.29
Bubbles in DPX mountant (Ziehl–Neelsen stain, original magnification ×20).

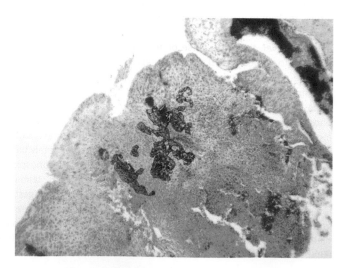

FIGURE 6.30
The effect of drying prior to section mounting.

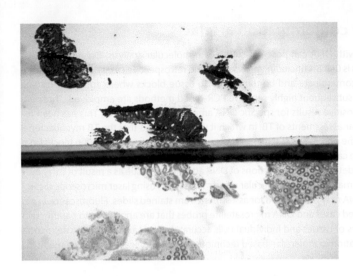

FIGURE 6.31
The effect on tissue of coverglass slippage or poor mounting practice.

Artefacts in coverslipping related to contamination by non-biological or biological material, excluding dye/reagent deposits, include squames, floaters, hair, tissue paper fibres, pencil/ink deposits, plant debris (e.g. algae spores), common dirt and grit, or insects (Figure 6.32).

6.4.8 Automated machine failures

In the modern histopathology laboratory, a growing number of the more routine or mundane tasks are performed through automated processes, the larger part of which are high-throughput and constant-production events. The equipment includes processing machines, embedding centres, staining machines and coverslipping machinery. While automated platforms are designed with a critical eye and are not prone to errors or the production of artefacts, one should always remember that they are programmed by the operator; if incorrect parameters are set then errors may occur. Some may be quite spectacular in consequence, as the automated process may not be questioned immediately and many samples may have been affected in any given run. Automated machine failures can result in defects in dehydration (processing machines), embedding (tissue embedding centres), staining (automated stainers) and coverslipping (automated coverslippers). Good examples of this are if a processing machine breaks down mid-programme, such that incomplete processing occurs, or if the wrong programme is selected, and in staining machines that may have run out of reagent in the middle of a run. Most of these will result in artefactual events. The point is that in a large number of cases they relate to human error at some point in the sequence of events. This is not exclusive as machines do fail, resulting in damage to samples; however, this is generally a rare event.

Automated machine failures can be reduced by considering the following:

- Ensure all service records for all machinery are in date.
- Keep good records of reagent management and know when reagents need to be changed.
- Ensure all logs of procedures are available to be assessed to enable error traceability.
- Clear training of staff in the use of automated equipment and the provision of adequate supervision for trainees using such equipment.
- Competence checks on staff using automated machinery.
- Attention to detail in manufacturer instructions about how to operate the equipment.
- Appropriate attention to in-house standard operating procedures.
- Robust internal and external quality control checks.

SELF-CHECK 6.5

What types of artefact can be produced from automated procedures? What measures should laboratory staff employ to minimize the incidence of such artefacts?

6.4.9 Molecular contamination artefacts

Contamination of tissues with DNA can pose difficulties with molecular analysis. Data indicate that the occurrence rate for this is 0–8.8% (including prospective and retrospective cases). Reports indicate that fragments can cross-contaminate and be transferred to tissue blocks where, following routine histological investigations, subsequent highly sensitive PCR-based methods are employed. These are then found to yield false-positive results for specific DNA amplification sequences. This has been reported in cases of molecular assessments of TB, in which it was discovered that the TB mycobacterial DNA can be transferred in the processing machine and become embedded within paraffin blocks from TB-negative patients. These cases are from TB endemic parts of the world; however, this indicates that a problem exists. Similarly, detecting minor portions of DNA attached to tissue as a result of carry over during staining procedures may also affect molecular assessments when using laser microscope dissection techniques, as such DNA may be removed for assessment from stained slides. Fluorescence *in situ* hybridization in sex-matched cases and DNA microsatellite probes that are applicable to paraffin sections can provide identifiers of tissues and individual cells accurately. They are extremely useful tools to identify tissue contamination in molecular-based techniques on histologically processed material.

6.4.10 Miscellaneous artefacts

Miscellaneous artefacts can occur throughout most of the stages of histological tissue evaluation, and may be caused by many different factors. Evaluation of nuclear detail is often critical in determining whether a tissue sample is benign or malignant in nature, and distortion of the nucleus or cytoplasm of the cells within tissue can be a big problem to overcome. Good examples of this miscellaneous group include:

- Excessive shrinkage of the cell nucleus and/or cytoplasm.
- Distorted staining characteristics of the nuclear detail.
- Cell nucleus breakdown.
- Intracellular vacuolization.
- Tissue fragmentation and architectural breakdown.

Dry out prior to fixation is particularly applicable to small specimens. To avoid this, specimens should be placed in fixative promptly. Excessive or rapid dehydration during processing will cause rapid cell shrinkage and can lead to perinuclear shrinkage. The use of graded alcohols on the processing machine, starting with 70%, then 90–95% followed by 99% alcohol, will facilitate gradual controlled shrinkage.

Water in xylene may affect the clearing step during processing and will prevent good penetration of paraffin wax. Alternatively, and more commonly, xylene contaminating the paraffin wax will adversely affect wax penetration rates into the tissues. This reinforces the importance of ensuring that reagent management procedures are followed and that solvents are changed before they become exhausted and contaminated (figure 6.33).

Similarly, overheating specimens, particularly small samples, will cause considerable cellular damage. This can occur during tissue processing, embedding, or on a hot plate or in an oven with cut sections on slides prior to staining. It is well known that ovens can suffer uneven heat distribution, and sections placed for several hours or overnight in a hot spot will be compromised by overheating. This affects some antigenic epitopes and thus subsequent immunocytochemical methods may be compromised (e.g. HER2 testing in breast tissue).

If there is inappropriate or incomplete removal of embedding medium prior to staining, whether paraffin wax or OCT, there will be compromised staining, particularly of the nucleus. Attention to ensure that this step is performed adequately for a suitable time is essential.

Finally, some comment should be made about artefacts in resin-embedded tissue sections. This usually involves electron microscopy evaluation or assessment of hard tissue such as bone/bone marrow trephines. Many of the key artefacts are similar to those seen in routinely processed tissue and involve incomplete removal of certain epoxy resins prior to staining, creating patchy staining. As resin-embedded tissue is harder than paraffin wax-embedded tissue, the knives used to cut them are often made from glass. However, these are prone to blunting more quickly than conventional disposable

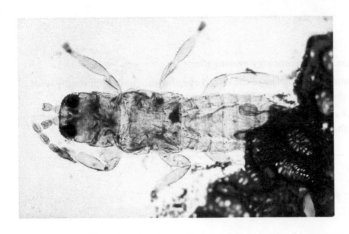

FIGURE 6.32
Insect trapped beneath
the coverslip.

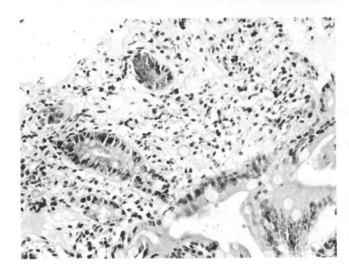

FIGURE 6.33
Incomplete dehydration
resulting in the presence
of water droplets
beneath the coverslip.

metal blades used in routine histopathology. Acrylic resins are not removed prior to staining and can absorb staining dyes, which increases the likelihood of background staining, particularly when using basic dyes. Careful preparation of the resin to ensure that the methacrylic acid is removed at the appropriate stage should reduce the incidence of this artefact.

 Chapter summary

This chapter has given you an insight into the key types of artefacts that can occur when we study tissue histologically. It is not an exhaustive summary but it is broad in content. It is also important to remember that the study of histopathology is, in reality, the study of artefact. This is because once tissue is removed from the body it is no longer in its natural state and every process we put the tissue through to evaluate it is by a means of induced artefactual change. The important point is that we are controlling all these steps and the artefacts we produce we are essentially standardizing. Therefore, there is consistency throughout, well at least in principle!

Key Points

■ Artefacts are common in histopathology investigations.

■ An appreciation of what they look like to the naked eye and also more importantly what they look like down the microscope is an acquired and very valuable skill.

■ An understanding of what causes these artefacts and also how to approach removing them or preventing them from occurring is essential.

 # Further reading

- The Royal College of Surgeons of England. *Good surgical practice*. London: RCS, 2014.

- Leica Microsystems (www.leica-microsystems.com/uploads/media/Artifacts_Handbook.pdf).

- Moore G, Knight G, Blann AD eds. *Haematology*. Oxford: Oxford University Press (ISBN 978-0-19-956883-3).

- Orchard GE, Nation BR eds. *Cell structure and function*. Oxford: Oxford University Press (ISBN 978-0-19-965247-1).

- Orchard GE. Immunocytochemical techniques in dermatopathology. *Curr Diagn Pathol* 2006: **12**; 292–302.

- Orchard GE. The use of positive controls in immunocytochemistry—some indicators of what is appropriate and what is not! *Immunocytochemistry* 2007; **6**: 11–2.

- Shambayati B ed. *Cytopathology*. Oxford: Oxford University Press (ISBN 798-0-19-953392-3).

- Suvarna SK, Layton C, Bancroft JD eds. *Bancroft's theory and practice of histological techniques* 7th edn. Edinburgh: Churchill Livingstone (ISBN-13-9780702042263).

- Freedberg IM, Eisen AZ, Wolfe K, Austen KF, Goldsmith LA, Katz SL, Fitzpatrick TB eds. *Fitzpatrick's dermatology in general medicine* 5th edn. Vol 1. New York: McGraw-Hill (ISBN 0-07-912938-2).

- Wheater PR, Burkitt HG, Daniels VG. *Functional histology: a text and colour atlas*. Churchill Livingstone (ISBN 0-443-01658-5).

- Williams JH, Mepham BL, Wright DH. Tissue preparation for immunocytochemistry. *J Clin Pathol* 1997; **50**: 422–8.

- Worsham MJ, Wolman SR, Zarbo RJ. Molecular approaches to identification of tissue contamination in surgical pathology sections. *J Mol Diagn* 2001: **3** (1):11–5.

 # Discussion questions

6.1 Discuss the various artefacts that can be generated as a result of fixation, and how their occurrence can be minimized.

6.2 Automation in histopathology: what impact does it have on the occurrence of artefacts?

6.3 Molecular techniques are gaining importance in histopathology. What artefacts are associated with this technology and how can they be minimized?

Answers to the self-check questions and tips for responding to the discussion questions are provided on the book's accompanying website:

 Visit www.oup.com/uk/orchard2e

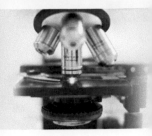

7

Mohs procedures

Guy Orchard and Mohammad Shams

Learning objectives

By the end of this chapter you should have:

- Developed an understanding of the process and procedures involved in Mohs techniques.

- A comprehension of the applications of Mohs in modern histopathology laboratories and the benefits it can bring to patient care.

- Developed an appreciation of troubleshooting and how to recognize clear technical failures.

- An understanding of what slow Mohs is and when its application is appropriate.

- An appreciation of the role of rapid immunocytochemical staining to aid in the assessment of frozen and paraffin sections in Mohs procedures.

- Developed an understanding of the new scanning devices used to improve the accuracy and precision of Mohs practice.

7.1 Introduction

Mohs represents a growing histological subspecialty, predominantly, although not exclusively, involving fresh frozen section preparations. Mohs has a growing application for the surgical removal of cancers. Its main application has been in the use of surgical removal of skin cancers. In the UK, Europe, and the antipodes it is used selectively for the removal of facial or head and neck skin cancers. Mohs procedures have the benefits of offering unparalleled accuracy for the total skin clearance of tumours without recurrence, with the majority of scientific literature quoting clearance rates for facial skin tumours without recurrence of 97–99.8%.

The technique is also sparing of tissue, only involving the removal of tissue with minimal clearance margins, thereby preserving patient's uninvolved surrounding skin tissue. This has clear advantage in the case of facial repairs and cosmetic benefits to the patient currently unequalled by any other procedure, whether surgical or involving radiation treatment regimes. Although sparing normal tissue is an important virtue of Mohs surgery, the one true goal of Mohs surgery is curing the cancer. It is the ability of properly performed Mohs surgery to achieve a high cure rate of 97–99.8%. This cure rate means that the Mohs procedure is the premier technique for the removal of skin cancer.

A video giving an overview of the Mohs technique can be found on the book's accompanying website: www.oup.com/uk/orchard2e

7.2 Historical perspective

There is a story to tell regarding the evolution of Mohs techniques, and as always the lessons learned and built on stand out like landmarks and act to guide us on how the technique has been refined and improved over time.

In 1933, a 23-year-old medical research assistant named Frederic Edward Mohs (Figure 7.1) was assigned to investigate the effects of injecting different chemicals into cancerous rat tissue to define the subsequent tissue reactions. One such chemical, zinc chloride, was found to 'fix' tissue in such a way that it would enable microscopic evaluation of the tissue without the disadvantage of effecting significant architectural change. Once combined with other substances, most notably sanguinarine, an alkaloid extract from bloodroot (the plant *Sanguinaria canadensis*), it could be made into a cohesive paste that, when applied to skin tumours, permitted excision without bleeding. Subsequently, Mohs found that frozen sections of the removed tissue could be prepared for examination under the microscope, and thus the first stage of the Mohs procedures was developed.

It was in 1936 that this approach to treating human skin cancers was first applied and the term 'chemosurgery' was coined as a name for the procedure. In practical terms, following a preliminary softening of keratin with dichloroacetic acid and subsequent scraping away, the paste would be applied to the tumour and often left on overnight. The tissue area would show evidence of necrosis and start to separate from the surrounding, unaffected tissue. This made the removal of the involved tumour area much easier the following day. The tissue would be excised in a saucer shape, which would then be sliced into numbered 1 cm square pieces with the adjoining edges inked with different coloured dyes and a map made of exactly where each piece of the jigsaw of skin tissue belonged in the overall excision.

Frozen sections were made of the under surface of each tissue piece and examined microscopically. If tissue was free of cancer cells then no further surgery would be performed. If cancer cells were detected then the patient would have the paste reapplied to the specific area corresponding to the tumour-involved tissue site and the process would be repeated. This process would continue until no further cancer cells were detected.

The key advantage of chemosurgery was that it proved to be 100% effective for the removal of cancer cells and at the same time facilitated preservation of normal, unaffected skin tissue. Neither of these advantages could be met equally successfully by any other conventional surgical procedure employed at the time.

Not uncommonly for innovative new procedures, whenever presenting his findings at national conferences, Mohs was met with resistance and general scepticism. There was a notion that dermatologists should not be surgeons and that in some way this process was 'a dark art' that should not be

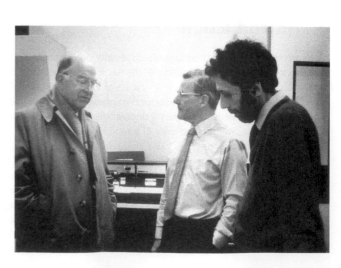

FIGURE 7.1
Frederic Mohs (pictured left) with Alex Hawkins and Dr Nick Gubbay in the histopathology laboratory at Cheltenham General Hospital.

trusted. There was also the fact that the majority of surgeons felt that this would be an uncomfortable and prohibitively long procedure for patients to endure.

The technique was modified over time with the key change being the removal of the use of the zinc chloride paste pretreatment and the use of fresh frozen tissue directly. Throughout the early 1970s, this modification of the original procedure gained increasing popularity and it was found to give comparable results with regard to the continued benefit of minimal tumour recurrence rates, but also having the advantage of reduced discomfort for the patients and improved speed and efficiency overall. Large cohort studies revealed over 97% cure rates for the procedure. Since these early reports and throughout the 1980s and 1990s, the technique has continued to expand in popularity and cure rates have risen to 98–99% in some of the very large US-based studies.

With the removal of the use of the zinc chloride paste, use of the term chemosurgery no longer seemed appropriate and in 1974 the term **micrographic surgery** was proposed by Dr Daniel Jones to reflect the fact that the procedure involved the use of maps and drawings in conjunction with microscopic evaluation. Eventually this was adopted by the American College of Chemosurgery in 1985.

Key Point

Micrographic surgery

A procedure used to treat skin cancers. It involves the removal of tissue layers for microscopic examination for tumour margin clearance, while the patient waits. The procedure is one of the most popularly employed methods for ensuring complete circumferential peripheral and deep margin assessment (CCPDMA). The technique largely employs fresh frozen tissue sections, but can be employed using formalin-fixed paraffin wax-embedded tissue (slow Mohs). The technique has the advantage over many other surgical procedures in the context that it permits removal of skin cancer with very narrow surgical margin clearance and with an extremely high cure rate.

7.3 Principle of Mohs micrographic surgery

The concept of complete circumferential peripheral and deep margin assessment (CCPDMA) may at first seem slightly daunting, but it is invaluable to understanding what Mohs actually delivers scientifically. The normal cut-up procedure for a skin ellipse of suspected cancer would involve inking the sample on its entire under surface and abutting to the epidermal layer all around. Sampling would then involve the transverse cutting and removal of both tips (apex) of the ellipse, to enable some comment on lateral excision margins when viewed under the microscope. One or two transverse sections from the centre (involved tumour area) will also be taken. The remainder of the tissue may then be reserved for future reference but not actually sampled.

Think of a medium sliced loaf of bread, in which the tips (each apex) are represented by the crust at either end, and the tumour is in one or two slices in the centre of the loaf. Normal tumour sampling would involve taking only four or five slices of this 30-pieced sliced loaf, and only the transverse face of each slice would be examined. Using the Mohs procedures and CCPDMA concept the complete circumference of the tissue is sampled (i.e. epidermal, lateral and deep tissue margins are examined in their entirety).

7.4 Mohs application in the removal of skin and mucosal tumours

The list of primary tumour types that can be treated using the Mohs approach is quite long, the main ones being basal cell carcinoma (BCC), squamous cell carcinoma (SCC), lentigo maligna melanoma (MM) and dermatofibrosarcoma protuberans (DFSP). Other, more unusual tumours that can be treated with Mohs include recurrent aggressive mutilating keratoacanthoma, malignant fibrous histiocytoma, atypical fibroxanthoma, verrucous carcinoma, microcystic adnexal carcinoma, neuroendocrine carcinoma (Merkel cell carcinoma), extramammary Paget's disease, and leiomyosarcoma.

CLINICAL CORRELATION

Lentigo maligna melanoma (LMM) is one of the four main catagories of malignant melanoma. The tumour is derived from the proliferation of atypical malignant melanocytes within the epidermal compartment. It is the slowest growing of all four main forms of malignant melanoma and typically begins as a patch of mottled pigmentation that is dark brown, tan, or black on sun-exposed skin sites, most notably, although not exclusively, on the facial area.

7.4.1 Recurrent tumours

In the majority of cases Mohs is advocated for recurrent cutaneous tumours in which more conventional treatments (i.e. surgery or radiotherapy) have proved unsuccessful and recurrence has occurred. The data on cure rates for recurrent tumours treated with Mohs have always shown the procedure to be consistently superior to conventional treatments.

7.4.2 Incompletely excised tumours

As well as advocating Mohs for incidences of recurrence, it can also be employed when there is incomplete excision of the tumour, particularly in cases where the deep margin is still involved. This may be because orientation of the primary tumour removal was not clearly indicated or where the anatomical site may have required minimal tissue removal in the first instance. Similarly, when using a skin flap repair to cover the surgically created defect for closure, there may be secondary movement of adjacent tissue over the surgical site which may make accurate correlation of involved margins difficult.

7.4.3 Tumour subtypes

There are many subtypes of certain cutaneous tumours, most notably BCC, SCC, and MM. In the case of BCC, tumours that are infiltrative, metatypical, keratinizing, multicentric, or morphoeic are all good candidates for Mohs treatment. These tumours may often be aggressive and also exhibit indistinct clinical margins. In the case of SCC, the undifferentiated or poorly differentiated and acantholytic forms of the tumour are good candidates for Mohs surgery. In addition, Mohs surgery should be employed where there is evidence of perineural invasion or perivascular invasion in BCC or SCC. In MM generally it is the removal of the lentigo maligna subtype for which Mohs finds most application. Of all the forms of MM, LMM is the slowest growing, affects predominately the elderly population, and most commonly, although not exclusively, occurs on the head and face areas.

7.4.4 Anatomical site

Primary tumours, particularly BCCs, occurring on the 'H' area of the face, are more likely to have higher recurrence rates than other sites (Figure 7.2). This area would include the nasolabial folds and walls, upper lip, across and underlying the lower eyelids (including the eyelid tissue), temples and around the ear or auricular areas, extending to the peripheral areas of the forehead.

In the case of SCC, sites of high risk for recurrence or metastatic spread (e.g. periorbital, auricular) and those occurring in and around mucosal sites (e.g. lips and nasal mucosa), or in cases of scarred tissue sites under investigation following primary treatment, are particularly problematic.

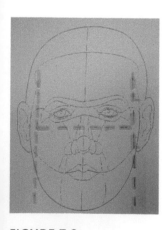

FIGURE 7.2
Anatomical facial map highlighting the key areas of the face that are affected ('H' zone and mask area).

SELF-CHECK 7.1

What are the main considerations for determining which patients should be selected for Mohs micrographic surgery?

7.5 The Mohs laboratory set up and key equipment

The concept of Mohs is based on the need for speed, accuracy, and efficiency. The laboratory should be the key to these requirements. The laboratory needs to be near the clinical theatres, ideally away from direct patient areas. It is often the room in which much discussion, both technical and medical, is likely to occur, and is the nerve centre for the process. Adjacent to the room containing the histological equipment, the laboratory ideally should have an annex with a dedicated viewing microscope for the surgical teams to assess slides. This should be a quiet area to encourage concentration and thinking. Ideally, the microscope should be multi-headed to enable discussion among medical staff and facilitate teaching and training. The multi-headed microscope is a fundamental teaching aid for medical and biomedical staff.

Laboratory layout should adhere to good, efficient, ergonomically orientated design. The design of Japanese car plants in the 1980s has seen the concept of efficient operative working station layouts become incorporated into modern laboratory design. This concept, termed 'Lean', is based on the key premise that we focus on testing samples in the most efficient way possible in terms of cost or speed (ideally both). There should be a clear sequential flow of operations with designated areas for specimen receipt, tissue embedding, microtomy, and staining. There should also be dedicated microscopes for quality control checking prior to slide submission to the medical teams (Figure 7.3 a–d).

Careful attention to the key operative requirements for performing Mohs should be made before the Mohs laboratory is built. These considerations include the obvious but often forgotten issues that can hinder Mohs operations, including not having:

- adequate external sunlight (windows)
- adequate ventilation and air flow

(a)

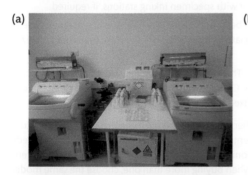

(b)

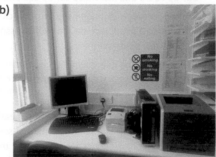

(c)

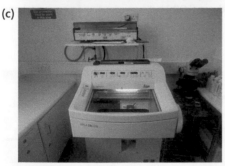

(d)

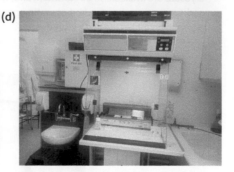

FIGURE 7.3

a) Mohs laboratory layout should follow Lean principles, with reception bench, cryostat and staining facilities in close proximity. b) Registration on laboratory information management system (LIMS) to assign the unique Mohs laboratory tracking number. c) Cryostat with linear staining machine positioned above for easy access, plus quality control microscope adjacent to the cryostat for easy access. d) Ventilated extraction hood for slide staining and mounting, if required.

- running tap water
- good overhead lighting
- appropriate shelving and cupboard space
- good non-slip flooring
- lockable doors with good general security (equipment is expensive and should be protected at all times)
- adequate health and safety indicators and supportive signage.

In addition to general laboratory layout, careful consideration needs to be employed to ensure that equipment purchased is adequate for purpose. There should also be consideration of back-up equipment for use in an emergency, which should also be in close proximity and readily available. Remember, if this is not readily available then patient care may be directly affected, due to subsequent delays in surgical completion of cases. Back-up plans that can be implemented without delay will be appreciated by the surgical team.

Key pieces of equipment include:

- *A receipt bench or slotted tray* to indicate the order of samples received, which will then allow prioritization of specimen samples into routine and urgent. All Mohs samples should be dealt with swiftly; however, there may be cases requiring complex surgical closure or repair. More time saved to allow the surgeons to complete these cases is facilitated by good planning.

- *A computer-based logging system* that will permit adequate tracking and auditing of the specimen process. It will also enable some laboratory-based accession number tracking systems to be installed. It is also an archive back-up, providing valuable information retrospectively should there be a need to revisit old cases.

- *Cut-up board and associated cut-up equipment* with specimen inking stations, if required.

- *A jeweller's eyepiece/magnifying lens.* This can be a simple eyepiece monocle or a magnifying lens attached to a headpiece device with an associated bright light shining down, to permit visualization of small tissue samples.

- *Tissue embedding and orientation equipment.* This may include simple glass slides and a freezing medium (e.g. optimal cooling temperature [OCT] medium), as well as a dedicated clamping device to secure orientation once the tissue is fixed in the appropriate position (Figure 7.4).

- *Cryostat.* You will have read about this in earlier chapters. If the microscope is a pathologist's tool of choice, the cryostat is the biomedical scientist's equivalent (Figures 7.5, 7.6a and b). It needs to be maintained, serviced regularly, and monitored carefully for performance issues. Different cryostats are available so be consistent and, when buying more than one, choose the same model and type, otherwise standard operating procedures (SOPs) will vary depending on model and type, which makes life complicated.

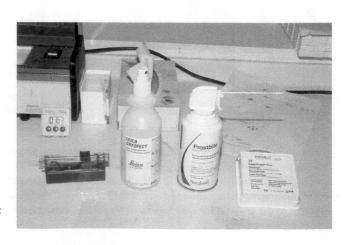

FIGURE 7.4
Preparation reception bench showing OCT, Cryofect disinfectant spray, microtome blade dispenser, and SuperFrost adhesive glass slides.

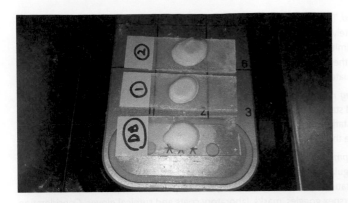

FIGURE 7.5
Part of the embedding
process of freezing tissue
onto a glass slide and
cooling the tissue down
to freeze within the
cryostat chamber.

(a)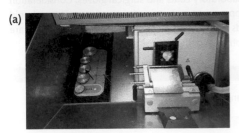

(b)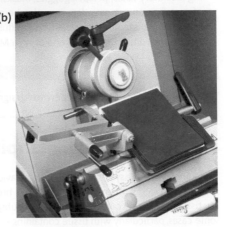

FIGURE 7.6
a) Inside the cryostat chamber showing the cooling plate (red arrow) and metal weight (black arrow). Both devices help with heat extraction from the sample and increase the speed of tissue freezing.
b) Tissue attached to the chuck/disc and secured within the chuck holder.

- *Cryostat chucks of various sizes.*
- *Staining equipment.* Although hand staining is acceptable, arguably it is not a productive way to spend time. A semi-automated, constant-feed platform such as a linear stainer is more appropriate. The larger the work volume the more important it is to embrace automated processes for non-critical steps in procedures (Figure 7.7).

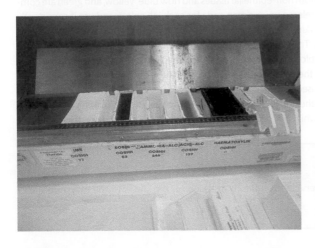

FIGURE 7.7
Linear staining machine for
rapid haematoxylin and eosin
(H&E) staining.

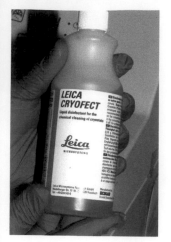

FIGURE 7.8
Cryofect disinfectant spray.
Ideal for decontamination of
equipment following Mohs
procedures.

- *Ventilated extraction hood.* This is necessary to reduce solvent fumes and ensure coverslipping is performed in an appropriately safe environment. If this is not available then coverslipping should be performed in close proximity to a window (which can be opened). A cautionary note is the infectious tissue sample. Whether these cases are dealt with routinely or occur as unexpected findings during Mohs procedures, adequate ventilation and protection for the biomedical scientific staff is essential.

- *Staining/quality checking microscope.* The checking microscope allows the evaluation of tissue orientation, section and staining quality. It takes a few seconds to do this, but it is time well spent and may save medical staff time if you are able to pre-empt the need for additional sections and start that process before the medical staff view the first sections.

- *Health and safety equipment.* This includes fire extinguishers and first aid boxes (adequately stocked and checked regularly); the inclusion of appropriate eye wash/irrigation bottles in case of eye splashes; hand sanitation and washing facilities; personal protective equipment (PPE) including laboratory coats, perspex goggles, masks, laboratory coats and surgical gloves. Consideration of metallic non-cut gauntlets may also be appropriate in certain circumstances. There should also be some adequate decontamination fluids (e.g. Cryofect) to ensure all working surfaces are cleaned and disinfected at the end of each Mohs session (Figure 7.8).

SELF-CHECK 7.2

What are the key factors to consider when designing and setting up a Mohs laboratory?

7.6 Tissue inking, mapping and cut-up

There are several dye systems available (e.g. Davidsons) for inking, which should not be excessive and should be applied with an orange stick, small brush or Q-tip. The important point is not to obscure key tissue margins by over-inking such that subsequent tissue orientation becomes problematic. In some cases, particularly with tissue containing cartilage (e.g. nose or ear) or tissue with a horseshoe appearance, use of a 'relaxing' incision to allow manipulation of the tissue for embedding purposes is advisable. Such tissues will simply not lie flat and therefore embedding will be difficult, and ensuring complete evaluation of CCPDMA will be compromised.

Generally, four inks are used for the removal of a circular saucer-shaped piece of tissue. The marginal surface of each quadrant is inked with a different colour. Tissue inking is the main key to preserving orientation of tissue on the slides to the map and the site of the excision. It is also important for ensuring that each subdivided specimen is labelled correctly on their separate slides. Each piece of tissue should have a distinct inking pattern, especially when several pieces are of the same size. For most cases inking is usually accomplished using two or three colours. In rare situations, for very large or complex-shaped specimens or specimens without epidermis, four colours may be required.

Red has been used as a tissue ink colour in the traditional Mohs procedure; however, many find red ink is more difficult to differentiate from non-epithelial tissues and now blue, yellow, and green are commonly used. It is very important to select a unique map code for each ink colour and use it consistently for all cases. All Mohs surgeons working in the same department are advised to agree on one colour-coding pattern protocol (Figure 7.9). The tissue should be placed in a secure flat transporting dish, ideally a Petri dish, with a piece of circular blotting paper on the base of the dish. Petri dishes are very good for this purpose as they have a lid and the tissue can be seen through the dish at all times. The white filter paper will allow marker pens to be used to indicate piece numbers and also to allow identification of the epidermal surface for each piece in the dish (Figure 7.10). This information should also be present on the associated anatomical Mohs map, which will accompany the tissue into the Mohs laboratory.

> ### Key Point
>
> **Inking is the main key to preserving orientation of tissue on the slides to the map and the site of tissue excision.**

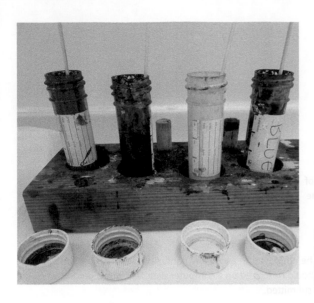

FIGURE 7.9
Marker dye set used to ink all Mohs tissue pieces before embedding and cryotomy.

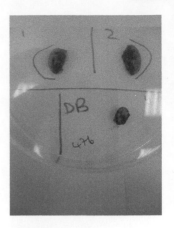

FIGURE 7.10
Mohs tissue received in the laboratory in a Petri dish. Information regarding tissue orientation can be made on the white filter paper to indicate epidermal surfaces.

The Mohs map will provide information on the exact anatomical location of the tissue removed, together with how many pieces of tissue have been inked and the number of rounds/layers of tissue removed from a revisited site (Figure 7.11). For example, in cases where four tissue pieces were inked in the first round, and the case remained positive for tumour cells, a second round/layer would be taken, perhaps involving removal of two more pieces of tissue, and this would continue numerically such that the second round/layer involved blocks 5 and 6. If the subsequent slides produced from these tissue blocks still contain tumour cells, then this process would continue until clearance for tumour cells is demonstrated for the entire tissue site. The use of the dyes and the anatomical map allows the medical team to identify where tumour cells are located and so it becomes possible to map the growth of the tumour deposits within the patient's tissue and to map out its surgical removal. Sometimes the surgical team may provide a saucer-shaped piece of tissue with the central clinically obvious tumour area removed and identified separately as 'debulk' tissue tumour site (Figure 7.12). These pieces of tissue do not need to be inked as they are not evaluated for margin clearance, but the surgical teams may request a vertical tissue section (transverse section) of this tissue to determine tumour presence and also possibly type the tumour histologically. As discussed earlier, BCCs have several clinical and histological appearances.

In cases of BCC it is not uncommon for patients to have more than one tumour on the face at any one time. In such cases, both sites may be treated using the Mohs procedure at the same time. However, each lesion would be distinguished on the anatomical map as lesion A and B accordingly.

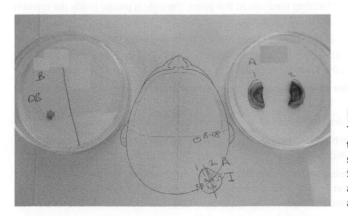

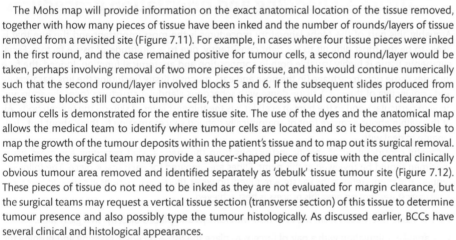

FIGURE 7.11
Two Petri dishes with tissue from two separate sites on the same patient. Sites are distinguished alphabetically as site A and site B.

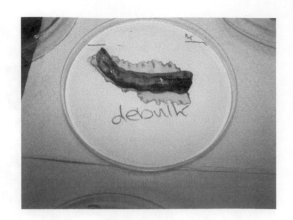

FIGURE 7.12
An example of the tissue 'debulk' representing the central portion of the initial first layer of Mohs tissue excision.

Separate Petri dishes should also be employed to avoid any confusion. For tracking and archiving purposes, all the tissues received should be logged on a computer database with a unique accession number associated with each case submitted.

7.7 Tissue embedding and orientation procedures

Arguably, this part of the Mohs laboratory procedures is the most important and the one that is likely to be the most difficult to get right consistently, due to a multitude of tissue factors. Facial cutaneous tissue is highly variable both in composition and anatomical function. Indeed, the face includes tissue rich in cartilage (in the nose and ear), mucosal tissue (including the lips, nasal cavity and conjunctiva of the eyes), tissue dense with sebaceous glandular structures (over the scalp and nose in particular), and in the human eyelid it has the thinnest layer of skin on the human body. All of this within about a square foot of anatomically defined space; amazing to think about but challenging to deal with.

Careful consideration of specific instructions from the medical staff regarding any given tissue specimen should be reviewed at this point. Slides are prepared for each tissue piece. The following sequence of events reflects the key steps required; however, there are variations in some steps as there is no clear statement on how this process is best achieved.

- The tissue is removed from the Petri dish with forceps and placed directly on a glass slide.

- Careful manipulation with a pair of forceps to place the tissue on edge, pressing and pushing the tissue to expand it to its full length while ensuring the tissue is on the epidermal edge.

- Tissue is frozen onto the slide or chuck using a cryo-freezing spray or liquid nitrogen aimed underneath the slide or chuck. OCT compound is then applied to cover the tissue entirely. After subsequent application of the cryo-freezing spray or liquid nitrogen, the tissue is effectively enveloped in a frozen embedding medium. At this point, the slide is placed inside the cryostat chamber to freeze down gradually, while dealing with the next tissue piece.

- Cover the entire surface of the cryostat chuck with OCT and invert the slide with the tissue attached to the chuck surface. Pressing down firmly either with a clamping device or by hand, apply the cryo-spray to freeze the tissue to the chuck.

- Place the chuck with slide attached inside the cryo-chamber and repeat the process with the next tissue piece.

- Within five minutes (or less) the tissue will have frozen securely to the cryostat chuck.

- Remove the chuck from the chamber and, applying heat from the palm of the hand, gently apply pressure to the slide, which will gradually become free and slide off the surface of the chuck.

- Essentially we have inverted the tissue such that the surface of the chuck now represents the outer portion of the tissue piece furthest from the centre of the tumour, so reflecting the true outer margins of the tissue removed (Figure 7.13a–d).

(a)
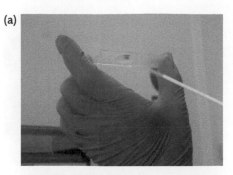

(b)
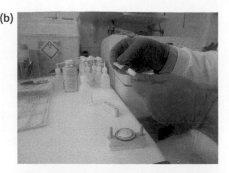

(c)
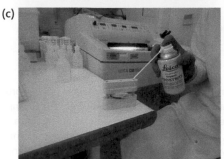

(d)
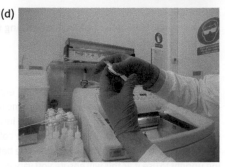

FIGURE 7.13
a) Freezing tissue onto a glass slide using cryospray. b) Once the tissue is frozen securely onto the glass slide, the tissue can be embedded using a clamping device such as a cryo-embedder. This ensures a uniformly flat surface for section cutting. c) Additional OCT can be applied and the clamp secured before freezing once again with cryospray. d) The slide and tissue is removed from the clamping device and, with heat from fingers or the back of the hand, the slide slides off the surface of the embedded block.

7.8 Tissue cryotomy

You will have read about cryostats in the earlier chapters of this book. The correct and effective use of a cryostat requires patience and practice in equal measure. Most biomedical scientists who have mastered the art of using a cryostat to cut a rapid frozen section may be under the impression that applying the same level of expertise to performing Mohs will be sufficient, but much greater expertise is required.

Mohs can be like doing an urgent frozen section procedure non-stop for anything up to eight hours depending on case volume, with precious few breaks. The degree of concentration, attention to detail, delicate touch, and general speed and efficiency required means that this is a demanding skill that takes time and practice to master.

Various types of cryostat are available, not all of which are suitable for Mohs procedures. The key points to look out for are:

- Adequate internal chamber space (you may have 20–30 blocks in the chamber at any one time).
- Appropriate size of the overall dimensions of the cryostat. Some modern cryostats have very rounded exteriors that can take up more space within the laboratory than is ideal. Space in the Mohs laboratory is a paramount consideration.
- An x/y axis. Not all cryostats have this feature. This enables you to re-orientate an embedded block in case one part of the tissue is being cut more deeply or unevenly than another. Adjustment of the x/y axis will enable the missing tissue block component to be cut following re-alignment.
- Adequate cooling plate (heat extraction device). This will speed the process of hardening and freezing the embedded tissue.
- Automated retraction of the object holder arm.
- Wheel lock to ensure there is no movement when placing or removing tissue from the object holder.
- Adequate lighting to illuminate all areas of the internal chamber.
- Provision of ultraviolet light options for rapid decontamination.

(a)
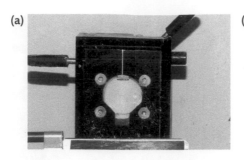

(b)
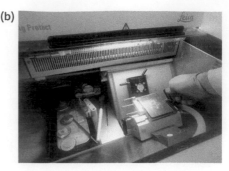

FIGURE 7.14

a) The cryostat chuck/disc holder. b) Clamping the knife holder securely to ensure there is no movement or vibration during sectioning.

Whatever your choice of cryostat, you should ensure that it is compatible with your embedding procedures. The **cryostat** is essentially a microtome in a freezer. Cryostat interior temperatures can range from –15°C to –30°C, which, if your hands are inside for long periods, can make it extremely cold and sometimes frankly uncomfortable. As well the cold, you should also be aware of body position when using the cryostat. It is a good idea to alternate between sitting and leaning over the cryostat to standing upright to use it as this will ensure you vary your body position and reduce back pain or repetitive strain injuries.

The knife and the knife angle set are crucial factors for good cryotomy. Nowadays, disposable blades have largely superseded the fixed knives in histopathology. They are cheap and can be bought in volume, reducing costs still further. They are quick and easy to fit into knife holders, and are very sharp.

The knife angle is critical to good section quality. If the angle is not correct then the tissue will compress when cut, or, worse still, not cut at all. Depending on composition (hardness/softness) of the tissue, the knife angle may need to be altered. As a general rule, the cryostat manufacturer should advise on knife angle, and, once set, in most cases it should not require adjustment. Altering other factors such as temperature or tissue section thickness in difficult cases can assist with the section cutting process.

Finally, the importance of ensuring that all movable, adjustable components of the knife holder and object holder are tightened to restrict any movement when cutting sections cannot be overstressed (Figure 7.14a and b). This can often be the cause of much frustration if not performed properly and will result in undesirable artefacts such as chatter or Venetian blind effects (see Chapter 6).

Key Point

Cryostat: a microtome contained within a freezer the interior temperature of which can range from –15°C to –30°C.

The use of brushes generally is highly recommended in Mohs procedures, specifically a coarse brush to remove roughly trimmed tissue, and then smaller, finer brushes to help with the delicate procedure of flattening sections as they come off the knife edge. Sometimes, trimming the brush edge so that it is angled can also help (Figure 7.15). Anti-roll plates can be used but generally need to be adjusted constantly as they can become misaligned quite easily. The process of resetting and aligning the anti-roll plate can be time-consuming and Mohs procedures require speed and efficiency; therefore, performing Mohs with the assistance of brushes but without an anti-roll plate is often more productive The key point is to ensure that all biomedical scientists in training practise this skill. They need to feel confident and to develop the delicate touch required to cut and lift sections from the knife edge correctly and safely.

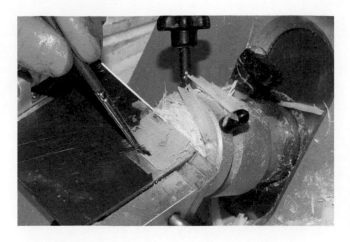

FIGURE 7.15
Section cutting using a brush to guide the section off the knife and to position the section for attachment to a glass slide.

There is no definition of what is required to cut a perfect cryostat section every time. There are a host of factors that come into play with any given tissue type. The key factors are:

- Tissue orientation (as a general rule the skin edge should be angled at 70–80° to the knife edge).
- Tissue composition:

    A) Factors to consider when cutting fat-containing tissues:

    i) cut with the fat component of the block being last to pass the knife

    ii) spraying the surface of the block with freezing cryo-spray, immediately prior to sectioning, will reduce the temperature of the tissue temporarily and enable a better section to be cut

    iii) increasing the thickness of the section

    iv) move the wheel with a swift, clean action

    v) change the disposable blade regularly.

    B) Factors to consider when cutting hard cartilaginous tissues:

    i) ensure you have a fresh disposable blade

    ii) ensure the knife holder and object holder are tightened

    iii) angle the tissue block in the holder so that the hard tissue component is in the long plane of the block face

    iv) move the wheel with a swift, clean action

    v) cut thinner sections (this will improve adhesion of the tissue to the adhesive slides).

SELF-CHECK 7.3

Name the key features of the cryostat that should be present for performing Mohs procedures adequately.

7.9 Tissue section slide mounting and staining

The most important point to raise first is that all frozen sections, whether they are to be stained with routine tinctorial methods (e.g. **haematoxylin and eosin** [H&E], toluidine blue) or used for immunocytochemical procedures, should all be placed on adhesive slides. There is a significant increase in the cost per slide as a result of using adhesive slides, but if the section becomes detached from the slide then you have lost valuable tissue that could be important in any given scenario.

Sections should be teased from the knife edge and flattened with the aid of fine brushes. The microscope slide is then placed directly over the top of the section and, with a steady hand, pressed

FIGURE 7.16
Positioning a glass slide at room temperature into the cryostat chamber and gently applying light force directly onto the section to secure attachment to the slide. The difference in heat between the room temperature slide and the cut section ensures the section attaches and melts the OCT directly onto the slide.

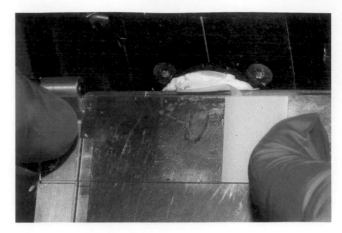

firmly down onto the section, resting on the knife plate while avoiding any lateral movement. As the slide has entered the chamber from room temperature, it is much warmer than the section temperature within the cryostat and so on contact with the slide the section sticks directly to the glass surface (Figure 7.16).

Slides should have a frosted end to permit prior labelling with the patient's name and unique accession number details using an indelible solvent-resistant pen. Depending on the block size, you may mount several sections on the slide or perhaps just one. In cases where there are numerous sections, ensure that the sections are located sequentially in a logical fashion, with the first section located at the top of the slide just below the frosted end, and so on down the slide.

Between each section an agreed volume of tissue should be trimmed before the next section is taken; this is usually agreed in the departmental protocol and with the surgical teams, and is generally around 50 microns (μm) between each section. It is also important to realize that the first sections taken represent the outer-most edge of the tissue block at the true margin. This is important because if tumour cells are seen in the first sections taken then tumour exists at the margins and the block is positive for tumour. However, if these early sections are free of tumour, but deeper tissue sections on additional slides reveal tumour on the same block, it indicates that the tumour has been cut through in the process of preparing the tissue sections and is effectively clear. Remember, in the process of embedding you have inverted the tissue!

Generally, two to three slides should be prepared per average block. In cases where only one section can be mounted on the slide then perhaps five to six slides will be required. Again, this can be agreed with the surgical teams (Figure 7.17).

Tinctorial staining is now almost exclusively H&E staining. Originally, **toluidine blue** was popular and indeed nuclear detail is well demonstrated with this stain; however, it is more susceptible to fading

FIGURE 7.17
Examples of the slides stained in Mohs cases to show the various tissue dimensions. The image demonstrates small tissue samples with multiple sections on a slide to large tissues with just one section per slide.

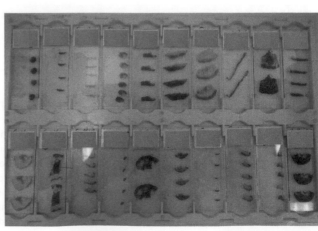

with time than is H&E staining. As all routine tinctorial staining is performed using H&E, it is logical that this is now the preferred stain of choice for Mohs procedures.

Key Point

Haematoxylin and eosin (H&E) is now used almost exclusively for the tinctorial staining of Mohs cases.

Key Point

Toluidine blue demonstrates nuclear detail well but is prone to fading over time.

Staining is often performed on either a linear staining machine or, if numbers of slides is small, by hand. The first step is to 'fix' the sections in 70% or 99% industrial methylated spirit (IMS) for two to three minutes, which ensures good preservation of nuclear detail. The slides should then be transferred to tap water. The following procedure reflects routine H&E staining on a linear staining machine and should act as a rough guide. This semi-automated staining procedure ensures that the biomedical scientist can continue cutting sections while sections are being stained, thereby improving general speed and efficiency. Adjusting this protocol to suit specific requirements from the medical teams can then be made.

Important points of which to be aware are factors that affect staining quality, including:

- sections are too thick or thin
- sections are excessively dried out before staining
- sections are not fixed or are inadequately fixed
- tissue thickness will affect fixation time and pre-wash time in tap water. The thicker the section the more OCT compound is present and the longer it will take to fix and wash the OCT out of the tissue prior to staining.

Once the slides have completed the staining process on the linear stainer or by hand, they can be cover-slipped or mounted. This also can be performed manually or using a dedicated coverslipper. Slides are then correlated with the anatomical map and placed in a slide tray, and the medical staff informed that tissue is ready to be viewed.

If the sections reveal tumour cells and are still positive, comments are made on the anatomical map to reflect where the tumour cells were seen. This will guide the surgical teams on exactly where more tissue needs to be removed, and essentially the tumour's growth pattern is being mapped for complete removal. The process then begins again until the patient's tumour is completely removed.

SELF-CHECK 7.4

Describe the factors that can cause aberrant staining outcomes, and how can they be avoided.

7.10 Troubleshooting

You will have read about artefacts in histopathology in Chapter 6, and some of these also pertain to frozen sections.

7.11 Basic microscope interpretation

For the biomedical scientist, there are several key interpretive concerns, as follows:

- What does good section and staining quality look like?
- Are you confident that the tissue is orientated properly?
- Have you demonstrated the entire block surface including the full epidermis (where appropriate) and, more importantly, the full inked tissue margins in the sections you have prepared?
- Understanding when you need to cut more sections and to pre-empt this for the benefit of the medical teams in order to save them time.
- An appreciation or basic understanding of what tumour cells look like in frozen sections is an advantage offered by the experienced biomedical scientist.

As a general rule, **tissue orientation** should be checked as soon as the first sections are cut. Placing the unstained slide under a microscope and increasing the light intensity will enable you to assess the fundamental tissue structures, and it should be possible to determine whether or not the full epidermis is present and the inked margins are fully displayed prior to staining. If this is not the case, it may be necessary to trim further into the block. More worryingly, you may have orientated the tissue incorrectly, in which case the block should be returned to room temperature and the tissue re-embedded following closer scrutiny. Generally, the first section may not show the full face of the block, but it will be evident that the tissue is orientated correctly and that simply cutting deeper into the block will reveal all that is needed.

Key Point

Tissue orientation should be checked as soon as the first sections are cut.

If, having stained and examined all the sections, a margin is still not fully exposed or a portion of the epidermis is not seen, then the experienced biomedical scientist should be able to recognize this, and will go back to the block to cut deeper tissue sections—sometimes the full margins may not be revealed until the block is nearly exhausted and very little tissue remains.

Although it is perhaps not the biomedical scientist's job to assess the presence of tumour in tissue sections, it is a great advantage to the surgical teams. This improves the working relationship and enables swifter decision-making among the surgical, biomedical, and nursing teams.

7.12 Slow Mohs

As the term slow Mohs implies, it is Mohs done slowly! But why would you do Mohs slowly? Does it not go against the whole principle of the procedure?

The answer lies in the interpretive complexity of any given case. You will have realized already, having read the earlier chapters, that the tissue morphology seen in frozen sections is not as good as that in formalin-fixed, paraffin wax-embedded tissue sections.

Cases selected for slow Mohs meet clearly defined criteria, as follows:

- Some tumours selected for Mohs may present with the requirement for improved morphological detail (e.g. lentigo maligna melanoma) and also a pathologist's input.
- Some tumours penetrate into the fat (e.g. dermatofibrosarcoma protuberans [DFSP]). Owing to the abundance of fat and the fact that these tumours can invade deep into the subcutaneous tissue, cutting sections of fat accurately and consistently is problematic when employing frozen sections. Processing tissue with abundant fat can still be problematic, even using conventional routine paraffin processing procedures. Consideration of extended processing schedules with extra exposure to the alcohol steps of the dehydration process should be employed. Fat contains a higher water content than most other tissues.

(a)

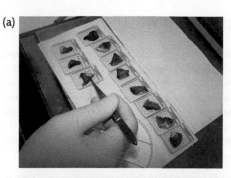

(b)

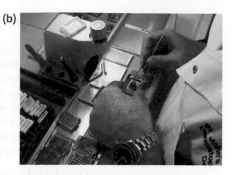

(c)

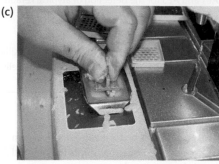

FIGURE 7.18

a) Organizing multiple tissue pieces received on a slow Mohs case into individual tissue cassettes for rapid fixation using formalin pre-warmed in an oven.
b) Orientating slow Mohs tissue into an embedding cassette and ensuring that the edges are pushed down flat.
c) Use of a damping iron to flatten the tissue to the base of the tissue cassette to ensure the entire periphery of the tissue can be sectioned accurately during microtomy.

- Sheer complexity of tumour removal. Large tumour sites requiring extensive surgery and subsequent microscopic examination will cause delays if booked in with routine frozen section service delivery.

- Complex patient-related issues (e.g. risks associated with patients who have known infections such as HIV and HBV). Fixing and processing the tissue through to paraffin wax negates that risk.

Slow Mohs procedures may result in patients staying in hospital overnight, and this increases the cost of treatment significantly, especially if the process continues over several days. In some cases, however, it cannot be avoided.

Slow Mohs is performed in the same way in terms of the basic principles of Mohs, with tissue inked and presented to the laboratory with the anatomical map. Any specific orientation issues are highlighted. The tissue is fixed overnight and processed the following day. All slow Mohs cases should be marked 'Urgent' and should be embedded and cut first. Once again, the principle of displaying the entire epidermis (where appropriate) and the full inked margins applies. One point of difference to note is that tissue processed and embedded into paraffin wax is often less flexible and malleable than frozen tissue. This can make tissue orientation and embedding difficult, and it often needs to be forced down in the paraffin embedding cassettes (Figure 7.18 a–c).

Key Point

Slow Mohs procedures may result in patients staying in hospital overnight, and this increases the cost of treatment significantly, especially if the process continues over several days.

CLINICAL CORRELATION

Dermatofibrosarcoma protuberans (DFSP) is a relatively uncommon tumour that arises within the dermis and underlying soft tissues. The tumour is relatively unresponsive to radiotherapy and therefore surgical excision is often the treatment of choice. This often requires relatively wide clearance margins (up to 3 cm or more). The slow Mohs procedure is often the preferred surgical approach for tumour removal as this process offers improved cure rates with maximal tissue conservation.

7.13 Immunocytochemistry and Mohs

The use of **immunocytochemistry** (ICC) in Mohs, whether on frozen sections or formalin-fixed, paraffin wax-embedded tissue sections, is a growing development and one that offers the medical teams the options of checking the final layers/rounds for tumour clearance. Sometimes, the detection of small tumour cell clusters in a frozen section may be problematic, particularly when approaching the final stages of surgical clearance, as such clusters may comprise just a few cells. In cases of LMM the implications of not removing all tumour cells could have quite significant consequences for the patient. Any additional laboratory-based investigation that can improve the likelihood of confirming tumour clearance therefore has merit. The main areas of ICC application include:

- Pan-cytokeratin antibodies such as MNF116 and AE1 and AE3 for the detection of atypical keratin-containing keratinocytes in cases of BCC and SCC (Figures 7.19a and b).
- Melan A antibodies for the detection of melanocytes in cases of LMM.
- CD34 antibodies for detection of the cell of origin in DFSP; this may also involve the use of FXIIIa antibodies to distinguish between associated reactive non-cancerous inflammatory spindle cells.

Key Point

Immunocytochemistry in Mohs, whether on frozen sections or formalin-fixed, paraffin wax-embedded tissue sections, is a growing development and one that offers the medical teams the options of checking the final layers/rounds for tumour clearance.

This is not an exhaustive list but does cover the main areas of application. The important thing to remember is that these antibodies allow the highlighting of residual tumour cells and allow the surgical teams to pinpoint and eliminate the residual tumour at the surgical margin. This is particularly useful when the tumour presents with subtle or non-specific histological features or when the tumour is masked by a dense cluster of inflammatory cells, making tumour distinction difficult morphologically.

The technique needs to be performed swiftly as in the ideal environment ICC should be completed within an hour, allowing visualization and subsequent closure of the Mohs case at the end of the surgical procedure, assuming the ICC results indicate that the tumour cells have been removed and all margins are clear.

In practical terms extra sections of the last layer/round should be sent for ICC staining while the routine H&E stains are performed. Ideally, the staining platform should be located in the Mohs laboratory if not in close proximity to a dedicated ICC laboratory. To ensure control protocols are established, the debulk tissue can be used as positive material for the assessment.

(a)
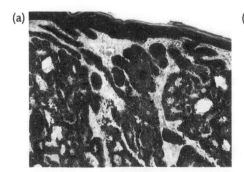

(b)
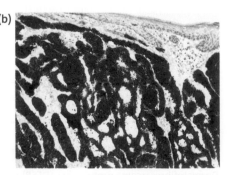

FIGURE 7.19
a) AE1, AE3 cytokeratin labelling of basal cell carcinoma (BCC) tumour cells in the dermal compartment of a piece of Mohs tissue (original magnification ×40). b) MNF116 cytokeratin labelling demonstrating BCC cells in the dermal compartment, but only basal dermal cell labelling in the epidermis (same case as in a; original magnification ×40).

The staff performing the ICC should be informed of the tissue being dispatched to them in advance so that the ICC machine can be prepared, thereby reducing the time required to complete the run. Once the H&E-stained sections have been assessed, the medical teams can then review the ICC slides, often with the input of a pathologist to confirm, or otherwise, that the case is clear of tumour cells.

The application of this methodology is increasing in Mohs surgery. With continued use and more cost-effective and faster staining methods, it is likely that ICC assessments as part of Mohs will become commonplace. Indeed, automated ICC platforms are available that offer staining times of just 15 minutes; however, in the authors' experience, these machines currently lack the consistency and accuracy required in this context.

7.14 Health and safety, and professional standards

Generally, health and safety within the Mohs laboratory is largely the same as in any other histopathology laboratory. The significant difference is that increased importance is placed on the health and safety issues associated with the assessment of fresh tissue.

Previous mention has been made of the necessary health and safety equipment required in a Mohs laboratory. What should also be encouraged is the regular auditing of the service with regard to health and safety checks. In this way, you will improve and develop the health and safety standards of your service and subsequently improve the working environment for staff.

Standards of professional accreditation will vary from country to country, and you will read more about this in Chapter 17. Currently in the USA, standards are set by Clinical Laboratory Improvement Amendments (CLIA) or Common Alerting Protocol (CAP), In Australia there is CAP-AU-STD 2012, developed by a CAP-AU-STD stakeholder group compromising federal agencies, Emergency Management Australia, GeoScience Australia, the Department of Agriculture, Fisheries and Forestry, and the Department of Health. In the UK there is the UK Accreditation Service (UKAS), which assesses laboratories to ISO 15189. These national or international standards agencies largely have a common goal, which should:

- advocate high quality and cost-effectiveness for patient care
- set global standards in laboratory quality
- promote continual education and continuous improvement
- inspect laboratories regularly
- work with professionals, particularly in relation to new technologies.

Despite this there is a need to ensure that Mohs procedures continue to be regarded as a specialty service, which has seen development of the American Society of Mohs Histotechnologists (ASMH) and more recently the British Society of Mohs Histologists (BSMH). Of equal importance is the development of a professionally recognized examination pathway for those biomedical scientists wishing to underpin their practical experience with formal examinations in the Mohs specialty. With this in mind, the BSMH, in conjunction with the Institute of Biomedical Sciences (IBMS) and the British Society of Dermatological Surgeons (BSDS), has developed the Expert Practice in Mohs Procedures examination for laboratory staff. This will act as the benchmark for professional standards of proficiency within the UK and possibly further afield.

7.15 Future developments

Imaging methodologies within Mohs procedures are currently under review. The basis behind these technologies is to improve the rapid intra-operative pathological margin assessment of patient tumours in order to guide staged cancer excisions. Examples of these methodologies include **optical coherence tomography** and **tri-modal confocal mosaics**. These methodologies represent an exciting development in terms of improving the accuracy and precision of tumour excision.

Currently, many of the methods are hampered by the science surrounding the ability of the scanning mechanisms to penetrate sufficiently deep below the epidermal surface to visualize tumour growth patterns. However, recent studies indicate that this technology is constantly evolving and the clarity of the images obtained is improving, as are the associated operating software packages.

(a)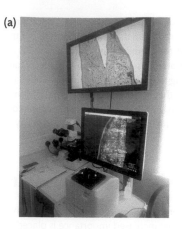   (b)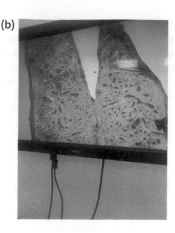

FIGURE 7.20
a) Confocal microscopy equipment for scanning tissue sections. b) Image of an H&E-stained slide demonstrating tumour cells on a large screen.

Key Point

Optical coherence tomography/tri-modal confocal mosaics represent exciting developments in terms of improving the accuracy and precision of tumour excision in Mohs procedures.

These new confocal scanning methodologies will increase the accuracy of surgical removal of skin tumours and facilitate the capacity to treat more patients. As the surgical removal of tumours becomes more precise, it will reduce the number of layers/rounds required of the procedure, saving time and increasing the capacity to treat more patients (Figures 7.20a and b).

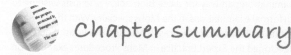 Chapter summary

This chapter has provided you with an understanding of a growing and more specialized branch of histopathology. Since its first inception in the 1930s, Mohs has expanded to become a widely practised technique worldwide.

The key points to remember are:

■ Mohs micrographic surgery is the most consistently accurate surgical method for the complete removal of skin tumours.

■ Mohs micrographic surgery offers the benefit of preservation of uninvolved normal tissue margins, providing minimal tumour clearance.

■ Mohs micrographic surgery techniques performed on facial areas provide benefits of improved cosmetic results.

■ Mohs is a higher skill, requiring prolonged concentration, with skill, understanding, and practical aptitude.

Further reading

- Coleman AJ, Richardson TJ, Orchard G, Uddin A, Choi MJ, Lacy KE. Histological correlates of optical coherence tomography in non-melanoma skin cancer. *Skin Res Technol* 2013; **19** (1): 10–19.

- Gareau D, Bar A, Snaveley N *et al.* Tri-modal confocal mosaics detect residual invasive squamous cell carcinoma in Mohs surgical excisions. *J Biomed Opt* 2012; **17** (6): 066018. Erratum in *J Biomed Opt* 2014; 19 (2): 029801.

- Gross KG, Steinman HK, Rapini RP. *Mohs surgery. Fundamentals and techniques.* St Louis, MO: Mosby, 1999.

- Lee S. *Introduction to Mohs cryotomy.* Fairfield, IA: First World Publishing, 2006.

- Orchard GE, Nation BR eds. *Cell structure and function.* Oxford: Oxford University Press, 2014.

- Orchard GE, Shams M. Dermatofibrosarcoma protuberans: dealing with slow Mohs procedures employing formalin-fixed paraffin wax-embedded tissue in a busy diagnostic laboratory. *Br J Biomed Sci* 2012; **69** (2): 56–61.

- Robins P. 44 years in dermatologic surgery: a retrospective. *J Drugs Dermatol* 2009; **8** (6): 519–25.

- Robins P, Ebede TL, Hale EK. The evolution of Mohs micrographic surgery. The single most effective skin cancer treatment. New York: Skin Cancer Foundation (www.skincancer.org).

- Suvarna SK, Layton C, Bancroft JD (eds). *Theory and practice of histological techniques* 7th edn. London: Churchill Livingstone.

- Trimble JS, Cherpelis BS. Rapid immunostaining in Mohs; current applications and attitudes. *Dermatol Surg* 2013; **39** (1 Pt 1): 56–63.

- Tromovitch TA, Stegman SJ. Microscope-controlled excision of cutaneous tumors: chemosurgery, fresh tissue technique. *Cancer* 1978; **41** (2): 653–8.

 Discussion questions

7.1 Discuss the key principles behind the benefits of Mohs micrographic surgery.

7.2 Discuss the key considerations required to set up a Mohs laboratory.

7.3 What is slow Mohs and what are the reasons for selecting this procedure over routine Mohs procedures?

Answers to the self-check questions and tips for responding to the discussion questions are provided on the book's accompanying website:

Visit www.oup.com/uk/orchard2e

8

Immunocytochemical techniques

Merdol Ibrahim and Guy Orchard

Learning objectives

After studying this chapter, you should be able to discuss:

- The concept of immunocytochemistry.

- Historical perspective.

- Role in diagnostic pathology.

- Tissue preparation.

- Antigen retrieval.

- Labelling methods.

- Automation.

- Quality control.

- Health and safety.

- Future developments.

8.1 Introduction

Immunocytochemistry (ICC) is not a tool to be used in splendid isolation. Like most methodologies utilized in cellular pathology, ICC is a complementary and often confirmatory investigative technique. As highlighted in previous chapters, ICC is used as a second string of investigations following conventional staining techniques. The role of the primary investigations is to demonstrate the morphological appearance of the cell and tissue architecture. This enables identification of the disease process, and in a substantial number of cases is adequate to formulate a final diagnosis. However, the demonstration of morphological detail alone may not enable a diagnosis to be made in all cases, and in such instances an assessment of the cell marker (**antigen**) expression on the cell membrane, cytoplasm or nucleus is required. This provides selective information that can be used to define certain cell types. This is the role of ICC, which, in some instances (e.g. lymphoma diagnosis), is closely allied to molecular diagnostics.

8.2 Historical perspective

'The further we can look back, the further we can look forward.'

Sir Winston Churchill

Immunocytochemistry was first used to evaluate pathological states in the early 1940s. A series of publications by Coons during this period reported the use of antibodies labelled with fluorescein, a fluorescent dye, which were employed to detect **antigenic epitopes** on tissue cells. This paved the way for the development of ICC and used fluorescein as an **antibody** label, which still forms the basis of immunofluorescence (IMF) investigations in pathology today.

Since the early work of Coons and colleagues, ICC techniques have developed and increased in both their **sensitivity** and **specificity** for demonstrating antibody–antigen interactions.

In terms of sensitivity, the technical advancements have focused on the ability to demonstrate ever smaller amounts of antigen. With regard to specificity, improvements in the nature and means of screening and producing antibodies (e.g. monoclonal versus polyclonal) has increased our understanding of the subtleties of the use of this technique.

SELF-CHECK 8.1

What is the definition of an antibody?

Major landmarks since Coons' early publications include:

1950s   Discovery and introduction of various chromogens.

1970   Sternberger *et al.*—development of the peroxidase-antiperoxidase (PAP) method.

1974   Taylor and Burns—first use in diagnostic pathology of formalin-fixed, paraffin wax-embedded (FFPE) material.

1975   Kholer and Milstein—monoclonal antibody production methodology.

1976   Huang *et al.*—first use of antigen retrieval techniques for paraffin sections with proteolytic enzyme digestion utilizing trypsin.

1981   Hsu *et al.*—avidin-biotin complex horseradish peroxidase (HRP) technique.

1983   Holgate *et al.*—colloidal gold label with silver enhancement.

1991   Hsu *et al.* and Shi *et al.*—heat-induced epitope retrieval, and the use of the microwave oven.

1993   Cattoretti *et al.*—citrate buffer systems for antigen retrieval.

SELF-CHECK 8.2

What is the definition of an antigen?

In 1994, Norton introduced the use of the pressure cooker as a means of applying heat for epitope retrieval (heat-induced epitope retrieval; HIER) and in so doing avoided the problems of variation in heat distribution (hot spots) in microwave ovens.

Pluzek *et al.* introduced polymer technology with the enhanced polymer one-step (EPOS) method, the basis of which has been refined several times over and is the foundation of most commercial detection methods employed to date.

Antigen or antigenic epitope
Antigen is the protein that interacts with an antibody complex. The epitope indicates the binding components that may be involved in this interaction.

Antibody
Proteins belonging to the immunoglobulin (Ig) group that arise in the blood of immunized humans and animals. There are five main subgroups (IgG, IgA, IgM, IgD, and IgE), which collectively form the basis of the body's humoral immune response mechanism.

Antibody sensitivity
A measure of the relative amount of antigenic epitope that a given ICC method is able to detect. The greater the sensitivity of any given ICC technique, the smaller will be the amount of antigenic epitope that may be detected.

Antibody specificity
A definition of the characteristics of an antibody to bind selectively to a given antigenic epitope. Specificity ultimately defines the labelling selectivity of any given antibody. It is important to remember that this is an absolute definition. Antibodies, when compared for labelling profiles, should not be stated to be more specific than each other. They may be more selective but not more specific.

The past 10 years have seen the widespread introduction of automation in ICC, with the production of fully automated machines with onboard antigen retrieval. These have been developed as a direct result of the increase in use and application of ICC and an associated increase in work volume. The strength of automation lies in the greater reproducibility of methods and its high-throughput capacity, as well as its ability to perform a wide range of ICC techniques (including double labelling methods and IMF). Further developments in ICC will include an attempt to achieve complete standardization of automated methodology, combined with direct digital image capture with subsequent image analysis for analysis and quantification of final reaction products.

It is clear that until the introduction of antigen retrieval techniques ICC was slow to take off as a widespread diagnostic tool in histopathology; it is now the most consistently utilized technique, providing a reproducible method of defining cell phenotypic profiles, and therefore is a cornerstone in our abilities to define pathological pathways and processes.

8.3 Immunocytochemistry in diagnostic histopathology

Immunohistochemistry has a wide range of applications in diagnostic histopathology. The key areas of application are:

- Defining cell types in tumour pathology.
- Defining cell types in inflammatory cell infiltrates.
- As prognostic indicators for a particular cancer type.
- As predictive indicators for potential targeted therapy strategies.
- Identifying infectious pathogens.
- Identifying defective proteins and providing evidence at the cellular level of defective gene transcription or translation.
- Evaluating immune complex deposition in autoimmune disease.
- Evaluating cell activation and apoptotic pathways.

Key Point

An understanding of the key terms and definitions used in ICC is essential (see Dabbs, 2013). These terms are used to define specific parameters and must be used in the correct context. One of the fundamental misconceptions in ICC is that these terms can be used interchangeably or loosely applied in a given context. This is wrong and should be avoided.

This list is not exhaustive but represents those areas in which ICC has a key role to play. However, although there are many selective research applications not covered above, the reader should be aware of the important role of ICC in the diagnostic setting.

Key Point

Immunocytochemistry is a widely used method that should be seen as a complementary technique used in conjunction with routine tinctorial methods (e.g. H&E staining) and molecular-based techniques.

8.4 Tissue preparation

The pre-analytic phase of histopathology includes stages of tissue handling, from sampling (surgical resections/biopsies) to fixation and processing, and represents a wide range of potential variables, all of which can have a detrimental effect on the final ICC result. The optimal result is determined by the need to standardize all such variables to provide consistency and reproducibility of the final product. From this base, consistency and accuracy in quantification and image analysis capture is also achievable. These represent new developments in ICC, particularly on the fully automated ICC machines currently being introduced.

Another very important factor which may be out of the hands of the histopathology laboratory includes ischaemia time (time that the sample is out of surgery and prior to placement in fixation). This has also been shown to have a dramatic effect on final ICC staining results. Ideally ischaemia time should not exceed one hour and it is imperative that there is good communication between the surgical team and histopathology department to communicate the need to have as low an ischaemia time as possible.

8.4.1 Fixation

Most tissue on which ICC is to be undertaken is fixed, although both ICC and immunofluorescence (IMF) may be applied to frozen tissue to accompany H&E-stained frozen sections used for rapid diagnosis or in the assessment of excision margins in certain specimens. However, with the advent of a wide range of antigen retrieval methods, the reality now is that frozen section work is almost completely obsolete in the diagnostic setting, although frozen sections are still cut from tissue submitted in some transport media (e.g. Michel's media in IMF).

Key Point

The objective is to achieve a balance between good morphological detail of tissue and cellular structures and appropriate preservation of antigenic epitopes. Adequate time in the appropriate fixative is paramount for optimal tissue/sample preservations. Inadequate fixation will lead to loss of antigenicity due to diffusion of antigens into surrounding tissue as a result of cellular lysis and degradation, resulting in poor localization of some antigens. While not a commonly encountered problem, excessive fixation may also compromise ICC methodology. A general guide for fixation includes six hours for core biopsies and 24–48 hours for surgical resections.

A consequence of poor fixation can be the demonstration of antigens normally localized to the nucleus, cytoplasm, or cell membrane in inappropriate cellular compartments. An example is oestrogen receptor (ER) detection, where this can sometimes be seen outside the nucleus in poorly fixed breast tissue.

A factor that has a significant impact on achieving good fixation is tissue sampling. Small core, needle or punch biopsies can be compressed and damaged by the inappropriate use of forceps during removal from the patient, or may dry out if fixation is not commenced immediately. This can produce artefactual changes and in the case of highly cellular tissue may result in areas of the biopsy being wholly inadequate for ICC evaluation (Figure 8.1).

The most widely used fixative in histopathology is formaldehyde, used as 10% neutral buffered formalin (NBF), formalin saline, or, less commonly, formalin calcium. Formalin, used as 10% NBF, has become the recommended fixative within ICC for all tissue types as it provides (when used correctly) acceptable morphological preservations and permits the full scope of histopathological and molecular investigations to be undertaken. Other fixatives are available and can be used in certain areas of ICC investigation, but none has gained widespread popularity possibly because there is not the long-term data that has been shown with 10% NBF. The process of fixation in

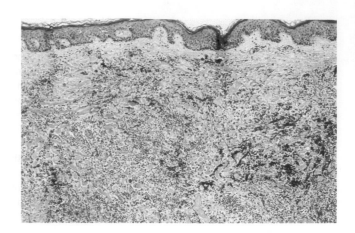

FIGURE 8.1
Crushing artefact, H&E.

METHOD 8.1 *Fixation: key facts*

1. Gross specimens (e.g. bowel or breast), and bloody or heavily keratinized samples need to be opened to allow penetration of the fixative.

2. Fixative type: generally, 10% neutral buffered formalin.

3. Fixative volume: 20× that of the specimen.

4. Block size: No more than 2 cm × 4 mm in size.

5. Fixative temperature: higher temperatures may increase fixation speed, while lower temperatures may slow fixation.

6. Fixative pH has an effect on the rate of fixation.

7. Time in fixative: core biopsies at least six hours; surgical resections 24–48 hours.

Chromogen

A compound that interacts with the final antibody–antigen complex to produce visualization of the coloured final reaction product at the site of the antibody–antigen interaction. Examples include diaminobenzidine tetrahydrochloride (DAB) or alkaline phosphatase.

formalin, changes protein structures by cross-linking amino acid side-chains. Excessive fixation of tissue samples can produce characteristic detrimental results, with the production of formalin pigment in some cases or, more significantly, masking of antigenic binding sites due to extensive cross-linking of amino acid side-chains. This normally arises after prolonged tissue exposure to the fixative. The issue of neutral pH for fixatives is important because acidic mixtures may induce undesirable changes to antigenic binding sites and therefore result in decreased ICC sensitivity. Furthermore, acid formalin is prone to producing formalin pigment, which could be confused with the 3,3'-diaminobenzidine tetrahydrochloride (DAB) **chromogen** used commonly in ICC methodology.

8.4.2 Processing

Having optimized tissue sampling and fixation, the next variable is tissue processing. Until fairly recently this was poorly understood in relation to ICC; however, it is now well documented that tissue processing temperature, duration of dehydration, and wax infiltration will all affect antigen preservation. It is important to ensure that tissue processing steps do not involve temperatures higher than 60°C, as excessive heating not only affects the preservation of antigenic epitopes, but may also result in destruction of tissue architecture. Although, more recently, the advent of micro-wave enhanced rapid tissue processing machines has enabled adequate processing for immunocytochemical techniques.

CASE STUDY 8.1 *Metastatic breast carcinoma*

The small bowel shows a tumour arranged in trabeculae and nests. The tumour infiltrates the entire bowel wall and extends to the serosal surface. Mitoses are conspicuous (33/10 high-power fields [HPF]). Perineural and vascular invasion are noted. One lymph node (1/1) shows metastatic carcinoma. The proximal and distal resection margins are free of tumour.

Immunostaining for synaptophysin, chromogranin, CK20, and GCDFP is negative. Staining for ER and CK7 is positive.

The immunoprofile supports a diagnosis of metastatic carcinoma of breast origin.

The patient is a 58-year-old female who presented with small bowel obstruction and a previous medical history of breast cancer (diagnosed 14 years previously) which had metastasized to the lung three years previously. The differential diagnosis included peritoneal nodules or adhesions due to previous surgery.

A laparoscopic small bowel resection revealed a nested tumour suggestive of neuroendocrine origin, which contained a few nucleolated cells (high-power H&E). Immunocytochemistry for neuroendocrine markers was performed, but this proved to be negative (low-power chromogranin). Cytokeratin staining was positive for CK7 but negative for CK20, suggesting a carcinoma of breast origin, and ER staining was then performed. This was strongly positive (low-power ER) and demonstrated that the tumour was indeed a metastatic breast carcinoma (Figure 8.2).

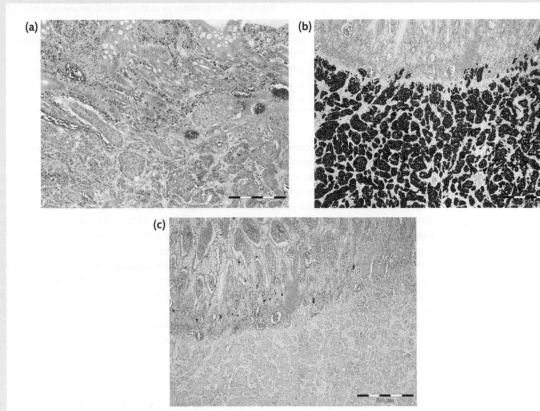

FIGURE 8.2
a) H&E stain. b) ER-positive tumour. c) Chromogranin-negative tumour.

TABLE 8.1   Limiting factors related to fixation which can affect ICC procedures.

Fixation/handling	Limiting factors
Ischaemia time	Time of removal of tissue and placement into fixative. Should ideally be no more than 1 hour.
Effect of crushing	Good biopsy practice. Ensure care when removing samples.
Specimen drying	Place specimens directly into fixative. Ideally 20× volume of specimen.
Excessive marker dyes	Some methylene-based dyes can affect hormone receptor marker labelling in ICC.
Heavily keratotic or fragmenting tissue The 'bloody' specimen The large mass	If necessary, ensure they are sliced open, fixed in an adequate volume of fixative, and for an adequate amount of time. When fragmented, wrap the specimen to preserve the sample volume.
Fixative pH	Neutral buffered formalin (NBF; pH 7.6) is the accepted standard. Avoids formalin pigment and improves preservation of antigenic epitopes.
Temperature	Room temperature or 37°C. Avoid fixation at temperatures above 45°C. Avoid low temperatures as these will slow the rate of fixation process.
Types of fixative	Wide range available. In practical terms, NBF is recommended. Others selective for ICC include B5, periodate lysine paraformaldehyde (PLP).
Time in fixative	• Core biopsies: at least 6 hours. • Surgical sections: 24–48 hours.

Once embedded in paraffin wax, sections should be cut at 3–4 microns. Thicker sections will contain multiple layers of cells and therefore ICC staining may become difficult to interpret. Cut sections should initially be allowed to drain and then 'dried/baked' ideally in a temperature-controlled oven (hot plates or hair dryers are not recommended!). At no time should cut sections be dried at excessive temperatures or for prolonged periods of time. Optimal drying temperature should be at around 40°C, normally for no more than 12–18 hours, or no more than 60°C for 1 hour. Commercially available charged/adhesive-coated slides are now used routinely for ICC investigation with the positively charged slides attracting the negatively charged tissue proteins.

A final consideration before undertaking ICC should be to ensure that tissue sections are appropriately dewaxed. The presence of residual paraffin wax is not a problem unique to ICC, and it is a surprisingly simple error to make. Heating the slide for a short time to soften the wax prior to immersion in the dewaxing solution of choice is a good practice to adopt. However, commercial epitope-retrieval solutions that simultaneously dewax the section are now available.

Tables 8.1 and 8.2 highlight the key areas of concern with regard to optimizing conditions of fixation and processing tissue samples.

TABLE 8.2   Limiting factors related to processing which can affect ICC procedures.

Processing and slide preparation	Limiting factors
Excessive dehydration during processing	Can cause: 1. Excessive tissue shrinkage. 2. Loss of antigenicity.
Paraffin wax temperatures	Wax temperatures should not exceed 60°C. Higher temperatures will cause loss of antigenicity.

TABLE 8.2 Limiting factors related to processing which can affect ICC procedures. (*Continued*)

Processing and slide preparation	Limiting factors
Section thickness	Should be 3–4 µm. Thicker sections will produce cell multilayers, making ICC interpretation difficult.
Microtomy: floating out sections	Ensure waterbath does not exceed 40°C.
Slide draining and drying	• Drain slides prior to drying • Dry slide in a temperature controlled oven for either around 40°C, for 12–18 hours, or no more than 60°C for 1 hour.
Storage of slides prior to ICC	This should ideally be avoided and clinical samples should be stained within 1–2 days of cutting or there may be a drop in antigenicity.
Dewaxing prior to ICC	Ensure slides are properly dewaxed prior to ICC. Failure to do so will severely affect the result.
Coated or charged slides	Now used commonly in ICC as sections may detach from the slide following antigen retrieval if not used.
Mounting medium and choice of haematoxylin counterstain	Some enzyme labels are alcohol labile (e.g. alkaline phosphatase) and require selective progressive haematoxylin staining (e.g. Mayer's) and an aqueous mounting medium (e.g. Faramount).
Storing IMF	IMF slides may show in increase in background autofluorescence over time so should be stored in the refrigerator (4–6°C) after or prior to analysis. Ideally the cover-slip should be sealed onto the slide using clear nail varnish to stop potential seepage of microscope objective oil onto the tissue section.

8.5 Antigen retrieval methods

Optimal tissue fixation followed by processing to paraffin wax has long been recognized as the most suitable means of preserving tissue morphology, but as ICC has developed it has become apparent that the process of fixation can result in the loss (if under-fixed) or masking of antigen immunoreactivity. There are many factors affecting ICC staining results that the investigator should be aware of, but may not have control over, and these include many of the pre-analytic stages mentioned including ischaemia time, fixative type, fixation time/pH processing, etc. Immunocytochemistry can only be correctly and confidently performed if the pre-staining factors are taken into consideration.

The number of antigenic determinants (epitopes) that comprise each antigen can vary enormously, as can the number of amino acids in each epitope. The three-dimensional structure of cellular proteins in FFPE material is determined in great part by protein denaturation, brought about by covalent bond formation between formaldehyde and amino groups present in the tissue. Formalin-induced cross-linking, due to methylene bridge formation, also occurs with subsequent folding of proteins. While some antigens remain unaffected by this process, others may be more susceptible to fixation, and the overall result then will be a loss of immunoreactivity due to masking of the epitopes. In general, because the degree of cross-linking is proportional to the time spent in fixative, tissue that has received prolonged fixation will require longer or more vigorous unmasking. Owing to the many variables that affect the extent of fixation-related cross-linking, it is necessary to find the optimum treatment time and technique for each antigen (see Box 8.1).

BOX 8.1

The ideal fixative should:

- Preserve morphological appearance.
- Preserve antigen immunoreactivity.
- Prevent antigen extraction during ICC.
- Not interfere with subsequent antigen–antibody interactions.

Heat-induced epitope retrieval

- Automated ICC platforms
- Microwave oven
- Pressure cooker
- Waterbath.

Various approaches have been used to recover this lost immunoreactivity by restoring the visibility of the antigenic sites to the antibody. Pretreatment is not necessary in tissues fixed and processed by methods which satisfactorily preserve the immunoreactivity of the antigen under investigation (e.g. alcohol fixation, which does not produce cross-links). Methodologies can be split into two main groups and are normally dependent on the ICC antibody under investigation:

- Those using proteolytic enzymes to cleave the formalin-induced cross-links.
- Those that use **heat-induced epitope retrieval**.

8.5.1 Proteolytic digestion

Proteolytic (enzyme) digestion

- Trypsin
- Chymotrypsin
- Pronase (now rarely used)
- Protease.

The use of **proteolytic enzymes** to improve the immunoreactivity of formalin-fixed material is well established but prone to variability. Selectively breaking protein links sufficiently to reveal masked/hidden epitopes without causing uncontrolled change to protein structure, particularly in cell membranes, requires a degree of standardization of fixation and processing which, on a day-to-day basis, may not be achieved. Adherence to protocol is essential if optimal staining and tissue preservation is to be maintained.

Trypsin

One of the most commonly used enzymes is trypsin, derived from porcine pancreas and consisting of a single-chain polypeptide of 223 amino acid residues. Protein digestion is achieved by cleavage of peptide bonds on the C-terminal side of lysine and arginine amino acid residues. The rate of hydrolysis is slower if an acidic residue is on either side of the cleavage site, and no cleavage occurs if a proline residue is on the carboxyl side of the cleavage site. In practical terms, this means that incubation of the tissue section with enzyme will need to vary depending on the antigen, and with some antigens will not work.

As well as removing cross-links brought about by fixation, the enzyme is thought to aid conversion of antigenic precursors to the immunoreactive form, and to digest protein aggregates, which may block access to the antigen. While the exact mechanism of proteolytic digestion is not fully understood at the macromolecular level it is accepted that this improvement in access to the antigen is at the heart of the increased antibody binding elicited by this approach. It would seem clear, therefore, that binding (and subsequent signal) should be proportional to the length of incubation in the enzyme solution; however, this is not the case in practice. The optimal time for each antibody must be determined using a range of incubation times on relevant control material showing expected positive and negative staining for the antibody being tested. However, the investigator should be aware that they may not have details of fixation of samples, especially those that are referred from other institutions, which may necessitate increasing or decreasing enzyme times accordingly. The effects of under-digestion and over-digestion are shown in Table 8.3.

The difference between under-digestion and over-digestion may only be a matter of two or three minutes. As discussed earlier, formalin-induced cross-linking is thought to be proportional to the duration of fixation, which may be unknown at the time of staining, and batch variation of the enzyme further complicates the picture. Consequently, optimal staining may require different digestion times, which hardly aids standardization of the technique.

TABLE 8.3 Issues affecting ICC following proteolytic enzyme digestion.

Under-digestion	Over-digestion
Failure to demonstrate any or all of the antigen.	Morphological damage (membrane disruption).
	Sections detach from slides.
	Excessive background staining.
	Cross-reactivity of antibody with inappropriate tissue components.
	Digestion of antigen under investigation.

Chymotrypsin

Chymotrypsin is another digestive enzyme used in immunocytochemistry for **antigen retrieval**. It is produced in the pancreas and exerts its proteolytic effect by cleaving peptides at the carboxyl side of tyrosine, tryptophan, and phenylalanine residues—three amino acids containing phenyl rings. Used on its own it is a much slower proteolytic agent than trypsin, but many commercial trypsin products actually contain a small amount of chymotrypsin to offer a wider spectrum of digestive activity.

Proteases

It is possible to make the above digestive approach more selective by utilizing specific families of enzymes (e.g. endopeptidases) in isolation. Many of the ready-to-use solutions available commercially will take this form, such as those manufactured for use on automated staining platforms. These solutions are often available in different concentrations such that the immunocytochemist controls digestion by choice of concentration and choice of incubation time—2.5 units of enzyme activity in solution incubated for two minutes is equivalent to 0.5 units incubated for 10 minutes, illustrating the fact that in a practical setting there is more opportunity for fine-tuning the enzymatic digestion when using a 'weaker' solution.

8.5.2 Heat-induced epitope retrieval

Historically it was shown that formaldehyde bound to fixed tissue can be removed by prolonged washing for two to three weeks in water, leading early researchers to investigate how increasing the temperature of the wash solution might affect the speed with which antigenicity could be restored in a tissue section. This entirely new approach to restoration of immunoreactivity was first reported by Shi *et al.* in 1991 using microwave heating of zinc sulphate or lead thiocyanate in solution. This produced greater sensitivity in subsequent ICC staining and the term antigen retrieval or heat-induced epitope retrieval (HIER) was used for the first time.

Subsequent studies focused on the pH of the solution as well as the type and duration of heating, and it was determined that a pH 6 citrate buffer was suitable for the demonstration of the majority of antigens under investigation. It had already been established that ICC staining could be improved by treating sections at room temperature with 5 mol/L urea or with mild detergent, but it soon became apparent that the time required for efficacious antigen retrieval could be shortened as the temperature of the solution increased. Subsequently, almost all studies have involved heating the solution to its maximum (i.e. 100°C) in a microwave oven or waterbath, or to 120°C in a pressure cooker. The commonly used approaches are described below, with a summary of the 'retrieval solutions' that may be used.

Antigen retrieval
A series of techniques that permit the controlled unmasking of antigenic epitopes, following the fixation of tissue and prior to subsequent demonstration of final reaction products with labelled antibodies. Conventionally, this relies on the application of heat (HIER) using a waterbath, microwave oven, or pressure cooker in conjunction with selective buffer systems, or the application of proteolytic enzyme digestion procedures using enzymes (e.g. chymotrypsin or protease).

Key Point

Sections must be fixed to charged/coated slides, drained, and then dried at either 40°C for 12–18 hours or no more than 60°C for one hour prior to dewaxing, hydration, and immersion in the chosen buffer.

Microwave oven

It was originally thought that microwaves broke the formalin-induced cross-links, but this notion has been called into question as domestic microwave cookers do not emit enough energy to achieve this, leaving the likelihood that it is purely the combination of temperature and buffer constituents that lead to antigen retrieval by one or more of the following:

- Removal of methylol groups allowing increased accessibility of antibody to epitope.
- Loss of 'blocking' proteins.
- Renaturation of protein molecules previously denatured by formalin.
- Removal of residual embedding medium (particularly with resin-embedded tissue).

Key Point

Although the optimum microwave oven retrieval time, as with proteolytic digestion, depends on length of fixation and other factors, 20 minutes appears to be sufficient for most protocols, and this is towards the upper limit of what many tissues will tolerate before becoming either damaged or detached from the slide. However, other factors which should be considered, and which may have impact on the retrieval times, include the 'wattage' of the microwave being used, and the possibility of 'hot/cold' spots in the microwave, which can result in variability of staining.

Heating needs to be followed by a cooling-down period of around 20 minutes before the slides can be washed in water and subsequently stained. It is essential that during the heating and cooling process the slides do not dry out, and the container in which the sections are microwaved must therefore be of sufficient size to keep the slides immersed at all times, even when the solution boils. A heatproof, loose-lidded container with venting holes is an essential piece of apparatus.

Pressure cooker

Pressure cookers allow the retrieval solution to be heated to 120°C, enabling a shorter antigen retrieval period (often just 2–4 minutes, once full pressure has been achieved) when compared to microwave retrieval. Pressure cookers also overcome hot and cold spots in the chamber that can lead to variation in the retrieval effect depending on the positioning of the specimen container. Pressure cookers are also able to treat larger batches of slides without evaporation of the buffer solution. The main drawback is the prolonged cooling period before the pressure cooker can be opened safely without causing rapid decompression. This can be minimized by rapid cooling in a sink of cold water, or use of a plastic pressure cooker heated in a microwave oven, the latter cooling much more rapidly than its metal counterpart.

There are now digitally controlled pressure cookers which allow for more accurate temperature and retrieval times. It is also important to have quality control measures in place, including using the same volume of retrieval buffer each time, and replacing the retrieval buffer as recommended by the commercial supplier. It is also important to always place the same number of slides into the pressure cooker so it is advisable to place blank slides alongside those slides which have the tissues being retrieved. Regular maintenance of the pressure cooker such as checking sealing rings is also important.

Waterbath

The use of a waterbath to incubate slides in a boiling buffer solution should, in theory, produce equivalent antigen retrieval to that obtained using a microwave oven. In practice, however, it is difficult to achieve reliable and reproducible results when using small-volume jars, which show marked change in temperature when inserting slides. Returning the solution to boiling is slow and can introduce

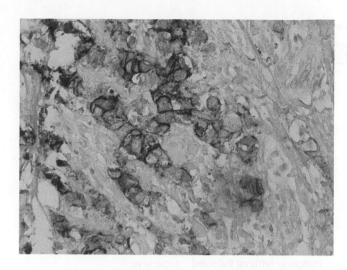

FIGURE 8.3
HER2 staining showing membrane disruption in breast tissue.

variability in the antigen retrieval achieved. Waterbaths are not a practical solution for treating large numbers of slides, but they have the advantage that it is possible to use them at whatever temperature is deemed best for the material being treated. Longer incubation (e.g. 40 minutes) at a lower temperature (e.g. 96°C) produces more consistent results, which is especially important for antigens that require semi-quantification (e.g. HER2). However, deviation from the temperature protocol required for some antibodies results in poor-quality staining with membrane disruption, leading to difficulty in interpreting the results (see Figure 8.3).

Ideally a waterbath with a heater–stirrer should be used to evenly distribute the heat and one with a digital temperature readout should be used. It is also important to make sure that the same volume of retrieval buffer is used and that the retrieval buffer is replaced as recommended by the commercial supplier. As with the pressure cooker method it is also recommended that the same number of slides is used during each retrieval session by placing blank slides alongside those slides which have the tissues being retrieved. Regular maintenance of the waterbath should be carried out.

It is also worth noting that semi and fully automated platforms for HIER are available. The majority of these systems rely on commercially manufactured optimal retrieval buffered systems. Some of these buffers will have specific applications with selective antigens. Those systems that have a digitally controlled process have the advantage of absolute reproducibility with each run.

Automated staining platforms

Fully automated stainers perform dewaxing, antigen retrieval, antibody incubation, and detection using proprietary reagents. These machines use a combination of heat and chemical solutions to achieve antigen retrieval and constant replenishment of buffer, which removes the risk of dried tissue sections.

The relative merits and pitfalls of HIER systems are summarized in Table 8.4.

8.5.3 Antigen retrieval solutions

The exact mechanism underlying HIER remains unclear. At least four features of these solutions are thought to be involved in their interaction with formalin-fixed tissue:

- hydrolysis of bonds between formaldehyde and tissue proteins
- metal cations
- chaotropic effects
- chelation of calcium ions.

TABLE 8.4 **Advantages and disadvantages of HIER systems.**

Antigen retrieval system	Merits	Disadvantages
Microwave	Low investment needed.	Time depends on microwave wattage.
		Hot and cold spots.
Pressure cooker	Few hot and cold spots.	Slow to heat up and cool down.
	No evaporation.	Cumbersome.
	Large number of slides.	Potentially hazardous to the user.
	Short incubation period at higher boiling point (120°C).	
Waterbath	Low investment needed.	Difficult to control temperature.
	Can perform sub-boiling point incubation.	Not suitable for large numbers of slides.
Automated platform	Walkaway retrieval followed by staining.	Expensive.
	Faster standardization of protocol.	Limited flexibility in optimizing retrieval time and buffer pH.
	User safety.	
	Very little inter-user variability.	
	Software to track workloads.	

Hydrolysis of bonds produced by formaldehyde

It is known that formaldehyde produces bonds between amino groups in tissue, as well as inducing the formation of methylene bridges, both of which are covalent in nature. The latter are more easily reversed but it is thought that heat and aqueous liquid together can break even the bonds between amino groups.

The pH of the incubating medium is known to have an effect on the degree of epitope unmasking, some being better revealed with acidic or with basic solutions. Again, the underlying mechanism is unclear but it seems likely that dependence on a particular pH is due at least in part to the amino acid constitution of each epitope.

Key Point

It has been proposed that 0.05% citraconic anhydride (2-methylmaleic anhydride) at pH 7.4 is the 'universal' antigen retrieval solution for the majority of antibodies, due to its ability to combine reversibly with amino groups and break the bonds between the formaldehyde-derived carbon atoms and nitrogen atoms in the protein molecules.

Metal cations

Early work in the field of antigen retrieval involved solutions containing metal salts such as zinc sulphate, lead thiocyanate, and aluminium chloride. These metal cations are protein coagulants but are not features of modern antigen retrieval methods as the conformational changes they produce in proteins are unpredictable and may counteract the heat-induced unmasking effects of the buffer.

Chaotropic effects

Water molecules cluster into groups of 280 molecules that have the ability to shift between an expanded and collapsed structure. In collapsed form the space between clusters is greater and allows more macromolecules to dissolve, but smaller molecules or ions in solution alter the equilibrium between the expanded and collapsed form—the term chaotrope (literally, disorder maker) refers to a solute that favours the latter. Chaotropic ions such as thiocyanate and molecules such as urea provoke the change from an expanded to a collapsed state, possibly allowing fixed proteins in a tissue section to be made to resemble proteins in solution, with a concomitant increase in epitope visibility.

Calcium chelation

Citrate buffer and EDTA solutions are the preferred retrieval medium for many antigens. The role of the citrate anion is primarily to stabilize the pH of the solution, but it will also form a soluble complex with calcium ions. EDTA also has a powerful chelating effect, and both of these anions are present in many decalcifying solutions. Their role in antigen retrieval is thought to be based on an ability to buffer the pH—thereby controlling protein hydrolysis—and remove Ca^{2+} from the tissue.

> ### Key Point
> A chelating agent reacts with a metal ion in solids or liquids, forming a compound of stable, unreactive and soluble rings of covalently bonded atoms.

Some antigen-antibody interactions are known to be inhibited by Ca^{2+} ions. One suggestion is that tissue-derived calcium bonds with protein side-chains and also with bound hydroxymethylene groups derived from formaldehyde, and therefore chelation improves epitope retrieval by removing the inhibitory calcium from the tissue.

It seems likely that the mechanism(s) of antigen retrieval will never be fully understood, but that it is likely to be a combination of all the factors discussed above. However, the key element, heat, remains universal throughout all the theories, both in facilitating the hydrolysis of the covalent bonds and methylene bridges induced by formaldehyde, and in speeding any chemical reactions between buffer constituents and protein residues in the tissue at the selected pH. The significant buffers are listed for reference in Table 8.5.

TABLE 8.5 Summary of key retrieval buffer solutes and suggested mechanisms of action.

Buffer solute	Suggested mechanism of action	Comments
Zinc sulphate (1%)	Zinc cation coagulates proteins.	Early work only—no longer studied.
Lead thiocyanate (1%)	Lead cation coagulates proteins (plus chaotropic effect).	Effective with tissue fixed in Bouin and methacarn.
Citrate (pH 6; 1 mol/L)	Control of pH, calcium chelation.	Most effective in routine use for a wide range of antigens.
Tris (pH 9, pH 10; 0.05 mol/L)	Alkaline protein hydrolysis.	Retrieval of over-fixed antigens when pH 6 citrate is ineffective.
EDTA (pH 8; 0.001 mol/L)	Calcium chelation.	Works best with pressure cooker.
Citraconic anhydride	Thought to reverse formaldehyde fixation by breaking carbon–nitrogen bonds.	Proposed 'universal' retrieval medium, as yet untested.

8.6 Immunocytochemistry detection methods

Affinity

A measure of the binding strength between an epitope and its specific antibody binding site.

Avidity

The combining strength of an antibody with its antigen is directly related to both the affinity of the antibody–antigen interaction and the valency of the antibody and antigen.

Polyclonal antibodies

These are produced by different antibody-producing cells and as such will be different in terms of how they recognize the various epitopes to which they are raised.

Monoclonal antibodies

These are the product of a single clone of chimaeric cells formed from an antibody-producing B cell and a myeloma cell line, and are immunologically identical and will react with the specific epitope to which they are raised.

Antibody titre

The highest dilution of an antibody that results in the maximum intensity and specificity of the final reaction product with minimal background staining.

Antibody dilution

Determined by antibody titre evaluation. Antibodies may be provided with recommendations for dilution or may be provided as ready-to-use (RTU) reagents. This should be viewed as a guide only, as antibody dilution may not be optimal and will depend on a host of variables.

Antibody label

A compound, usually an enzyme such as peroxidase, attached to the final linking complex, which reacts to allow the visualization of a final reaction product at the site of the antigen–antibody reaction.

Developments in ICC have led to the increasing sensitivity of labelling systems so that lower levels of antigen can be demonstrated, with the ultimate goal of complementing cellular and tissue analysis with molecular information.

The principles behind all these techniques are fundamentally quite simple. It is a question of physical chemistry. Ideally, the larger the final reaction product the more obvious it is under the microscope. The more layers of antibody with associated enzyme **labels** that can be attached to the binding site via the target antigen and the primary antibody, the larger the final reaction product will be. The more layers in the sandwich, or the more label molecules attached to each layer, the more appealing the end product will appear to be. If we replace the word 'appealing' with 'improved sensitivity' we have a workable analogy. Equally important, however, is antibody **affinity** and **avidity**.

Antibodies belong in the immunoglobulin (Ig) family of proteins and are present in all immunized animals. There are five major Ig classes (IgG, IgA, IgM, IgD and IgE), each of which is composed of two heavy (H) and two light (L) chains. It is the H chain that differs from class to class and determines structural properties. The L chain is designated either kappa (κ) or lambda (λ). In terms of ICC antibodies, most are derived from IgG and a few from IgM. Digestion techniques reveal that cleavage of the N-terminal side of the inner H-chain disulphide bridges results in the formation of three fragments, two monovalent antigen binding (Fab) fragments and one crystalline fragment (Fc). See Figure 8.4.

It is worth considering in a little more detail the two key forms of antibody: **polyclonal** and **monoclonal**.

An understanding of the structural features of antibodies will be essential in the following section on methods of labelling in ICC.

All current commercially produced detection systems have been optimized for use on FFPE tissue. However, earlier systems were also widely used on frozen sections and to this day direct immunofluorescence labelling is still used on frozen tissue. The most important factors to consider with a primary antibody are the **antibody titre** and **antibody dilution**.

8.6.1 Direct ICC method

Direct ICC is the very earliest technique and relies on an enzyme-labelled primary antibody. It is a one-step procedure in which antibody binds to antigen and the final reaction is visualized by the appropriate substrate–chromogen reaction.

This technique is limited in terms of sensitivity and is simply not adequate for work with FFPE tissue (Figure 8.5).

8.6.2 Indirect ICC method

Indirect ICC is a two-step procedure. First, an unconjugated primary antibody is applied and binds to the antigen if present. The tissue section is then rinsed in a buffer, usually Tris-buffered saline (TBS) or phosphate-buffered saline (PBS), often at neutral pH. A second enzyme-labelled antibody, raised against the primary antibody, is then applied. If the primary antibody binds to the secondary antibody, a two-layered complex is produced, which can be visualized using the appropriate substrate–chromogen final reaction product. This procedure is more sensitive than the direct method as more secondary antibodies are likely to react with different epitopes of the primary antibody, thus amplifying the signal as more enzyme molecules will be attached to the target site. See Figure 8.6.

At this point, mention should be made of IMF methods. These continue to be used for diagnostic purposes in the fields of skin and renal pathology. The methodology involves the direct technique for analysis of tissue samples and the indirect technique for determination of circulating antibody in patients' serum. The enzyme link is replaced with a fluorochrome compound; for example, in single fluorescence techniques it is fluorescein isothiocyanate, which emits green light when excited with the correct wavelength of light. Fluorochromes have the property of absorbing light of one colour (wavelength) and then emitting light of a different colour. This characteristic enables the compounds

(a) Immunoglobulin structure

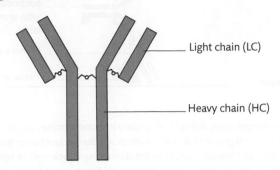

— Light chain (LC)

— Heavy chain (HC)

(b) Immunoglobulin molecule

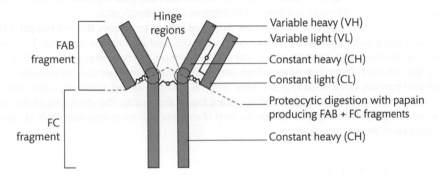

Hinge regions

FAB fragment

FC fragment

— Variable heavy (VH)
— Variable light (VL)
— Constant heavy (CH)
— Constant light (CL)
— Proteocytic digestion with papain producing FAB + FC fragments
— Constant heavy (CH)

(c) IgM immunoglobulin molecule

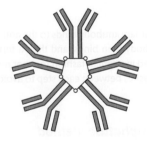

FIGURE 8.4
a) Basic antibody structure, b) IgG antibody structure, c) IgM antibody structure.

Immunocytochemistry staining methods

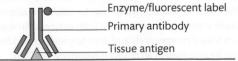

— Enzyme/fluorescent label
— Primary antibody
— Tissue antigen

FIGURE 8.5
Direct ICC technique.

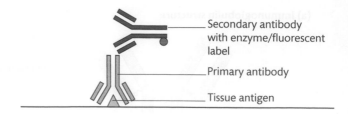

FIGURE 8.6
Indirect ICC technique.

to glow or fluoresce. In most cases, IMF is used to study immune complex deposition along the basement membrane of the renal glomerulus or at the dermoepidermal junction in the skin. Fluorescence detection may fade with continued exposure to the stimulating wavelength of light (photobleaching) or prolonged storage, or samples may develop background fluorescence (autofluoresence) again with increased storage. Sections are therefore stored in the dark or are photographed to preserve a permanent record. Immunofluorescence remains popular because it is a simple and effective method, if performed properly. Propidium iodide or DAPI can be used as an orange or blue counterstain, respectively, to identify the cell nuclei and therefore facilitate structural identification.

Despite the relative lack of sensitivity of the direct and indirect techniques, IMF still compares favourably with paraffin-processed ICC techniques in skin and renal autoimmune pathology. The most likely explanation for this is that the antigenicity of IMF specimens is better preserved than in FFPE tissue. Specimens are often either delivered fresh directly to the laboratory or are transported in Michel's transport medium, which helps to preserve the antigenic epitopes. Indeed, specimens can be stored for long periods in this medium without significant loss of antigenicity. Therefore, despite the improved sensitivity offered by ICC methods, the level of antigenicity is lower than that in IMF samples, due to fixation and processing effects.

8.6.3 Three-step methods

There are several variations on the three-step method. Essentially, a larger complex is produced for visualization by virtue of the presence of the three layers.

Peroxidase–antiperoxidase method

In the peroxidase–antiperoxidase (PAP) method the primary antibody binds to the antigenic epitope, a secondary antibody raised against the primary antibody then binds, and then a tertiary enzyme-labelled PAP complex is applied, which can be visualized in a similar fashion to other methods.

It is important to realize the importance of buffer washes between each step to avoid non-specific antibody binding.

Alkaline phosphatase–anti-alkaline phosphatase method

The alkaline phosphatase–anti-alkaline phosphatase (APAAP) method is similar in many ways to the PAP method above. The first and third layers of antibody must be produced in the same animal species. The linking secondary antibody is directed against immunoglobulins of the species producing the primary and tertiary layers. The secondary antibody is applied in excess and one of the Fab sites binds to the primary antibody, leaving the second site open to bind with the tertiary immune complex.

Both peroxidase and alkaline phosphatase occur naturally in many cell types. In order to ensure that cells already containing the enzyme used as the final reaction product do not produce a 'false-positive' reaction, it is important to block these pre-existing enzymes. In peroxidase-based systems, this 'quenching' or 'blocking' is achieved using a 3% methanol/hydrogen peroxidase step, while in the case of alkaline phosphatase this is achieved using 5 mmol/L levamisole in the substrate solution. Another consideration is the final reaction product, which may be soluble in alcohol; however, there are alcohol-fast and alcohol-soluble chromogens available for both enzymes. An appropriate counterstain is Mayer's haemalum, which is used progressively and does not need to be differentiated in acid/alcohol. If necessary, sections can be mounted in an aqueous mounting medium.

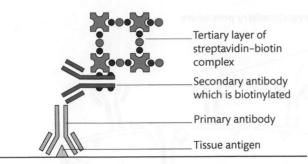

Tertiary layer of streptavidin–biotin complex

Secondary antibody which is biotinylated

Primary antibody

Tissue antigen

FIGURE 8.7
StABC technique.

Avidin–biotin methods

The rationale behind the avidin–biotin methods is the fact that avidin (derived from chicken's egg) or streptavidin (derived from *Streptomyces avidinii*) have a strong affinity for the vitamin co-factor biotin. Avidin and streptavidin have four binding sites for biotin. The primary antibody is applied, followed by a secondary biotinylated antibody raised against the primary. The tertiary layer consists of either an avidin–biotin complex (ABC) or a streptavidin–biotin complex (StABC). The most commonly used enzyme labels are horseradish peroxidase or alkaline phosphatase. The tertiary complex has the ability to capture numerous enzyme molecules, resulting in a larger final reaction product and therefore much greater sensitivity than other methods.

Variations on the ABC method include the labelled avidin–biotin (LAB) method and the labelled streptavidin–biotin (LSAB) method.

The one significant drawback with biotin-based systems is the fact that endogenous biotin is present in a wide variety of tissue, and high levels are found in the liver, kidney, and paracortical histiocytes in lymphoid tissue. This can be blocked by sequential 10–20-minute incubations of sections with 0.01–0.1% avidin, followed by 0.001–0.01% biotin prior to performing the ICC procedure. See Figure 8.7.

An amplification step based on the use of tyramide has gained limited popularity when used in conjunction with StABC systems. Various names have been given to this amplification process, such as catalysed signal amplification (CSA) or tyramide signal amplification. The rationale is essentially the same and is based on the fact that phenolic compounds can become oxidized to highly reactive and unstable intermediates (free radicals) that have a very short half-life. The phenolic compound is biotinylated tyramide, which, when added to the StABC complex, becomes catalysed by the peroxidase enzymes on the bound antibodies to form insoluble biotinylated phenols. These short half-life compounds must bind almost instantly to the tissue surface at the site of their production. Deposited biotin then reacts with the StABC complex to produce a much larger final reaction product at the primary antibody binding site. The end result is a 50-fold increase in sensitivity over conventional StABC methods (Figure 8.8).

CSA immunocytochemistry procedure

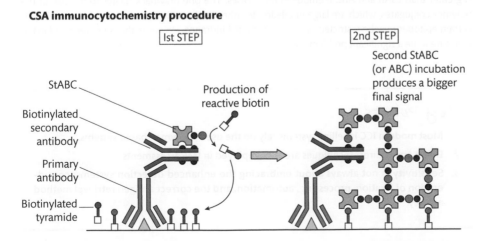

1st STEP

StABC

Biotinylated secondary antibody

Primary antibody

Biotinylated tyramide

Production of reactive biotin

2nd STEP

Second StABC (or ABC) incubation produces a bigger final signal

FIGURE 8.8
CSA amplifications.

Polymer-based immunocytochemistry procedure

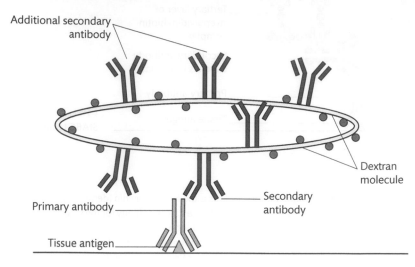

FIGURE 8.9
Polymer technique.

Polymer-based methods

Polymer-based systems are now the most widely used methods in ICC. These systems rely on a concept that involves the use of a polymer backbone that permits multiple antibodies and enzyme molecules to be conjugated, an early example being the enhanced polymer one-step system (EPOS). However, this has been superseded by two-step and enhanced polymer methods. An alternative and more commonly used option is to produce a polymer backbone that contains only enzyme molecules, which can react with secondary antibodies and which are universal in that they contain anti-mouse and anti-rabbit Ig specificity. This universal second layer therefore permits use with both monoclonal and polyclonal antibodies and gives the user greater flexibility.

The major advantage of this system is that it does not involve the use of biotin and therefore avoids the need for elaborate blocking steps. It is also apparent that polymer-based systems are faster to perform than StABC methods simply because there are often fewer steps or layers. The primary antibody incubation is followed by the polymer with the conjugated anti-rabbit and anti-mouse secondary antibodies and attached multiple enzyme molecules. The sensitivity of these methods is greater than LSAB and ABC methods in most cases. The one drawback relates to the size of the polymer conjugates, which are large in relation to other final reaction products, and accessibility to certain epitopes may be restricted as a result of steric hindrance. However, this is not reported in the literature to be a significant problem (Figure 8.9).

Key Points

1. Most modern ICC labelling systems rely on the use of polymer-based systems.

2. Direct and indirect techniques are still employed in IMF assessments.

3. Sensitivity is not always about embracing the enhanced detection systems; consideration of fixation, processing, automation, and the correct antigen retrieval method are key.

8.7 Automation in immunocytochemistry

The development of automation in ICC has expanded exponentially over the past 10 years and this has been complemented by advances in detection system technology. The key driver for expansion in automation has been increasing workload. In many large histopathology departments in the UK, ICC workload has increased five-fold, on average. Although much of this increase is due to demands made on the routine ICC service, it is also true to say that the expansion and increasing complexity of ICC testing has had a significant impact. In addition to the increasing number of antibodies available for diagnostic use, there is now greater scope for application due to improved antigen retrieval methods and a wider range of ICC tests that can be performed on the same machine.

Most modern automated machines permit these tests to be performed on the same platform. With the advent of automation, laboratories have had to consider not only work volume, but also staff skill mix, cost implications and ICC turnaround times. The benefits of automation are that, once standardized, automated procedures allow for greater reproducibility, encompassing standardization of all the critical steps in the staining process. It provides slide reading and reagent management systems, and options for continuous flow automation, so that urgent ICC cases can be loaded at any time during an analyser run.

Onboard antigen retrieval is standard for the more up-to-date automated platforms. Many of the new machines also offer an integrated IT system for monitoring workflow and audit purposes. These systems have freed the biomedical scientist from performing some of the more labour-intensive and tedious pipetting and multiple washing steps required by manual ICC staining.

Some of these developments have involved a 'closed system' approach, and are generally used by clinical laboratories where specific antibodies and associated protocols have been pre-defined for the automated platform being used. This may restrict choice and has the added risk of increasing test costs. On the other hand, it does ensure optimal performance; as such equipment is often tailored for use with dedicated reagents.

Automated staining platforms described as being 'open systems' are mainly used by research laboratories where greater flexibility in staining procedures are required.

Furthermore, certain automated systems are capable of running multiple staining procedures simultaneously, including double labelling and *in situ* hybridization methods, and therefore offers full versatility. With all automation options there is a caveat: all parameters and performance will be determined and established by the operator, and therefore optimization of the final product will be determined by the skill of the biomedical scientist.

A laboratory must therefore consider numerous points that they would like to achieve when deciding to implement an automated platform into their laboratory.

Key Points

1. Automation in ICC has arisen as a result of increasing workload and advances in the complexity and range of ICC tests now available.

2. Benefits include slide reading and reagent management, onboard antigen retrieval, integrated IT systems, continuous flow automation, and options for digital image capture and transfer.

3. Optimization of the final product will be determined by the skill of the biomedical scientist.

8.8 Quality control and immunocytochemistry

As with all diagnostic laboratory investigations, quality control (QC) is critical to the process. Quite simply, without it there is little validity to the test. The use of controls in ICC provides a tool to establish whether or not substandard results have been achieved and therefore help to determine if the test should be deemed invalid and repeated. Adequate QC provides a benchmark of performance and more significantly acts as a guide to staff members, both scientific and medical, who asses the end result. The reasons for substandard ICC performance are multifactorial: fixation parameters, processing issues, temperature, and pH variation all have cumulative effects on the result achieved. As control material should be prepared under optimal conditions, it can be regarded as an accurate indicator of test performance. Control sections allow the user to evaluate failures objectively, narrowing the field of investigation to pinpoint specific failings in any given procedure. Controls for ICC fall into two groups:

- The reagents used, which can be positive and negative.
- Use of tissues, which again can be positive and negative, but also internal.

In evaluating the primary antibody, the user should establish the optimal dilution by first employing a range of tissue known to contain the target antigen. In addition, the specificity of the antibody can be addressed in a number of ways. Replacing the antibody with an affinity absorbed antiserum or Ig fraction will mean that the primary antibody will be absorbed by highly purified antigen and therefore produce a negative test result, proving the specificity of the primary. This method can also be applied to the secondary antibody. In practical terms, however, as affinity purified antigen is hard to obtain, most laboratories will use either an Ig fraction from the same species as the primary or omit the primary and replace it with buffer. This last method is the most widely applied means used to determine the specificity of primary monoclonal antibodies.

Although determination of the primary antibody dilution factor and specificity is the fundamental requirement, the user should also take precautions to ensure that all buffers used for dilution, antigen retrieval, or washing are optimal. All can contribute to undesirable non-specific background staining or weak specific staining.

Tissue controls can be positive, internal or negative. In most cases, normal tissue should be used for tissue controls. In the case of the positive tissue control, fixation and processing should be optimized and be comparable to that used to prepare the test material. In doing so, complete standardization of these variables will have been established and this will permit the optimization of the final staining outcome. The most commonly used normal tissues include lymph node or appendix as they are suitable for the application for a wide range of antibodies. Such material will also allow some assays to demonstrate a spectrum of staining (from weak to strong) according to the presence of the epitope and will allow the assessment of sensitivity as well as specificity (Figure 8.10).

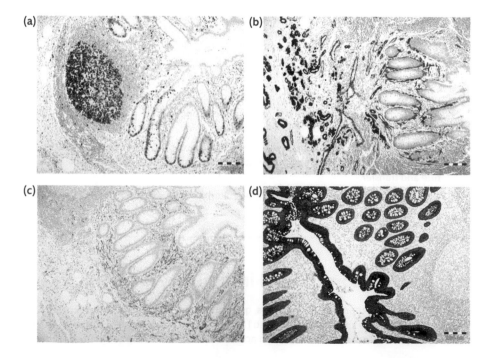

FIGURE 8.10
Appendix a) Ki67/MIB1.
b) Smooth muscle action
(SMA). c) CD56. d) Cytokeratin
MNF116.

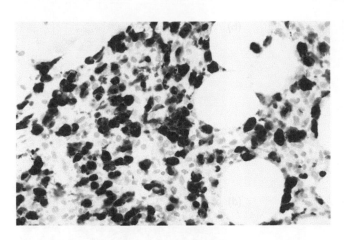

FIGURE 8.11
CD246 (ALK-1)-positive labelling.

Some laboratories prefer the use of the multi-block concept to positive tissue controls. Such blocks contain small portions of a wide range of tissue types (e.g. lymph node, appendix, muscle, pancreas, kidney, skin, etc.). This increases the options for use with a wider assortment of antibodies. The only drawback is size, as cells containing the antigen under evaluation may be sparse under certain circumstances in very small tissue blocks. In some cases, the use of normal tissue as a positive control material will not be appropriate. An example of this is CD246 (ALK-1), which requires a known nodal large-cell anaplastic CD30-positive lymphoma (Figure 8.11).

Use of multi-block control material may also be appropriate when using antibodies that show a wide selectivity of staining (e.g. S100 protein in malignant melanoma). In such a case the selected material should contain not only S100-positive tumour cells, but also the presence of internal normal target antigen (e.g. nerves and dendritic reticulum cells). A different type of control involves the use of an antibody to, for example, vimentin, as this antigen can be used as an internal control because it is found in most tissue types.

An important point to remember when using tumour material as a control is that malignant tissue may arise from more than one clonal population. Molecular genetic studies indicate that protein expression at the cellular level will vary from one clone to another. This means that ICC may not demonstrate universal expression of antigen throughout the tumour, as some areas may stain less intensely or not at all. Thus, the issue of antigen expression is not necessarily one of sensitivity but more appropriately reflects the lack or variability of protein expression in the tumour cells (Figure 8.12).

This point should be remembered in a control setting and has implications in the use of tissue microarrays (TMAs) or cell lines. In some cases it is necessary to prepare controls composed of tissues

(a) 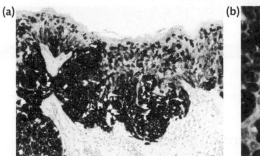 (b)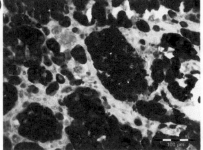

FIGURE 8.12
Superficial spreading malignant melanoma demonstrating double labelling with Melan A (red) and HMB45 (brown). a) Low power, b) high power. Note different proportions of tumour cells labelling with either antibody.

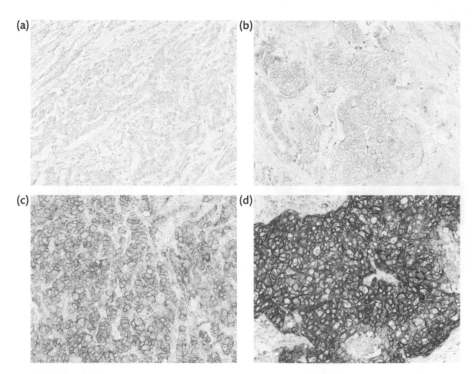

FIGURE 8.13
HER2 staining. a) Negative, b) 1+, c) 2+, d) 3+.

that express the target antigen at various levels, from negative to moderate to strong expression, and three appropriate cell lines on one control slide is ideal for assessment in this context. This approach is adopted with HER2 testing in breast pathology, and enables use of an assessment scoring system that is an absolute test of the technique's sensitivity (Figure 8.13).

Negative tissue controls ideally should indicate the lack of specificity of an antibody or determine the presence of non-specific background staining. The negative tissue control should not contain the specific target antigen under evaluation. If positive staining is achieved, then the results obtained with the test case should be deemed unacceptable and the test should be repeated.

Background staining in ICC can be a common problem and may arise due, for example, to natural variation in antibody production, contamination with unwanted antibody, and cross-reactivity. In addition, variation in Fc receptors, and undesirable hydrophobic, ionic or electrostatic interactions also contribute to the problem of background staining (Table 8.6).

SELF-CHECK 8.3

What causes background staining in ICC?

8.8.1 External quality assessment programmes

External quality assessment (EQA) programmes allows laboratories to make sure that their produced staining is up to the expected standard for the antibody or area of pathology that the user subscribes to. EQA is not solely a means to identify poor performance; more importantly, it is a tool to be used to educate users and improve performance by learning and implementing change to existing practice to meet good laboratory standards.

TABLE 8.6 The main sources of background and other technical problems in ICC with possible remedies.

Cause of technical problem	Preferred remedy
1. Tissue preparation issues, including fixation and processing	
(a) Over-fixation leading to masking of epitopes.	(a) Standardize routine fixation times to achieve desired effect.
(b) Inadequate sampling of tissue or specimen. Poor biopsy technique resulting in tissue damage and the leaching of enzymes and antigens into surrounding tissue.	(b) Apply good biopsy practice. Handle tissue carefully.
(c) Drying tissue before fixation leading to diffuse antigen presence in surrounding tissue.	(c) Immerse tissue in fixative promptly following removal from the patient.
(d) Necrotic areas of tissue result in autolysis, and background staining will be seen with all reagents.	(d) Largely unavoidable. Try to ensure sample tissue also contains viable areas for analysis.
(e) Inadequate permeation of fixative results in unfixed areas with loss of antigenicity.	(e) Slice large specimens and create a 'wick' to ensure fixative reaches deep into the tissue. The larger the sample, the longer the fixation time required.
(f) Excess dehydration during processing reduces antigenicity and causes excessive tissue shrinkage.	(f) Optimize the processing schedule to standardize this variable.
(g) Temperature of wax above 60°C, leading to reduced antigenicity.	(g) Ensure processing temperature does not exceed 60°C.
2. Slide preparation issues	
(a) Section adhesives applied incorrectly, either in excess, leading to undesirable antibody binding to the slide surrounding the section, or too little, resulting in section detachment.	(a) Optimize application of section adhesive and ensure it is adequate for purpose. Use commercially available charged slides. Make sure purchased slides are in date.
(b) Section too thick, resulting in the presence of more than one layer of cells and subsequent difficulties in interpretation.	(b) Sections should be cut at 3–4 μm for routine ICC procedures. Make sure microtome is regularly serviced.
(c) Contaminants picked up from the waterbath (e.g. bacteria or yeasts).	(c) Ensure the waterbath remains clean and the surface is wiped between each block cut.
(d) Sections not dewaxed adequately before ICC, resulting in patching, uneven or no staining.	(d) Optimize dewaxing procedures to ensure appropriate section preparation. Make sure dewaxing solutions if used are changed regularly or as per the supplier's recommendations.
(e) Poor intensity of staining with some antibodies on sections cut and stored for some time before use. Antigenicity of some epitopes in cut sections will 'tail off' with time.	(e) It is best practice to cut sections from blocks as required, and not use stored slides.
3. Antigen retrieval issues	
(a) Inappropriate antigen retrieval, resulting in weak or no staining.	(a) Ensure standard operating procedure (SOP) for antigen retrieval is followed for each antibody used.
(b) Excessive proteolytic digestion, resulting in loss of antigenicity and poor morphology.	(b) Always follow SOP. Use correct times for proteolytic digestion.
(c) Excessive HIER, resulting in loss of antigenicity and inappropriate staining, antigen localization and poor morphology.	(c) As (b) above.
(d) Inappropriate use of HIER buffer system or incorrect pH, resulting in poor antigen retrieval and weak, uneven staining or no staining.	(d) As (b) and (c) above. Ensure pH of retrieval buffer does not drift with time. Make fresh and check regularly.

continued

TABLE 8.6 The main sources of background and other technical problems in ICC with possible remedies. (*Continued*)

Cause of technical problem	Preferred remedy
4. Blocking endogenous enzymes or biotin	
(a) Blocking can affect ICC reactivity (e.g. CD4 with H_2O_2/methanol blocking for endogenous peroxidase).	(a) Reduce length of blocking step if required to improve staining intensity.
(b) Inadequate blocking of cells rich in endogenous peroxidase (e.g. plasma cells, eosinophils) or alkaline phosphatase (e.g. kidney, liver).	(b) Extend blocking steps to overcome this problem or use detection system that best suits the tissue type under investigation.
(c) Endogenous biotin present in tissues (e.g. liver, kidney) can give non-specific staining.	(c) Always use a biotin block if employing an ABC or StABC system. Alternatively, use a polymer detection system.
5. ICC antibody issues	
(a) Substandard primary antibody, resulting in weak or no staining.	(a) Repeat the procedure, checking that the SOP is followed. Refer to the manufacturer's recommendations. If necessary, return the antibody to the manufacturer for assessment.
(b) Inappropriate dilution of the primary antibody, either too dilute, resulting in weak staining, or too strong, leading to excessive non-specific staining.	(b) Follow the manufacturer's guide on dilution and be prepared to perform a checkerboard titration to optimize this variable.
(c) Inappropriate buffers used in substrate–enzyme detection system, resulting in weak, non-specific, or no staining.	(c) Check SOP. Read manufacturer's recommendations. Repeat with freshly prepared reagents.
(d) Detection system sensitivity not adequate to demonstrate antigen present at low levels. This may be due to loss of antigenicity or the fact that the selected antigen is expressed at low levels in a given case.	(d) Use a more sensitive detection system, employ amplification procedures, increase incubation times in the primary antibody, or increase length of antigen retrieval.
(e) Excessive incubation with substrate–chromogen reagents, resulting in excessive non-specific staining.	(e) Reduce the incubation time with the substrate–chromogen reagents.
(f) Inadequate rinsing of slides between antibody incubation steps, leading to non-specific staining.	(f) Always rinse thoroughly between steps with the appropriate rinse buffer. Results will improve with the use of a mild detergent in the buffer.
(g) Hydrophobic and ionic interactions with immunoglobulin and lipid substances can cause undesirable background staining.	(g) This is largely unavoidable.
(h) Binding of the Fc portion by the Fc receptor on the cell surface of cells (e.g. macrophages and some lymphocytes) can cause background staining.	(h) Use F(ab') 2 of Fab fragments for primary and secondary antibodies.
6. Counterstaining issues	
(a) Excessive counterstaining will mask the ICC label.	(a) Ensure counterstaining times are appropriate.
(b) Inappropriate counterstain steps can result in some reaction products being dissolved prior to mounting.	(b) Ensure that the appropriate counterstain is used for the detection system employed.
7. Mounting media	
(a) Inappropriate mounting medium use, resulting in fading of the final reaction product.	(a) Use the appropriate mounting medium for the detection system employed.

In the UK, affiliation to an EQA is now mandatory for all laboratories wishing to obtain UKAS 15189 accreditation (previously Clinical Pathology Accreditation UK [CPA]).

There are a number of external quality assessment (EQA) ICC programmes available such as UK NEQAS ICC & ISH and all diagnostic laboratories in the UK performing ICC must be affiliated to the UK National External Quality Assessment Scheme for Immunocytochemistry and In Situ Hybridization (UK NEQAS ICC & ISH), which is an international accredited assessment scheme with representation from laboratories from around the world. Similar schemes are available in Europe and the USA.

CASE STUDY 8.2 *Anaplastic large cell lymphoma*

A 38-year-old man presented to his GP with a lump in his groin which initially was thought to be a hernia. He was referred to his local hospital, but in the meantime the lump became inflamed and was lanced in the hospital out-patient clinic. The wound failed to heal and a biopsy suggested undifferentiated carcinoma, sarcoma or melanoma, although there was no obvious primary lesion.

A staging computed tomography (CT) scan at another hospital revealed ilio-inguinal node enlargement, and the patient underwent node dissection. The patient subsequently mentioned that he had been suffering from 'drenching night sweats'.

Immunocytochemistry on the original biopsy and subsequent skin and node dissection specimens performed at the referral hospital showed that all markers for carcinoma, sarcoma and melanoma were negative. Haematoxylin and eosin (H&E)-stained sections of the tumour showed sinus infiltration (Figure 8.14) and evidence of hallmark cells with kidney-shaped nuclei (Figure 8.15).

The tumour was positive for the lymphocytic markers CD45RO (Figure 8.16) and CD30 (Figure 8.17), which, combined with the morphological appearances (Figures 8.14 and 8.15), suggested anaplastic large cell lymphoma (ALCL).

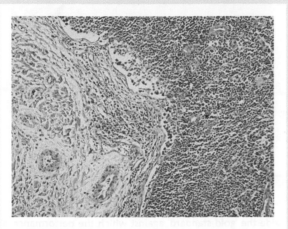

FIGURE 8.14
Sinus involvement.

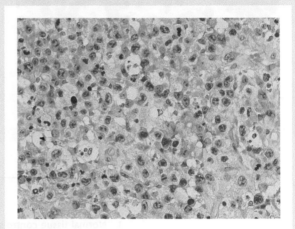

FIGURE 8.15
Hallmark cells.

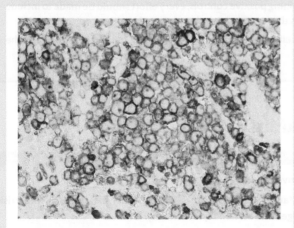

FIGURE 8.16
CD45RO staining.

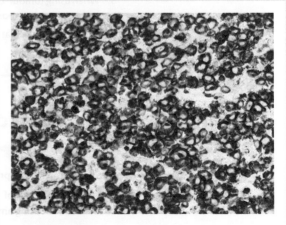

FIGURE 8.17
CD30 staining.

Around 70% of ALCL cases are positive for the marker CD246 (ALK-1), which helps to differentiate this disease from CD30-positive B-cell lymphoma. Figure 8.18 shows the tumour cells staining strongly with CD246 (ALK-1), while Figure 8.19 illustrates the sinus involvement of the tumour.

With regard to prognosis, the three-year progression-free survival rate for ALCL is around 75–80%, which is considerably higher than that for most of the other tumours that comprise the differential diagnosis.

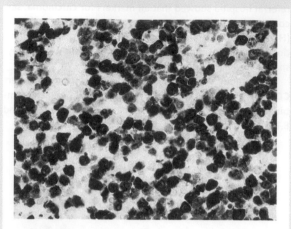

FIGURE 8.18
CD246 (ALK-1) staining.

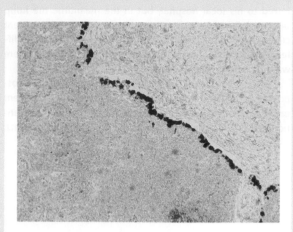

FIGURE 8.19
CD246 (ALK-1) positivity in sinus.

Key Points

1. Normal tissue controls provide the 'gold standard' against which the performance of most antibodies can be assessed.

2. The use of tumour cell lines or tissue microarrays is now mandatory with certain antibodies.

3. When using tumour-containing positive controls, every effort should be made to include normal tissue components that contain intrinsic or internal positive control material.

4. Epitope expression at the cellular level in any given malignant tumour may vary with the sample field.

8.9 Health and safety in the ICC laboratory

HEALTH & SAFETY 8.1

- Always wear personal protective clothing (PPC).
- Always read Control of Substances Hazardous to Health (COSHH) data sheets on the risks associated with using any reagents in immunocytochemistry.
- Always be alert to the dangers of handling hot or boiling buffer systems.
- Always follow the local health and safety regulations and departmental health and safety policies and procedures.

All standard health and safety procedures and policies apply in the ICC laboratory. As many of the reagents used in ICC will be hazardous, it is important to remember the importance of personal protective clothing (PPC) and the use of gloves and goggles if transporting or moving hot buffer fluids. The immunocytochemist should at all times abide by the employer's local health and safety regulations and also the departmental safety policy.

8.10 The value of ICC in multidisciplinary team meetings

Over the past few years there has been significant expansion and development of multidisciplinary team (MDT) meetings to discuss the care of patients who have cancer. This initiative has been driven by the need to improve clinical management, from the point of diagnosis through the clinical management to eventual completion of treatment. Cancer testing turnaround times for pathology departments are now key indicators of performance and are measured accordingly. This has resulted in an increased burden on histopathology staff, as all cases of cancer ideally should be reviewed at MDTs on a regular weekly basis. This involves retrieving slides for presentation to the MDT, with input from pathologists and biomedical scientists. Immunocytochemistry is pivotal in many instances of cancer diagnosis, management and prognosis. In certain areas of pathology, ICC is the main diagnostic tool, a prime example being lymphoma classification where ICC remains the most useful technique in this area of pathology. Standards of quality performance need to be assured and the biomedical scientist must be able to demonstrate and communicate knowledge to this effect at such meetings.

CASE STUDY 8.3 *Lymphoma*

A 64-year-old female, who presented with a lesion on the forehead, had a previous history of mantle cell lymphoma treated with chemotherapy, but subsequently relapsed.

Flow cytometry showed CD3+ T cells as 3% of leucocytes, with B cells as 88% of leucocytes, of which <5% were negative for surface immunoglobulins (sIg). Surface immunoglobulin-positive B cells were monoclonal (kappa-negative and lambda-positive) with the phenotype CD19+, CD5+, CD20+, CD10–, CD23–.

Immunocytochemistry (Figure 8.20) showed a mantle cell lymphoma phenotype with cyclin D1+, CD20+, CD5+, CD3– and CD23–.

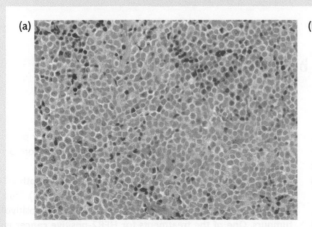

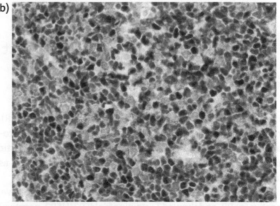

FIGURE 8.20

a) Haematoxylin and eosin stain

b) Cyclin D1-positive

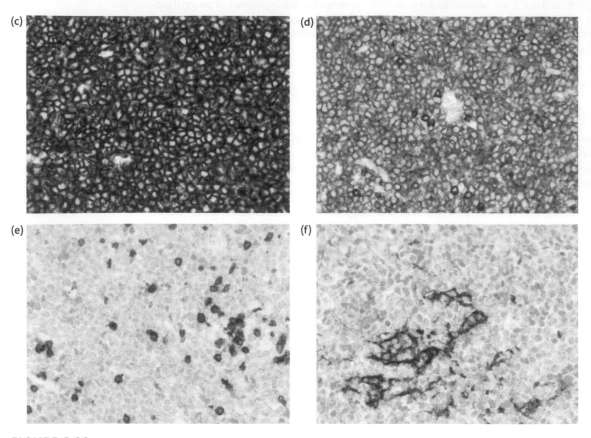

FIGURE 8.20
(*Continued*)

c) CD20-positive

d) CD5-positive

e) CD3-negative; only non-neoplastic T cells are stained

f) CD23-negative; only dendritic cells are stained.

CASE STUDY 8.4 *Breast biomarkers as prognostic and predictive markers*

Immunocytochemistry of breast markers for oestrogen (ER), progesterone (PR) and HER2, along with conventional histopathology (H&E), can be used as predictive and prognostic markers to select patients for specific treatment regimes, as illustrated in the following two patients.

Patient A: Breast tumour found to be very strongly ER-positive, negative for PR, and showed 1+ staining for HER2 (HER2-negative) (Figure 8.21). This patient is quite possibly a good candidate for hormone therapy (e.g. tamoxifen or aromatase inhibitors). The choice of hormone treatment will, however, depend on a number of other factors such as patient age (pre- or postmenopausal) and whether treatment is prescribed before or after surgery.

Patient B: Breast tumour found to be negative for both ER and PR, but strongly positive for HER2 (3+) (Figure 8.22). This patient's tumour is more aggressive than the ER/PR-positive tumours. One of the treatments for HER2-positive cancer is trastuzumab (Herceptin), which may be given in early or metastatic HER2-positive cancers and may be given with chemotherapy, either before or after surgery and radiotherapy.

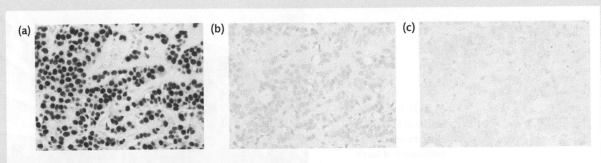

FIGURE 8.21
a) ER-positive; intense nuclear staining in the majority of tumour cells
b) PR-negative; not all ER-positive tumours express PR
c) HER2-negative; very faint HER2 membrane staining but the sample is interpreted as 1+ (negative for HER2).

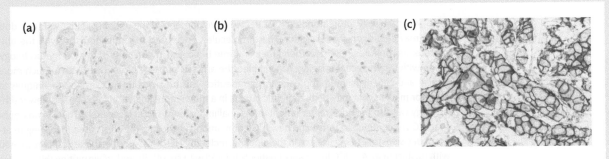

FIGURE 8.22
a) ER-negative
b) PR-negative
c) HER2-positive (3+); there is complete, intense membrane staining in the majority of the tumour cells.

8.11 Future developments in immunocytochemistry

Ever since its earliest introduction as a diagnostic tool, ICC has become an integral element of the diagnostic pathology process. It was one of the first techniques to elevate histopathology to a more analytical platform, and it is in this respect that the introduction of automation has had the biggest impact. It is the global expansion of ICC usage, coupled with the comparative inexpense of the methodology, that has accounted to some extent for its longevity and expansion. The advent of automation has enabled complete hands-free staining, optimal standardization of staining protocols, complete logging systems for the analysis of each step of the procedure, and subsequent options for error logging, and the effect this has had in reducing the impact of human error. The introduction of image analysis, capture and transfer systems has meant that projecting or sending final images for use in national or international meetings is now a realistic option. As mentioned in the opening paragraph of this chapter, ICC has trodden a path for the growing emergence of molecular pathology. It has complemented the developments of *in situ* hybridization and more recently fluorescence *in situ* hybridization (FISH). A glance through the scientific literature provides a clear indication that ICC is still widely used to investigate the pathological process, now often accompanied by molecular-based investigations such as the polymerase chain reaction (PCR), cDNA arrays, and cytogenetics.

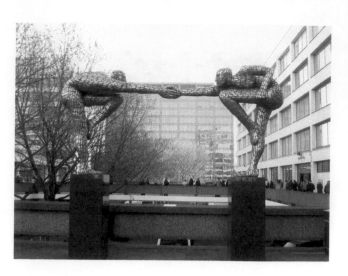

FIGURE 8.23
Statue at St Thomas'
Hospital reflecting the
unification of Guy's
and St Thomas' NHS
Trusts, akin to the
complementary role
of molecular and ICC
techniques.

So, what are likely future trends in ICC? Recent developments in the use of colloidal quantum dots (QDs) may be a significant indicator. These molecules, once used in semiconductors with the ubiquitous fluorophores, have now found their way into biological investigations. This QD methodology, along with hyperspectral imaging, has enabled the analysis of tissue biomarkers with a much more critical and patient-tailored approach to therapeutics. It is now possible to develop techniques to monitor markers that may be therapeutic targets in a much more analytical fashion. This new methodology will also provide greater insight into signalling pathways to assess cancer. There is no doubt that ICC will continue to thrive and new ICC 'companion' diagnostics (ICC tests used in making treatment decisions) are being used or in the pipeline, including HER2 ICC-positive breast cancers treated with trastuzumab, ALK ICC lung cancer patients treated with crizotinib, and, while writing this chapter, novel immunotherapy drugs in the lung setting identified by ICC for programmed cell death antibodies such as PD1 and PDL-1; however, molecular-based techniques seem set to have become the new benchmark for future advances in the understanding of pathology (Figure 8.23).

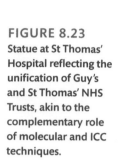 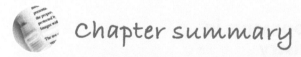

Chapter summary

In summary, the key points to remember are:

- Immunocytochemistry is a widely employed histological technique which can help to differentiate a wide spectrum of cancerous and inflammatory states.

- As techniques, ICC and IMF rely on the use of antibodies raised against specific antigens which, when bound to tissue sections, can be visualized under the microscope using various chromogenic or fluorogenic agents.

- A wide range of labelling techniques are employed in ICC and IMF procedures.

- Immunofluorescence techniques are used largely to assess inflammatory or autoimmune states in the skin and kidney.

- Broadly speaking, antibodies can be classified using the 'cluster of differentiation' (CD) system. This classifies antibodies according to stringent assessments that outline the labelling profiles of each antibody.

- Immunocytochemistry techniques have paved the way for the development of *in situ* and molecular techniques.

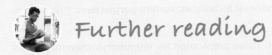

Further reading

● Bobrow MN, Harris TD, Shaughnessy KJ, Litt GJ. Catalyzed reporter deposition, a novel method of signal amplification. Application to immunoassays. *J Immunol Methods* 1989; **125**: 279–85.

● Cattoretti G, Pileri S, Parravicini C *et al.* Antigen unmasking on formalin-fixed paraffin embedded tissue sections. *J Pathol* 1993; **171**: 83–98.

● Chaplin M. *Water structure and behaviour* 2004 (www.lsbu.ac.uk/water/index.html).

● Coons AH, Leduc EH, Connolly JM. Studies on antibody production: a method for the demonstration of specific antibody and its application to the study of the hyperimmune rabbit. *J Exp Med* 1955; **102**: 49–60.

● Dabbs DJ. *Diagnostic immunohistochemistry: Theranostic and genomic applications*, 4th edn. Chichester, Elsevier, 2013.

● Hsu SM, Raine L, Fanger H. Use of avidin–biotin peroxidase (ABC) in immunoperoxidase techniques: a comparison between ABC and unlabeled antibody (PAP) procedures. *J Histochem Cytochem* 1981; **29**: 577–80.

● Institute of Biomedical Science. *Training logbook for the diploma of expert practice in immunocytochemistry*. London: Institute of Biomedical Science, 2006.

● Jasani B, Morgan JM, Navabi H. Mechanism of high temperature antigen retrieval: role for calcium chelation. *Histochem J* 1997; **29**: 433.

● Medintz IL, Mattoussi H, Clapp AR. Potential clinical applications of quantum dots. *Int J Nanomed* 2008; **3**: 151–67.

● Namimatsu S, Ghazizadeh M, Sugisaki Y. Reversing the effects of formalin fixation with citraconic anhydride and heat: a universal antigen retrieval method. *J Histochem Cytochem* 2005; **53**: 3–11.

● Norton AJ, Jordan S, Yeomans P. Brief, high-temperature heat denaturation (pressure cooking): a simple and effective method of antigen retrieval for routine processed tissues. *J Pathol* 1994; **173**: 371–9.

● Orchard G. Immunocytochemical techniques and advances in dermatopathology. *Curr Diagn Pathol* 2006; **12**: 292–302.

● Orchard G. The use of positive controls in immunocytochemistry—some indicators of what is appropriate and what is not! *Immunocytochemistry* 2007; **6**: 11–12.

● Orchard G. Detecting antigenic epitopes using immunocytochemistry in tumour pathology—is it really all about sensitivity? *Immunocytochemistry* 2008; **6**: 116–18.

● Pluzek KJ *et al.* A major advance for immunocytochemistry: enhanced polymer one-step staining (EPOS). *J Pathol* 1993; 169 (Suppl.): Abstr. 220.

● Sabattini E, Bisgaard K, Ascani S, Poggi S, Piccioli M, Ceccarelli C. The Envision system: a new immunohistochemical method for diagnostics and research. Critical comparison with the APAAP, ChemMate, CSA, LABC, and SABC techniques. *J Clin Pathol* 1998; **51**: 506–11.

● Sahni D, Robson A, Orchard G *et al.* The use of LYVVE-1 antibody for detecting lymphatic involvement in patients with malignant melanoma of known sentinel lymph node status. *J Clin Pathol* 2005; **58**: 715–21.

● Shi SR, Key ME, Kalra KL. Antigen retrieval in formalin-fixed, paraffin-embedded tissue: an enhancement method for immunohistochemical staining based on microwave oven heating of tissue sections. *J Histochem Cytochem* 1991; **39**: 741–8.

- Shi SR, Cote RJ, Taylor CR. Antigen retrieval techniques: current perspectives. *J Histochem Cytochem* 2001; **49**: 931–7.

- Williams JH, Mepham BL, Wright DH. Tissue preparation for immunocytochemistry. *J Clin Pathol* 1997; **50**: 422–8.

 Discussion questions

8.1   What is meant by the terms sensitivity and specificity in immunocytochemistry (ICC)?

8.2   What is the meaning of the abbreviation CD, and how is it employed in classifying antibody characteristics?

8.3   What are the key areas of application for ICC in histopathology?

8.4   What is meant by the term antigen retrieval and what are the key methods used to achieve it in ICC?

8.5   What is meant by the term chromogen in ICC?

8.6   List the main ICC labelling systems currently available.

8.7   Explain internal quality control and external quality assessment in ICC.

8.8   What are the advantages of automated ICC in the modern laboratory?

Answers to the self-check questions and tips for responding to the discussion questions are provided on the book's accompanying website:

 Visit www.oup.com/uk/orchard2e

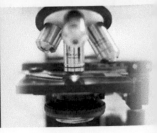

9

Analytical immunocytochemistry

Guy Orchard, David Muskett and Anne Warren

Learning objectives

After studying this chapter, you should be able to:

- Discuss the difference between benign and malignant cells.

- Discuss the features of the key malignant tumour groups.

- List the most common forms of cancer.

- Describe the difference between *in situ* and invasive disease.

- Discuss the use of the key antibodies for diagnostic use.

- Describe the use of the key antibodies in the investigation of breast cancer.

- Describe the use of the key antibodies in lung cancer.

- Describe the use of immunocytochemistry (ICC) in the investigation of lymphoma.

- Discuss how ICC can contribute to the identification of tumours of an unknown primary malignancy.

- Discuss the role of ICC in the investigation of autoimmune skin disease.

- Discuss the complementary role of ICC in a diagnostic setting.

- Comprehend the role of ICC in the strategy of patient management targeted therapies.

9.1 Introduction

In the previous chapter you will have read about immunocytochemistry (ICC) as a laboratory technique. You will have learned about the technical aspects of the procedures involved and the key issues to consider. The key terms and definitions should now be familiar to you.

In this chapter we build on this in order to consider how the technique can be employed in the investigation of pathological states.

Key Point

Immunocytochemistry has a major role in the diagnosis of malignancy, but also contributes to the investigation of other types of pathological condition.

Despite the ever-advancing role of molecular techniques in pathology, ICC remains widely popular and extensively used. Indeed, in certain significant areas of histopathology it remains the key investigative technique. An example in point will be lymphoma classification. Why ICC remains the most popular investigative technique in histopathology, and why its longevity has spanned five decades when so many other techniques have faded, may be explained in the following list:

- As a technique, ICC is remarkably sensitive and specific. Advances in antigen retrieval procedures and the development of ever more sensitive detection systems have ensured that the technique continues to expand its role in histopathology.

- It is a consistent and highly reproducible procedure that can be taught and mastered with dedicated training. In essence, ICC is a technique that can be standardized relatively easily.

- It does not rely on fresh tissue and is therefore useful for retrospective studies. This means that it can be employed on archival material. In reality, arguably it is more successful than molecular methods because such procedures are more susceptible to variations in fixation and processing, which can result in an inability to amplify DNA sequences successfully.

- As a technique, ICC represents an almost limitless opportunity to study almost any antigen at the light microscope level. This is due to the fact that the principle of the methodology in linking an antibody to a chromogen molecule is almost boundless in its application. As new antigenic molecules are identified so new antibodies can be raised to identify their presence, distribution and association with any given pathological state.

- As a technique, ICC complements molecular investigations. It enables the identification of protein expression in any population of cells at the light microscope level, which can then be used in tandem with molecular techniques to determine genetic defects.

- In recent years there has been an increased ability to quantify the final reaction products produced from ICC studies. A good example of this is the quantification of prognostic marker expression in tumour pathology.

- In real terms, ICC is a highly cost-effective investigative technique. With the increasing use of automated platforms, the 'cost per slide' has invariably been driven downwards as workloads increase and increased volumes have resulted in more competitive reagent or equipment rental packages.

SELF-CHECK 9.1

What features make immunocytochemistry a valuable tool to aid diagnosis?

9.2 Key principles in the diagnostic use of immunocytochemistry

The key principles of ICC can be listed thus:

- Tissue morphology remains the key diagnostic tool despite the use of ICC.

- No marker is perfect and thus diagnosis by a single marker is not valid without correlation to the H&E.

- The correlation of ICC results, H&E findings, and clinical history is essential for high-quality patient management.
- Immunocytochemistry is a tool within an interpretive science.

9.3 Reasons for immunocytochemical investigations

There are many reasons for ICC investigation, the key ones being:

- Confirmation of tumour type suspected on H&E.
- Identification of adjacent tumour spread.
- Identification of distant metastases.
- Confirmation of tumour subtype.
- Identification of tumours of unknown aetiology.
- Predictive information about the likely response of the tumour to drug treatment, and subsequent changes to patient drug regimes and therefore overall patient management.
- Evaluation of inflammatory states and autoimmune diseases.
- Identification of aetiological agents.

9.4 What is malignancy?

Malignancy is defined by a change in the normal cell biology of cells. It results in an abnormal growth or tumour that can then spread (metastasize) to other body sites. Growths (tumours) that do this are termed malignant. There are genetic alterations within the cells that stimulate both rapid proliferation and atypical maturation.

In contrast, however, sometimes tumours may grow locally and not spread (metastasize) to other parts of the body and are termed benign. See Figures 9.1 and 9.2.

Key Points

Benign tumours are characterized by slow growth patterns and are localized to the original site of production, growing by expansion rather than invasion.
Malignant tumours grow rapidly and will often metastasize.

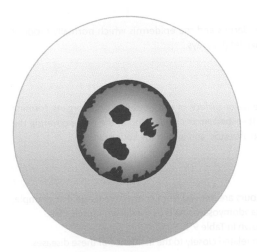

FIGURE 9.1
A normal cell. The nucleus is relatively small compared to the cytoplasm and has a smooth edge. Chromatin is discretely clumped.

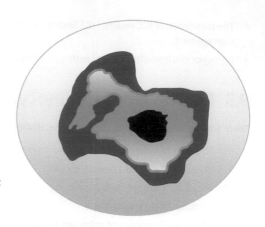

FIGURE 9.2
A malignant cell. The nucleus is larger and has an irregular edge. There is a prominent nucleolus (mauve) and the chromatin shows irregular clumping.

SELF-CHECK 9.2

What differences can be seen on routine histopathology between a benign cell and a malignant cell?

9.5 Introduction to tumour groups

Within histopathology there are recognized key malignant tumour groups. Broadly speaking, these include the following types.

9.5.1 Carcinoma

These tumours are malignant and are derived from cells of epithelial origin (e.g. squamous cell carcinoma). A variation of this group is adenocarcinoma, a tumour derived from glandular epithelium (e.g. gastrointestinal tract or breast).

9.5.2 Lymphoma

These are derived from lymphoid tissue (e.g. Hodgkin's disease). Variations include leukaemia, a tumour derived from haemopoietic elements that arise from blood cells, but which can form solid tumour masses (e.g. chronic lymphocytic leukaemia [CLL] or acute lymphoblastic leukaemia [ALL]).

9.5.3 Melanoma

A cancer of melanocytes, cells present in the dermis and the epidermis which normally produce pigment to protect the skin from harmful ultraviolet (UV) rays.

9.5.4 Mesothelioma

Mesothelioma

A cancer of mesothelial cells that line internal body cavities. Most cases of mesothelioma are related to exposure to asbestos.

A cancer of mesothelial cells, which cover the outer surface of most internal body organs, forming a lining sometimes called the mesothelium. **Mesotheliomas** can develop in the tissue covering the lung (pleura), often associated with exposure to asbestos, and also in the abdomen.

9.5.5 Sarcoma

Generally, although not exclusively, these tumours are derived from connective tissue. For example, liposarcoma is derived from adipose tissue. Rhabdomyosarcoma is derived from muscle cells.

The most common cancers in the UK are shown in Table 9.1.

The workload of the ICC laboratory will thus be related closely to the incidence of these diseases.

TABLE 9.1 The most common types of cancer seen in the UK. Note how the list is dominated by different types of carcinoma (source: CRUK cancer statistics).

Cancer type	Incidence	Main tumour type
Breast	15%	Carcinoma
Lung	13%	Carcinoma
Colorectal	13%	Carcinoma
Prostate	12%	Carcinoma
Non-Hodgkin's lymphoma	4%	Lymphoma
Malignant melanoma	4%	Melanoma
Stomach	3%	Carcinoma
Oral	2%	Carcinoma
Mesothelioma	1%	Mesothelioma

SELF-CHECK 9.3

What are the most common types of cancer?

9.6 Key antibodies used in immunocytochemistry

Many antibodies are available and no laboratory will stock them all. Some are purely for research yet many are used diagnostically.

Carcinomas comprise the largest group of malignancies investigated using ICC, with **cytokeratin** the key molecule for distinguishing different types of epithelium. See Table 9.2.

SELF-CHECK 9.4

How might the use of cytokeratins help in the diagnosis of types of carcinoma?

Cytokeratins

These are structural cytoplasmic proteins expressed in epithelial tissue. Cytokeratins are divided into around 20 categories based on molecular weight.

9.6.1 Cluster of differentiation

In the previous chapter you read about **cluster of differentiation** (CD). In order to appreciate antibody labelling profiles for cell surface molecules, a form of stringent classification is required. In 1982 such a classification system was introduced at the International Workshop and Conference on Human Leucocyte Differentiation Antigens (HLDA). This conference focused on the classification of antibodies raised against epitopes expressed on the surface of leucocytes. This system has since expanded to encompass a host of other cell types. The classification process involves evaluations of data on all aspects of epitope characterization. It allows cells to be defined based on the molecules that are expressed on the cell surface. Any assigned CD number is only given if at least two specific monoclonal antibodies can be shown to bind to the molecule. The CD system is most effectively employed to help establish immunophenotyping of any given population of cells. In effect CD markers on specific cell populations will provide evidence of these cells' immune functions and thus provide evidence for typing/classifying cells. It is this very concept that is employed in diagnostic immunocytochemistry, most significantly in the typing of atypical/pleomorphic and malignant tumour cells. In lymphoma classification ICC still remains the most effective tool in sub-classifying such a wide variety of lymphoma types that exist. Currently, there are around 350 CD numbers in use. The large majority of antibodies used in histopathology are assigned a CD number. At the very least, this classification system enables

Cluster of differentiation (CD)

This represents the characterization and subsequent classification of human leucocyte antigens. The cluster number relates to different antibodies that have been found to have the same specificity as defined by at least two or more antibody-based techniques.

TABLE 9.2 The key cytokeratins used to investigate carcinomas. Note that no single cytokeratin (CK) antibody provides a magic bullet marker to identify a tumour type.

Marker	Normal use	Pathological use	Staining pattern
MNF 116 (CK5, 6, 8, 17 and 19)	**Broad-spectrum cytokeratin** used to identify epithelium. Identifies normal epithelium.	Useful in the primary investigation of carcinoma.	Cytoplasmic
CK 5/6	Recognizes cells expressing cytokeratins 5 and 6. It labels mesothelioma and epithelial cells in prostate (basal cells) and tonsil.	Low-level expression in adenocarcinoma. Can be used to distinguish mesothelioma and adenocarcinoma.	Cytoplasmic
CK 7	Found in columnar and glandular epithelium of the lung, cervix, breast, bile duct, and larger collecting ducts of the kidney. It is present in the urothelium of the bladder, in ovarian and lung epithelia, and occasionally in endothelial cells.	Useful in differentiating the site of origin of poorly differentiated carcinoma in conjunction with other antibodies (e.g. gynae tract adenocarcinomas are usually positive and colonic adenocarcinomas are negative).	Cytoplasmic
Cytokeratin 20	Found on normal gastric and colonic epithelium. Found on bladder urothelium (surface umbrella cells). Reacts with a 46 kDa protein corresponding to cytokeratin 20. Positive in colon and stomach.	Labels most adenocarcinomas of the colon and stomach, and urothelial and Merkel-cell carcinomas. It is mostly negative in squamous cell carcinoma and adenocarcinomas from other sites (e.g. breast, lung and endometrium).	Cytoplasmic

Broad-spectrum cytokeratin

A solution of a number of monoclonal antibodies to cytokeratins. The purpose of a broad-spectrum cytokeratin in diagnosis is to label all tissues that express cytokeratins. This can be useful in the identification of a carcinoma or the extent of invasion.

consistency in defining antigen/antibody binding. It gives assurance that antibodies used with a given CD number have been classified stringently and defined for their labelling characteristics.

9.6.2 CD marker antibodies

As the number of antibodies with CD numbers steadily increases there is an ongoing need to ensure that those antibodies used for diagnostic purposes are the most relevant in any given situation. In reality, it can be a challenge to ensure that any given 'panel' of antibodies used is the best panel to employ, especially in light of the need to interpret all subsequent labelling profiles in a constructive fashion. In reality, many antibodies are never characterized by CD classification but are still employed widely. The majority of these antibodies are often valued in specifically defined areas of pathology. Their popularity often derives from supportive research publications demonstrating their application in selected areas of the discipline.

Immunocytochemistry performed in any histopathology laboratory will not only vary in terms of the technical aspects of how such procedures are performed, but also in the numbers and types of antibody employed in the diagnostic armoury of the service. Appendix 9.1 at the end of this chapter lists some of the most widely employed CD classified antibodies used in diagnostic histopathology. This is not an exhaustive list but it does demonstrate the length and breadth of the system in practice and how it can be used to delineate a wide spectrum of disease processes.

In addition to the list of markers in Appendix 9.1, many more CD markers exist (Appendix 9.2). They are of particular use in the investigation of lymphomas—a very heterogeneous group of tumours.

9.6.3 Other antibodies

Other commonly used antibodies that are not CD markers are outlined in Appendix 9.3 at the end of this chapter.

In what different cellular components can antibodies be detected?

9.7 Use of antibody panels

The use of antibody panels to help define a disease is employed widely. The most important point is an appreciation of the fact that ICC panels aid in making a series of diagnostic decisions that confirm or refute original deductions based on H&E and/or special stains.

Defining what constitutes an appropriate panel of antibodies for a given area of pathology is not always universally clear, the reasons for which fall under three main areas of consideration:

- cost-effectiveness
- consistency and reliability of use
- laboratory-based procedural issues.

9.7.1 Cost-effectiveness

This relies on an appreciation that all antibodies are relatively expensive. In selecting a panel of antibodies, careful consideration of cost is prudent. In addition, purchase of antibodies only rarely used is not always appropriate, and thus referral to another centre may be a better option. Antibodies have a clearly defined shelf-life and appropriate storage of such antibodies is essential. The modern ICC laboratory must employ automated procedures in order to minimize the cost per slide.

9.7.2 Consistency and reliability

This relates to the final results and the fact that some antibodies will work more effectively in one laboratory compared to another. Such variation is well demonstrated by UK NEQAS Immunocytochemistry data for a wide range of diagnostic antibodies. This variation may indicate that in certain hands the results achieved may not be reliable or reproducible.

9.7.3 Laboratory-based procedural issues

These encompass a wide spectrum of factors, most of which have been mentioned in the previous chapter. These would include adequacy of fixation and processing, appropriate antigen retrieval procedures, antibody dilution factors, and issues surrounding the efficiency of antigen–antibody detection systems. An additional variable will be introduced with the use of automated platforms for immunostaining.

Whatever the decision made relating to the composition of an antibody panel, the notion that each panel should contain as many antibodies as possible is not the ideal. This can result in confusing and counter-productive information in certain situations. An ideal panel would include antibodies that are reliable and produce consistent results in a given laboratory. It should be remembered that difficult cases can be referred to specialist centres for more extensive ICC investigations.

Key Point

Immunocytochemistry is a very cost-effective way of typing cancer, producing permanent preparations that can be reviewed and audited at **multidisciplinary team meetings**.

9.7.4 Multidisciplinary team meetings

You will have read about the role of multidisciplinary team meetings in Chapter 1. You will by now understand the role of these meetings with regard to patient management. ICC often provides integral information on tumour typing which is often discussed at such meetings. It involves medical professionals from differing backgrounds and disciplines, including surgeons, nurses, oncologists, radiologists and pathologists who meet to discuss patients and establish a treatment plan. For example, a patient who has a breast cancer diagnosed on a core biopsy will have the results correlated with the radiology and then go forward for surgery to remove the cancer.

9.8 Antibody panels in diagnostic practice

Panels generally are composed of those antibodies that broadly assist in defining cell histogenesis. Malignant disease falls into various groups that can be identified by ICC. In cases where the cancer is of unknown origin, the tumour group can be identified by using just four antibodies: a broad-spectrum cytokeratin, vimentin, S100 and leucocyte common antigen (LCA). See Table 9.3.

TABLE 9.3 **An algorithm to identify the main groups of tumour using just four antibodies.**

	Broad-spectrum cytokeratin	Vimentin	S100	LCA
Carcinoma	+	–	–	–
Lymphoma	–	+	–	+
Melanoma	–	+	+	–
Sarcoma	–	+	±	–
Nerve-derived tumours	–	+	+	–

However, for full elucidation of the source of a tumour, panels of antibodies are used because no single marker is 100% accurate in the identification of a tumour. There are many examples of antibody panels, some of which are listed below:

- cytokeratin(s) and epithelial membrane antigen (EMA), for epithelial derivation
- desmin and smooth muscle actin, for muscle
- CD68 and factor XIIIa, for fibrohistiocytes
- HMB 45 and Melan A, for melanocytes
- FVIII, CD34 and CD31, for endothelial and perivascular cells
- leucocyte common antigen (LCA), CD3, CD20, and CD30 for haematopoietic cells
- neuron-specific enolase (NSE), chromogranin and synaptophysin, for neuroendocrine cells.

Key Point

No single antibody is able to identify a tumour. Diagnosis must be made in conjunction with H&E morphology.

Antibodies which help to classify an undifferentiated malignant tumour may add to information already compiled from a primary panel of antibodies. Examples include the subtyping of a lymphoma into T-cell or B-cell lineage using T-cell-selective antibodies such as CD4 (T-helper) and CD8 (T-cytotoxic), or the B-cell markers CD10 and CD21 (follicular B-cell lymphoma).

Antibody panels may be employed to identify the origin of a tumour, as in the case of cancer that is diagnosed initially by the presence of metastasis. Examples include carcinomas from the colon, stomach, prostate or lung, and panels would include antibodies to selected molecular weight cytokeratins, often in conjunction with tissue or organ-selective markers such as prostate-specific antigen (PSA) or thyroid transcription factor (TTF1).

Panels may also be employed to assist in distinguishing metastatic adenocarcinoma (gross cystic disease fluid protein 15 [GCDFP-15], CK20, CK7, ER, CA125, mesothelin, lysozyme), mesothelioma from carcinoma (B72.3, calretinin, Ber-EP4, placental alkaline phosphatase, carcinoembryonic antigen [CEA], EMA, thrombomodulin), or bladder from prostate carcinoma (PSA, PSAP, CK20, CK7, p63, 34BetaE12).

Some mention of the introduction of antibody cocktails should be made. There is a growing number now available for diagnostic use. As the name implies, they represent a mixture of two or three antibodies in one product. Examples include melanoma cocktails, composed of Melan A, tyrosinase and HMB45; prostate adenocarcinoma cocktails, composed of P504S (α-methylacyl coenzyme A racemase) with p63 and/or 34βE12; breast carcinoma cocktails, composed of ER and GCDFP-15; and endocrine carcinoma cocktails, composed of chromogranin A, synaptophysin and NSE. Many other cocktails are available which have gained some popularity as a result of increased workloads and the attraction of applying a panel approach using one product. They have the advantage of requiring fewer sections, which is useful when tissue is limited, and have relevance in specifically defined areas; they should not necessarily be seen as a primary antibody screen.

SELF-CHECK 9.6

Why are panels of antibodies used rather than a single marker?

9.9 Investigation of breast cancer

Breast cancer is the most common cancer in the UK and is a major contribution to the immunocyto-chemistry workload of most routine laboratories.

CLINICAL CORRELATION

Breast cancer affects mainly women aged 40–70. In the UK, breast cancer is screened by mammography. Women (aged 45–65) are invited to be screened to investigate radiologically suspicious lesions. These are biopsied and sent to the laboratory for investigation.

Investigation of breast disease aims to answer four questions:

- Is it malignant?
- If it is malignant, is it invasive?
- What type of cancer is involved?
- How will the cancer respond to drug therapy, and will the patient be suitable for Herceptin?

The initial investigation of malignancy is undertaken by H&E staining. The key histological features are the presence of abnormal breast ducts and, if identified, myoepithelial cells present within these glands. This indicates *in situ* disease (see Figures 9.3 and 9.4, and Case study 9.1). Absence of myoepithelial cells indicates an invasive component to the disease. The amount of invasion can be as little as a single breast duct, so the sample provided makes a huge difference to the final report.

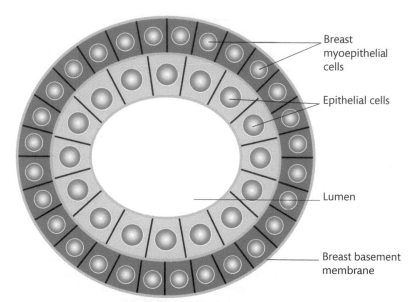

Breast myoepithelial cells

Epithelial cells

Lumen

Breast basement membrane

FIGURE 9.3
Diagram showing normal breast gland structure.

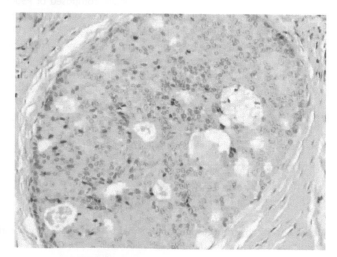

FIGURE 9.4
H&E staining showing ductal carcinoma *in situ* of the breast.

TABLE 9.4 Staining pattern of breast myoepithelial cells.

	SMA	p63	SMM	S100
Myoepithelial cells	+	+	+	+

To this end, investigations to confirm the presence of myoepithelial cells are performed. Their staining profile is characterized in Table 9.4.

Key Point

The identification of myoepithelial cells in neoplastic breast disease is important to determine whether breast carcinoma is *in situ* or invasive.

Breast cancer can be subcategorized into three groups (Table 9.5).

The tumour may be frankly malignant, in which case diagnosis can be made on H&E staining alone. In cases where there is doubt about whether the tumour is invasive or not, markers for myoepithelial cells are performed. Case study 9.2 is of a woman with invasive breast disease. Once invasive breast cancer is diagnosed, patient treatment is then discussed. Breast cancer patients whose tumours are oestrogen receptor (ER)-positive and HER2-positive are suitable for monoclonal antibody therapy using trastuzumab (Herceptin). Case study 9.3 illustrates a case of lobular carcinoma.

TABLE 9.5 Incidence of the various types of breast cancer.

Cancer	Incidence
Ductal	80%
Lobular	10%
Other type	10%

CASE STUDY 9.1 *Ductal carcinoma in situ* (DCIS)

A woman aged 48 attended a breast screening appointment for mammography. Initial radiological investigation suggested a suspicious lesion, and a breast core biopsy was taken. Figure 9.5 shows a diagram of DCIS.

Initial H&E staining (Figure 9.6) indicated a differential diagnosis of ductal carcinoma or ductal carcinoma *in situ*.

Immunocytochemistry was requested for SMM and p63 (Figures 9.7 and 9.8 show ICC for SMM and p63, respectively, in benign breast ducts), both of which are markers for breast myoepithelial cells, along with S100 (not shown).

The presence of myoepithelial cells around the tumour would confirm ductal carcinoma *in situ*.

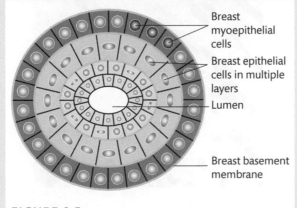

Breast myoepithelial cells

Breast epithelial cells in multiple layers

Lumen

Breast basement membrane

FIGURE 9.5
Diagram of *in situ* disease.

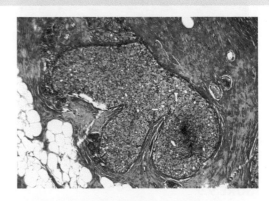

FIGURE 9.6
H&E staining of DCIS.

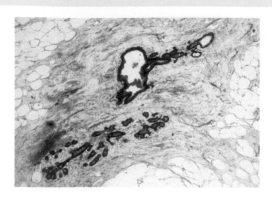

FIGURE 9.7
SMM immunostaining of benign breast ducts.

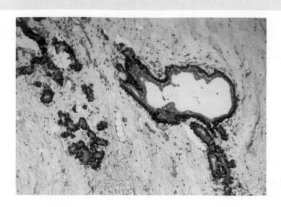

FIGURE 9.8
p63 immunostaining of benign breast ducts.

CASE STUDY 9.2 Invasive breast cancer

An asymptomatic female, aged 53, attended a breast screening appointment and had a radiologically suspicious lesion identified. Two needle core biopsies were taken and sent to the laboratory for investigation.

Initial H&E findings (Figure 9.9) suggested focal stromal infiltration by invasive ductal carcinoma. Microcalcific bodies were seen within the tumour vicinity.

Immunocytochemistry was performed for MNF116, SMA and p63 (Figures 9.10, 9.11 and 9.12, respectively) to investigate the presence of myoepithelial cells.

Note the absence of normal breast structure on H&E staining and the strong staining for MNF116, showing the tumour cells to be of epithelial origin. Staining for SMA and p63 are both negative, confirming invasive ductal breast cancer.

A subsequent lumpectomy was performed and ER staining (Figure 9.13) was performed on this sample to confirm the patient's suitability for tamoxifen treatment.

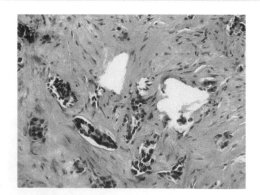

FIGURE 9.9
Invasive carcinoma of breast (H&E). Note absence of normal gland structure.

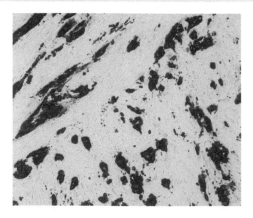

FIGURE 9.10
MNF116.

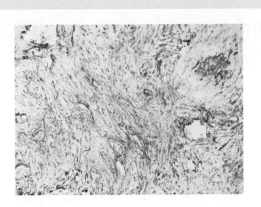

FIGURE 9.11
SMA.

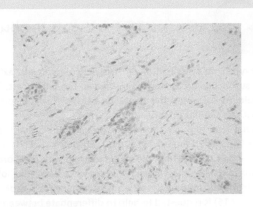

FIGURE 9.12
p63.

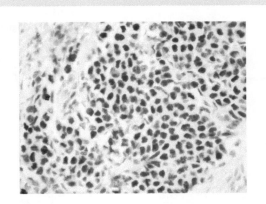

FIGURE 9.13
Positive ER staining.

CLINICAL CORRELATION

Ductal carcinoma of breast is the most common type of breast cancer. The introduction of the breast screening programme has helped to detect **asymptomatic** cancer. This has allowed earlier clinical intervention and an improvement in survival rates.

Asymptomatic

Without clinical signs or symptoms. Early cancers often grow unknown to the patient.

SELF-CHECK 9.7

Why is the identification of myoepithelial cells by immunocytochemistry important in the diagnosis of breast disease?

E-cadherin

A cell adhesion molecule.

CASE STUDY 9.3 *Lobular carcinoma*

A 46-year-old female attended breast screening and extensive suspicious areas were identified in the left breast. The radiologist suggested this might be cancer. A single core of breast was sent for investigation.

Initial H&E findings showed an absence of normal breast ducts (Figures 9.14 and 9.15) and no obvious two-cell layer in the glands. Columns of single malignant cells within the breast stroma (also known as Indian filing) are seen, suggesting lobular carcinoma. Immunocytochemistry staining for E-cadherin (Figure 9.16) is requested to help to differentiate between the possibility of ductal or lobular carcinoma, the latter usually being E-cadherin-negative.

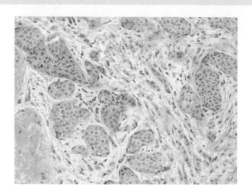

FIGURE 9.15
Columns of malignant cells seen in the stroma (H&E).

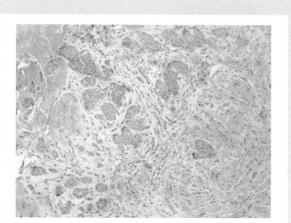

FIGURE 9.14
Lobular breast carcinoma (H&E).

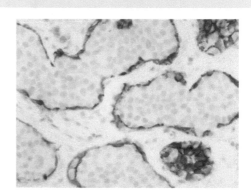

FIGURE 9.16
E-cadherin.

9.10 Investigation of lung cancer

Primary lung cancers consist of a number of different types, the most common being:

- squamous cell carcinoma
- small cell carcinoma
- adenocarcinoma
- mesothelioma (arising from the pleura that lines the thoracic cavity).

A panel of antibodies is required to distinguish the various types of lung cancer. Table 9.6 shows the reaction of each tumour type with lung cancer markers (see Case studies 9.4, 9.5 and 9.6).

CLINICAL CORRELATION

Carcinomas of the lung

The lung may be a source of metastatic deposit from tumours in many different organs, so care must be taken with ICC to confirm the lung as the primary site.

Key Point

TTF-1 and CK7 can be used to confirm malignancy as a lung primary.

Key Point

Mesotheliomas show positive staining with calretinin and negative staining with epithelial markers.

TABLE 9.6 Antibody algorithm for identifying tumours of the lung and pleura.

	CEA	CK 5/6	CK 7	Ber- EP4	EMA	Calretinin	TTF-1	CD56	Synaptophysin
Squamous cell carcinoma		+	+	+	–		+	–	–
Small cell carcinoma							+	+	+
Adenocarcinoma	+	+	+	+	+	–		+	–	–
Mesothelioma	–		+	–	–	+			

CASE STUDY 9.4 *Adenocarcinoma of the lung*

A 73-year-old man who smoked 30 cigarettes a day presented with vocal cord palsy. After chest X-ray he had a biopsy removed from a suspicious region in the left lower lobe.

Three small grey/brown tissue fragments, the largest measuring 0.3 cm, were received. Two of the fragments appeared normal but the third showed absence of normal glands. The lining epithelium exhibited pleomorphism and the enlarged hyperchromatic nuclei contained prominent nucleoli, and an accumulation of mucus was seen in the cytoplasm. The H&E (Figure 9.17) suggested a well-differentiated adenocarcinoma.

Immunocytochemistry for TTF-1, CK7 and CK20 (Figures 9.18, 9.19 and 9.20, respectively) is used to confirm a primary lung tumour.

Supplementary report:

As stated in the body of the original report, in order to confirm the presence of a probable adenocarcinoma of lung, primary additional immunocytochemical stains were requested as follows:

TTF-1: Strong nuclear positivity in all cells in the focus of tumour.

CK7: Strongly positive on cytoplasmic membranes of tumour focus.

CK20: Negative in tumour.

These findings support the original interpretation of this biopsy and exclude a potential metastatic lesion to the lung.

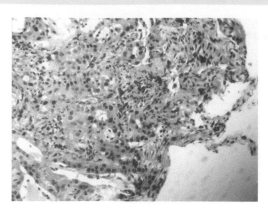

FIGURE 9.17
Lung adenocarcinoma (H&E).

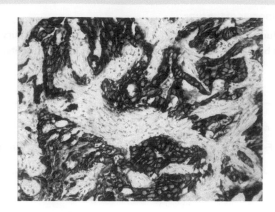

FIGURE 9.19
CK7. Note strong cytoplasmic staining.

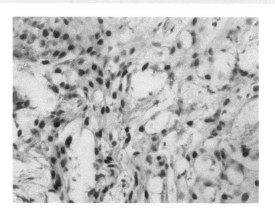

FIGURE 9.18
TTF-1. Note intense nuclear staining.

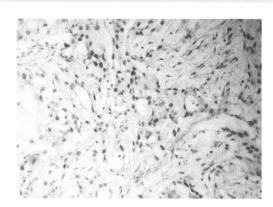

FIGURE 9.20
CK20. Note absence of positivity.

CASE STUDY 9.5 Mesothelioma

A 68-year-old female presented with exudative unilateral pleural effusion. Fragments of fibrofatty tissue and striated muscle fibres obtained from the fluid showed the presence of atypical mesothelial cells predominantly as solid sheets (Figure 9.21). On ICC staining the cells showed strong positivity for calretinin and CK7 (Figures 9.22 and 9.24, respectively).

Positive staining, probably spurious, was also seen with CK20 (Figure 9.23), but no staining was seen with Ber-EP4 and CEA (epithelial markers).

Note the positive staining for calretinin and CK7 and the lack of staining with the other epithelial markers, confirming a diagnosis of mesothelioma.

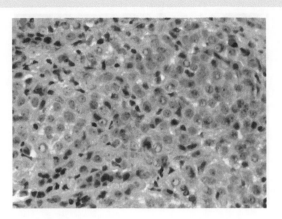

FIGURE 9.21
Mesothelioma (H&E).

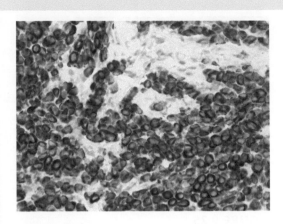

FIGURE 9.23
CK20.

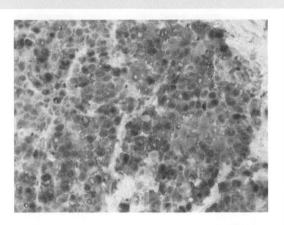

FIGURE 9.22
Calretinin.

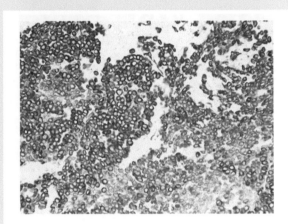

FIGURE 9.24
CK7.

CASE STUDY 9.6 Small cell carcinoma

A male, aged 78, presented with a left pulmonary mass and enlarged hilar nodes. These were PET-positive on imaging and he was presumed to have a primary lung carcinoma.

Needle cores were taken from the pulmonary mass which showed neoplastic tissue composed of medium-sized very **pleomorphic** cells showing a **high nuclear:cytoplasmic ratio** and hardly any cytoplasm. Numerous mitoses were present and abundant apoptosis was seen (Figure 9.25).

Immunocytochemistry showed strong positive reactions with CK7, CAM5.2 and TTF-1 (Figures 9.26, 9.27 and 9.28,

respectively). Cytokeratin 20 was negative, excluding a metastatic deposit from the colon, and LCA was also negative, excluding lymphoma. TTF-1 was strongly positive. CD56 and synaptophysin (neuroendocrine markers) were also very strongly positive (Figures 9.29 and 9.30, respectively).

Note the tumour cells are medium-sized with small amounts of cytoplasm. The ICC profile shows positivity for the neuroendocrine markers CD56 and synaptophysin, which, in conjunction with CK7 and TTF-1 (markers for lung tissue), confirms a diagnosis of small cell carcinoma of the lung.

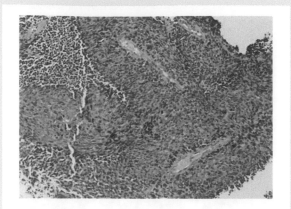

FIGURE 9.25
Small cell carcinoma of the lung (H&E).

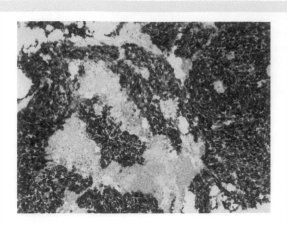

FIGURE 9.28
TTF-1.

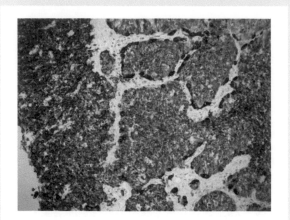

FIGURE 9.26
CK7.

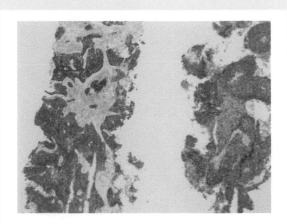

FIGURE 9.29
CD56.

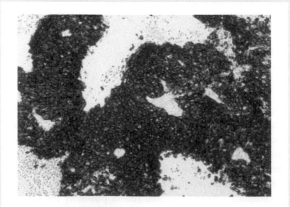

FIGURE 9.27
CAM 5.2.

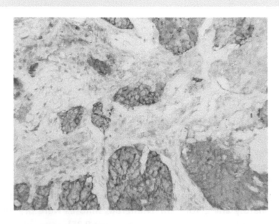

FIGURE 9.30
Synaptophysin.

Which markers are used to distinguish lung carcinomas from mesothelioma?

9.11 Investigation of prostate cancer

The prostate gland is an accessory sexual organ situated around the urethra in males (Figure 9.31). The function of the prostate is to secrete nutrient-rich fluids that form part of the male ejaculate in sexual intercourse. Cancer of the prostate is common among older men (usually over 50), and by the age of 80 years 80% of men have some form of prostate cancer, although this may be small and does not necessarily require treatment.

The initial stages of prostate disease often involve enlargement of the gland. This change may be benign, as in prostatic hyperplasia that commonly occurs with increasing age, or show some *in situ* neoplastic change in prostatic glands, or be frankly malignant.

Symptoms of prostatic cancer are very similar to those for benign prostatic hyperplasia. These are:

- a need to urinate frequently, especially at night
- difficulty starting urination or holding back urine
- weak or interrupted flow of urine
- painful or burning micturition (urination)
- blood in urine or semen.

Initial histological examination is by needle core biopsy. The biopsy gun is inserted through the anus and the prostate is biopsied through the rectal wall (i.e. transrectal and usually ultrasound guided). It is common for six cores to be taken from each lobe of the prostate, and these are known as sextant cores. Transperineal skin approaches are also becoming more common, to enable more systematic extensive sampling of the prostate and to target any lesions seen on a MRI scan.

Figure 9.32 shows a diagram of prostate biopsy sampling.

Under normal circumstances prostate glands have two cell layers, an outer basal cell layer and an inner epithelial (secretory) cell layer, very similar to the two epithelial cell layers seen in a breast gland (Figure 9.33). In prostatic intraepithelial neoplasia (known as high grade PIN) there is malignant change in the prostatic epithelium, but the tumour remains *in situ* and does not breach the basal cell layer or prostatic basement membrane (Figure 9.34). In invasive prostatic disease the basement membrane is effaced and prostatic epithelial cells are seen to breach the basement membrane and invade the stroma of the prostate (Figure 9.35; see Case studies 9.7 and 9.8).

High nuclear:cytoplasmic ratio

Describes the morphology of the cells. Malignant cells tend to have a higher nuclear: cytoplasmic ratio than normal cells. In small cell carcinoma the ratio seen in these cells is particularly high when compared to adenocarcinoma or mesothelioma.

Pleomorphic

Describes the varied shapes and sizes of cells within the tumour. The more varied the cell size the more pleomorphic it is said to be. Greater pleomorphism generally indicates a higher-grade tumour and a worse prognosis.

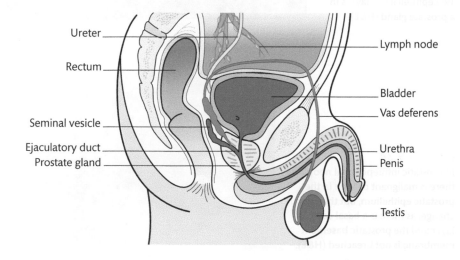

FIGURE 9.31
Anatomy of the prostate gland.

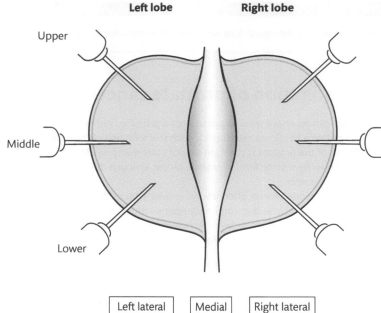

FIGURE 9.32
Diagram of prostate biopsy sampling.

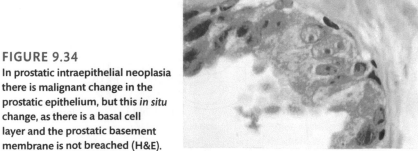

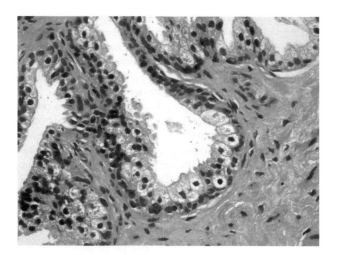

FIGURE 9.33
Two epithelial cell layers in a prostate gland (H&E).

FIGURE 9.34
In prostatic intraepithelial neoplasia there is malignant change in the prostatic epithelium, but this *in situ* change, as there is a basal cell layer and the prostatic basement membrane is not breached (H&E).

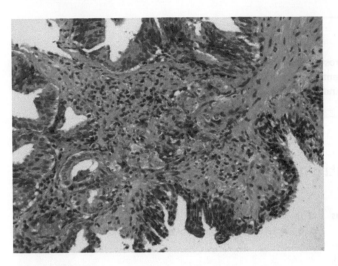

FIGURE 9.35
In invasive prostatic disease the basement membrane is effaced and prostatic epithelial cells are seen to breach the basement membrane and invade the stroma of the prostate (H&E).

Prostate-specific antigen (PSA)

A protein secreted by the prostate. When the gland is enlarged, inflamed and/or malignant the level of PSA is seen to rise above the normal reference range. The normal PSA reference range in healthy men under 60 is 0–3 ng/mL, rising to 0–5 ng/mL in men over 70 years of age. A raised PSA level will trigger further investigation by biopsy.

CASE STUDY 9.7 *Prostatic intraepithelial neoplasia*

A patient aged 58 underwent repeat biopsies as his **prostate-specific antigen** (PSA) level had risen to 6.9. Clinically, the prostate was large but benign.

A series of sextant biopsies was taken from each lobe of the prostate. In the right base core biopsy, a small focus of high-grade prostatic intraepithelial neoplasia (PIN) was found towards one edge on the H&E (Figure 9.36). Immunocytochemistry was performed for 34βE12 and p63 (Figures 9.37 and 9.38, respectively) which confirmed the presence of an intact basal cell layer. The diagnosis of high-grade PIN on a biopsy specimen, if multifocal, will usually lead to re-biopsy as there is a risk that the prostate will have an associated prostate cancer.

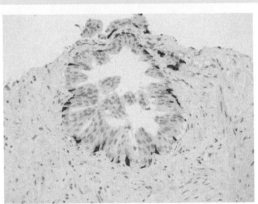

FIGURE 9.37
34βE12. Note strong basal cell cytoplasmic staining.

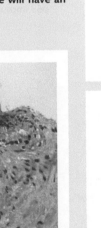

FIGURE 9.36
Prostatic intraepithelial neoplasia (H&E).

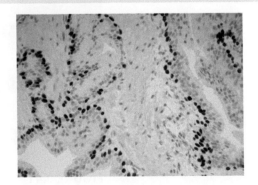

FIGURE 9.38
Note strong p63 nuclear staining.

CASE STUDY 9.8 *Prostatic adenocarcinoma*

A 69-year-old man had a raised PSA of 12 mg/L, which was investigated with 12-core transrectal prostate core biopsies.

Two of the cores contained small foci of invasive adenocarcinoma, Gleason score 3+3 = 6 (Grade Group 1) (Figure 9.39).

This was confirmed with immunocytochemistry for p63 (Figure 9.40), CK5/6 (not shown) and AMACR (Figure 9.41).

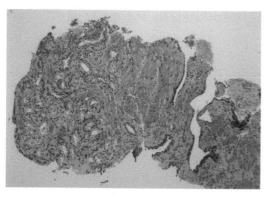

FIGURE 9.39
Invasive prostate cancer (H&E).

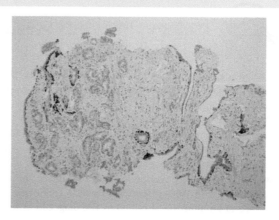

FIGURE 9.40
p63 immunostaining of invasive prostate cancer.

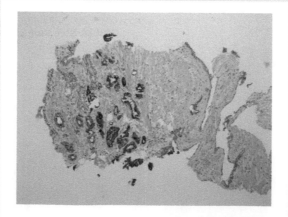

FIGURE 9.41
AMACR immunostaining. Note absence of staining in the normal glands, which act as an internal control.

9.12 Distinguishing lymphoma types

Lymphoma is a malignant tumour of the haematological cells within lymph nodes and commonly requires the use of ICC for diagnosis. On H&E staining, many lymphomas exhibit very similar morphology and thus accurate distinction of the cell types present is not possible.

The various subdivisions of lymphoma are based on the types of cell involved and their maturity. The initial division is between Hodgkin's lymphoma and non-Hodgkin's lymphoma. Figure 9.42 shows a simplified algorithm for categorization of lymphomas. The presence of Reed–Sternberg (RS) cells distinguishes the two tumours (Figure 9.43). Hodgkin's lymphoma is characterized by the presence of RS cells, which are absent from non-Hodgkin's lymphoma. Clinically, the most common symptom of both is painless swelling in a lymph node, usually in the neck, axilla or groin (see Case studies 9.9, 9.10 and 9.11).

Symptoms of advanced lymphoma include:

- unexplained tiredness or fatigue
- night sweats
- unexplained weight loss
- fever
- trouble getting rid of infections

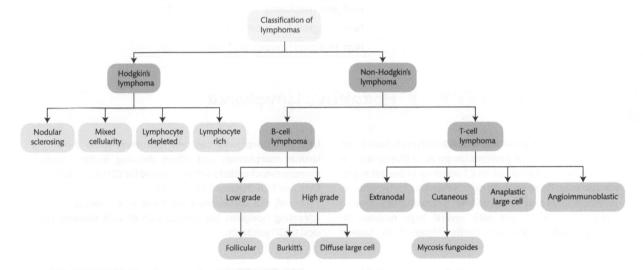

FIGURE 9.42
Simplified algorithm for the categorization of lymphomas.

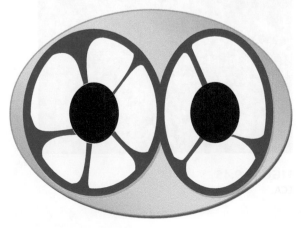

FIGURE 9.43
Diagrammatic representation of a Reed–Sternberg (RS) cell.

- persistent cough or feeling of breathlessness
- persistent itching of the skin all over the body.

Key Points

Immunocytochemistry allows accurate diagnosis of lymphoma.

The presence of Reed–Sternberg cells distinguishes Hodgkin's lymphoma from non-Hodgkin's lymphoma.

As you can see from Figure 9.42 there are many different types of lymphoma. Immunocytochemistry plays a very important part in identifying subtypes of lymphoma. See also Table 9.7.

TABLE 9.7 Incidence of lymphoma.

Lymphoma	%
Hodgkin's lymphoma	10
Non-Hodgkin's lymphoma—B cell	80
Non-Hodgkin's lymphoma—T cell	10

CASE STUDY 9.9 Hodgkin's lymphoma

An 81-year-old male presented with a large lymph node in the region of his shoulder. A previous lymph node biopsy was necrotic. A node was identified on CT scanning in the left supraclavicular fossa. There was high clinical suspicion for lymphoma.

A lymph node was removed and histopathology showed an abnormal architecture with several large nodules focally separated by sclerotic bands (Figure 9.44). Several large pleomorphic RS-like cells were seen, some showing a lacunar morphology and others showing multinucleation. Immunocytochemistry was performed for CD15, CD20, CD30, EMA and LCA (Figures 9.45 to 9.49).

Overall, the appearances are those of a classical nodular sclerosing Hodgkin's lymphoma, with RS cells showing classical CD30 positivity.

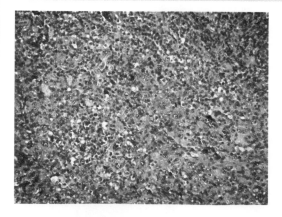

FIGURE 9.44
Hodgkin's disease (H&E).

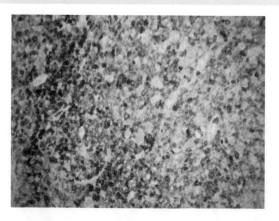

FIGURE 9.45
LCA.

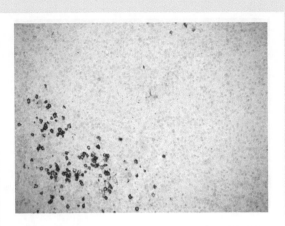

FIGURE 9.46
CD20.

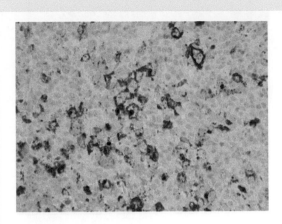

FIGURE 9.48
CD15.

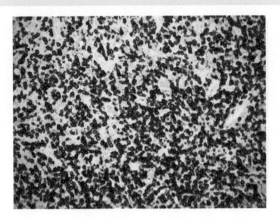

FIGURE 9.47
CD3.

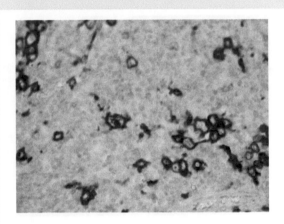

FIGURE 9.49
CD30.

CASE STUDY 9.10 *Multiple myeloma*

A 68-year-old woman presented with a pulmonary mass and bone lesions. Metastatic disease was suspected, possibly a lung primary, but lung lesions were not typical.

To confirm metastasis and identify the primary if possible, slender needle cores of tissue were taken for investigation. Routine H&E staining (Figure 9.50) showed a monomorphic tumour composed of small cells with abundant cytoplasm.

There was only mild nuclear pleomorphism and the mitotic rate was low. Immunocytochemistry was performed for S100 and MNF 116 (both negative) and CD38, CD138, kappa and lambda (Figures 9.51 to 9.54). The ICC confirmed the cells to be plasma cells demonstrating light chain restriction and therefore a malignant clone.

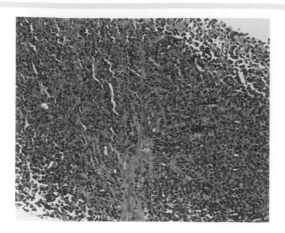

FIGURE 9.50
Multiple myeloma (H&E).

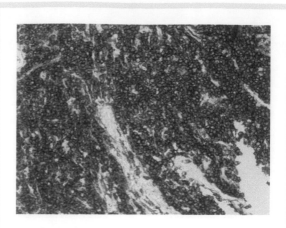

FIGURE 9.52
CD138.

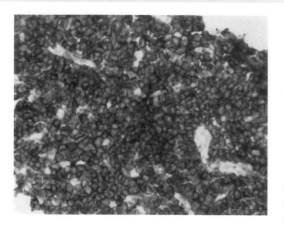

FIGURE 9.51
CD38.

FIGURE 9.53
Kappa.

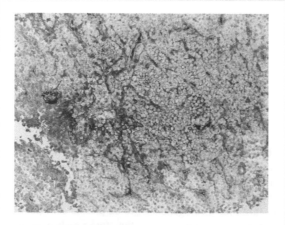

FIGURE 9.54
Lambda.

CASE STUDY 9.11 Confirmation of lymphoma metastases

A male, aged 69, with known non-Hodgkin's lymphoma (NHL) presented at endoscopy with gastric ulcers, which were biopsied. Initial H&E findings suggested B-cell lymphoma (Figure 9.55). The previous lymph node specimen histopathology report was examined and the findings compared to the gastric biopsy, which showed a similar pathology. Immunocytochemistry was performed for CD20 and Ki-67 (Figures 9.56 and 9.57) to confirm B-cell lymphoma.

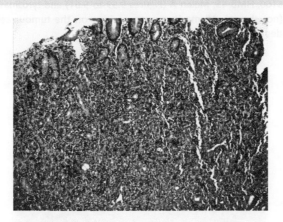

FIGURE 9.55
Gastric biopsy (H&E).

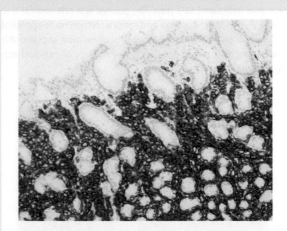

FIGURE 9.56
CD20.

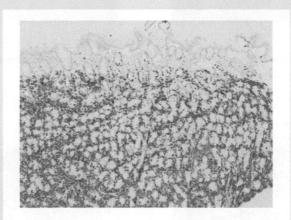

FIGURE 9.57
Ki-67.

9.13 Assessment of sentinel lymph nodes

The sentinel lymph node is the closest lymph node (or group of nodes) to a tumour. It is the node first affected by metastases from a tumour. Identification of tumour in the closest lymph node has a significant impact on patient treatment and management (see Case study 9.12).

CASE STUDY 9.12 *Sentinel lymph nodes*

This case exemplifies the use of antibody panels to assess **sentinel lymph nodes**.

A 34-year-old woman had a melanoma removed from her right lower leg. The melanoma was classified as a superficial spreading malignant melanoma and the **Breslow** depth of invasion was measured as 7 mm. The patient was referred for **secondary wide local excision** and sentinel lymph node appraisal.

On H&E examination, the wide local excision showed skin containing scar tissue only and no evidence of residual malignant melanoma.

On examination of the sentinel lymph node, metastatic tumour deposits were identified in the subcapsular sinus (Figure 9.58).

In order to confirm a diagnosis of metastatic malignant melanoma, a panel of melanoma markers was employed, including S100, HMB 45, Melan A (Figures 9.59 to 9.61) and tyrosinase (not shown). All markers were positive on the tumour cell deposit.

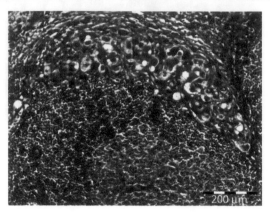

FIGURE 9.58
Malignant melanoma deposits in the lymph node subcapsular sinus (H&E, original magnification ×40).

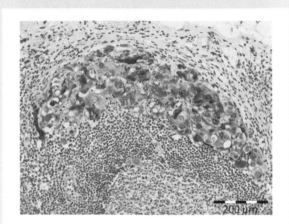

FIGURE 9.60
Melan A -positive tumour cells (original magnification ×30).

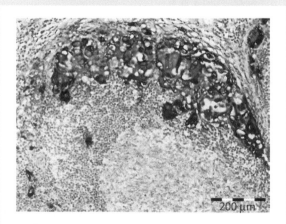

FIGURE 9.59
S100-positive tumour cells (original magnification ×40).

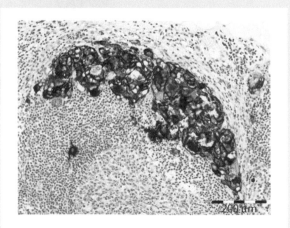

FIGURE 9.61
HMB 45-positive tumour cells (original magnification ×30).

TABLE 9.8 The link between viruses and cancer.

Cancer	Associated virus
Hepatocellular carcinoma	Hepatitis B
Kaposi's sarcoma	HIV and herpes type 8 (HHV8)
Burkitt's lymphoma	Epstein–Barr virus
Squamous cell carcinoma of the neck	Human papillomavirus
Cervical carcinoma	Human papillomavirus

CLINICAL CORRELATION

Metastatic melanoma has a very poor prognosis.

9.14 Identification of aetiological agents

Viral and bacterial agents may be detected by immunocytochemistry. There is a growing body of literature linking incidence of viral infection with cancer. Identification of viral agents can be useful for the management of patients with malignant disease. See Table 9.8 and Case study 9.13.

Sentinel lymph node

The first draining lymph node away from the primary lesion site.

Breslow thickness

Named after Alexander Breslow, this is a direct measurement of the depth of tumour invasion of a primary malignant melanoma. It is measured (in mm) using a microscope and represents the distance from the granular cell layer in the epidermis to the deepest invasive melanoma cell identified.

Secondary wide local excision

The standard surgical treatment following the diagnosis of cutaneous malignant melanoma. Patient management involves a wider excision of the primary melanoma site to remove any residual tumour and any further cutaneous spread that may have occurred.

CASE STUDY 9.13 p16

A 61-year-old patient presented to his GP with a neck lump and was referred to the head and neck clinic of the local hospital. The initial FNA proved inconclusive so a day surgery appointment was arranged. The lump was excised and initial clinical diagnosis indicated a cyst.

On H&E examination (Figure 9.62) there was a lymph node containing a metastatic tumour deposit. It consisted of epithelial cells in solid sheets showing proliferative activity with nuclear pleomorphism and mitotic figures. An expert referral was sought and a diagnosis of previously undiagnosed oropharyngeal carcinoma was made. Immunocytochemistry confirmed the presence of p16 (Figure 9.63) and *in situ* hybridization confirmed the presence of human papillomavirus (HPV) subtype 16.

The clinical presentation made the patient unsuitable for radical neck dissection but subsequent tonsillectomy confirmed the presence of further deposits of tumour.

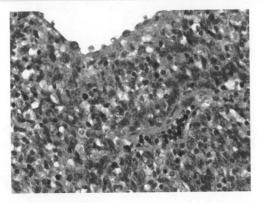

FIGURE 9.62
Squamous cell carcinoma (H&E).

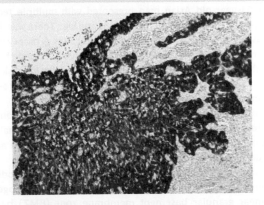

FIGURE 9.63
p16.

CLINICAL CORRELATION

Ninety per cent of oropharyngeal cancers are squamous cell carcinomas and typically affect patients aged over 60 years. Factors affecting incidence of oropharyngeal cancer are drinking and smoking. Recently, an HPV-positive subtype has been identified which generally affects younger patients in their thirties and forties. Only about half of the patients diagnosed with oropharyngeal cancer survive for five years.

Key Point

Viral agents integrate with human DNA and can cause malignant change.

9.15 Identifying autoimmune states

Immunocytochemistry is not just about the investigation of malignant conditions; it can also play an important role in the identification of autoimmune conditions (see Case study 9.14).

The key autoimmune conditions of interest in the laboratory are:

- Pemphigus: autoimmune reaction with the desmosomes of the epithelium.
- Pemphigoid: autoimmune reaction with the hemidesmosomes of the dermo-epidermal junction.
- Dermatitis herpetiformis.
- Adverse drug reactions.

CASE STUDY 9.14 Pemphigoid

The following case exemplifies the use of antibody panels against immunoglobulins to evaluate autoimmune disease.

A 63-year-old Asian man presented with multiple tense fluid-filled blisters over his back, arms and legs. There was also an associated erythema around the blister sites. A biopsy was taken of a blister from the arm which involved sampling both involved and uninvolved skin (lesional and perilesional skin). The biopsy was placed in Michel's transport medium and sent for immunofluorescence investigation.

On H&E examination (Figure 9.64) of a frozen section, a blister was identified which appeared to be subepidermal in nature. Numerous associated eosinophils were seen in and around the blister.

Following the use of a panel of FITC-labelled antibodies to immunoglobulins (IgM, IgA, IgG) plus C3 and fibrinogen, a linear granular basement membrane zone (BMZ) band with IgG, C3 (Figures 9.65 and 9.66) and fibrinogen was demonstrated.

The immunofluorescence profile confirmed a diagnosis of pemphigoid.

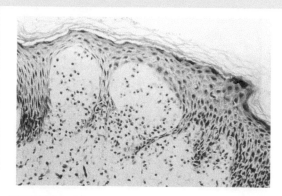

FIGURE 9.64
Subepidermal blister (H&E, original magnification ×20).

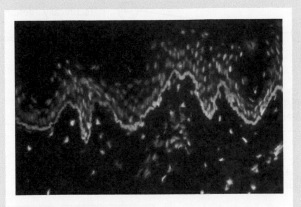

FIGURE 9.65
Anti-IgG linear granular basement membrane labelling (original magnification ×40).

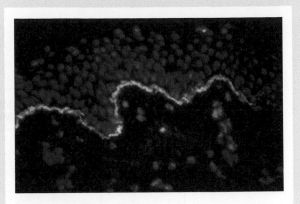

FIGURE 9.66
Anti-C3 linear granular basement membrane labelling (original magnification ×30).

Key Points

H&E demonstration will only determine whether a blister is intraepidermal or subepidermal. Classification of blistering disease is largely determined by immunofluorescence or immunoperoxidase studies of immunoglobulin, C3 and fibrinogen deposition.

Immunofluorescence studies are widely employed in the study of autoimmune disease in kidney and skin.

CLINICAL CORRELATION

The classification of autoimmune diseases in kidney and skin is heavily reliant on the immunofluorescence or immunocytochemical profiles achieved in conjunction with careful clinicopathological correlation.

9.16 Algorithmic approach to the use of antibody panels

This approach uses panels of antibodies to solve a diagnostic problem. At each round of investigation, the production of a positive or negative result directs the path towards a final diagnosis. The panel of antibodies employed should be based on the morphological appearance of the tissue, in conjunction with the patient's clinical history. All algorithmic panels should be followed by selective markers for subtyping/classifying any given tumour. There are many examples of the use of algorithms in diagnostic settings. An example of one is highlighted in Figure 9.67. It is, however, important to remember that reliance on this approach to aid classification of tumours should not be adopted as a standalone strategy. As with all histopathological interpretation, defining the morphology of tumour cells by conventional H&E staining remains the most effective reference point, supported by ICC data.

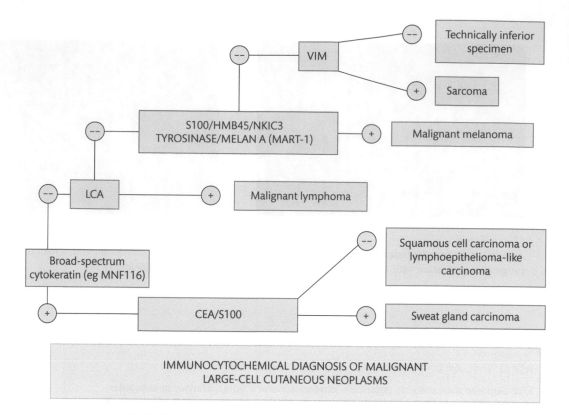

FIGURE 9.67

An algorithmic approach to using antibody panels. Modified from DeYoung BR, Wick M. Immunohistologic evaluation of metastatic carcinomas of unknown origin: an algorithmic approach. *Semin Diagn Pathol* 2000: **17** (3): 184–93.

9.17 Identification of tumours of unknown aetiology

CASE STUDY 9.15 *Metastatic malignant melanoma*

An 87-year-old man reported to his GP with symptoms of general tiredness and complaining of chest and back pain. On examination, a large subcutaneous nodule was identified on his abdomen. The GP suspected a metastatic tumour deposit but was unclear as to the origin of the primary tumour. A 2 mm punch biopsy was performed on the subcutaneous mass and sent for histopathological assessment.

Figure 9.68 (original magnification ×20) shows a flattened epidermis overlying a dense dermal infiltrate composed of nests of single cells with pink, abundant cytoplasm.

Figure 9.69 (original magnification ×40) shows nests of cells displaying large hyperchromatic nuclei and prominent nucleoli. Mitoses are not frequent and no pigmentation is seen.

At this point, a metastatic tumour deposit of unknown origin was suspected and ICC was performed. Based on the H&E findings, a metastatic carcinoma was suspected and a pan-cytokeratin marker was requested (MNF116). Figure 9.70 shows a negative result for MNF116, excluding a diagnosis of carcinoma (original magnification ×20).

To rule out a lymphoma, CD45 (LCA) was requested. Figure 9.71 shows a negative result for CD45, excluding lymphoma (original magnification ×20).

Now suspecting a diagnosis of malignant melanoma, S100 protein was requested. Figure 9.72 shows S100-positive labelling of dermal tumour cells, which supports a diagnosis of malignant melanoma (original magnification ×20).

For further confirmation, a panel of melanocyte-selective antibodies was requested (HMB 45, Melan A, tyrosinase).

Figure 9.73 shows focal HMB 45-positive labelling of dermal tumour cells (original magnification ×20). Figure 9.74 shows positive Melan A labelling of all the tumour cells (original magnification ×20). Figure 9.75 shows positive tyrosinase labelling of all tumour cells. Of note is the demonstration of tumour cells invading lymphatic vessels (circled, original magnification ×40).

The overall findings confirm a diagnosis of metastatic malignant melanoma.

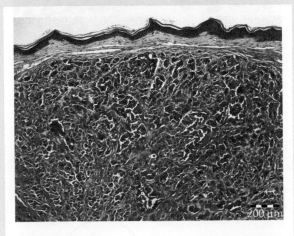

FIGURE 9.68
Flattened epidermis overlying a dense dermal infiltrate composed of nests of single cells with pink, abundant cytoplasm (H&E).

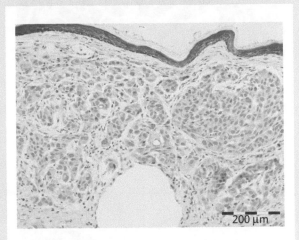

FIGURE 9.70
Negative result for MNF116, excluding a diagnosis of carcinoma.

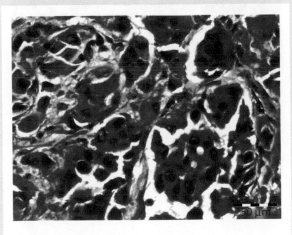

FIGURE 9.69
High-power view of Figure 9.68. Nests of cells displaying large hyperchromatic nuclei and prominent nucleoli. Mitoses are not frequent and no pigmentation is seen (H&E).

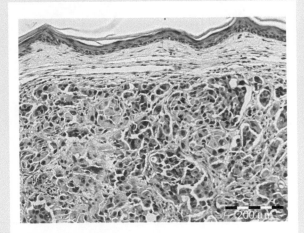

FIGURE 9.71
Negative result for CD45, excluding lymphoma.

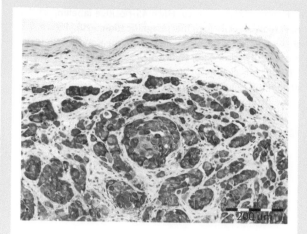

FIGURE 9.72

S100-positive labelling of dermal tumour cells, supporting a diagnosis of malignant melanoma.

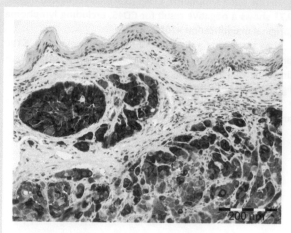

FIGURE 9.74

Positive Melan A labelling of all the tumour cells.

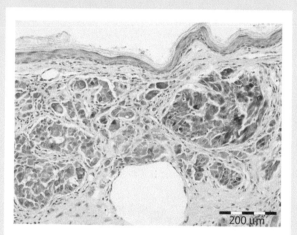

FIGURE 9.73

Focal HMB 45-positive labelling of dermal tumour cells.

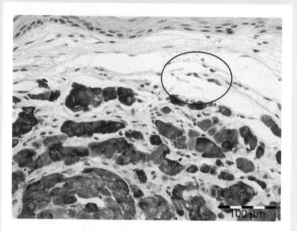

FIGURE 9.75

Positive tyrosinase labelling of all tumour cells.

Key Points

HMB45, S100, tyrosinase and Melan A can be used to identify malignant melanoma.

Malignant melanoma will metastasize if not identified early. Patient outcome is improved significantly by early detection.

Malignant melanoma

The incidence of melanoma is linked directly to excessive sun exposure in paler skin types and has been on the rise for the past 50 years. Government encourages people to adopt the 'slip, slap, slop' approach with regard to the application of sunscreens, in order to limit exposure to the sun's rays and to help prevent melanomas.

9.18 Immunocytochemistry as an indicator of suitability for therapy

Immunocytochemistry is playing an increasing role in evaluating patient suitability for monoclonal therapy. More recently we have seen the introduction of terms such as 'Personalized medicine'. Broadly speaking, this concept attempts to separate patients into groups with defined medical decisions, practices and interventions which are 'tailored' to the individual patient needs and are based on predictive responses or disease risk factors. As a concept it is not new and dates back to Hippocrates himself. We can appreciate that modern therapies are based on a number of factors and most significantly with regard to these is genetic information; you will read more about these in the following chapters encompassing *in situ* and molecular techniques. However molecular-based techniques are detecting genetic mutations and associated defects at the DNA or RNA level; they do not provide information on protein expression at the light microscope level. A wide variety of antigens that are prognostically significant and that can provide valuable information for therapeutic regimes are detected using ICC methodology, including those summarized in Table 9.9.

Although this information can be extremely valuable it is also important to realize that many of these approaches are looking at single individual genetic mutations within a cellular pathway in any given lesion and, based on the results obtained, these patients are categorized for different treatment regimes. Unfortunately, many diseases and especially cancers are often far more complex and involve multiple cellular pathways in their activation, proliferation and maturation, thus 'life is never that simple!' Sequencing of patient genomes on an individual by individual basis will provide a much greater insight and will undoubtedly contribute significantly to future clinical practice, but for the time being this is still awaited.

TABLE 9.9 Therapeutic regimes employed following ICC detection techniques.

ICC antibody	Cancer	Drug name
HER2	Breast	Trastuzumab (Herceptin)
HER2	Stomach (gastric)	Trastuzumab (Herceptin)
CD20	B-cell lymphoma	Rituximab
CD117	Gastrointestinal stromal tumour	Glivec/sunitinib
EGFR	Metastatic colorectal cancer	Cetuximab and panitunumab

CASE STUDY 9.16 Breast cancer

A patient (aged 41) attended breast screening where the mammogram showed clusters of calcification in the upper half of the right breast. A Stereocore biopsy was performed in the craniocaudal position. Six cores were taken, three of which showed calcification (Figure 9.76).

A lumpectomy was performed and invasive ductal breast cancer confirmed. HER2 testing (Figure 9.77) was requested to investigate the patient's suitability for Herceptin treatment.

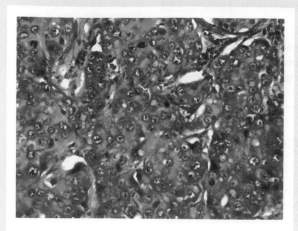

FIGURE 9.76
Invasive ductal breast cancer (H&E).

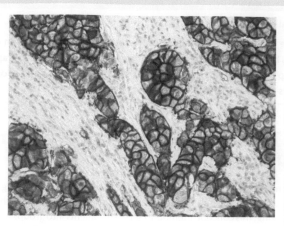

FIGURE 9.77
HER2 positivity.

CASE STUDY 9.17 *Urothelial carcinoma in situ*

A 67-year-old man with a history of carcinoma *in situ* (CIS) of the bladder, previously treated with intravesical (instilled into the bladder) BCG, had a six-month check cystoscopy at which a red patch was seen on the bladder mucosa and was biopsied. On microscopy, the biopsy showed granulomatous inflammation consistent with the BCG treatment and an abnormal area of surface urothelium with atypical discohesive cells.

There was no associated invasive malignancy. Immunocytochemistry for CK20 showed all of the atypical cells to be strongly positive, in contrast to the adjacent normal urothelium, thus supporting a diagnosis of recurrent CIS.

In normal urothelium, only the surface umbrella cells are CK20 positive, whereas diffuse full-thickness staining is typical of CIS. A proliferation marker (e.g. Ki-67) may be used in conjunction with the CK20, to highlight the raised proliferation index also seen in CIS. This is illustrated in a section of ureter, where sharply demarcated areas of CIS (Figure 9.78) show a contrasting CK20 and Ki-67 staining pattern with normal urothelium (Figures 9.79 and 9.80).

A knowledge of the usual distribution of staining with any antibody is vital to accurate interpretation of immunocytochemistry.

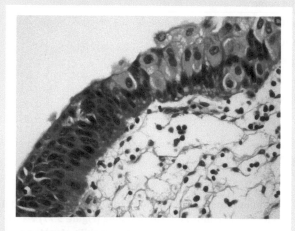

FIGURE 9.78
Ureter, H&E staining: normal urothelium (left) and CIS (right).

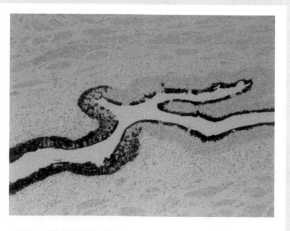

FIGURE 9.79
Ureter, CK20 staining: CIS (left), normal urothelium (right).

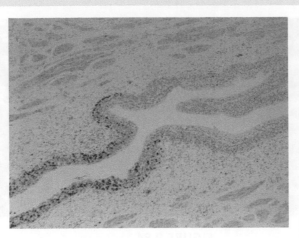

FIGURE 9.80
Ureter, Ki-67 staining: CIS (left), normal urothelium (right).

CASE STUDY 9.18 Metastatic renal cell carcinoma

A 70-year-old woman presented with large bowel obstruction. Gross examination of the resected segment of obstructed colon revealed a tumour located within the submucosa and muscular wall, rather than the mucosal lining, thus suggesting a metastasis. On microscopy, the tumour was composed of trabecular arrangements of cells with clear cytoplasm and round nuclei with prominent eosinophilic nucleoli (Figures 9.81 and 9.82). Further clinical history obtained was of a previous nephrectomy for malignancy.

Immunocytochemistry was performed to establish suspected renal original and the tumour type. The tumour was positive for Pax-8 (Figure 9.83), vimentin (Figure 9.84), RCC, Ca-IX and cytokeratin AE1/3, and negative for CK7, confirming this to be metastatic clear cell renal cell carcinoma. This tumour typically co-expresses both vimentin and cytokeratin, unlike many carcinomas.

Knowledge of relevant clinical history is important in directing appropriate panels for immunocytochemistry.

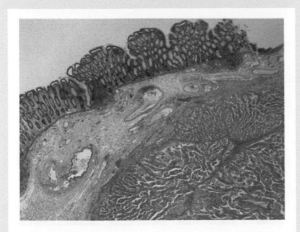

FIGURE 9.81
Bowel wall with normal mucosa (top) and mass in the bowel wall (bottom) (H&E).

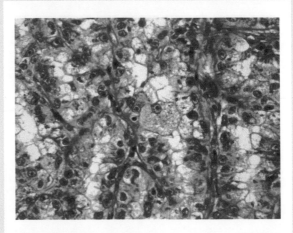

FIGURE 9.82
Tumour, high power (H&E).

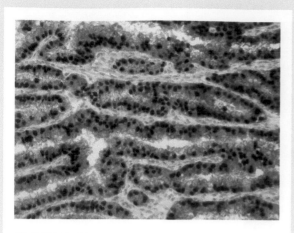

FIGURE 9.83
Pax 8 staining.

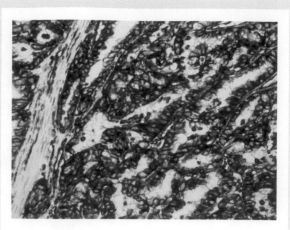

FIGURE 9.84
Vimentin staining.

CASE STUDY 9.19 *Testicular tumour typing*

A 29-year-old man had an enlarged, firm right testis, which was removed as clinically suspicious of malignancy. A 45 mm tumour was present, confined to the testis, which had a variegated gross appearance, with solid cream areas and foci of haemorrhage and necrosis.

On histopathology, this was a mixed malignant germ cell tumour. There were two distinct tumour patterns: pleomorphic tumour cells arranged in sheets with occasional glandular spaces (embryonal carcinoma—Figure 9.85) and more uniform loosely cohesive tumour cells with clear cytoplasm, separated by fibrous bands containing lymphocytes (seminoma—Figure 9.86).

Immunocytochemistry was used to confirm the different tumour types present. As expected, both were OCT 3/4 positive (Figure 9.87—seminoma only shown). The embryonal carcinoma was also CD30 (Figure 9.88) and cytokeratin positive. The seminoma was negative with those markers but positive for CD117 (Figure 9.89).

Testicular germ cell tumours are often a mixture of tumour types. Confirmatory immunocytochemistry is frequently used, because different germ cell tumours may show overlapping morphological features on H&E. The distinction is important, as treatment may vary, depending upon the combination present.

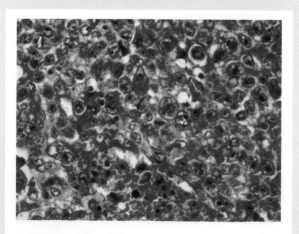

FIGURE 9.85
Embryonal carcinoma, H&E staining.

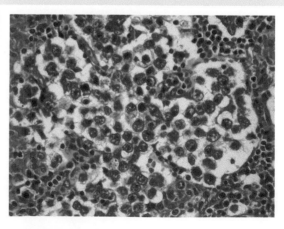

FIGURE 9.86
Seminoma, H&E staining.

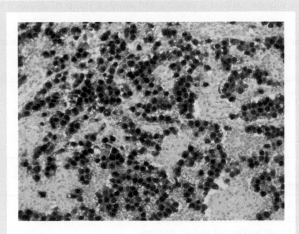

FIGURE 9.87
Seminoma, OCT 3/4 (nuclear stain).

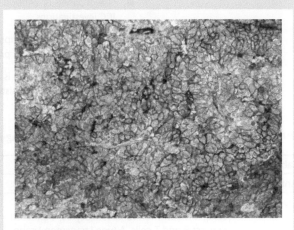

FIGURE 9.88
Embryonal carcinoma, CD30 staining.

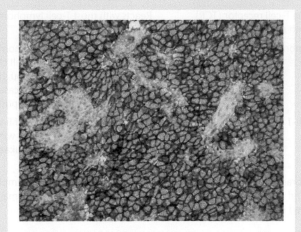

FIGURE 9.89
Seminoma, CD117 staining.

Chapter Summary

Immunocytochemistry is an integral part of modern histopathological diagnosis. No single antibody provides a 'magic bullet' approach to diagnosis and thus panels of antibodies are used in diagnostic practice.

Although many well-differentiated tumours bear a likeness to the tissue from which they arise, reporting by H&E alone is not sufficient and in most cases the tumour type needs to be investigated further.

The key facts to remember are:

■ Immunocytochemistry is an extremely useful complementary technique in histopathology but should never be used in isolation. Consideration of morphological features is paramount.

■ Use of panels of antibodies to subtype tumours is valuable and avoids a 'shotgun' approach to ICC investigations.

■ Use of an algorithmic approach to delineate tumours has value in diagnosis and directs investigations in a logical and progressive fashion.

■ Immunocytochemistry is a valuable technique in determining prognostically significant data for tumour staging and assisting in defining patient therapy strategies.

APPENDIX 9.1   Key CD marker antibodies used in the diagnostic laboratory.

Labelling profile			
Antibody	Normal	Pathological	Staining pattern
CD45	Also known as leucocyte common antigen (LCA), it is common to all leucocytes, expressed on most B and T cells. A type I transmembrane protein present on all haematopoietic cells except erythrocytes. Assists in cell activation.	LCA is expressed in lymphoma, B-cell chronic lymphocytic leukaemia, hairy cell leukaemia and acute non-lymphocytic leukaemia. Useful as a primary marker to distinguish lymphoma from carcinoma.	Membrane
CD3	A component of the T-cell receptor (TCR) complex. Reacts with most T cells.	Reacts with most T-cell lymphomas.	Membrane
CD20	A type III transmembrane protein found on B cells.	It is expressed in B-cell lymphomas, hairy cell leukaemia and B-cell chronic lymphocytic leukaemia. In roughly a quarter of Hodgkin's disease cases, Reed–Sternberg cells will be CD20-positive.	Membrane
CD79a	Encoded by the *mb-1* gene. Expressed on most B cells.	Expressed on the full range of B-cell neoplasms and co-expressed with CD3 in 10% of T-lymphoblastic leukaemia/lymphoma.	Membrane
CD5	A type I transmembrane protein found on T cells, thymocytes and some B cells. A ligand for CD72 and is involved in cellular activation or adhesion.	Expressed in B-cell chronic lymphocytic leukaemia and T-cell lymphoma.	Membrane
CD10	A type II transmembrane protein found on pre-B cells, germinal centre B cells, some neutrophils, kidney cells, T-cell precursors and epithelial cells. It acts as a zinc metalloprotease, cleaving peptide bonds on the amino side of hydrophobic amino acids.	It is expressed in acute lymphocytic leukaemia, multiple myeloma and follicular centre cell lymphomas. Sometimes called common acute lymphoblastic leukaemia antigen.	Membrane
CD15	A carbohydrate adhesion molecule (not a protein) that mediates phagocytosis and chemotaxis. It is found on neutrophils.	It is expressed in patients with Hodgkin's disease, some B-cell chronic lymphocytic leukaemias, acute lymphoblastic leukaemia and most acute non-lymphocytic leukaemias.	Membrane and Golgi apparatus in the cytoplasm
CD30	A type I transmembrane protein present on activated T and B cells. It may play a role in cell activation and/or differentiation.	It is expressed in Hodgkin's disease, some T-cell lymphomas and anaplastic large cell lymphoma.	Membrane and Golgi apparatus in the cytoplasm
CD21	A type I transmembrane protein found in the cytoplasm of pre-B cells and on the surface of mature B cells, follicular dendritic cells, pharyngeal and cervical epithelial cells, some thymocytes and some T cells. It plays a role in signal transduction.	It is expressed in hairy cell leukaemia, B-cell lymphoma and some T-cell acute lymphocytic leukaemias. Receptor for complement (C3d) and Epstein–Barr virus (EBV). Mainly used to define follicular dendritic cell networks in follicular lymphoma.	Membrane

APPENDIX 9.1 Key CD marker antibodies used in the diagnostic laboratory. (*Continued*)

Labelling profile

Antibody	Normal	Pathological	Staining pattern
CD23	A type II transmembrane protein found on mature B cells, monocytes, activated macrophages, eosinophils, platelets and dendritic cells.	It can help to distinguish B-cell chronic lymphocytic leukaemia from other entities.	Membrane
CD56	A 140 kDa isoform of neural cell adhesion molecule (NCAM). It is a marker for natural killer cells and some subsets of CD4+ and CD8+ T lymphocytes.	Useful in the identification of tumours of neuroendocrine origin.	Membrane
CD138	Also known as syndecan-1, a transmembrane proteoglycan expressed in stratified and simple epithelia. In haemopoietic tissue, it is expressed in late-stage B cells.	A marker for myeloma cells, useful for terminally differentiated plasma cells. It is associated with multiple myeloma and subclasses of diffuse large B-cell lymphoma.	Membrane
CD246	80 kDa NPM-ALK chimaeric and the 200 kDa normal human ALK proteins.	Recognizes the hybrid gene *NPM-ALK* created by the t(2;5)(p23;q35) chromosomal translocation found in a proportion of anaplastic large cell lymphomas.	Predominantly nuclear but can also be cytoplasmic

APPENDIX 9.2 Additional CD markers used to fine-tune laboratory investigations, particularly for lymphoma diagnosis.

Labelling profile

Antibody	Normal	Pathological	Staining pattern
CD1a	A transmembrane antigen, expressed on cortical thymocytes and Langerhans cells.	Expressed on a subset of precursor T-lymphoblastic lymphoma/leukaemia. Marker for Langerhans cell histiocytosis.	Membrane
CD2	A type I transmembrane protein found on thymocytes, T cells and some natural killer cells.	Expressed in the large majority of T lymphoma and natural killer cell lymphomas.	Membrane
CD4	The CD4 molecule interacts with HLA class II in antigen recognition. It defines T-helper subsets of T cells. It is also expressed on various monocytes.	Most mature T-cell lymphomas are positive.	Membrane
CD7	A type I transmembrane protein found on thymocytes, some T cells, monocytes, natural killer cells and haematopoietic stem cells.	Expressed in patients with mycosis fungoides, some patients with T-cell acute lymphoblastic lymphoma, and a few patients with acute non-lymphocytic lymphoma.	Membrane
CD8	A co-receptor for MHC class I, it defines the T-cytotoxic subset of T cells. It is also found on a subset of myeloid dendritic cells.		Membrane
CD 25	A type I transmembrane protein present on activated T cells, activated B cells, some thymocytes, and myeloid precursors. It recognizes the interleukin 2 (IL-2) receptor.	It is expressed on hairy cell leukaemia and T-cell leukaemia/lymphoma.	Membrane
CD31	Also known as platelet endothelial cell adhesion molecule-1 (PECAM-1), a 130 kDa glycoprotein. Labels endothelial cells.	Useful in demonstrating vascular tumours and to aid confirmation of vascular space invasion by tumours.	Membrane

continued

APPENDIX 9.2 Additional CD markers used to fine-tune laboratory investigations, particularly for lymphoma diagnosis. (*Continued*)

Labelling profile			
Antibody	Normal	Pathological	Staining pattern
CD34	A stem cell marker expressed on haematopoietic stem cell precursors, capillary endothelium and embryonic fibroblasts.	The antibody is also used to identify vascular and lymphatic tumours.	Membrane
CD38	Cyclic ADP ribose hydrolase glycoprotein found on many immune cells. Also functions in cell adhesion, signal transduction and calcium signalling.	Used as a prognostic marker in leukaemia and can also identify plasma cells.	Membrane
CD68	A 110 kDa highly glycosylated transmembrane protein which is mainly located in lysosomes. Present in macrophages in many human tissues, including Kupffer cells and macrophages in the red pulp of the spleen, in lung alveoli, in the lamina propria of the intestine, and in the bone marrow. Used as an immunocytochemical marker for monocytes/macrophages.	Useful where there is a need to distinguish macrophages (positive) from other cells, such as tumour cells, in an inflamed area.	Cytoplasmic and membranous
CD99	Fas receptor—receptor for Fas ligand, an extrinsic apoptotic signal *MIC2* gene product (p30/32mic2).	Strongly expressed on cell membranes in Ewing's sarcoma and primitive peripheral neuroectodermal tumours.	Membrane
CD117	Recognizes the proto-oncogene *c-kit*, the receptor for stem cell factor. A glycoprotein that regulates cellular differentiation, particularly in haematopoiesis.	Often employed for gastrointestinal stromal tumours and small-cell lung carcinomas.	Membrane

APPENDIX 9.3 Other commonly used antibodies that are not CD markers.

Labelling profile			
Antibody	Normal	Pathological	Staining pattern
Smooth muscle actin (SMA)	It can also be used for myoepithelial cells.	Positive for smooth muscle cells and tumours derived from them. Myoepithelial cells are absent in ducts and glands in foci of invasive breast cancer.	Cytoplasmic
Androgen receptor	Labels cells containing the androgen receptor.		Nuclear
Bcl-2	Labels cells involved with the t(14;18) translocation. It is important in inhibiting the apoptopic pathway.	It is used mainly to demonstrate follicular lymphomas.	Nuclear
Bcl-6	A transcriptional regulatory protein. It demonstrates a nuclear staining pattern.	Expressed in a variety of B-cell lymphomas including follicular, diffuse large B-cell lymphoma and Burkitt's lymphoma.	Nuclear
β-amyloid		Labels β-amyloid in senile plaques in brain tissue from patients with Alzheimer's disease.	Extracellular
34βE12	Reacts with cytokeratin 1, 5, 10 and 14. Labels normal squamous, ductal and other complex epithelia.	Labels ductal carcinoma of the breast, pancreas, bile duct and salivary gland. Used to label urothelial carcinoma of the bladder, nasopharyngeal carcinoma, thymoma and epithelioid mesothelioma.	Cytoplasmic

APPENDIX 9.3 Other commonly used antibodies that are not CD markers. (*Continued*)

Antibody	Normal	Pathological	Staining pattern
	Labelling profile		
CA 125	Labels a mucin glycoprotein.	Labels adenocarcinoma of the colon, breast and lung, bronchoalveolar carcinoma, uterine adenomatoid tumours, ovarian endometrioid and serous carcinomas.	Cytoplasmic
Calcitonin	A 32 amino acid peptide hormone found in thyroid C-cells.	Used mainly to identify medullary thyroid carcinoma and related metastatic deposits.	Cytoplasmic
Caldesmon	A smooth muscle-specific protein involved with muscle contraction.	Useful in labelling smooth muscle-derived tumours.	Cytoplasmic
Calponin	A developmental regulatory protein in smooth muscle and myoepithelial cells.	Useful for tumours of smooth muscle derivation.	Cytoplasmic
Calretinin	Also known as 29 kDa calbindin. A vitamin-dependent calcium-binding protein.	Stains mesothelioma and is useful in the differentiation of lung tumours.	Cytoplasmic
CAM 5.2	Labels cytokeratin 8. Often paired with cytokeratin 18.	Used to differentiate lobular from ductal carcinoma of the breast. Labels neuroendocrine carcinomas (Merkel-cell carcinoma) with a characteristic 'perinuclear dot' staining pattern.	Cytoplasmic
Carcinoembryonic antigen (CEA)		A 180 kDa glycoprotein. The antibody can react with ductal carcinomas of the breast in addition to lung and colorectal carcinomas.	Cytoplasmic
Chromogranin A	Labels normal neuroendocrine cells.	Derived from the C-terminal half of chromogranin A isolate from patients with carcinoid tumours. Useful for demonstrating neuroendocrine tumours.	Cytoplasmic
Collagen IV	An important protein of the basement membrane zone.	Can be useful in the interpretation of peripheral nerve sheath tumours.	Extracellular
Cyclin D1		A 36 kDa protein encoded by the *CCND*1 (*bcl*-1) gene. Cyclin D1 is mainly used for the identification of mantle cell lymphoma.	Nuclear
D2-40	Reacts with a 40 kDa sialoglycoprotein expressed in a variety of tissues. It labels lymphatic endothelium but not vascular endothelium.	Useful in the investigation of Kaposi's sarcoma.	Membrane
Desmin	Reacts with smooth and striated muscle cells.	It can be used to label tumours derived from such cells.	Cytoplasmic
E-cadherin	Reacts with a 120 kDa transmembrane cell adhesion molecule. It is an important molecule in intercellular adhesion of epithelial cells.	It labels the majority of ductal breast carcinomas, whereas lobular carcinomas are weak or negative.	Membrane
Epithelial growth factor receptor (EGFR)	Recognizes a 170 kDa variant of wild-type EGFR and EGFRvIII variant.	It labels simple and squamous epithelium and is expressed in a variety of tumours.	Membrane
Epithelial membrane antigen (EMA)	Reacts with normal and neoplastic epithelium.	Useful for demonstrating epithelial derived tumours.	Cytoplasmic

continued

APPENDIX 9.3 Other commonly used antibodies that are not CD markers. (*Continued*)

Labelling profile			
Antibody	**Normal**	**Pathological**	**Staining pattern**
Epstein–Barr virus latent membrane protein 1 (LMP-1)		Labels the Epstein–Barr virus latent gene product. Useful for demonstrating latent EBV, often used in the assessment of Hodgkin's disease.	Cytoplasmic
Estrogen (oestrogen) receptor (ER)	Reacts with oestrogen receptor-α. Labels epithelial and myometrial cells of the uterus.	Neoplastic cells of the breast.	Nuclear
Factor VIII (von Willebrand factor)	Reacts with von Willebrand factor, present in endothelial cells of blood vessels. It is also present in megakaryocytes.	Antibody used to identify tumours derived from endothelial cells or megakaryocyte proliferation.	Membrane and cytoplasmic
Factor XIIIa	Labels dermal dendrocytes.	Useful in the delineation of some cutaneous neoplasms, such as distinguishing dermatofibromas from dermatofibrosarcoma protuberans.	Membrane and cytoplasmic
Glial fibrillary acidic protein	Recognizes a 50 kDa intracytoplasmic filamentous protein present in astrocytes.	Astrocytomas.	Cytoplasmic
Granzyme B	Labels a 29 kDa serine protease localized to cytotoxic T cells and natural killer cells.	The antibody has application in assessing cytotoxic and natural killer cell lymphomas.	Cytoplasmic
Gross cystic disease fluid protein 15 (GCDFP15)	Labels a 15 kDa secretory glycoprotein and is a marker of apocrine differentiation. The protein is expressed in breast cystic fluid, apocrine, lacrimal, ceruminous and eccrine glands.	Used to assess primary and metastatic tumours of the breast, occasionally in cases of salivary, sweat gland and prostate tumours.	Cytoplasmic
HER2		Labels the HER2 protein. Used to assess over-expression of HER2 in breast carcinomas. Over-expression occurs in 10–40% of invasive breast carcinomas.	Membrane
HMB-45		Recognizes the gp100 antigenic epitope. This antibody is a melanocyte-selective antibody, although it is not specific. Its main application is in the assessment of melancytic lesions.	Cytoplasmic
Kappa	Recognizes the kappa light chain in B cells.	It represents one of the only markers which can prove clonality and malignancy.	Cytoplasmic, membrane and extracellular
Ki-67	Recognizes a huge nuclear protein (345–396 kDa in size). It is expressed during all stages of the cell cycle (G_1, S, G_2 and M phases), but absent in resting cells (G_0 phase).	It is a useful antibody to assess proliferation rates in normal and neoplastic states.	Nuclear
Lambda	Labels lambda light chains in B cells.	It represents one of the only markers which can prove clonality and malignancy.	Cytoplasmic, membrane and extracellular
Laminin	Recognizes a 380 kDa laminin α5-chain. It has application in the assessment of the basement membrane, blood vessels, muscle, fat and nerves.		Extracellular

APPENDIX 9.3 Other commonly used antibodies that are not CD markers. (*Continued*)

Labelling profile			
Antibody	Normal	Pathological	Staining pattern
Lysozyme	Labels histiocytes and malignancies derived from such cells.	Useful in assessing monocytic leukaemias.	Cytoplasmic
Melan A	Melanocyte-selective marker. A transmembrane protein expressed in skin and the retina.	Used to identify melanocytic neoplasms.	Cytoplasmic
MUM1	Recognizes the MUM1 protein in a subset of light zone germinal centre B cells.	It has application in assessment of the transition of germinal centre B cells (BCL6+) to immunoblasts and plasma cells (CD138+).	Nuclear
MyoD1	Recognizes a 45 kDa nuclear protein associated with myogenesis in muscle tissue. Its expression is restricted to skeletal muscle.	It has application in the assessment of rhabdomyosarcoma.	Nuclear
Myogenin	Myogenin is a regulatory protein involved in muscle development. It is restricted to cells of skeletal muscle.	The majority of rhabdomyosarcomas and Wilms' tumours are positive.	Nuclear
Neuron-specific enolase (NSE)	Reacts with normal and neoplastic cells of neuronal and neuroendocrine derivation.	It has application in the identification of neuroendocrine tumours, neuroblastomas, retinoblastomas, desmoplastic malignant melanoma and small-cell lung carcinoma.	Cytoplasmic
p16	Cyclin-dependent kinase inhibitor 2A. Also known as CDKN2A. Recognizes a gene involved in tumour suppression.	Regulates cell cycle mutations in p16 and is increased in a variety of cancers, notably melanoma. Also seen in cervical intraepithelial neoplasia (CIN).	Nuclear
p53	Labels wild and mutant type of the *p53* oncogene.	Increases in p53 expression occur in numerous malignant tumours.	Nuclear
p63	Transformation-related protein 63. This is a protein encoded by the *TP63* gene.	p63 is useful in differentiating prostatic adenocarcinoma and benign prostatic tissue, as it highlights basal cells in the latter. It distinguishes poorly differentiated squamous cell carcinoma (strongly expressed) from small-cell carcinoma or adenocarcinoma (negative).	Nuclear
Human papillomavirus		Reacts with non-conformational, internal and linear epitopes of a major capsid protein of HPV-1. It has been shown to label cells infected with HPV types 6, 11, 16, 18, 31, 33, 42, 51, 52, 56 and 58. It predominantly labels nuclei of infected cells.	Nuclear
Progesterone receptor (PR)		Labels cells containing the steroid hormone receptor in breast carcinoma. It is often used in conjunction with ER as a prognostic breast carcinoma marker.	Nuclear
Prostate-specific antigen (PSA)	Recognizes a 33 kDa protein produced by prostatic epithelium and epithelial cells lining the periurethal glands.	Used to assess normal and neoplastic prostatic tissue. Helpful in verifying the prostatic origin of a metastasis.	Membrane and cytoplasmic
Smooth muscle myosin (SMM; myosin heavy chain)	Reacts with smooth muscle cells and myoepithelial cells, but not myofibroblasts.	Useful in labelling myoepithelial cells in breast tumours, helping to distinguish benign lesions and carcinoma *in situ* from invasive tumours.	Cytoplasmic

continued

APPENDIX 9.3 Other commonly used antibodies that are not CD markers. (*Continued*)

Labelling profile			
Antibody	Normal	Pathological	Staining pattern
S100	Recognizes S100 protein in cells derived from the neural crest. Labels myoepithelial cells.	It has wide application and is positive in malignant melanoma, chondroblastoma and schwannomas. It is also useful for labelling tumours of histiocytic/dendritic cell lineage.	Cytoplasmic and nuclear
Synaptophysin	Present on nerves and neuroendocrine cells.	Reacts with cells of neuroendocrine origin. It has application in identifying such cells and tumours derived from such cells.	Cytoplasmic
Thrombomodulin	Recognizes a transmembrane glycoprotein lining blood and lymphatic vessels, mesothelial cells macrophages, synovial cells, megakaryocytes and platelets.	It has application in the assessment of vascular tumours and aids the differentiation of mesothelioma from pulmonary adenocarcinoma.	Membrane and cytoplasmic
Thyroid transcription factor-1 (TTF-1)	Lung and thyroid cells.	Lung and thyroid tumour cells.	Nuclear
Vimentin	Reacts with the intermediate filament vimentin found in cells of mesenchymal origin.	Identifies sarcomas and melanomas.	Cytoplasmic

 Further reading

- Adams GP, Weiner LM. Monoclonal antibody therapy of cancer. *Nat Biotechnol* 2005; **23**(9): 1147–57.

- Amin MB, Epstein JI, Ulbright TM *et al*. Best practice recommendations in the application of immunohistochemistry in urological pathology: report from the International Society of Urological Pathology consensus conference. *Am J Surg Pathol* 2014; **38**: 1017–22.

- Dabbs D. *Diagnostic immunohistochemistry* 3rd edn. Chichester: Elsevier, 2010.

- Dennis JL, Hvidsten TR, Wit EC *et al*. Markers of adenocarcinoma characteristic of the site of origin: development of a diagnostic algorithm. *Clin Cancer Res* 2005; **11**: 3766–72.

- De Young BR, Wick MR. Immunohistologic evaluation of metastatic carcinomas of unknown origin: an algorithmic approach. *Semin Diagn Pathol* 2000; **17**: 184–93.

- Gutierrez C, Schiff R. HER2: biology, detection and clinical implications. *Arch Pathol Lab Med* 2011; **135**: 55–62 (www.archivesofpathology.org/doi/pdf/10.1043/2010-0454-RAR.1).

- Matutes E. New additions to antibody panels in the characterisation of chronic lymphoproliferative disorders. *J Clin Pathol* 2002; **55**: 180–3.

- Paner GP, Luthringer DJ, Amin MB. Best practice in diagnostic immunohistochemistry: prostate carcinoma and its mimics in needle core biopsies. *Arch Pathol Lab Med* 2008; **132**: 1388–96 (www.archivesofpathology.org/doi/pdf/10.1043/1543-2165[2008]132 [1388:BPIDIP]2.0.CO;2).

- Yeh IT, Mies C. Application of immunohistochemistry to breast lesions. *Arch Pathol Lab Med* 2008; **132**: 349–58 (www.archivesofpathology.org/doi/pdf/10.1043/1543-2165 [2008]132[349:AOITBL]2.0.CO;2).

- Sutton K. How 'personalised' is personalized medicine? What are the challenges for pathology in delivering this for patients? www.pathsoc.org. 2013.

Useful websites

- Cancer Research UK (**www.cancerresearchuk.org/**)
- The Royal College of Pathologists (**www.rcpath.org**)
- Prostate Cancer Research Institute (**www.prostate-cancer.org/pcricms/**)
- The Prostate Cancer Charity (**www.prostate-cancer.org.uk/**)
- The Lymphoma Association (**www.lymphomas.org.uk/**)
- Herceptin (**www.herceptin.com**)
- Glivec (**www.glivec.com**)

 Discussion questions

9.1 Describe the use of antibody panels in immunocytochemistry to identify tumours.

9.2 Explain the value of CD nomenclature in antibody classification.

9.3 Explain the main tumour groups in which immunocytochemistry is used to assist in determining diagnosis.

9.4 Explain why the demonstration of basal cells and myoepithelial cells is significant in prostate and breast disease, respectively.

9.5 Describe the use of immunofluorescence in the study of autoimmune disease.

Answers to the self-check questions and tips for responding to the discussion questions are provided on the book's accompanying website:

 Visit www.oup.com/uk/orchard2e

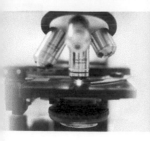

10

In situ hybridization: key concepts and applications

Anthony Warford and Emanuela Volpi

Learning objectives

After studying this chapter, you should have:

■ An understanding of the principles of *in situ* hybridization for the microscopic localization of nucleic acids in cell and tissue preparations.

■ An appreciation of the key technical aspects of the methodology and factors that promote the achievement of successful results.

■ An overview of recent developments and advances for improved sensitivity.

■ Examples where *in situ* hybridization is being used to assist in diagnosis and to answer research questions via the demonstration of DNA, mRNA, and microRNA target sequences.

10.1 Introduction

In situ hybridization
An integrated experimental approach which combines cell-by-cell microscopic visualization with high-resolution analysis of nucleic acids (DNA and RNA).

As described in Chapters 8 and 9, immunocytochemistry allows for the specific localization of proteins in cells and tissues. The subject of this chapter is ***in situ* hybridization** (ISH), a method that relies on base pair complementarity to enable specific localization of nucleic acids in cellular pathology samples. The two methods share many technical similarities, including fixation and pre-treatment steps to optimally conserve then reveal targets for antibodies or nucleic acid probes to bind to. Detection methods, to allow visualization of the interaction of these reagents, can also be similar. However, as will be noted, there are important distinctions. Both methodologies are widely employed in research studies and are used in the diagnostic setting in a complementary fashion to assess the molecular status of cancers as a prerequisite to targeted therapy.

ISH was first described in 1969 by two independent research groups (Gall and Pardue, 1969, John *et al.*, 1969) and was amongst the first in the collection of methods that have since been grouped under the heading of molecular biology. In Figure 10.1, the principles of fluorescent and chromogenic ISH are outlined. There are many other variations of the method and the acronyms used for these together with a brief explanation for each is provided in Table 10.1.

While the application of ISH to demonstrate specific DNA and RNA sequences in a variety of cell and tissue preparations had been described by the early 1970s, the potential for its widespread use in cytology, histology, pathology, and genetics had to wait for the next decade with the transition from radioactive probe labelling to non-radioactive chromogenic and fluorescent methods of probe detection (Herrington *et al.*, 1989; Pinkel *et al.*, 1988). Today ISH, in all its permutations, is widely employed in both diagnostics and research. In the pathology setting it can be successfully applied as an adjunctive, powerful diagnostic, prognostic and predictive tool to detect a variety of specific DNA changes within tissue sections and inform 'personalized' therapeutic approaches. This began with the application of non-radioactive fluorescence ISH (FISH) to demonstrate HER2 gene copy number change or 'amplification' in breast carcinoma (Wang *et al.*, 2000). ISH has also found a niche diagnostic application in the demonstration of mRNA as an indicator of specific changes in gene expression in cases where immunocytochemistry (ICC) does not provide unequivocal results (Akhtar *et al.*, 1989). In research applications ISH presently complements high-throughput microarray analysis outputs by providing evidence of dysregulation of gene expression, at mRNA and microRNA level, on an individual cell basis (Sempere, 2014, Weil *et al.*, 2010). With the introduction of methodological variants that have potential for the demonstration of very low copy number mRNA species (Cassidy and Jones, 2014) the technique is set to further the understanding of the molecular basis of human disease and to become more widely used for practical applications in 'precision' medicine.

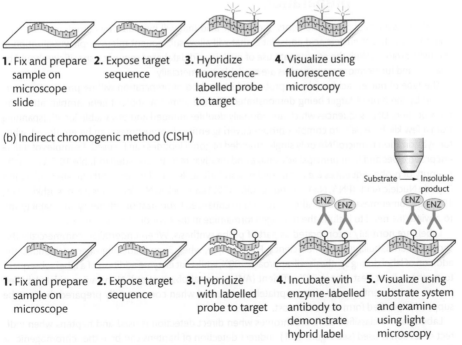

(a) Direct fluorescence method (FISH)

1. Fix and prepare sample on microscope slide   **2.** Expose target sequence   **3.** Hybridize fluorescence-labelled probe to target   **4.** Visualize using fluorescence microscopy

(b) Indirect chromogenic method (CISH)

Substrate → Insoluble product

1. Fix and prepare sample on microscope   **2.** Expose target sequence   **3.** Hybridize with labelled probe to target   **4.** Incubate with enzyme-labelled antibody to demonstrate hybrid label   **5.** Visualize using substrate system and examine using light microscopy

Note: Fluorescein hapten labels can be used in indirect methods

FIGURE 10.1
Examples of direct and indirect *in situ* hybridization methods.

TABLE 10.1 Abbreviations and acronyms used for *in situ* hybridization methods.

Chromosome 'painting': Methodology that provides differential fluorescent colouring of entire chromosomes or chromosome arms. It is used to show gross chromosomal alterations.

CISH (Chromogenic ISH): Indirect detection of probe label with antibody or other enzyme labelled reagent/s. Visualization using substrate system producing an insoluble end product for bright field microscope examination.

DISH (Double ISH): Two nucleic acid targets demonstrated simultaneously (using fluorescent labelled probes) or sequentially using chromogenic detection.

FISH (Fluorescence ISH): End point is fluorescent. Can be direct when probe is fluorescently labelled or indirect when last step in the detection method introduces a fluorescent molecule.

M-FISH (Multiplex FISH): ISH applied to metaphase spread preparations for simultaneous detection of multiple fluorescent probes.

RISH (Radioactive ISH): Radiolabel incorporated into the probe nucleic acid sequence. Detection is by autoradiography. Resolution is dependent on radiolabel used. 32p provides for low resolution, 33p and 35s for moderate resolution and 3h for best resolution.

SISH (Silver-enhanced ISH): Relies on the deposition of metallic silver as the end point for the method. It Is suitable for bright field microscopy.

SELF-CHECK 10.1

What type of molecules can be demonstrated using ISH and to what type of preparations can the method be applied?

10.2 **Technology**

10.2.1 **Probe preparation**

A probe is composed of two elements; the nucleic acid that will hybridize by complementary base pairing to the target nucleic acid and a label that will allow subsequent microscopic visualization of this hybridization. With the appropriate use of nucleic acid databases sequence specificity should be assured, and furthermore many probes are available commercially.

The type of nucleic acid used as a probe and its method of preparation will be principally determined by the type of target being demonstrated. For the demonstration of gene amplification and translocation, DNA sequences which are normally double-stranded and of variable length (spanning from a few kilobase pairs to complex probes covering entire chromosomes) can be employed, while for hybridization to microRNA only single-stranded oligonucleotides can be used. Examples of different probe types and their principal advantage and disadvantage are provided in Table 10.2. Whilst the majority of probe sequences are composed of standard nucleic acid bases, synthetic alternatives like Peptide Nucleic Acids (PNA, Nielsen and Egholm, 1999) and Locked Nucleic Acids (LNA, Koshkin *et al.*, 1998) are sometimes used. Both alternatives claim enhanced hybridization efficiency and stability and to obviate the need to include the teratogen formamide in the hybridization solution.

Labels are normally incorporated as part of probe synthesis. When undertaken commercially this should assure labelling at high efficiency. For example, when 3' end labelling oligonucleotides, the addition of label during synthesis will approach 100%, whilst Tdt enzyme addition of a label subsequent to synthesis is, at best, about 50% efficient (AW, personal observation). Non-radioactively labelled probes are inherently stable, if appropriately stored, and when commercially prepared they can be supplied in purified form at modest cost.

Labels can be classified as fluorochromes when direct detection is used and haptens when indirect detection is used (see Figure 10.1). Indirect detection of haptens can be either chromogenic or fluorescent.

TABLE 10.2 Examples of nucleic acid probe types used in ISH.

	Recombinant sequences		Oligonucleotides	PCR
	Double-stranded DNA	Single-stranded RNA	Single-stranded DNA	Double-stranded DNA
Application	Demonstration of DNA and RNA targets.	Demonstration of mRNA targets.	Demonstration of DNA, mRNA, and microRNA targets.	Demonstration of DNA and mRNA targets.
Principal advantage	Probes can be very long and incorporate many hapten labels. Ideal for gene visualization.	Very high hybridization efficiency.	High hybridization efficiency due to short length. Must be used for microRNA visualization.	Length can be precisely controlled and produced when needed.
Principal disadvantage	Probe requires denaturation before hybridization.	Difficult to produce and store without degradation.	Multiple sequences may be needed to raise sensitivity levels.	Potential batch variation.

A wide variety of fluorescent labels are available and their use has been associated with the demonstration of DNA targets in metaphase and interphase preparations (Fauth and Speicher, 2001, Langer *et al.*, 2004). Previous disadvantages of the quenching of fluorescent labels during microscopy and slide storage have largely been overcome and semi-permanent mountants are available. This method is known as fluorescence *in situ* hybridization (FISH).

In research applications the use of fluorescent-labelled probes or fluorescent end points to indirect ISH methods is favoured for the simultaneous (multiplex FISH) demonstration of nucleic acids as, by simple change of excitation and emission filter combinations, it provides ready discrimination between targets co-located in the same region of a cell or tissue (Sempere *et al.*, 2010). Quantum dot technology offers an alternative means of introducing a fluorescent label and can, in theory, provide for many spectral end points dependent on the diameter of the 'dot' (Gao *et al.*, 2005). This technology results in permanent non-quenching preparations and its use in multiplex FISH has been described (Byers *et al.*, 2007).

As stated, hapten labels provide a means for indirect demonstration of hybridization. In its most commonly used methodology the hapten label is detected using an antibody to which is conjugated an active enzyme. Using an appropriate substrate an insoluble coloured precipitate is formed, thereby localizing the target of hybridization. This ISH method is known as chromogenic ISH or CISH and is outlined in Figure 10.1.

Hapten labels invariably include a carbon chain 'spacer' between the nucleotide analogue and the label itself. This spacer ensures that the label is not hidden in hybridized helix and so is available to bind efficiently to the reagent that recognizes it at the commencement of the detection procedure.

Biotin was introduced as the first hapten label and has the advantage of being able to react very efficiently with avidin/streptavidin that in turn can react with fluorochrome-conjugated avidin or streptavidin/biotin/enzyme complexes to amplify the demonstration of the hybrid. However, when using biotinylated probes in tissues, blocking steps must be undertaken to suppress the demonstration of endogenous biotin due to its abundant presence in liver and kidney and to a lesser extent in other tissues.

The most commonly used hapten label is digoxigenin (Herrington *et al.*, 1989). This label has no endogenous tissue distribution. In FISH, digoxigenin is detected by a fluorochrome-conjugated anti-digoxigenin antibody. Fluorescein and its derivatives are less frequently employed as hapten labels for CISH. Fluorescein is not considered to have an endogenous distribution, but peptide-producing endocrine cells in the gastrointestinal tract can stain non-specifically when this label is used (AW, personal observation).

Key Point

Probe preparation

A probe is composed of two elements: a nucleic acid sequence that has a complementary base sequence to the target and a label to allow visualization of the nucleic acid hybrid.

10.2.2 Sample preparation

As with all technologies that are based on the microscopic examination of cells and tissues there is a necessity to retain, in as an unaltered form as possible, the target to be demonstrated whilst also preserving cytology or morphology. Inevitably this means that the sample must be chemically fixed or undergo a process of molecular stabilization that renders proteins and nucleic acids insoluble. As there is no ideal fixative that is able to fulfil the criteria of absolute target and cytology/morphology conservation, allowance must be made for the limitations imposed by this necessary process. Consideration must also be given to the native stability of nucleic acids where DNA is more stable than mRNA. Interestingly microRNA evidence suggests that such sequences are more stable than mRNA (Hall *et al.*, 2012).

Fixation can be broadly categorized by type and application. Non-additive (precipitating) fixatives (e.g. methanol and ethanol) act by disrupting hydrophobic interactions and effectively 'congealing' the cytoplasm, and are frequently used for cytological preparations. Nucleic acid conservation is typically very good and the sequences are not masked by the fixation process. Brief paraformaldehyde fixation is also employed for cytological preparations. This tends to protect the cells better than non-additive fixation through the rigours of the ISH procedure. However, due to its additive (cross-linking) interaction with nucleic acids and surrounding proteins it introduces some degree of target masking. Target masking is exacerbated when formalin-fixed and paraffin-embedded (FFPE) sections are used for ISH (Illig *et al.*, 2009). The cross-linking properties of formaldehyde and the conditions imposed during paraffin processing also fragment nucleic acids (Klopfleisch *et al.*, 2011). This tends to reduce the sensitivity of ISH when using FFPE preparations, but sufficient nucleic acid sequence identity is usually present to allow for complementary hybrids to be formed.

Due to formalin-induced target masking, pre-treatment is required at the beginning of the ISH procedure to 'open up' the preparations to allow subsequent hybridization to occur efficiently. This is usually done by incubating preparations with Proteinase K. This enzyme can be applied for a set time at 37°C, but at variable concentrations, according to the type of nucleic acid target and duration of fixation (Mostegl *et al.*, 2011, and Table 10.3). When the fixation conditions are not consistent or unknown, it is sensible to pre-treat with Proteinase K at a minimum of two concentrations to establish optimal unmasking conditions or, at least, to point to what these may be. When using commercial ISH kits, especially when coupled to their use on automated platforms, proteolytic digestion can be combined with the pre-treatments that mimic those employed for heat-mediated antigen retrieval in ICC.

TABLE 10.3 Proteinase K pre-treatment concentrations according to preparation and target nucleic acid following formaldehyde-based fixation.

Target	Fixation time	Preparation	Proteinase K range (μg/mL)
DNA	2–15 min	Cell culture, ThinPreps*, fine-needle aspirations, frozen sections.	0.5–10
	6–168 h	FFPE.†	25–50
RNA†	2–15 min	Cell culture, ThinPreps, fine-needle aspirations, frozen sections.	0.5–5
	6–168 h	FFPE.	2–15

Key:
*Applies to all similar preparations
'Formalin-fixed, paraffin-embedded
'Applies to mRNA and microRNA

Other pre-treatments can be included. When a biotin/avidin-based detection system is used the blocking of endogenous biotin is required. Acetylation, that has been claimed to enhance ISH sensitivity and reduce non-specific staining (Hayashi *et al.*, 1978), may also be included as a pre-treatment. In both situations these step are undertaken after proteinase digestion. A further important consideration is that all solutions used for pre-treatment and during hybridization must be nuclease free to avoid degradation of the target nucleic acid. This is particularly the case when demonstrating RNA, which is more sensitive to nuclease degradation than DNA.

Finally, for the labelled probe to recognize and bind its complementary 'target' both probe and target nucleic acids must be single-stranded. For this purpose, both specimens and probes will normally undergo a heat denaturation step when DNA is being demonstrated and/or when a DNA probe is being used.

Key Point

Sample preparation

Fixation is necessary to preserve the target nucleic acid together with cytology or morphology during the ISH process.

What are the key criteria for optimal cell and tissue preparation of samples for ISH?

10.2.3 Hybridization

This step is central in the ISH procedure as it is here that the principles of base pair complementarity are applied to hybridize the labelled probe to its target sequence. The aim is to obtain hybridization only between the probe and its target and thus to achieve absolute specificity. Providing due care and attention are paid to the conditions used during this step this can be achieved.

Factors that affect the specificity of hybridization are typically discussed under the heading of stringency. Principal amongst these factors are probe concentration, temperature and time of hybridization, and the concentration of monovalent cations present in the hybridization solution. The effects of these factors along with those that make a secondary contribution are summarized in Table 10.4.

A distinctive feature of many hybridization solutions used for ISH is the inclusion of formamide. It acts as a helix destabilizing reagent and thereby allows hybridization to be undertaken at temperatures significantly below that of the melt temperature of potential hybrids and thus helping to preserve the cytology/morphology of the samples. However, formamide is a teratogen. It has been shown that when LNA probes are used it can be removed from the hybridization solutions as the temperature of hybridization is 55°C (Jørgensen *et al.*, 2010).

Many ISH procedures include a pre-hybridization step where the preparations are *equilibrated* in a solution that is identical to that of the hybridization solution, but without the presence of the probe. Also it is common to include post-hybridization stringency washes to remove any excess probe and/or probe that may have non-specifically hybridized to sequences other than that of the target because of partial sequence match. Here it should be noted that the stability of hybrids will be determined by the type of nucleic acid used as a probe and its *target*, with RNA/RNA hybrids being most stable and DNA/DNA hybrids being least stable.

TABLE 10.4 Hybridization solution components and conditions and their effects.

Component/condition	Purpose	Comment
Probe	Hybridization to target sequence	Concentration influences sensitivity and of hybrid formation
Monovalent cation (sodium chloride)	Regulation of specificity and sensitivity of hybrid formation	Concentration will regulate charge repulsion between nucleic acid probe and target sequence. Higher concentration negates charge repulsion, enhancing hybrid formation, but potentially allowing non-specific hybridization.
Temperature		Higher temperatures will favour specific hybridization, but without use of formamide the temperature used may compromise cell/tissue preservation.
Formamide		As a helix destabilizing reagent it introduces repulsion between probe and target sequence thereby allowing hybridization to be undertaken at lower temperatures where cell/tissue preservation should be maintained.
Macromolecules (dextran sulphate)	Rate of hybrid formation and regulation of non-specific hybridization	Negates charge repulsion between probe and target and locally concentrate the hybridization solution thereby increasing rate of hybrid formation.
Divalent anions	Inhibition of nuclease activity	Should not be used as a substitute for nuclease-free preparation of hybridization solution.
Buffer	Maintains pH	

Key Point

Hybridization

Hybridization relies on complementary base pairing between the probe and target nucleic acid sequence.

SELF-CHECK 10.4

How do probe concentration, temperature of hybridization, monovalent cation concentration, and formamide interact to affect the specificity of hybrid formation?

10.2.4 Detection

When fluorescence-labelled probes have been employed this step can be as simple as completing any post-hybridization washes, counterstaining nuclei with 4',6-diamidino-2-phenylindole (DAPI), a fluorescent staining with high affinity for A–T rich DNA, and anti-fade mounting. This is followed by microscopic examination using a fluorescence microscope fitted with appropriate excitation and emission filters. This approach is widely used in cancer diagnosis for the demonstration of gene amplification and translocation (Caria and Vanni, 2014; Perner *et al.*, 2008; Wang *et al.*, 2000). Fluorescent end points can also be obtained via the application of indirect detection methods where signal amplification, as discussed in Section 10.2.6, can provide a means of demonstrating low copy target sequences.

Chromogenic detection of ISH hybrids is usually based on the interaction of digoxigenin probe label with an alkaline phosphatase-tagged antibody against the label followed by demonstration of the enzyme using a nitroblue tetrazolium, 5-bromo-4-chloro-3-indolyl phosphate (NBT/BCIP) substrate system. This gives a deep blue to purple end product that requires aqueous mounting. A distinct advantage of the use of the NBT/BCIP is that the formation of the precipitate does not prevent the continuing activity of the enzyme. Accordingly, this simple detection system can result in considerable signal amplification. CISH methods reliant on the detection of fluorescent labels usually use an alkaline phosphatase-labelled antibody and NBT/BCIP substrate.

As an alternative chromogenic detection method, the peroxidase/diaminobenzidene end point provides for a permanent mounted preparation. However, the enzyme–substrate reaction, whilst intense, is very short lived. Accordingly, when this chromogenic end point is employed, the amplification of signal is provided by using multistep detection methods.

Silver enhanced ISH (SISH) detection relies on the deposition of metallic silver as the end point of the ISH procedure. A variety of methodologies have been described that usually involve multistep detection of a hapten-labelled probe with gold or horseradish peroxidase catalysed deposition of silver (Powell et al., 2007). This method has been automated and is available for the bright field assessment of HER-2 gene amplification.

Key Point

Detection

The end point of modern non-radioactive ISH methods can be fluorescent or chromogenic.

SELF-CHECK 10.5

What chromogenic end point options are available for the completion of an ISH technique?

10.2.5 Controls

As with all analytical methods the inclusion of appropriate controls to validate sensitivity and specificity during technology workup and run controls to verify the subsequent performance of the method are vital.

During probe validation the expected distribution of the target can be confirmed using cultured cell lines and/or relevant tissue samples. When cell cultures are used consideration should be given to using artificially manipulated cells that express a range of target copy numbers and/or a range of cell lines so as to assess the copy number sensitivity of the probe/detection system as well its specificity. If the probe is to be applied to tissue sections then it will also be important to conduct a workup on the relevant tissue/s and again to explore sensitivity by using preparations containing a range of target copy numbers. During this process, an assessment of potential non-specific interactions can also be made and addressed by attention to stringency of hybridization, and/or modification of the ISH procedure, such as post-hybridization washes.

Labelled 'sense' (identical to the target sequence) or scrambled ('nonsense') nucleic acids, prepared in exactly the same way as the specific ('antisense') probe, are often used as controls to highlight non-specific hybridization. The omission of the probe from the hybridization solution will also provide a gauge of any non-specific interactions intrinsic to the procedure itself. For example, this could highlight an issue with the demonstration of endogenous enzyme activity when using a CISH method or show regions of auto-fluorescence when FISH is used. The inclusion of (a) positive control(s) in ISH runs offers an assessment of the consistency of results from run to run. When the positive control contains low or moderate quantities of the target then early warning of sub-optimal performance of the ISH procedure is provided.

> ## Key Point
>
> **Controls**
>
> All new probes must be validated for specificity and sensitivity. In each ISH run, positive and negative controls should be included.

SELF-CHECK 10.6

What type of sample preparation could be used as a positive control for assessment of ISH runs?

10.2.6 Advanced technologies

Several technologies have now been described that offer ISH results of exquisite sensitivity. Amongst these, the tyramide signal amplification (TSA) and branched DNA methods are now making a significant impact in research applications where the demonstration of low copy number mRNA targets is required. It is probable that these will be adopted in diagnostic settings when the demonstration of low copy target sequences is required.

- The TSA method (Yang *et al.*, 1999) is based on the catalytic local deposition of a reporter molecule via the action of tyramide with horseradish peroxidase. Originally introduced with biotin as the reporter, and requiring considerable skill to produce amplification without high non-specific cell/tissue interactions, the system is now offered in kit form using alternative reporters such as dinitrophenol or fluorescent dyes. The procedure, which has been automated, is outlined in Figure 10.2.

- The branched DNA method (Wang *et al.*, 2012), offered commercially as RNAscope (Advanced Cell Diagnostics) and ViewRNA (Affymetrix), is a technique for amplifying mRNA hybridization.

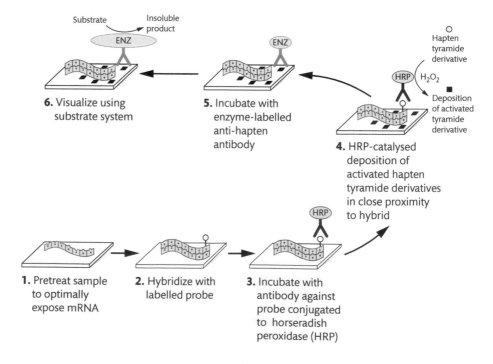

FIGURE 10.2
Tyramide signal amplification for chromogenic ISH.

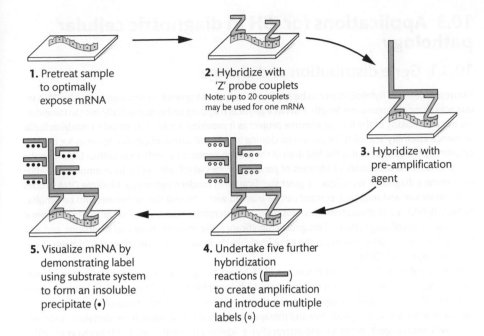

1. Pretreat sample to optimally expose mRNA

2. Hybridize with 'Z' probe couplets
Note: up to 20 couplets may be used for one mRNA

3. Hybridize with pre-amplification agent

4. Undertake five further hybridization reactions (⌐▬) to create amplification and introduce multiple labels (○)

5. Visualize mRNA by demonstrating label using substrate system to form an insoluble precipitate (•)

FIGURE 10.3
Branched DNA method for chromogenic ISH.

Its use allows very low copy number (<10) of mRNA targets to be demonstrated in cell preparations and low copy number targets in FFPE preparations. The technology is based on the hybridization of couplets of oligonucleotides to target sequences that are in close proximity to one another. Each oligonucleotide has a short linking sequence attached and, at their distal ends, base sequences that will hybridize to the pre-amplification reagent. Due to their configuration the probes are usually referred to as 'Z probes'. Following initial hybridization, that may involve up to 20 'Z probe' couplets, the distal probe sequences are hybridized to the pre-amplification reagent that is, in turn, repetitively hybridized to labelled DNA sequences for visualization of the mRNA target. Using this technology, specificity is assured as it is necessary for both 'Z probes' of a couplet to hybridize to the target for subsequent interaction with the detection system to be initiated. Furthermore, by using several 'Z probe' couplets for hybridization a measure of redundancy is built into the system whereby sensitivity is still achieved even when some of the probes fail to hybridize. As with TSA this methodology has also been automated. A schema describing the branched DNA method is provided in Figure 10.3.

Key Point

Advanced technologies

The tyramide signal amplification and branched DNA are novel approaches that permit very low copy number target sequences of mRNA to be demonstrated.

SELF-CHECK 10.7

What are the chief distinguishing features of TSA and branched DNA methods in comparison with standard CISH as illustrated in Figure 10.1?

10.3 Applications for ISH in diagnostic cellular pathology

10.3.1 Gene distribution and change

Fluorescence *in situ* hybridization can be applied to metaphase spreads to visualize and order DNA sequences along chromosomes length. FISH as a physical mapping technique initially rose to fame during the undertaking of the human genome project as it provided a reliable method to establish initial sequence assembly 'scaffolds' for positional cloning and for validation of candidate genes for disease. Conversely, the completion of the first draft of the human genome has led to a wealth of bioinformatic resources and the availability of 'libraries' of genomic probes which altogether have empowered FISH to become a diagnostic technique of great significance in modern pathology. Multiple DNA probes of disparate size and sequence content can be labelled with different fluorochromes and be simultaneously hybridized to metaphase chromosomes and interphase nuclei to 'mark' gross chromosomal rearrangements of diagnostic and prognostic significance, like translocations and inversions, and also to visualize specific DNA changes at the gene level, like duplications and deletions (Mühlmann, 2002; Rondón-Lagos *et al.*, 2014).

In combination with ICC, FISH is used on FFPE breast and gastric cancer preparations to identify *HER2* oncogene copy number on chromosome 17 in interphase nuclei (Figure 10.4). In cases where gene amplification is demonstrated targeted therapy with Herceptin (trastuzumab) is indicated. As this assessment is linked to predictive and therapeutic decisions, FISH must be undertaken in accordance with strict reagent, protocol, and interpretive guidelines (Bartlett *et al.*, 2011; Rakha *et al.*, 2015; Wolff *et al.*, 2014). Establishments offering this procedure must also participate in national external quality assessment schemes and obtain satisfactory scores to be allowed to continue to provide this high value test in diagnostic situations.

Interphase FISH is also currently used to assess patients with non-small cell lung cancer for EML4-ALK fusions resulting from a small inversion within chromosome 2p. In this situation two probes of differing colour are simultaneously applied. When fusion has occurred these are brought into juxtaposition to produce a 'new' colour. Such tumours are suitable for therapeutic intervention with ALK inhibitors (Morán *et al.*, 2013). As with HER-2 ISH, the link between gene change and therapy demands that the hybridization procedure is undertaken under controlled conditions (Demidova *et al.*, 2014).

Chromogenic demonstration of gene copy number change, amplification, and fusion may soon replace FISH in critical diagnostic settings. For these applications several chromogenic end-point methods, which are usually linked to automation, have now been described. These claim to provide equivalent diagnostic sensitivity and specificity to FISH whilst allowing pathologists to readily identify diseased areas for assessment and counting (Gruver *et al.*, 2010; Wagner *et al.*, 2014).

FIGURE 10.4
HER2 **significant amplification (red dots) in SKBR3 cultured cells demonstrated using FISH. Note also copy number gain of the control chromosome 17 centromeric targets (green) due to chromosomal instability in this cell line. Nuclei are counterstained with DAPI (blue). Image courtesy of AstraZeneca, Innovation Center China.**

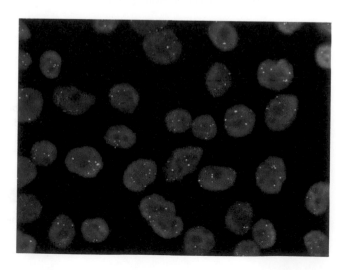

It is very likely that other prognostic and predictive ISH procedures will be introduced (Betts *et al.*, 2014; Park *et al.*, 2015), but in every instance their place alongside the use of ICC and molecular analysis for gene mutations will determine their eventual importance in cancer diagnosis, assessment, and therapeutic intervention.

10.3.2 Infective agents

Due to its ability to visualize nucleic acid sequences in their cellular location, ISH has been extensively used to investigate the association of viruses with disease and their tissue distribution. This has been particularly prominent in locating the epitheliotropic low and high risk human papilloma (HPV) viral subtypes associated with cervical and head and neck cancer and their precursor lesions (Kelesidis *et al.*, 2011; Venuti and Paolini, 2012; Figure 10.5). Epstein–Barr virus (EBV) targets such as latent EBNA and lytic BHLF are very highly expressed and can be demonstrated with equivalent sensitivity and timeliness as when employing ICC methods (Gulley and Tang, 2008; Figure 10.6). Bacteria (Bjarnsholt *et al.*, 2009; Kirketerp-Møller *et al.*, 2008) and fungi (Shinozaki *et al.*, 2012) have also been demonstrated using ISH.

With the exception of EBV demonstration, ISH is usually confined to research applications. For rapid and sensitive diagnosis, PCR methods are often used to identify the infective agent. However, an ISH-based method has been described that may make a significant diagnostic impact when rapid identification of an infective agent is required. This method is based on the use of peptide nucleic acid probes with a fluorescent end point and can provide results within 20 minutes (Forrest *et al.*, 2006). It is commercially available and is known as AdvanDX QuickFISH (Advandx).

10.3.3 mRNA demonstration

As the intermediary between genes and protein expression the selective transcription of mRNA is absolutely vital to the function of cells in health and gene expression levels are frequently altered in disease. As cell function is ultimately controlled by proteins there is a view that change in mRNA expression, whilst of research interest, is not important for diagnosis. However, some examples may be given where ISH for mRNA can provide valuable diagnostic information.

In distinguishing between reactive B-cell hyperplasia and malignant B-cell proliferations it is important to establish if light chain restriction is present. This is normally done using ICC by demonstrating the kappa/lambda immunoglobulin light chain ratio by ICC. In a reactive condition this will be in the order of 6/4 in favour of kappa light chain immunoglobulin, but in a malignant proliferation the ratio will be skewed to greatly favour one of the light chains. A problem can arise when immunoglobulins are being secreted from proliferations as substantial background staining may occur making it difficult to establish a ratio. As mRNA is never exported from cells the demonstration of kappa and lambda light chain mRNA by ISH can be valuable in these situations as no background staining should be present (Akhtar *et al.*, 1989; Lang, 2010). Using standard chromogenic ISH methods light chain restriction has also been reported in lymphoproliferative disease in situations where immunoglobulin

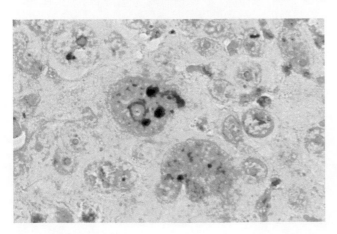

FIGURE 10.5
HPV 16 (dark blue staining) within the nucleus of a cancer cell. Fluorescein-labelled oligonucleotide probe and indirect detection using anti-fluorescein antibody labelled with alkaline phosphatase followed by NBT/BCIP substrate demonstration.

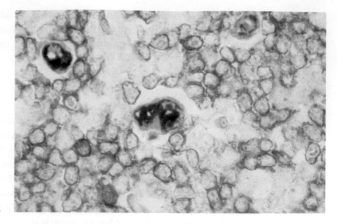

FIGURE 10.6
Staining of EBER RNA
(blue) in Reed–Sternberg
cells in Hodgkin's
lymphoma by ISH and
surrounding lymphocytes
for CD3 (brown) using ICC.

synthesis does not occur, for example in follicular lymphoma (McNicol *et al.*, 1998). However, in routine diagnostic situations this would appear to be the exception rather than the rule (AW, personal observation). Using the branched DNA method, light chain restriction at the mRNA level has been demonstrated with ease in lymphoproliferative disease in which no active immunoglobulin synthesis is being undertaken (Tubbs *et al.*, 2013; Figure 10.7). A further example of where ISH may be preferable to ICC, due to high background staining associated with the latter, is in the demonstration of albumin in cholangiocarcinoma (Ferrone *et al.*, 2014).

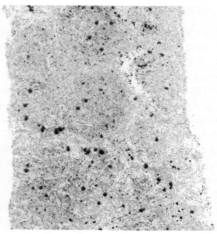

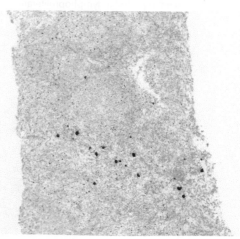

FIGURE 10.7
Demonstration of mRNA
immunoglobulin light
chain restriction using
the RNAscope branched
DNA method in core
biopsy FFPE sections of
follicular lymphoma. Top:
Kappa immunoglobulin
mRNA. Bottom: Lambda
immunoglobulin mRNA.
Note the predominance
of kappa mRNA in the
malignant follicles.

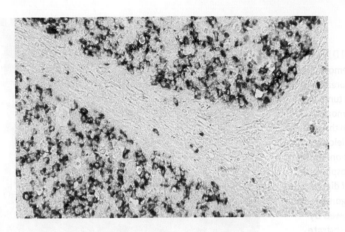

FIGURE 10.8

Demonstration of proliferating lymphocytes (dark blue) concentrated in germinal centres of a reactive tonsil. Indirect alkaline phosphatase detection of fluorescein-labelled histone oligonucleotide probe cocktail. Indirect detection using anti-fluorescein antibody labelled with alkaline phosphatase followed by NBT/BCIP substrate demonstration.

The establishment of cell proliferation indices for cancers is frequently used to provide prognostic information in cancer assessment (Patani et al., 2013) and the demonstration of Ki-67 (Mib1) by ICC is extensively used for this purpose. Cell proliferation indices can also be established by demonstrating the mRNA of histone genes that are only transcribed in the S phase of the cell cycle. As they are expressed at very high levels they can easily be demonstrated using standard CISH methods (Figure 10.8). The ISH demonstration of histone mRNA has been shown to give almost identical cell proliferation indices to Brdu labelling (Alison et al., 1994). As the gene sequences for histones are highly conserved their demonstration by ISH can be applied to other species without alteration of probe sequence (Muskhelishvili et al., 2003).

Using standard ISH methods, many mRNA species cannot be routinely demonstrated due to their low copy expression level. However, with the introduction of ultrasensitive ISH technologies this is changing with reports of the application of branched DNA (Bishop et al., 2012; Chae et al., 2011; Kang et al., 2012) and TSA methodologies (Kiflemariam et al., 2012). Accordingly, it is possible that the demonstration of mRNA will play a greater role in understanding the regulation of transcription in health and disease and find further diagnostic application in the near future.

10.3.4 microRNA

MicroRNA (miR) was first discovered in 1993 in *Caenorhabditis elegans* (Lee et al., 1993) and then identified in humans in 2000 (Pasquinelli et al., 2000). MiRs are very short (15–22 nucleotide) non-coding RNA sequences that regulate the translation of mRNA and thus influence protein expression. Applying molecular analysis methods to homogenates of cell line and tissue preparations, it has become clear that a complex pattern of expression of miRs is required to regulate mRNA in health and that in disease significant perturbations occur (Raisch et al., 2013). In contrast to mRNA, microRNA is never translated and, accordingly, microscopic localization is solely reliant on the use of ISH. The requirement to use ISH has been highlighted by the initial misinterpretation of the role of miR-143 and miR-145 in normal colon and colonic cancer using homogenate sample analysis only (Chivukula et al., 2014; Kent et al., 2014).

With 1881 miRs being deposited in the human miR database (University of Manchester) as of June 2015 there is obviously scope for extensive investigation. As many miRs are expressed at high copy number and conserved in FFPE tissue (Hall et al., 2012), ISH can be undertaken with a high expectancy of success. An extended working day protocol for the demonstration of miR targets using locked nucleic acids probes has been described (Jørgensen et al., 2010; Nielsen and Holmstrøm 2013; Nielsen et al., 2014) (Figure 10.9). It would appear that ISH is poised to make a very positive contribution to identifying specific microRNA expression for cancer diagnosis (Sempere, 2014).

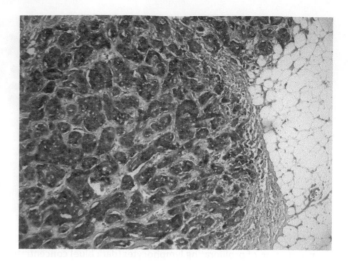

FIGURE 10.9
miR-205 demonstrated in invasive breast cancer. The tumour islands are more darkly stained than the stroma. Locked nucleic acid demonstration. Indirect alkaline phosphatase detection of digoxigenin-labelled oligonucleotide probes followed by NBT/BCIP substrate demonstration.

10.4 Future directions

Owing to its unique characteristics of a combined molecular and cytological approach enabling DNA and RNA visual analysis in single cells, *in situ* hybridization retains a central role within research and diagnostics many decades since its introduction. ISH should be viewed as an established complementary technology to other molecular methods of analysis for the demonstration of nucleic acids and to ICC for protein expression. Applied appropriately to hypothesis-driven research questions ISH will continue to contribute to the understanding of the relationship between gene and protein expression in health and disease. As the applications of ISH to identify HER2 amplification and EML4-ALK fusions for targeted therapeutic intervention have shown, ISH now has an important place in diagnostic cellular pathology. It is reasonable to predict that ISH-based mRNA and microRNA diagnostic, prognostic, and predicative biomarkers may be introduced in the near future.

As will be explored in Chapters 11 and 12, polymerase chain reaction (PCR) and microarray methods for the analysis of nucleic acids in homogenates of cellular pathology samples offer both qualitative and quantitative readouts. In the diagnostic setting PCR technology is employed to demonstrate single point gene mutations that can influence therapeutic choice. In the research context microarray analysis continues to provide information on the regulation of gene expression at the mRNA and microRNA level. However, the application of ISH and ICC is an absolute requirement to determine exact cellular localization and thus assist in understanding perturbations of gene expression in disease. ISH and ICC, at present, provide a semi-quantitative end point. That these read outs could be automatically microscopically scanned and sorted in terms of relative abundance of target is possible. However, this technology needs to be made more robust before the claim of a 'digital readout' being available is made.

CASE STUDY 10.1 A recommendation for HER2-targeted therapy for breast cancer

A 55-year-old female was shown to have 'spiculated margins' at a routine screening mammogram. A core breast biopsy was requested and the formalin-fixed sample embedded in paraffin wax and processed for histopathological investigation.

A diagnosis of invasive ductal carcinoma was made from the haematoxylin and eosin section and immunocytochemistry was requested to establish hormone and HER2 status.

The controls for the immunocytochemistry revealed satisfactory performance of the test and the tumour was negative for hormone receptors. In the HER2-stained slide positive staining was present and this was scored as 2+ as the number of cells with strong complete membrane staining was less than 10% of the tumour cell population. In accordance with recommendations for HER2 testing this result was equivocal and fluorescence *in situ* hybridization was requested to clarify gene amplification status.

The FISH result revealed two copies of the control centromeric chromosome 17 (CEP17) probe in the 20 intact tumour cell nuclei that were counted. In these cells there was no frank amplification of HER2 present and a count was made in each nucleus of the number of positive HER2 signals present. The HER2/CEP17 ratio was then calculated as 2.5. As this ratio was above 2, the tumour was reported as HER2-positive and suitable for HER2-targeted therapy.

CASE STUDY 10.2 Broken bone and lymphoproliferative disease

A 60-year-old male presented with a fractured femur, but with no history of a recent fall or other trauma that would account for the condition. Blood and urine tests revealed an increase in gamma globulins and the presence of Bence-Jones protein, respectively. A bone marrow trephine biopsy was requested. The biopsy was fixed for 24 hours in neutral buffered formalin and then decalcified for a further 24 hours in EDTA to conserve morphological and molecular reactivity. It was then processed for paraffin wax embedding.

On review of the haematoxylin and eosin section a proliferation of plasmacytoid cells was apparent. Combined with the clinical presentation and the blood and urine test results, a diagnosis of multiple myeloma was suggested. To confirm this immunocytochemistry was requested for kappa and lambda light chains to determine if light chain restriction was present. Although appropriately undertaken, the results of the immunocytochemistry were uninterpretable due to the presence of high background staining. It was considered that the most likely reason for this was that the cells were bathed in immunoglobulin secreted by the plasmacytoid cells.

The pathologist then requested *in situ* hybridization for kappa and lambda light chain mRNA to further assess for light chain restriction. As mRNA is not secreted from its cell of origin it was anticipated that background staining would be absent. This indeed proved to be the case and the stained slides showed cytoplasmic staining for kappa light chain mRNA in 90% of the plasmacytoid cells. The demonstration of the light chain restriction by *in situ* hybridization had assisted in confirmation of a diagnosis of multiple myeloma.

Chapter summary

- The principle of *in situ* hybridization (ISH) is outlined and its unique contribution as a tool to demonstrate nucleic acids in their cellular localization highlighted.

- The various types of ISH technology are explained and the principles of ultrasensitive tyramide signal amplification and branched DNA detection methods to detect low copy nucleic acid targets in cells are provided.

- The concepts underlying the key technical steps of ISH are discussed under the headings of probe preparation, sample preparation, hybridization, detection, and use of controls.

- With an emphasis on diagnosis, applications of ISH are considered for the demonstration of genes, infective agents, mRNA, and microRNA.

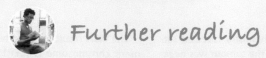 **Further reading**

The field of ISH is fast-moving and for the latest technological advances the pathology-orientated journals should be consulted for research and diagnostic applications. However, some books and book chapters do provide robust protocols and background information that will greatly assist in establishing the method in the laboratory. The following can be recommended:

● Bridger JM, Volpi EV eds. *Fluorescence in situ hybridization (FISH) protocols and applications.* Springer, 2010.

● Hauptmann G ed. *In situ hybridization methods.* Springer, 2015.

● Nielsen B ed. *In situ hybridization protocols.* Springer, 2014.

● Parker A, Bain B, Devereux S *et al. Best practice in lymphoma diagnosis and reporting.* British Committee for Standards in Haematology, Royal College of Pathologists 2010.

● Suvarna KS, Layton C, Bancroft JD eds. *Bancroft's theory and practice of histological techniques* 7th edn. Edinburgh: Churchill Livingstone, 2013.

References

Akhtar N, Ruprai A, Pringle J H, Lauder I, Durrant S T. *In situ* hybridization detection of light chain mRNA in routine bone marrow trephines from patients with suspected myeloma. *Br J Haematol* 1989; **73**: 296–301.

Alison M, Chaudry Z, Baker J, Lauder I, Pringle H. Liver regeneration: a comparison of *in situ* hybridization for histone mRNA with bromodeoxyuridine labeling for the detection of S-phase cells. *J Histochem Cytochem* 1994; **42**: 1603–8.

Bjarnsholt T, Jensen PØ, Fiandaca MJ, *et al. Pseudomonas aeruginosa* biofilms in the respiratory tract of cystic fibrosis patients. *Pediatr Pulmonol* 2009; **44**: 547–58.

Bartlett JM, Starczynski J, Atkey N, *et al.* HER2 testing in the UK: recommendations for breast and gastric in-situ hybridisation methods. *J Clin Pathol* 2011; **64**: 649–53.

Betts G, Valentine H, Pritchard S, *et al.* FGFR2, HER2 and cMet in gastric adenocarcinoma: detection, prognostic significance and assessment of downstream pathway activation. *Virchows Arch* 2014; **464**: 145–56.

Bishop JA, Ma XJ, Wang H, *et al.* Detection of transcriptionally active high-risk HPV in patients with head and neck squamous cell carcinoma as visualized by a novel E6/E7 mRNA *in situ* hybridization method. *Am J Surg Pathol* 2012; **36**: 1874–82.

Byers RJ, Di Vizio D, O'Connell F, *et al.* Semiautomated multiplexed quantum dot-based *in situ* hybridization and spectral deconvolution. *J Mol Diagn* 2007; **9**: 20–9.

Caria P, Vanni R. FISH molecular testing in cytological preparations from solid tumors. *Mol Cytogenet* 2014; **7**: 56.

Cassidy A, Jones J. Developments in *in situ* hybridisation. *Methods* 2014; **70**: 39–45.

Chae BJ, Bae JS, Yim HW, *et al.* Measurement of ER and PR status in breast cancer using the QuantiGene2.0 assay. *Pathology* 2011; **43**: 248–53.

Chivukula RR, Shi G, Acharya A, *et al.* An essential mesenchymal function for miR-143/145 in intestinal epithelial regeneration. *Cell* 2014; **157**: 1104–16.

Demidova I, Barinov A, Savelov N, *et al.* Immunohistochemistry, fluorescence *in situ* hybridization, and reverse transcription-polymerase chain reaction for the detection of anaplastic lymphoma kinase gene rearrangements in patients with non-small cell lung cancer: potential advantages and methodologic pitfalls. *Arch Pathol Lab Med* 2014; **138**: 794–802.

Fauth C, Speicher MR. Classifying by colors: FISH-based genome analysis. *Cytogenet Cell Genet* 2001; **93**: 1–10.

Ferrone CR, Ting DT, Shahid M, *et al.* The ability to diagnose intrahepatic cholangiocarcinoma definitively using novel branched DNA-enhanced albumin RNA *in situ* hybridization technology. *Ann Surg Oncol* 2016; **23**: 290–6.

Forrest GN, Mehta S, Weekes E, *et al.* Impact of rapid *in situ* hybridization testing on coagulase-negative staphylococci positive blood cultures. *J Antimicrob Chemother* 2006; **58**: 154–8.

Gall JG, Pardue ML. Formation and detection of RNADNA hybrid molecules in cytological preparations. *Proc Natl Acad Sci USA* 1969; **63**: 378–83.

Gao X, Yang L, Petros JA, *et al. In vivo* molecular and cellular imaging with quantum dots. *Curr Opin Biotechnol* 2005; **16**: 63–72.

Gruver AM, Peerwani Z, Tubbs RR. Out of the darkness and into the light: bright field *in situ* hybridisation for delineation of ERBB2 (HER2) status in breast carcinoma. *J Clin Pathol* 2010; **63**: 210–19.

Gulley ML, Tang W. Laboratory assays for Epstein–Barr virus-related disease. *J Mol Diagn* 2008; **10**: 279–92.

Hall JS, Taylor J, Valentine HR, *et al.* Enhanced stability of microRNA expression facilitates classification of FFPE tumour samples exhibiting near total mRNA degradation. *Br J Cancer* 2012; **107**: 684–94.

Hayashi S, Gillam IC, Delaney AD, Tener GM. Acetylation of chromosome squashes of *Drosophila melanogaster* decreases the background in autoradiographs from hybridization with [^{125}I]-labeled RNA. *J Histochem Cytochem* 1978; **26**: 677–9.

Herrington CS, Burns J, Graham AK, Evans MF, McGee JO'D. Interphase cytogenetics using biotin and digoxigenin-labelled probes I: relative sensitivity of both reporter molecules for HPV16 detection in CaSki cells. *J Clin Pathol* 1989; **41**: 592–600.

Illig R, Fritsch H, Schwarzer C. Breaking the seals: efficient mRNA detection from human archival paraffin-embedded tissue. *RNA* 2009; **15**: 1588–96.

John HA, Birnstiel ML, Jones KW. RNA–DNA hybrids at the cytological level. *Nature* 1969; **223**: 582–7.

Jørgensen S, Baker A, Møller S, Nielsen BS. Robust one-day *in situ* hybridization protocol for detection of microRNAs in paraffin samples using LNA probes. *Methods* 2010; **52**: 375–81.

Kang YG, Jung CK, Lee A, Kang WK, Oh ST, Kang CS. Prognostic significance of S100A4 mRNA and protein expression in colorectal cancer. *J Surg Oncol* 2012; **105**: 119–24.

Kelesidis T, Aish L, Steller MA, *et al.* Human papillomavirus (HPV) detection using *in situ* hybridization in histologic samples: correlations with cytologic changes and polymerase chain reaction HPV detection. *Am J Clin Pathol* 2011; **136**: 119–27.

Kent OA, McCall MN, Cornish TC, Halushka MK. Lessons from miR-143/145: the importance of cell-type localization of miRNAs. *Nucleic Acids Res* 2014; **42**: 7528–38.

Kiflemariam S, Andersson S, Asplund A, Pontén F, Sjöblom T. Scalable *in situ* hybridization on tissue arrays for validation of novel cancer and tissue-specific biomarkers. *PLoS One* 2012; **7** (3): e32927.

Kirketerp-Møller K, Jensen PØ, Fazli M, *et al.* Distribution, organization, and ecology of bacteria in chronic wounds. *J Clin Microbiol* 2008; **46**: 2717–22.

Klopfleisch R, Weiss AT, Gruber AD. Excavation of a buried treasure—DNA, mRNA, miRNA and protein analysis in formalin fixed, paraffin embedded tissues. *Histol Histopathol* 2011; **26**: 797–810.

Koshkin AA, Singh SK, Nielsen P, *et al.* LNA (Locked Nucleic Acids): Synthesis of the adenine, cytosine, guanine, 5-methylcytosine, thymine and uracil bicyclonucleoside monomers, oligomerisation, and unprecedented nucleic acid recognition. *Tetrahedron* 1998; **54**: 3607–30.

Lang G. Demonstration of kappa and lambda light chains by dual chromogenic *in situ* hybridization of formalin-fixed, acid-decalcified, and paraffin-embedded bone marrow trephine biopsies. *J Histotechnol* 2010; **33**: 9–13.

Langer S, Kraus J, Jentsch I, Speicher MR. Multicolor chromosome painting in diagnostic and research applications. *Chromosome Res* 2004; **12**: 15–23.

Lee RC, Feinbaum RL, Ambros V. The C. *elegans* heterochronic gene lin-4 encodes small RNAs with antisense complementarity to lin-14. *Cell* 1993; **75**: 843–54.

McNicol AM, Farquharson MA, Lee FD, Foulis AK. Comparison of *in situ* hybridisation and polymerase chain reaction in the diagnosis of B cell lymphoma. *J Clin Pathol* 1998; **51**: 229–33.

Morán T, Quiroga V, Gil M de L, *et al.* Targeting EML4-ALK driven non-small cell lung cancer (NSCLC). *Transl Lung Cancer Res* 2013; **2**: 128–41.

Mostegl MM, Richter B, Dinhopl N, Weissenböck H. Influence of prolonged formalin fixation of tissue samples on the sensitivity of chromogenic *in situ* hybridization. *J Vet Diagn Invest* 2011; **23**: 1212–16.

Mühlmann M. Molecular cytogenetics in metaphase and interphase cells for cancer and genetic research, diagnosis and prognosis. Application in tissue sections and cell suspensions. *Genet Mol Res* 2002; **30**: 117–27.

Muskhelishvili L, Latendresse JR, Kodell RL, Henderson EB. Evaluation of cell proliferation in rat tissues with BrdU, PCNA, Ki-67(MIB-5) immunohistochemistry and *in situ* hybridization for histone mRNA. *J Histochem Cytochem* 2003; **51**: 1681–8.

Nielsen BS, Holmstrøm K. Combined microRNA *in situ* hybridization and immunohistochemical detection of protein markers. *Methods Mol Biol* 2013; **986**: 353-65.

Nielsen BS, Møller T, Holmstrøm K. Chromogen detection of microRNA in frozen clinical tissue samples using LNA probe technology. *Methods Mol Biol* 2014; **1211**: 77–84.

Nielsen PE, Egholm M. An introduction to peptide nucleic acid. *Curr Issues Mol Biol* 1999; **1**: 89–104.

Park YS, Na YS, Ryu MH, *et al.* FGFR2 assessment in gastric cancer using quantitative real-time polymerase chain reaction, fluorescent *in situ* hybridization, and immunohistochemistry. *Am J Clin Pathol* 2015; **143**: 865–72.

Pasquinelli AE, Reinhart BJ, Slack F, *et al.* Conservation of the sequence and temporal expression of let-7 heterochronic regulatory RNA. *Nature* 2000; **408**: 86–9.

Patani N, Martin L-A, Dowsett M. Biomarkers for the clinical management of breast cancer: international perspective. *Int J Cancer* 2013; **133**: 1–13.

Perner S, Wagner PL, Demichelis F, *et al.* EML4-ALK fusion lung cancer: a rare acquired event. *Neoplasia* 2008; **10**: 298–302.

Pinkel D, Landgent J, Collins C. Fluorescence *in situ* hybridization with human chromosome-specific libraries: detection of trisomy 21 and translocations of chromosome 4. *Proc Natl Acad Sci U S A* 1988; **85**: 9138–42.

Powell RD, Pettay JD, Powell WC, *et al.* Metallographic *in situ* hybridization. *Hum Pathol* 2007; **38**: 1145–59.

Raisch J, Darfeuille-Michaud A, Nguyen HT. Role of microRNAs in the immune system, inflammation and cancer. *World J Gastroenterol* 2013; **19**: 2985–96.

Rakha EA, Pinder SE, Bartlett JM, *et al.* National Coordinating Committee for Breast Pathology. Updated UK Recommendations for HER2 assessment in breast cancer. *J Clin Pathol* 2015; **68**: 93–9.

Rondón-Lagos M, Verdun Di Cantogno L, Rangel N, *et al.* Unraveling the chromosome 17 patterns of FISH in interphase nuclei: an in-depth analysis of the HER2 amplicon and chromosome 17 centromere by karyotyping, FISH and M-FISH in breast cancer cells. *BMC Cancer* 2014; **14**: 922.

Sempere LF, Preis M, Yezefski T, *et al.* Fluorescence-based codetection with protein markers reveals distinct cellular compartments for altered microRNA expression in solid tumors. *Clin Cancer Res* 2010; **16**: 4246–55.

Sempere LF. Tissue slide-based microRNA characterization of tumors: how detailed could diagnosis become for cancer medicine? *Expert Rev Mol Diagn* 2014; **14**: 853–69.

Shinozaki M, Okubo Y, Sasai D *et al.* Development and evaluation of nucleic acid-based techniques for an auxiliary diagnosis of invasive fungal infections in formalin-fixed and paraffin-embedded (FFPE) tissues. *Med Mycol J* 2012; **53**: 241-5.

Tubbs RR, Wang H, Wang Z, *et al.* Immunoglobulin light chain mRNA in B-cell lymphoproliferative disorders. *Am J Clin Pathol* 2013; **140**: 736–46.

Venuti A, Paolini F. HPV detection methods in head and neck cancer. *Head Neck Pathol* 2012; **6**: S63–74.

Wagner F, Streubel A, Roth A, Stephan-Falkenau S, Mairinger T. Chromogenic *in situ* hybridization (CISH) is a powerful method to detect ALK-positive non-small cell lung carcinomas. *J Clin Pathol* 2014; **67**: 403–7.

Wang F, Flanagan J, Su N, *et al.* RNAscope: a novel *in situ* RNA analysis platform for formalin-fixed, paraffin-embedded tissues. *J Mol Diagn* 2012; **14**: 22–9.

Wang S, Saboorian MH, Frenkel E, Hynan L, Gokaslan ST, Ashfaq R. Laboratory assessment of the status of Her-2/neu protein and oncogene in breast cancer specimens: comparison of immunohistochemistry assay with fluorescence *in situ* hybridization assays. *J Clin Pathol* 2000; **53**: 374–81.

Weil TT, Parton RM, Davis I. Making the message clear: visualizing mRNA localization. *Trends Cell Biol* 2010; **20**: 380–90.

Wolff AC, Hammond ME, Hicks DG, *et al.*; American Society of Clinical Oncology; College of American Pathologists. Recommendations for human epidermal growth factor receptor 2 testing in breast cancer: American Society of Clinical Oncology/College of American Pathologists clinical practice guideline update. *Arch Pathol Lab Med* 2014; **138**: 241–56.

Yang H, Wanner IB, Roper SD, Chaudhari N. An optimized method for *in situ* hybridization with signal amplification that allows the detection of rare mRNAs. *J Histochem Cytochem* 1999; **47**: 431–45.

Useful websites

- Advandx (**www.advandx.com**)
- Advanced Cell Diagnostics (**www.acdbio.com**)
- Affimetrix (**www.panomics.com/products_rna-in-situ-analysis_view-rna-overview**)
- University of Manchester (**www.mirbase.org/cgi-bin/mirna_summary.pl?org=hsa**)

 Discussion questions

10.1 With reference to Chapter 8 compare and contrast the key steps of chromogenic *in situ* hybridization and immunocytochemistry.

10.2 A series of FFPE sections from a head and neck cancer biopsy have been received to identify HPV status and subtypes present. How should the optimal proteinase K concentration be determined for the test sections? What internal quality controls should be run to ensure that the HPV probes are capable of detecting the virus?

Answers to the self-check questions and tips for responding to the discussion questions are provided on the book's accompanying website:

 Visit www.oup.com/uk/orchard2e

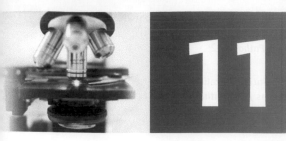

11

Molecular diagnostics: techniques and applications

Brendan O'Sullivan and Philippe Taniere

Learning objectives

After studying this chapter, you should have:

- Knowledge of the essential theory and concepts of DNA replication and translation.

- An understanding of the basic principles, organic or semi-synthetic, which underlie the broad range of techniques utilized in the molecular pathology laboratory. By necessity, this will focus largely on the properties of and methods to manipulate nucleic acids derived from cell and tissue preparations, which may not have already been discussed in sufficient length in earlier chapters.

- Insight into the wide variety of pre-, intra- and post-processing factors that impact upon the range and quality of information derived by molecular analysis of pathological tissues.

- An appreciation of how these factors influence the technologies employed within the laboratory; and the fundamental roles and responsibilities of the biomedical scientist in determining when, how and by what means to implement different analytical processes.

- Some awareness of contemporary developments at all stages of molecular diagnostic processing and testing, and the benefits and challenges that these will bring.

11.1 Introduction

Molecular diagnostics has developed over recent years as a catch-all phrase with a multitude of different intended meanings and interpretations. Wikipedia, that great online repository of knowledge, defines the term as '...a technique used to analyse biological markers in the genome and proteome—the individual's genetic code and how their cells express their genes as proteins—(for) medical testing'.

While perhaps a little vague, this illustrates brilliantly one key point, that molecular diagnostics covers a vast repertoire of laboratory processes both novel and historical. After all, if we are to include (quite correctly) the assessment of protein expression within this repertoire, any scientist performing routine tinctorial stains or immunocytochemistry (ICC) is involved in molecular diagnostics. Hence, we should bear in mind that molecular testing is not, and has not been for some time, the domain of a few highly specialized laboratories with uniquely trained staff. Against that realization we should perhaps weigh the momentum of current trends favouring a centralization of molecular pathology, as proposed in, for example, the 2012 Department of Health (DH) report 'Building on our inheritance: Genomic technology in healthcare' (Bell, 2012); and the more recent Personalized Medicine Strategy Board Paper (Keogh, 2015). In this chapter, and the next, we will try to bring an understanding not only of the technical methods and applications of molecular diagnostics, but also of the 'state of play' so far as test provision in the UK, and to some extent internationally, is concerned.

To return to the rudiments of molecular diagnostics, once we exclude the analyses and interpretation of protein expression and DNA structure/sequence dealt with elsewhere in this book, we are left largely to focus on the analysis of nucleic acids (NAs), most often by some means in conjunction with the classical polymerase chain reaction (PCR) or one of its variants. Our ability to manipulate NAs for analytical purposes does, of course, pre-date the discovery of PCR, with the development of first Southern and later Northern blotting over the second half of the 1970s (Nicholas and Nelson, 2013). However, an array of more sensitive, less complex high-throughput techniques has now rendered blotting techniques largely redundant outside a small number of specialist applications. The fundamental advantage of PCR lies in the ability to rapidly, cheaply, and with great specificity reproduce vast numbers of new copies of target sequences, factors which caused a paradigm shift in molecular biology upon its development in 1983 by Kary Mullis and subsequent description in the literature a little over 30 years ago (Saiki et al., 1985).

With the limitations of initial sample size removed, and scientists able to continuously reproduce NAs for analysis as and when required, focus shifted to exploitation of the PCR by modification of the components to allow post- or mid-amplification analysis. DNA sequencing, in its various forms, pre-dated the development and dissemination of PCR methods (Maxam and Gilbert, 1977; Sanger et al., 1977) but their utility was vastly increased with this breakthrough; many reviews on the variants and applications of the techniques for those seeking greater detail may be found in the literature (e.g. Franca et al., 2002). Less than a decade after PCR was first described came initial publications regarding real-time and quantitative PCR (VanGuilder et al., 2008); a few years later, in 1996, came the concept of pyrosequencing (Ahmadian et al., 2006); and just a little over 20 years on from Mullis's 'game-changing' discovery, the landscape was once more dramatically altered by the birth of so-called next-generation sequencing (Pareek et al., 2011). We will come to each of these, in turn, as we explore their wide-ranging benefits, applications, and limitations. Bear in mind, however, that no single one of these techniques can meet the needs of every analytical process; and that the vast majority of laboratories continue to utilize many or all of these variants in their day-to-day workflow. Through these various techniques, the delivery of molecular diagnostics (which in reality tends to include diagnostic, prognostic and predictive marker testing) allows the laboratory increasingly to provide what we tend to refer to as 'precision' or 'stratified' medicine, concepts that we will expand upon throughout the next two chapters.

Key Points

Molecular diagnostics

Molecular diagnostics is a multifarious concept, acting as an umbrella term to include:

- the use of widely varied techniques and platforms
- to profile variation in a broad array of biomolecules
- supporting medical decisions regarding the diagnosis of disease, patient prognosis and prediction of response to treatments and interventions.

SELF-CHECK 11.1

What is the key property of the polymerase chain reaction (PCR)? When we talk about a 'PCR-based' test, what variations might we be utilizing?

11.2 Essential background knowledge

11.2.1 Nucleic acids

Deoxyribonucleic acid (DNA) is the genetic blueprint of the cell, containing genes that can be switched on and off to enable cellular functions. The sequence, position and faithful replication during cell division of a gene at its particular chromosomal location play a fundamental role in pathology, as alterations have the potential to alter protein function and result in disease. Ribonucleic acid (RNA) acts as the molecular go-between, translating the genetic code of DNA into the proteins that control cell physiology.

Basic structure and function of nucleic acid

Nucleic acids comprise a backbone of nucleotide bases. In RNA, the single strand folds in on itself to give a three-dimensional shape. In DNA, the bases form pairs between two strands, which then form a right-handed double helix. Complementarity of these bases is the most important concept to understand, as it is the basis for all molecular diagnostic techniques. In the DNA double helix, adenine (A) pairs with thymine (T) using two hydrogen bonds, and guanine (G) pairs with cytosine (C) using three hydrogen bonds. In RNA, thymine (T) is replaced by uracil (U).

Denaturation and hybridization

Under physiological conditions, DNA is a double-stranded duplex, formed by the hydrogen bonds between A and T, and between G and C. The duplex can be denatured, or 'melted', into two single strands either by heating or exposure to alkaline pH. The higher the proportion of GC pairs (GC content) in the duplex, the more stable the bonding and the greater the heat (the melt temperature) required for denaturation. On cooling, DNA strands re-associate (anneal) to reform the duplex. Only complementary strands anneal, and this hybridization can take place between complementary strands of DNA, RNA, or one of each. Denaturation and hybridization form the core of all molecular diagnostics techniques.

Replication of DNA

Replication of DNA is an enzymatic process. Following denaturation, which allows each single strand to be used as a template, DNA polymerases add A, T, G or C bases according to the complementarity rule, and the replicon elongates. Eventually, two new identical double-stranded molecules are formed (see Box 11.1). This process occurs in cell division, where whole chromosomes are duplicated. It also forms the basis of the PCR method, which will be discussed in Section 11.3.

BOX 11.1 Replication of DNA

First, a section of the double helix (blue in Figure 11.1) is unwound by the enzyme helicase to form two template strands. DNA synthesis can only occur in a 5' to 3' direction so one strand (leading) is synthesized continuously as DNA polymerase enzyme (orange) binds and moves along it, adding complementary bases and producing a complete strand (green). Another DNA polymerase molecule binds to the second strand (lagging) and the complementary strand is synthesized in small stretches as Okazaki fragments. To complete the sequence DNA ligase (purple) then joins these together.

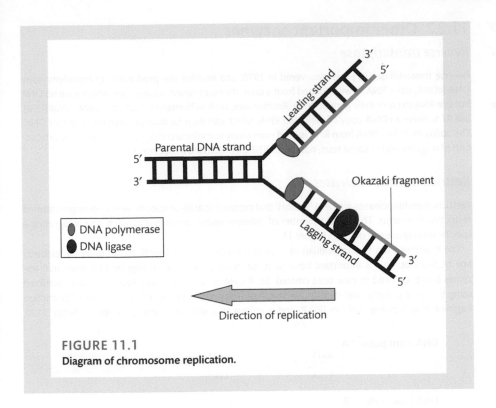

FIGURE 11.1
Diagram of chromosome replication.

Transcription (making RNA from DNA)

The cell uses separated single strands of DNA as a template to make different RNA types. RNA polymerase recognizes a start sequence and synthesizes RNA by adding the complementary bases G, C, A and U until the enzyme reaches a stop region. This signals that the RNA is complete, and is ready to be exported out of the nucleus for modification into one of a number of different types of functioning RNA. Messenger RNA (mRNA) then provides the template for the cell to make a protein product.

Translation (making proteins from RNA)

The mRNA template carries information from DNA as a three-letter genetic code of nucleotide triplets (codons). Each codon has a complementary anti-codon on a tRNA molecule. Each anti-codon corresponds to a specific amino acid; for example, the anti-codon G-C-U codes for alanine, while G-U-U codes for valine. In this way, the cell manufactures proteins comprised of a specific amino acid sequence that directly relates to the sequence of DNA. The proteins are then used by the cell, act as signals for further steps in a process, or are exported from the cell. Messenger RNA molecules may remain in the cytoplasm for several days after translation, allowing their detection long after the protein product has gone (Figure 11.2).

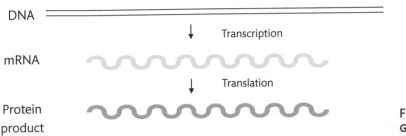

FIGURE 11.2
Genetic information in DNA.

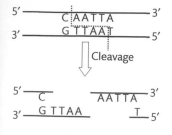

FIGURE 11.3

EcoR1, a restriction endonuclease enzyme, will cleave the DNA every time it recognizes the sequence AATT.

11.2.2 Other important enzymes

Reverse transcriptase

Reverse transcriptase (RT) was discovered in 1970, and enables the production of complementary DNA (cDNA) from RNA. It was isolated from a class of viruses called retroviruses, which have no DNA but use RNA to carry their genetic code. Retroviruses, such as human immunodeficiency virus (HIV), use RT to make a cDNA copy of their own RNA, which can then be incorporated into the host DNA. The ability to make cDNA from RNA is used extensively in molecular diagnostics, both in the production of reagents and in some tests, notably in RT-PCR (discussed in Section 11.3.8).

Restriction endonucleases

Restriction endonucleases are DNA 'scissors' that cut nucleic acids at specific sites into lengths termed restriction fragments. There are a number of different restriction enzymes, each one recognizing a specific short sequence of bases (Figure 11.3).

The genomes from two individuals of the same species are not identical, but differ by relatively few nucleotides. This is important because it can result in the sites recognized by restriction enzymes being removed or new ones created. So, if DNA is taken from two individuals and restricted using the same enzyme, variation in the length of fragments is produced. This is termed restriction fragment length polymorphism (RFLP) and is unique to a specific restriction enzyme (Figure 11.4).

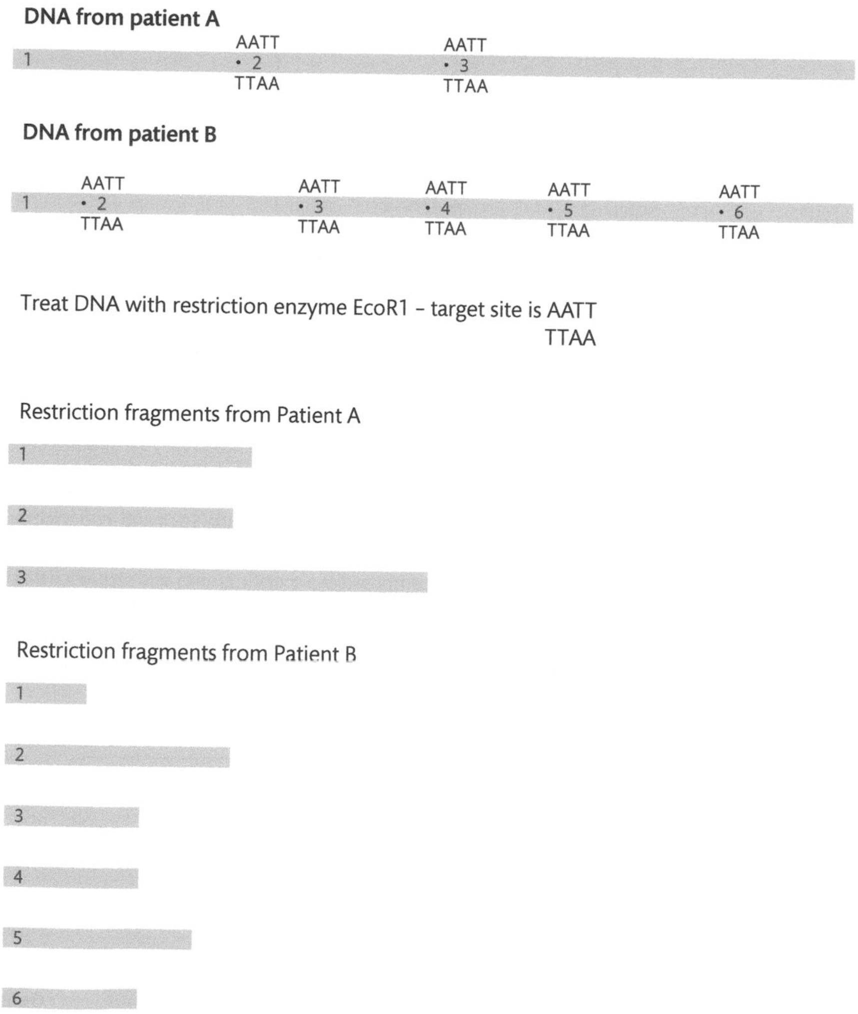

DNA from patient A

```
                    AATT              AATT
1                   • 2               • 3
                    TTAA              TTAA
```

DNA from patient B

```
      AATT              AATT        AATT        AATT          AATT
1     • 2               • 3         • 4         • 5           • 6
      TTAA              TTAA        TTAA        TTAA          TTAA
```

Treat DNA with restriction enzyme EcoR1 – target site is AATT
                                                              TTAA

Restriction fragments from Patient A

1

2

3

Restriction fragments from Patient B

1

2

3

4

5

6

FIGURE 11.4

An illustration of the difference in restriction fragments produced when DNA from patient A and patient B is cut by the same restriction enzyme.

Some polymorphisms are associated with inherited diseases (e.g. Huntington's chorea, sickle cell anaemia and cystic fibrosis) and can be used as genetic markers for those conditions.

Key Points

Nucleic acids

- DNA is usually referred to in terms of size, measured in numbers of base pairs (nucleotides): 15 nucleotides would be denoted as 15bp; 1500 would be abbreviated to 1.5 kb (kilobase).

- The chemical and physical properties of DNA and RNA are exploited in all molecular diagnostic tests. Key among these are:
  - **Replication**: a template is used to duplicate the genetic sequence by enzymatic addition of complementary bases.
  - **Complementarity**: base pairs form only between G and C, A and T or A and U.
  - **Denaturation**: the separation of a DNA duplex into single-stranded DNA.
  - **Hybridization**: nucleic acids, be they cellular genomic DNA or a synthetic probe, bind or hybridize to their complementary sequence (which may be DNA:DNA or DNA:RNA).

11.2.3 Variations in DNA structure

Variations in DNA sequence are seen in healthy individuals, benign changes to normal tissue, and in overtly malignant abnormalities. While the sequence of the human genome is long established and much studied, databases and repositories of variants are constantly evolving and growing to accommodate newly described alternations (e.g. the National Centre for Biotechnology Information's short genetic variation database dbSNP [www.ncbi.nlm.nih.gov/SNP/] or the Manchester National Genetics Reference Laboratory's Diagnostic Mutation Database DMuDB [www.ngrl.org.uk/Manchester/projects/informatics/dmudb]). Although these are frequently revised and updated, the most contemporary and clinically relevant information on alterations is usually found in journal articles. How we define and classify a variant depends on many factors. Simply finding a genetic alteration in a diseased cell does not prove causality; cancerous cells often show hundreds or thousands of genetic variants, many of which may not influence pathogenicity whatsoever. Similarly, some variants seen frequently in apparently healthy individuals may have pathogenic potential; the influence of common small alterations upon disease predisposition, for example, is still being unravelled.

Polymorphisms

Variations at a particular position found among individuals in a population, frequently inherited, are often referred to as single nucleotide polymorphisms (SNPs, pronounced 'snips'). When these do not result in a mutation—the change in DNA coding does not alter the protein product—these are said to be 'synonymous' changes. Inherited, pathogenic SNPs are not always referred to as mutations because they are not sporadic alterations to germline DNA sequences.

Mutations

Changes to the sequence of bases in a gene can alter the transcribed RNA and subsequent protein production, and therefore cellular activity. Remember that synonymous changes do not alter the ultimate translation product because DNA codons have some redundancy. This means that different combinations of nucleotides can encode the same amino acid; glycine, for example, is encoded by any triplet of nucleotides in which the first two positions are 'GG', and so a change to the DNA sequence from 'GGT' to 'GGC' has no impact on the protein translated. Mutations that do alter the downstream protein structure can cause disease and deformity; however, they are also responsible for inherited genetic variation and can convey survival advantages by, for example, conferring resistance to certain infections, or increasing enzymatic activity. There are various types of mutation, some involving alteration to a single nucleotide (base), termed point mutations, some that involve thousands of nucleotides, and any variation in between.

Translocation

The abnormal positioning of sections of chromosomes by rearrangement is termed translocation. In an inherited condition, each cell in the body will have the same translocation. In certain acquired diseases, a characteristic translocation occurs in each cell of the diseased tissue. This means that genes within the region where the specific translocation is found are affected by the disease. Translocations can result in one or more genes within the new 'fusion' region having their usual activity altered. One classic example is chronic myeloid leukaemia (CML), in which the breakpoint cluster region (BCR) of chromosome 22 is brought into conjunction with the *ABL1* gene of chromosome 9 (this forms the so-called Philadelphia chromosome). This translocation is said to be diagnostic for CML. Analysis of the fusion product, *BCR-ABL*, is used to test for and monitor CML because ≥ 90% of patients have this particular translocation. Functionally, this is oncogenic because the fusion product results in constitutive activation of the ABL tyrosine kinase with a cascade of upregulated downstream activity. Convention dictates that translocations are always abbreviated in a similar way; for example, that for the Philadelphia chromosome is t(9;22).

Amplification

Amplification is an increase in the number of copies of a particular gene. This may occur naturally during cell differentiation; for example, a cell producing a hormone may have many copies of the appropriate gene to enable it to function. Alternatively, it may arise as the result of a disease process, or even cause the disease.

Deletion and insertion

Deletions can range in size from a single base to large chromosomal losses, affecting whole or multiple genes. Insertions involve the addition of bases within an existing sequence; this can be an entirely novel sequence or a repetition of an existing sequence in the gene, known as a duplication. The impact of this kind of mutation is not necessarily dependent on the length of the affected sequence; the position of the mutation within the sequence is more important, as this will affect function. It may stop DNA replication altogether (a 'nonsense' mutation which terminates transcription) and subsequently produces RNA that is non-functional; or produce a new RNA that translates into a pathogenic protein product, most commonly by reducing or enhancing enzymatic activity.

SELF-CHECK 11.2

When investigating a new disease and/or developing a new test, how would you determine what variations need to be analysed? How could you ensure that a test is fit for purpose in light of the latest relevant findings?

11.3 The polymerase chain reaction

Since its inception more than 30 years ago, the polymerase chain reaction (PCR) has revolutionized gene analysis. It was adopted into histopathology soon after, at last making it possible to analyse genes in routinely fixed and processed samples. All types of sample can provide DNA or RNA, from large resection specimens to the tiniest biopsies, cytological fluids and aspirates, and even archival stained sections. Before a PCR assay can be developed we need to know:

- the area of the DNA that we want to amplify
- the sequences that flank this region, as the primers will be designed to anneal here
- the sensitivity required, since different forms of PCR have different limits of detection (LODs).

11.3.1 Specimen requirements

Many different samples can provide DNA, including paraffin sections, frozen tissue sections, bodily fluids such as effusions, and blood and bone marrow. DNA fragmentation due to fixation and processing tends to render such samples less suitable (or indeed entirely unsuitable) for more demanding techniques such as comparative genomic hybridization (CGH) and Southern blotting. The beauty of the PCR reaction lies in the fact that the fragments of DNA to be amplified can be deliberately restricted in size, permitting use not only on frozen tissue, but also on formalin-fixed, paraffin wax-embedded (FFPE) samples.

11.3.2 What is PCR?

The polymerase chain reaction is an *in vitro* method for the amplification of specific short fragments of DNA or cDNA. This so-called target DNA can be a whole gene's sequence, individual coding segments of a gene (exons), or short sections of a particular exon which are of interest. For the reaction to be successful, five basic components are required: DNA (or cDNA), reaction buffer, oligonucleotide primers, nucleotide triphosphates and polymerase enzyme.

11.3.3 DNA/cDNA

The genetic sequence to be amplified is called the target or template and in classical PCR it must be in the form of DNA. If RNA from the sample is the target template, it is possible to prepare cDNA from the RNA using an enzyme called reverse transcriptase (RT). See section on RT-PCR within Section 11.3.8.

11.3.4 Oligonucleotide primers

Oligonucleotide primers are short sequences of single-stranded DNA that anneal to the template, flank the region of interest, and initiate polymerization. Primers are generally between 18 and 30 bases in length, and available cheaply and commercially from a variety of manufacturers. Simply submitting the sequence online can result in your primers being synthesized and delivered by post a few days later. In a basic PCR method, two primers are required, one for each strand of the template available after denaturation.

11.3.5 Reaction buffer

The reaction buffer contains detergent, salt, magnesium chloride and other ingredients needed for the reaction to occur, and each polymerase has individual buffer requirements. Magnesium chloride concentration in the buffer is critical as it modulates the activity of the polymerase enzyme, affects the melting temperature of the hybrids that are formed during the reaction, and ensures the optimal reaction pH of around 8.4. Since DNA from FFPE is often degraded, modest increases in magnesium chloride can be useful in enabling amplification.

11.3.6 Nucleotide triphosphates

Nucleotide triphosphates (dNTPs) provide the energy and the nucleotides needed to copy the DNA template by incorporation into the new strand. These dNTPs may be added manually to the reaction buffer, although frequently now they are sourced pre-mixed as solutions of reaction buffer and dNTPs, known commercially as 'mastermixes'.

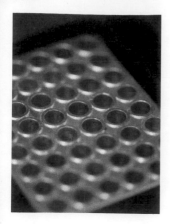

FIGURE 11.5

A PCR thermocycler 'block' comprising multiple identical wells to accommodate individual PCR tubes or PCR plates. The 'Peltiers' in the block strictly regulate the temperature in each well, and can change temperatures at a rate of several degrees centigrade per second with great accuracy.

11.3.7 Polymerase enzyme

The DNA polymerase adds nucleotides to the template. The most widely used enzyme is *Thermus aquaticus* (*Taq*) DNA polymerase because it is stable at high temperature and tolerates a broad range of pH conditions. A wide variety of variants are employed for varying PCR applications; polymerases with higher fidelity may be used, for example, when the lowest possible error rate of replication is needed. These enzymes can be more fastidious and less efficient when amplifying poorer quality template, meaning they may not be a good choice for use with FFPE specimens. 'Hot-start' *Taq* is a popular choice when working with poorer quality template because of the greater specificity it offers. The enzyme is supplied bound to an inhibitory antibody that prevents activity until such time as a high temperature (usually ≥95°C) environment is generated, the antibody denatures and the enzyme is released. Re-association of antibody and enzyme below 72°C prevents activity below the optimal temperature for primer extension.

11.3.8 Principles of the technique

All components are added to the reaction tube; it is common practice to create a 'working' mastermix of all components using the formula R(1.1n) to calculate the volume of each reagent needed, where R is the volume of reagent per reaction and n is the number of samples tested (including controls). This 10% excess allows for pipetting errors or wastage; the enzyme in particular is often relatively viscous, although the use of low binding pipette tips can reduce the impact of this issue. Many laboratories will now employ filter-tipped pipettes throughout the process to help reduce contamination. In the past, contents could be overlaid with a small amount of mineral oil to prevent evaporation as the reaction proceeded; however, the vast majority of PCR machines (thermocyclers) now have a heated lid which can be set to maintain a temperature above the maximum reached within the reaction tube (Figure 11.5), therefore preventing the reagents condensing and the reaction ceasing.

The basic reaction is the same no matter what the target and consists of three steps: denaturation, primer annealing and primer extension.

Denaturation

The reaction mix is heated to around 95°C, causing denaturation (melting) of the template DNA into two separate strands and activation of the *Taq* enzyme, if a hot-start form is in use. Denaturation is essential because DNA cannot be copied while it is in the form of a double helix.

Primer annealing

The tube is then cooled, usually to 50–60°C. At this temperature the primers bind to their complementary sequences, one on each strand, in a process called primer annealing. Small drops in the temperature used can reduce the specificity of annealing, potentially leading to non-specific amplification of non-target regions; increasing temperature above the ideal point will reduce or eliminate annealing altogether, impacting on overall yield of PCR product. When setting up a PCR protocol for the first time, running optimization reactions over a range of annealing temperatures is good practice, allowing the ideal temperature to be established. PCR machines may have a 'gradient' function available, whereby different annealing temperatures across a selected range are applied to a set of reaction tubes on the same heating block, so a single round of PCR can provide this optimization information.

Primer extension

Once added, the polymerase enzyme begins to create the new strand of DNA. It does this by taking dNTPs from the solution and adding them to the ends of the primers (primer extension). The DNA polymerase needs a short double-stranded region in order to start copying so it will only add nucleotides where the primers are annealed, as this is the only place where double-stranded DNA is available. In line with normal DNA replication, the new strand comprises a sequence complementary to that of the template. Many PCR programmes employ a final, 'extended extension' phase which aims to maximize the overall yield of amplified products.

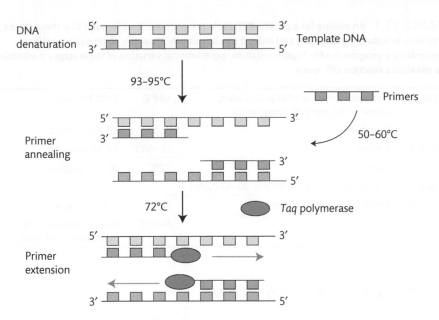

FIGURE 11.6

Template DNA is denatured into single strands by heating to 93–95°C. Primers in the reaction mix anneal at their complementary sites at 50–60°C. *Taq* polymerase begins to work at 72°C, adding nucleotides from the reaction mixture to produce a duplicate copy of the original template. This sequence of events is repeated, doubling the amount of DNA in every cycle.

The PCR cycle

The three steps of denaturation, primer annealing and primer extension are called a PCR cycle (Table 11.1). Theoretically, in one cycle the amount of the target sequence is doubled. Thus, two strands of DNA (four single strands after denaturation) can be used in the next cycle, and so on. These three steps are usually repeated 25–30 times. Doubling the target sequence each cycle will lead to an exponential increase in the sequence of interest (see Figure 11.6).

RT-PCR

Reverse transcriptase PCR is an important addition to the PCR repertoire as analysis of mRNA permits the examination of gene transcription. The basic technique is the same but an extra step is inserted after extraction of RNA, producing DNA for the PCR. This involves the incubation of mRNA with reverse transcriptase enzyme to produce complementary DNA (cDNA).

Key Points

The polymerase chain reaction

The PCR technique requires several key components to work; without these it cannot function:

- DNA (or cDNA), from the specimen being tested.
- Reaction buffer, to provide a stable environment and promote amplification.
- Oligonucleotide primers, to dictate the region being amplified.
- Nucleotide triphosphates, 'building blocks' for synthesis of new strands.
- Polymerase enzyme (*Taq*), to perform primer extension and chain synthesis.

TABLE 11.1 An outline for a generic PCR cycle programme. Bear in mind that these stages can vary in nature considerably and indeed can be entirely absent in some variants. When optimizing a programme for implementation, experimental variation of these stages is essential to maximize reaction efficiency.

Step 1	Denature template DNA and, if used, activate 'Hot-start' *Taq* polymerase	>94°C	5–10 minutes
Step 2	Denature	95°C	20–60 seconds
Step 3	Anneal	50–60°C	20–60 seconds
Step 4	Extend	72°C	30–90 seconds
Step 5	Repeat steps 2–4 for a total of 30–40 cycles		
Step 6	Additional extension phase	72°C	5–10 minutes
Step 7	Hold	4–15°C	Usually between a few hours and indefinitely

11.4 Laboratory workflow

A consideration of the key steps in the laboratory workflow, their optimization, and limitations is worthwhile before moving on to the physical techniques and processes involved. Most biomedical scientists would consider themselves *au fait* with their own laboratory's fundamental processes, and how they integrate into the overall flow of work, but they may not necessarily appreciate the impact of traditional practices and approaches upon downstream applications used in molecular diagnostics. Few laboratory scientists remain unaware of Lean working, for example, and its principles have broadly been adopted, to some extent, in both day-to-day and prospective practices (Clark *et al.*, 2013). A fine tuning of Lean may be needed, however, for laboratories to adapt to and support molecular diagnostics processes; standardization of laboratory processes to ensure a robust molecular diagnostic service brings constraints previously unseen or less relevant to the histopathology practitioner, including but not limited to:

- More strictly regulated measurement of specimen handling parameters, with time and temperature variations impacting to an extent not apparent in traditional histopathology.

- Rationalization of specimen 'wastage' to ensure that the usage of tissues and cytological fluids is maximized, potentially through coalescing of traditionally disparate pathways, in order that the demand for testing material is accommodated with as little impact upon other clinical pathways as is possible.

- Careful consideration of whether staffing, technologies and specimen numbers within each workflow allow a laboratory to provide a particular analysis in a timely, safe and quality-assured manner.

- Essential evolution of resulting and reporting processes to accommodate an ever-increasing quantity and complexity of information derived from the patient specimen, ensuring that the laboratory continues to deliver data to the clinician in a valuable, succinct and, most importantly, relevant form.

11.4.1 Specimen handling metrics

Most laboratory information management systems (LIMS) allow the recording of key specimen handling time points, but may not have provision for wider metrics such as specimen fixation/processing start and end times (and from this the calculation of process durations). With specimen fixation times increasingly acknowledged as a fundamental influence upon biomolecule preservation (Hicks and Boyce, 2012), a laboratory cannot guarantee quality control and reproducibility in its techniques without adequate processing controls. For many years, traditional guidelines have emphasized (with good cause) minimum fixation times as the basis of robust specimen processing (Qizilbash, 1982).

However, the exceptionally detrimental effects of *over*-fixation (Nam *et al.*, 2014) are now clear; the laboratory should question whether fixation times of greater than 24 hrs are necessary, in view of data in the literature. Counterbalancing this argument, molecular diagnostics are largely worthless without fundamental microscopic analysis and any approach undertaken to optimize specimen preservation must still prioritize the needs of 'traditional' histological and cytological methods.

11.4.2 Pre-analytical processes

Traditional histopathological processing methods, without doubt, have the potential to be seriously deleterious to the integrity of many biomolecules and in particular DNA (Srinivasan *et al.*, 2002). Since we approach specimen processing with the key aim of 'fixing' and preserving tissues for future analysis, it is unsurprising that the chemical and thermal methods used for this will alter their relatively labile natural state. Unfortunately for the molecular diagnostician this can often limit or, at worst, completely ablate their usefulness in analyses; more worryingly still, they can lead to serious errors in molecular profiling of which the reporter may not be aware (Kapp *et al.*, 2015). Key contributing elements to this pre-analytical degradation are as follows.

Pre-fixation and specimen transport times

From the moment tissue is removed from the patient, indeed from the moment of induced hypoxia which may precede the excision, tissues enter a phase of altered molecular expression. This can not only alter their molecular profile (altering the results of analysis) but ultimately and rapidly trigger biomolecule degradation through apoptotic pathways, rendering them entirely unsuitable for testing. Alterations may impact on both molecular diagnostics and classical analyses; hypoxic times have been shown to impact directly upon factors ranging from RNA expression to mitotic figure counts (Cross *et al.*, 1990).

Formaldehyde

The key property of formaldehyde is its protein cross-linking activity (Figure 11.7) that is so vital to tissue preservation. A side-effect of this is that proteins interacting with DNA, such as histones, are involved also and there is resulting physical disruption of DNA strands. This fragmentation results in specimens

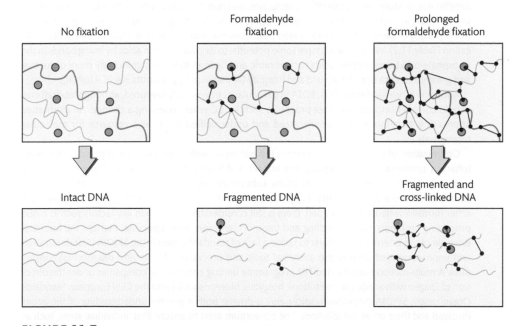

No fixation   Formaldehyde fixation   Prolonged formaldehyde fixation

Intact DNA   Fragmented DNA   Fragmented and cross-linked DNA

FIGURE 11.7
Formaldehyde molecules form 'cross-linking' chemical bonds between proteins during the fixation process. As fixation progresses, and during subsequent processing, this leads to NA fragmentation.

TABLE 11.2   Impact of decalcifying agents upon DNA yield and integrity (Singh *et al.*, 2013). DNA concentration is given in nanograms (ng); integrity, as measured by qPCR, is a function of the number of PCR cycles (C) required to reach a significant threshold (t) of PCR product (the Ct value). The lower the Ct, the greater the DNA template integrity.

Decalcification solution	DNA yield (mean ng)	RNA yield (mean ng)	DNA integrity (mean Ct)	RNA integrity (mean Ct)
Strong (HCl, Nitric)	6.15	121.53	35.79	33.03
Weak (Formic, EDTA)	68.68	288.89	30.16	26.5
Significance	$P < 0.001$	$P = 0.003$	$P < 0.001$	$P < 0.001$

yielding only short (typically <300–400 base pair) DNA segments for analysis, limiting the maximum length of DNA amplicons (the regions amplified in the PCR reaction) which can be produced and reducing the overall numbers of DNA copies which can be successfully amplified (since fragments terminating in the region between primers will limit overall amplification rates). Furthermore, although now less relevant with widespread use of neutral buffered formalin (NBF) and improvements in specimen handling and processing times, formaldehyde ultimately oxidizes to provide an acidic environment, which will over time degrade NAs. RNA, too, is highly susceptible to formalin-induced fragmentation, and the natural lability of these single-stranded molecules is further compounded when utilizing RNA derived from fixed tissue (Evers *et al.*, 2011).

Temperature, pressure, radiation and chemicals

These components of the processing pathway can all impact upon biomolecule integrity; introducing alterations to existing processing pathways should always include a consideration of their impact on downstream molecular analyses. The use of high temperature and microwave processing, modified paraffin wax mixtures and/or paraffin alternatives, and non-formaldehyde fixative agents may all severely impact upon NA integrity and their influence when used in high-throughput tissue processing is not yet clearly understood. One widespread process with a clear deleterious impact is that of decalcification (Table 11.2). While all acids have some potential to degrade nucleic acids by lysing bonds in the phosphate backbone, 'strong' acids such as nitric and hydrochloric are significantly more disruptive and greatly decrease both DNA yield and integrity (as measured by quantitative PCR [qPCR]).

Adoption of 'weak' decalcifiers, EDTA in particular, is now widely favoured, although laboratories should consider impacts on other processes such as ICC when assessing a change. An alternative approach is to retain frozen, unprocessed and undecalcified tissue as a resource for molecular testing only.

Optimization of pre-analytical processes is a hot topic, with many public and private institutions (often in combination) investigating the impact and imposed limitations of different processing approaches upon downstream applications. Laboratory network surveys have revealed that while laboratories have adopted standard approaches in many areas (use of neutral buffered saline over other formalin variants, for example), there is still considerable variation in key factors such as tissue processing protocols, tissue handling and transport, and specimen sampling. Perhaps the foremost example of the international efforts to tackle a lack of standardization is the SPIDIA (**S**tandardization and improvement of generic **p**re-analytical tools and procedures for *in vitro* **dia**gnostics) consortium. A multi-million Euro-funded FP7 programme uniting commercial companies under the direction of Qiagen with academic institutions, hospitals, biorepositories and the CEN European Standards Organization, SPIDIA (http://www.spidia.eu/) is driving both a greater understanding of the issues involved and their potential solutions. The consortium aims to ensure that 'individual steps, such as sample handling, stabilization and storage, will be standardized and integrated in one holistic process combining classical and molecular diagnostics', recognizing that molecular diagnostics are inextricably linked to and co-dependent upon current pathology processes.

11.4.3 Specimen consumption

The rapid sectioning through a tissue block to reach and section a next 'level', with the intervening sections cast aside to clear the blade holder, is a practice that may appear confusing to the molecular diagnostician; why is valuable clinical material being disposed of and not utilized? For those unfamiliar with the high-throughput nature of histopathological processing, this apparently casual 'wastage' of tissue can seem shocking. However, without a paradigm shift in funding and practices, the rapid processing of tissue blocks for standard microscopy while at the same time retaining all unused tissue is an impossibility. Instead laboratories must begin to consider how they can rationalize processes to meet both needs. 'Saving' intervening sections between preparation of initial levels, for example, is becoming more popular; by reserving these for ICC or molecular analysis, at least in the short term until diagnosis and molecular classification is complete, a temporary storage burden can prevent far more serious long-term consequences, need for re-biopsy being a worst-case scenario. Many molecular diagnostic techniques inform treatment for patients with advanced, metastatic disease who can no longer benefit from surgery or undergo more aggressive investigations; the initial diagnostic sample may be all that the laboratory can work from. The pathology community itself has acknowledged and looked to tackle wastage of material, not least in beginning to address the use of specimens by reporting pathologists as detailed, for example, in The Royal College of Pathologists 2014 dataset for lung cancer histopathology reports (Nicholson, 2014).

The molecular diagnostician must contribute to this process also, always considering how to offer 'more for less' to the clinician in order that patients with limited specimen volume or quality are not denied standard-of-care testing. This could be something as simple as pre-emptive sample preparation, simply increasing initial NA extraction quantities so that potential future testing demands can be met; by eliminating the need to return to the block for duplicate sectioning, extraction and other handling, staff time and material efficiencies are greatly increased. Excess cytological fluids could be processed to an archival cell block, even if not required for immediate diagnostic work. At the other end of the processing pathway, optimizing the amount of data that can be retrieved from a given specimen could take the form of extracting DNA from previously stained histopathological (Figure 11.8) or cytological diagnostic or molecular testing sections (Ulivi *et al.*, 2013).

11.4.4 Demand versus quality

The histopathology community needs no reminding of the serious consequences it faces should laboratories attempt to undertake service provision that falls outside their experience and competence. Particular incidents have illustrated that poor practice, once engrained, is difficult to spot and eliminate (CQC, 2012); and that unmanaged adoption of novel or unfamiliar techniques to meet new clinical demands can be compromised by poor quality management (Bartlett *et al.*, 2009). There are still relatively few guideline documents regarding the provision of molecular diagnostic testing and no official Department of Health (DH) or Royal College of Medicine (RCM) guidelines; where suggested guidelines exist they often cover one particular indication only and vary between countries and services (Bellon *et al.*, 2011; Lindeman *et al.*, 2013). Taken together, this situation has the potential to create a toxic mix of unregulated testing in the face of rapidly evolving clinical demands and the

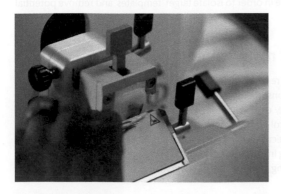

FIGURE 11.8
Dedicated microtomy areas assist the biomedical scientist in maintaining high levels of cleanliness, reducing the likelihood of contamination. Dedicated microtomy protocols can help minimize wastage and improve continuity and consistency of processes.

absence of mandatory guidelines; and yet a highly proactive collaboration between laboratory leads, EQA providers and, in some cases, pharmaceutical and companion diagnostics manufacturers has moved to head off this issue (Deans *et al.*, 2013).

Laboratory managers and clinical leads must consider whether demand in their individual institution or network will provide high enough sample throughput to ensure that they can not only meet essential turnaround times (TATs), but also maintain the requisite levels of experience and understanding to ensure quality of service. And, to refer back to our previous discussion of specimen consumption, a laboratory without access to diverse platforms and technologies should consider the detrimental impact this might have upon specimen handling. Should samples need to be routed through multiple laboratories in order to perform, for example, requisite PCR, fluorescence *in situ* hybridization (FISH) and ICC testing, specimen consumption becomes excessive and may compromise basic testing requirements; it can certainly jeopardize the ability to later access trial and novel therapies.

SELF-CHECK 11.3

Why might samples submitted for molecular analysis be of limited size and volume? And what might limit the possibility of obtaining further specimens?

11.5 Processing the sample

In very simple terms, the molecular diagnostics workflow can be broken down into a series of fundamental steps, the technical aspects of which will be dealt with in subsequent individual sections.

11.5.1 Specimen preparation and assessment

Production of tissue- or cytological fluid-derived materials in a form suitable for processing varies widely, depending upon local preferences, availability of material, and requirements of downstream processes. Formalin-fixed, paraffin-embedded (FFPE) tissue is typically prepared as mounted or unmounted sections, or tissue cores; while cytological fluids may be used 'as-is' or centrifuged to form cell pellets or precipitates, helping to concentrate target populations of cells. Laboratories increasingly favour preparing sections for assessment of tumour content (both overall cellularity and relative tumour:non-tumour cell ratio); data published in the UKNEQAS for Molecular Genetics scheme reports highlight this trend among their many international and UK users (www.ukneqas-molgen.org.uk/annual-report).

11.5.2 Extraction and/or isolation of target molecules

One key contrast between classical histological and cytological techniques and a significant proportion of molecular diagnostic procedures is the dissociation of targets from their environment. Setting aside *in situ* hybridization, most tests for the analysis of NAs require amplification for analysis; NA extraction is fundamental to the procedure in order to isolate target 'templates' and remove potential inhibitors.

11.5.3 Amplification and measurement

Amplification of target molecular regions results in a pool of replicate molecules more easily and accurately analysed than the initial tissue constituents alone. Measurement (as a process distinct from data analysis itself) can take a wide variety of forms, from simple sequencing of NA chains, through relative quantification of target and control NA regions, to absolute quantification for the purposes of stratifying fluctuations in levels of molecular expression or transcription. These two steps are not always co-employed; classical sequencing involves temporally distinct stages of amplification, purification, molecular labelling, and sequencing, whereas quantitative methods more often combine the two for a 'real time' analytical procedure.

11.5.4 Analysis and interpretation

Data in isolation is of limited value. Qualitative data, such as the DNA sequence variants detected by Sanger sequencing, should be interpreted using published disease-specific data and/or relevant variant databases such as the Welcome Trust Sanger Institute's Catalogue of somatic mutations in cancer (COSMIC, http://cancer.sanger.ac.uk/cosmic). While this applies to quantitative data also, this should be further interpreted in the context of the technical parameters which determine 'significance' of data; this can allow highly sensitive methods to be used without fear of over-interpretation and the possibility of false-positive calls in resulting.

11.5.5 Reporting of findings

There is undoubtedly some overlap between this step and the last, as again any findings require interpretation in the context of the specimen assessment and clinical details. Qualitative data giving results over a range can relate directly to specimen quantity and quality, and, as such, 'outlier' results may indicate not a technical failure but a reflection of specimen properties. This can guide interpretation of results, such as when specimens rich in tumour cells show evidence of mutation at very low levels only, indicating clonal evolution. Or it may indicate that further processing would be useful in obtaining a result, for example by repeating a procedure with more or less starting template, or that repeating DNA extraction is needed to eliminate PCR inhibitors. Both the interpreter of data (usually an experienced scientist) and the reporter of results should have an appreciation of both the analytical and reporting processes in order that there be bi-directional communication on findings. Clinical context, as detailed more extensively in Chapter 12, is also essential; the same mutation can have vastly different prognostic and predictive significance in different types of malignancies.

Key Points

Processing the sample

- The PCR workflow should be organized in a linear fashion, with specimens moving from pre-processing (i.e. sectioning) to extraction, PCR set-up, amplification and analysis.

- Failure to do so can have catastrophic consequences; movement of amplified products backwards through the workflow to PCR set-up or extraction laboratories is the main source of PCR contamination.

- As well as preventing physical movement of amplified products, laboratory staff should change their gloves and lab coats when moving between rooms to minimize transfer.

- Laboratory items such as pipettes and racks should be restricted to use at a designated stage of the process; allocate items for use in each laboratory. If moving specimens between areas (e.g. the transfer of extracted DNA to the PCR set-up area, or reaction mixes to the PCR cycler) try to ensure movement is unidirectional, 'forwards' through the processing chain.

11.6 Pre-extraction sample handling and assessment

Once a molecular diagnostic test is ordered, the laboratory must ensure that the sample is appropriate for use and render it into such a form that it can be then moved through the analytical pathway, the initial phase of which will be nucleic acid extraction.

11.6.1 Assessment

Although a diagnosis (preliminary in the case of diagnostic tests, often final when asking for predictive testing) will usually have been made prior to test requisition it cannot be assumed that any given tissue specimen still contains sufficient, *or indeed any*, representative tumour material upon which

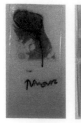
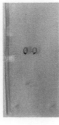

FIGURE 11.9

Two examples of slides labelled for macrodissection: Left: A section of colorectal tumour with the area richest in tumour highlighted. Note that deeper invasive areas have not been selected in order to help exclude surrounding 'normal' stromal and inflammatory cells. Right: Scanty cores from a lung biopsy which have small regions only of tumour selected. Despite utilizing only this small volume of tissue, sufficiently sensitive assays will be capable of detecting mutations. Normal tissue has still been excluded to decrease the possibility of a false-negative result.

to perform analysis. It is now considered good standard practice to obtain a new H&E section of the tissue before proceeding with analysis; at minimum this allows confirmation that the tumour population is still present, but should further guide the laboratory in judging suitability for a given analytical process, in view of relative and absolute tumour population. Where sectioning a significant depth (i.e. greater than 50 µm, or at the assessor's discretion) through the block, just as with classical diagnostic processing, it is sensible to take an additional section for H&E staining and assessment at the end of the process, ensuring the tumour has not 'cut-out'.

The H&E sections produced are usually then both assessed and 'marked' by either a pathologist or a suitably experienced scientist to highlight the area of interest. Essentially this should best isolate the area of tumour within the section to enable technical/scientific staff to select it easily during macrodissection (Figure 11.9). There is some discrepancy between laboratories as to exactly how stringent this selection should be; for example, there is a widely adopted dogma that necrotic areas of tumour should be excluded since they are unlikely to contribute viable DNA and may introduce PCR inhibitors to the reaction. However, certain studies suggest that high levels (>50%) of tumour necrosis are not a significant source of analytical variability when sufficiently sensitive assays are employed (Fisher *et al.*, 2014). The level of sensitivity is a key consideration at this stage; are the assays that will be employed later in processing sensitive enough to detect alterations in the proportion of tumour cells present, even if the tumour is accurately macrodissected? Laboratories may wish to stipulate a minimum % of required tumour nuclei to ensure sensitivity of testing and/or a threshold of tumour content below which sensitivity is not guaranteed.

The growing digitization of tissue microscopy is expanding to allow not only recording, but also assessment and analysis of tissue. Many larger commercial tissue processing and microscopy companies now offer some sort of digital microscopy system; while initially intended for high resolution image capture to archive or share sections digitally, quantitative or even analytical software is becoming widespread. This can take the form of *in vitro* diagnostic (IVD) use scoring algorithms, such as Leica's ERsight and PRsight applications (www.leicabiosystems.com/digital-pathology/image-analysis-solutions/details/product/ariol/) or Ventana's Companion Algorithm software (www.ventana.com/product/page?view=companionalgorithm); digital software 'plug-ins' which supplement the manufacturer's own hardware or tests, providing (semi-)quantitative data on staining patterns. Other companies are taking an alternative approach, producing software scoring algorithms (sometimes platform agnostic) only, which are for use in conjunction with other manufacturers' hardware. One such company, Definiens, offers a bespoke companion diagnostic software service which analyses clinical and digital image data, producing algorithms of clinical significance to be used prognostically or predictively (www.definiens.com/clinical-and-dx). Another application highly relevant to molecular pathology is use of digital image sharing for teaching and assessment of tissue assessment skills; PathXL, which offers a broad range of digital tissue recording and analytical services, are now supporting UKNEQAS in a module evaluating the participant's ability to assess tissue for molecular pathology applications (www.ukneqas-molgen.org.uk/tissue-i-histopathology-assessment).

11.6.2 Macrodissection and the associated removal of unwanted specimen constituents

Macrodissection is essentially the process of manually removing slide-mounted target tissue areas from the whole section for their subsequent analysis, and should not be confused with microdissection, where cells are usually removed individually or in very small numbers using 'real-time' microscopic assessment and guidance. It typically involves using solvents or a specifically designed deparaffinization solution to remove paraffin wax, and subsequent use of a scalpel blade or pipette tip to loosen tissue from the slide surface and transfer it to a receptacle for tissue digestion. A marked, stained section cut immediately before or after the section for macrodissection is used as a guide to inform the procedure. Some laboratories prefer to remove tissue prior to deparaffinization, but most histologists will be aware of the difficulties of carefully handling static-charged, 'free' paraffin wax-embedded tissue that is no longer adhered to a slide. Alternatively, a transfer medium (such as 70% ethanol solution) can be used to cover tissue sections, and once scraped loose into suspension in the medium the embedded material can be moved safely, then deparaffinized. While more specific, microdissection does not necessarily improve the yield of the target cell population (Leong *et al.*, 2013); use of sufficiently sensitive detection methods renders any benefits of microdissection minimal and is more practical to implement.

Deparaffinization is itself essential; paraffin waxes will physically inhibit PCR. Both deparaffinization solutions and the classical stepwise dewaxing-to-rehydration process will eliminate not only wax, but also residual solvents; again, this is essential for downstream processing since both xylene and alcohol are PCR inhibitors—alcohols in particular will rapidly precipitate nucleic acids. However, as we will see in the next section, some manufacturers have simplified this area by combining the removal of paraffin, rehydration of tissue and digestion of tissue to release nucleic acids in a single step.

Key Points

Pre-analytical processes

The biomedical scientist has a duty to consider various factors when assessing whether and how to analyse a sample. These include but are not limited to:

- What the specimen has been subjected to prior to submission for testing.
- The quantity and quality of specimen available for testing.
- Whether the technique(s) employed for testing will be appropriate.
- What additional demands could be made of the specimen for further molecular or routine histopathological testing.

11.7 Nucleic acid extraction

Extraction of DNA (and to a lesser extent RNA, given the smaller number of common applications) from FFPE tissue has transformed radically in the past decade. A proliferation of molecular pathology tests essential (and indeed mandatory) for patient management; new commercially available products designed specifically to enhance NA retrieval from FFPE tissue; the desire to derive purer, less fragmented NAs which will improve analytical success rates and allow application of more demanding tests; and the need to do more (a greater breadth of testing) for less (with relatively smaller specimens), have all influenced this move. At the turn of the century many laboratories still employed simpler 'home brew'/'laboratory developed test' extraction methods, often based on chemical lysis techniques, such as classical phenol:chloroform phase separation (Sengüven et al., 2014), these were more hazardous and unpleasant for the practitioner and yielded a crude NA isolate of relative impurity. While classical Sanger sequencing was the mainstay of analytical processes this perhaps represented less of an obstacle; with the increasing adoption of more sensitive, qualitative assays a better alternative was needed.

Many commercial companies had already addressed the issue of NA retrieval from low volume/quality samples in the research (for example in low cell population proliferation assays or small volume animal samples) or forensic (where NAs were often poorly preserved) settings, and laboratories made initial progress with FFPE samples by exploiting these kits. We'll look in this section at some of the main approaches to extraction, their advantages and limitations, and how laboratories can best integrate them into their overall specimen workflow. There are no strict or even informal guidelines on how nucleic acid extraction should be performed—it is very much determined at local level on an 'as-needs' basis to meet the requirements of the assays employed by the laboratory. However, this arrangement may already be changing in response to various pressures. As laboratories move towards greater standardization, in order to obtain ISO 15189 accreditation, for example, commercial kits offer a simpler alternative to self-regulated methods. Increasing adoption of commercial CE IVD assays (the Conformité Européene IVD standard that must be met in order to provide clinical devices or tests commercially within the European Union) often comes hand-in-hand with specified pre-analytical processes; a particular assay may require in-house validation if the laboratory does not use the manufacturer's specified extraction protocol. And NHS England, in association with Genomics England (GEL), has, for the first time, provided some guidance, albeit in a limited form; the publication of guidelines for specimen processing within the 100,000 Genomes Project includes detailed protocols on how participating laboratories should extract DNA for submission to its central biorepository and sequencing laboratory (www.genomicsengland.co.uk/ and www.genomicsengland.co.uk/wp-content/uploads/2015/03/GenomicEnglandProtocol_030315_v8.pdf).

11.7.1 Spin-column purification and 'on-membrane' DNA isolation

Many commercial manufacturers offer a variation of this now long-established extraction technique; digested cellular material in suspension is passed over a membrane to isolate free NAs from solution, and subsequent chemical 'washing' removes other cellular constituents before a final elution stage releases purified NAs into a buffer or sterile water solution. In Figure 11.10 we can see the component parts of one of Qiagen's extraction-spin column units. Both automated and manual methods are available; for a more in-depth explanation of automated systems such as the Qiagen Qiacube, visit Qiagen's YouTube channel for a Qiacube guide (https://www.youtube.com/watch?v=egHqZqkLkAc).

A tissue isolate, deparaffinized on the section prior to removal and transfer to a sample tube, or deparaffinized in the sample tube itself, is mixed with key components to the tissue digestion process: a cell-membrane disrupting agent such as a detergent, a buffer which provides a mildly alkaline pH and ensures acidic degradation and depurination of nucleic acids is inhibited, and a proteolytic enzyme, typically proteinase K. In conjunction these degrade cellular constituents that would otherwise render nucleic acids inaccessible and allow them to pass freely into solution. This process is performed at above ambient temperature to enhance enzymatic activity and accelerate digestion, usually at around 56°C; it can be further enhanced by agitation to promote mixing and physical disruption. The complete digestion of tissue is heavily dependent upon the starting volumes used, and laboratories should tailor protocols to standardize input for optimization of the process; incompletely digested constituents can severely impair the downstream membrane-isolation stage. Addition of buffer, to reduce saturation, and proteinase K, to aid proteolysis, can both be used mid-process to promote more rapid completion.

Once fully digested, the suspension is usually subjected to a short high-temperature incubation phase ≤90°C. While historically this acted to deactivate proteinase K and prevent proteolytic activity in the downstream PCR reaction, it is now understood to assist in formalin-protein cross-linking reversal and enhanced nucleic acid retrieval. The entire digest is then transferred to the spin column and centrifuged to isolate cell constituents on the column membrane; if large quantities of digested material are to be used, this process can be usually be repeated until all the suspension has been passed through the column. The unwanted solution is discarded and 'clean-up' of the NA performed by one or more 'washing' stages; a wash buffer containing, typically, a guanidinium salt such as guanidinium thiocyanate is passed over the membrane by further centrifugation to remove other constituents—mainly proteins—and leave the NA *in situ* on the membrane. Once complete, a dedicated elution buffer (or simple sterile water, depending upon the user preference) is used to release the NA into solution and elution into a sterile dedicated specimen tube for storage and further use.

An adapted version of the standard Qiagen method for FFPE extraction (for more information and specific protocols see www.qiagen.com/gb/shop/sample-technologies/dna/dna-preparation/qiaamp-dna-ffpe-tissue-kit/) was endorsed by GEL as an approved process for retrieving DNA of sufficient quality to be utilized in downstream DNA-hungry whole-genome sequencing. Spin column

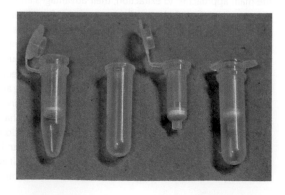

FIGURE 11.10

On the right is a complete unit, comprising the spin column and elution tube; these two component parts can be seen separated, centrally. The white band of the filter is clearly visible; when the digest is added to the upper compartment then passed across the filter by centrifugation, NAs bind to the filter while waste and wash buffers collect in the elution tube, and can be discarded. In the final stage, the spin column is inserted into a permanent storage tube (as shown on the left) and the NAs are washed from the filter with an elution buffer and collected for downstream use.

methods are versatile and scalable, allowing for fluctuations in throughput without compromising delivery by requiring batching to remain cost efficient. Where automatable, many of the same kit components can be used in both manual and mechanical processes, allowing flexibility of application and continuity of service during machine downtime. However, they are perhaps more liable to loss of NAs during processing when compared to other popular methods, and manual processing is labour intensive, repetitive and more prone to human error.

11.7.2 Magnetic bead isolation

Nucleic acids are inherently charged, due to their phosphate backbone, and this property can be easily exploited to assist in isolation. By following an identical initial processing pathway to that described in Section 11.7.1 a crude tissue lysate can be prepared, but instead of opting to perform multiple fluid transfers with associated centrifugation the NA itself can be transferred from solution to solution in order to achieve the same process. In order to do so, magnetically charged beads are added to the lysate and DNA present therein will rapidly bind to these. A magnetic rod is then immersed into the solution and the DNA–bead complexes in turn bind to this. Risk of cross-contamination and NA carry-over is reduced by employing thin disposable rod covers; these prevent direct binding of DNA to rods but do not interfere with magnetic interactions to the extent that valuable material is lost. Once the isolation–purification process is complete the rod covers are detached from the rod and rapidly agitated within a specimen tube containing suspension fluid; the DNA–bead complexes, free from any attraction, are released in to suspension.

By minimizing pipetting in the processing chain, bar the initial addition of prepared tissue lysate and any post-processing (see Section 11.8), the risk of cross-contamination and carry-over of material is much reduced when compared to spin-column type methods. The loss of liquid and material by residual binding to pipette tips is no longer a concern. The final DNA suspension is not, in fact, absolutely ready for use since the magnetic beads used for isolation remain present and can cause interference with molecular application. They are, however, relatively easily removed in a subsequent precipitation to leave pure DNA, but these methods are not entirely without some manual processing stages. These methods usually employ sealed, single use, 'per-sample' kits containing all necessary reagents in discrete compartments. As such, without the automated system to process them, they are entirely redundant; unlike many spin-column methods they cannot be hand-processed as a back-up method should equipment failure occur. To ensure continuity of service a laboratory using magnetics bead isolation will need to maintain and support an alternative method if downtime is to be avoided.

11.7.3 Ultrasonication methods

Although perhaps less widespread than the aforementioned methods, ultrasonication is worthy of consideration for some of its novel features and advantages. The theoretical basis of the method is that exposure of a liquid medium to ultrasonic waves will agitate and disrupt cells or tissues therein. Practically, tissue—often in the form of cores or fragments rather than sections—is immersed in buffer and subjected to bursts of ultrasonication which dissociate the tissue from the paraffin and rehydrate the tissue. Subsequent proteinase digestion, cross-linkage reversal, and purification is then carried out similarly to spin-column methods. Advantages include the use of an aqueous medium, eliminating organic solvents and other hazardous chemicals, and one-step single stage dissociation of paraffin and tissue, including tissue disruption. It is also possible to use far greater volumes of starting material; larger volumes of paraffin wax, which are slow to dissolve chemically and easily block spin-columns if not fully disrupted, are easily rendered into emulsion by sonication. This capacity to increase tissue input and resulting DNA output, along with more even yield of DNA fragments from across the genome, make this form of extraction popular with some users of DNA-hungry next-generation sequencing (NGS) methods.

SELF-CHECK 11.4

What are the key variables in deciding on a DNA extraction method to employ, and which sorts of samples are most suitable for the different methods described?

11.8 PCR analysis methods

At the beginning of the chapter we looked at the fundamentals of the PCR reaction and variables to be considered when designing a protocol. Manipulating the amplified DNA (our PCR products) post-PCR or as a real-time process during the PCR itself allows us to obtain qualitative and quantitative data. A wide variety of PCR variants exist which vary the fundamental cycling parameters previously discussed to different effects. Cold PCR exploits the subtle differences in melting and annealing temperatures which are caused by small variations in the sequence of a given region; by identifying these and adjusting accordingly, the PCR reaction can be biased to favour amplification of a mutant sequence over the wild-type variant and allow variants present at very low levels to be more easily identified. Touchdown PCR employs a graduated decrease in the annealing temperature of each cycle, usually descending incrementally for around 10 cycles, before settling at a low annealing temperature for the remaining 20–30 cycles. The lower temperature employed for the later cycles means that primer sets with different annealing temperatures can be amplified simultaneously and a dedicated thermocycler is not needed for each protocol; however, the initial higher annealing temperatures ensure the first few rounds of amplification are specific, and the later lower temperature does not lead to non-specific amplification as might be expected, because multiple copies of specific product are already amplified, favouring their reproduction. Below, however, we consider a few of the fundamental PCR-analysis methods.

11.8.1 Sanger sequencing

The Sanger method has been a mainstay of laboratories for more than 30 years, and has only recently begun to lose its status as the gold standard of analysis. Amplified PCR products are subject to a second round of PCR over a shorter series of cycles, utilizing a series of fluorescently tagged dideoxy-nucleotides (ddNTPs) which terminate chain extension in the reaction when incorporated. These labelled products are then subjected to a purification process which removes excess of fluorescent tags and nucleotides, vital in ensuring that background noise is reduced and a more specific sequence is given. Finally, labelled products are run through a polymer-filled capillary and subjected to electrophoresis to separate them on the basis of size. Since the chain is terminated by ddNTP inclusion, both the type of nucleotide incorporated (ddATP, ddGTP, ddCTP and ddTTP are each labelled with a different fluorophore) and the length of fragment can be determined, and the nucleotide present at each position of the chain determined.

11.8.2 Real-time PCR

This variant involves PCR with subsequent quantification/analysis of PCR products; this quantification usually employs fluorescent probes or DNA-philic molecules. As such the amount of fluorescence emitted equates to the amount of PCR product and allows (semi-) quantitation. The amount of PCR product measured after each PCR cycle is used to generate a plot of PCR product against time. Real-time PCR was born from a desire to try to quantify the products of amplification, and the realization that end-point PCR was not always accurate enough to be fit for purpose. End-point PCR relies upon running a PCR to its completion then performing a measurement of the total product, for example by fluorimetry or gel-based methods. However, variables such as the starting template quality, quantity, length and the reaction efficiency itself far too easily skew this measurement; real-time PCR, to some extent, eliminates the impact of these factors.

Classic examples of real-time PCR applications usually involve quantitation of products to some extent; this could involve measuring levels of a gene of interest vs a control gene (i.e. expression); increase or decrease in levels of a given variant (such as monitoring of disease response or progress); and calculating the copy number of an agent (i.e. viral load). The high degree of sensitivity the technique provides makes it highly attractive; this can make it routinely employable where low overall quantity or quality of starting template mean that other visualization techniques might fail. The technique is best suited to analysis of restricted-region point mutations, small deletions and insertions, and methylation; larger 'in-dels' or genes and regions where mutations are randomly distributed over a wide area are harder to assess because of the number of reactions that would be needed to assess longer regions of DNA.

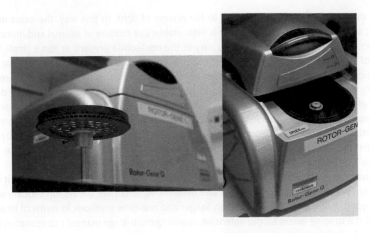

FIGURE 11.11
The Qiagen Rotorgene-Q (RGQ) 5-plex real-time PCR system. Microtubes containing PCR
reaction mixes are loaded into the slots lining the outer wall of the disc (left). The disc is then
mounted onto the central podium within the system (right); continuous spinning of the disc
throughout the PCR programme maintains constant temperatures across the disc.

Most real-time PCR methods can be said to fall under one of the following two strategies, although
variations in the format of reagents and conditions and automation (Figure 11.11) can be used to
enhance specificity or sensitivity. Intercalating assays employ a DNA-philic molecule, added to the
PCR mix, which fluoresces when bound to DNA; as the quantity of PCR product increases exponentially so does the level of fluorescence. Although simple and usually relatively cheap, and theoretically
applicable to any existing PCR assay, these agents are relatively unselective; non-specific amplification products and primer-dimers will also contribute to fluorescence levels and decrease accuracy.
Molecular beacons and Taqman probes are primer-like sequences which have been tagged with both
a fluorophore that emits light and a quencher that blocks this fluorescence when in close proximity.
The probe binds to a target sequence lying between the two standard PCR primers and, when amplification occurs, extension from the primer physically lyses the probe; the fluorophore and quencher
are released and the former begins to emit light. Each round of amplification increases overall levels
of fluorescence; because the emission is strictly linked to amplification of the targeted region it is
much more specific than intercalation. However, in order to design your probe, you must first know
the sequence at your region of interest; furthermore, this synthesis, particularly the fluorescent dyes
used, is relatively expensive.

11.8.3 Pyrosequencing

This is what we often refer to as a 'sequence-by-synthesis' method; instead of synthesizing a product which is then measured, the nucleotides incorporated during extension from the primer are
analysed as each is added in turn. As with Sanger sequencing, an initial round of PCR is used to
amplify up a region of interest, before a second stage using a modified form of PCR is used for the
analytical process. One of the primers used in the first round is tagged with biotin and this is used to
subsequently isolate the strand (forward or reverse) into which these biotin tags have been incorporated; streptavidin beads are mixed with the PCR product, precipitated with ethanol, and denatured
with sodium hydroxide to leave only the tagged strand bound to the beads. These isolated single
strands are then subject to primer extension of a modified form. A sequencing primer is annealed
to the unidirectional strands, and these are then incubated with the enzymes DNA polymerase, ATP
sulphurylase, luciferase, and apyrase, as well as the substrates adenosine 5' phosphosulphate (APS)
and luciferin.

In simple terms, each individual nucleotide is then added one at a time rather than as a pool of
all four nucleotides (as in Sanger sequencing); when a nucleotide is incorporated and phosphate

released, this enzyme combination leads to the release of light. In this way, the exact nucleotide present at a given position *and* its quantity is measurable; in a mixture of normal and mutated DNA, where two different copies of a gene may vary in the nucleotide present at just a single base, the addition of the two nucleotides at different points in time means that the amount of light given off by each incorporation is independently measurable. Since we can quantitatively compare the light emitted for any/each nucleotide incorporated at any point in the chain, it is possible to determine not only whether a variation is present, but what percentage of the DNA carries the variant. The apyrase mops up any excess nucleotides and ATP present by degradation, so each incorporation gives a distinct, brief light signal; once a given position in the chain has been extended by addition of the different nucleotide variants, the process repeats so that each subsequent position can have its composition 'interrogated'.

While pyrosequencing has a distinct advantage over real-time PCR in one sense, since it is not essential to know the target sequence in full and different variants over the region sequenced can be precisely typed, it falls somewhere between Sanger and real-time methods in terms of its sensitivity and speed. It is to some extent labour-intensive, requiring multi-stage manual manipulation to isolate the biotin-labelled strands; furthermore, these biotin-tagged primers are somewhat labile and require careful handling with minimal freeze–thaw cycling when used. For greater detail on the specifics of the method and a visual overview, see Qiagen's technology pages (www.qiagen.com/gb/resources/technologies/pyrosequencing-resource-center/technology-overview/ and www.qiagen.com/gb/resources/e-learning/videos/pyrosequencing%20cascade%20reaction/).

11.8.4 Next-generation sequencing

The complexity and diversity of NGS methods render it difficult to summarize the many benefits and limitations they bring. It is certainly fair to say that implementation of an NGS workflow requires a tailored approach to all stages of the workflows already discussed; extraction methods employed need to meet the more demanding quantity and quality of NAs required; and specimen handling and PCR workflows remain more complex and intricate than traditional methods, although much focus on their development has concentrated on streamlining this phase. Additionally, and putting aside the need to access requisite sequencing platforms, interpretation of data requires a complex and robust bioinformatics pipeline to ensure accurate and reproducible analysis. In very general terms, NGS workflows utilize:

- **Library preparation**

  During library preparation DNA is either fragmented and/or synthesized (e.g. by PCR) to a specific length; production of double-stranded DNA copies of the target regions; ligation or other attachment of oligonucleotide adapters to the end of fragments to be sequenced; and quantification of this final 'library' prior to sequencing, to ensure efficient and—as far as possible—unbiased sequencing.

- **Sequencing**

  Various sequencing methods have been used for this phase; combinations or variations of pyrosequencing, PCR amplification, ion semiconduction, and many other technologies can be used to produce multiple 'reads' of target regions. The product of this is multiple (tens to thousands) or individual sequence results for a given gene or region which can be individually analysed; potentially this provides a method with greater specificity than Sanger sequencing and greater sensitivity than real-time PCR.

- **Bioinformatic interpretation**

  One issue with this quantity of data is the need for a robust interpretive method; while a trained interpreter can easily and quickly analyse Sanger sequences, the output from most NGS runs is simply far beyond accurate interpretation without computational support. Each of the 'reads' produced requires alignment against a reference sequence—the consensus 'normal' sequence for a region; small, genuine variations in the sequence or errors introduced during the sequencing (and PCR, if performed) process make this highly difficult for such a huge number of sequences. Discriminating between genuine variants and errors, and doing so consistently at high throughput is a key requisite of a bioinformatics solution.

Key Points

PCR analysis methods

■ Different PCR analyses have benefits and limitations, making an evaluation of the best method to use a part of any test development.

■ Most methods require some form of highly specialized equipment and access to platforms is an important consideration.

■ There is often a balance to be struck between specificity and sensitivity; both must be relevant to the investigation and should be considered in the interpretation of data.

■ Whether or not a method provides the clinical information required is the key factor in any decision.

CASE STUDY 11.1 Unknown artefacts

● With an increase in workload, a previously reliable pyrosequencing assay began to show intermittently an artefact in signal profile at a particular position in the sequenced region.

● Troubleshooting was employed to try to determine the source of the issue: sequentially the laboratory exchanged all reagents used and any semi-permanent consumables (such as filters, probes and hard plastics); staff members performing analysis were rotated through the set-up and processing, and had their practical performance checked against competency standards; and a maintenance check was performed by the system manufacturer.

● When these steps failed to elucidate the issue, senior scientific staff assessed the entire handling process for the specimens and reagents employed in an 'end-to-end' fashion. This revealed two key handling errors:

– The commercial kit contained multiple components requiring different storage conditions, some provided as a considerable excess. Since appropriate storage meant any given kit

was split and components stored separately, staff had been exchanging the reagents provided in excess volumes only when they were exhausted and not when the limited components were fully consumed. As a result, reagents from the kit were used at different rates, their expiration not monitored, and different lots of kits were being mixed. Logging and tracking of reagents was amended to address this.

– The additional stock ordered and held in storage to meet demand was being placed in a monitored refrigerator within the post-PCR area. The bulky stock to the rear of the refrigerator showed freeze–thaw artefact and it was discovered that the sheer volume of stock was inhibiting air circulation and causing temperature pockets within the refrigerator; the monitor placed at the front of the refrigerator did not detect these. As well as redistributing stock to enable cooling, individual kit components were moved to stock holders to reduce the volume of packaging present.

Introduction of these measures eliminated the issue, and these practices were applied universally where applicable.

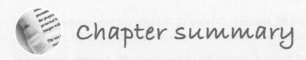

Chapter summary

■ The growth in molecular diagnostics, particularly in recent years, has been driven by growing numbers of diagnostic, prognostic and predictive markers.

■ Most molecular diagnostic applications exploit the biological properties of nucleic acids, in particular their replication, to generate sufficient quantities of specimen template to allow use in other analytical processes.

■ The nature of the patient groups requiring molecular diagnostic tests means that routinely obtained pathological specimens are often most pertinent for patient testing. Consequently, the quality and quantity of material available may be relatively limited.

■ Pre-analytical processing and histopathological analytical pathways can further compromise specimens. It is a priority for any biomedical scientist working with these specimens to reduce wastage and optimize all aspects of specimen handling to ensure downstream processes are not compromised.

■ Analytical techniques across a breadth of different techniques are now requisite for a 'complete' panel of molecular diagnostic techniques. Laboratories should consider how they can best offer these, if not independently, to best minimize specimen wastage and transport times.

■ A wide variety of LDT and commercial options exist for every stage of the molecular analytical pathway. These should be carefully selected on the basis of how best to meet demands for testing, primarily to meet clinical requirements for the largest possible patient population.

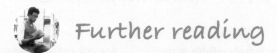 Further reading

● Ahmadian A, Ehn M, Hober S. Pyrosequencing: history, biochemistry and future. *Clin Chim Acta* 2006; **363**: 83–94.

● Bartlett JM, Ibrahim M, Jasani B, *et al.* External quality assurance of HER2 FISH and ISH testing: three years of the UK national external quality assurance scheme. *Am J Clin Pathol* 2009; **131** (1): 106–11.

● Bell J. *Building on our inheritance. Genomic technology in healthcare*. A report by the Human Genomics Strategy Group. Department of Health White Paper, January 2012. (www.gov.uk/government/uploads/system/uploads/attachment_data/file/213705/dh_132382.pdf)

● Bellon E, Ligtenberg MJ, Teijper S, *et al.* External quality assessment for KRAS testing is needed: setup of a European program and report of the first joined regional quality assessment rounds. *Oncologist* 2011; **16** (4): 467–78.

● Clark DM, Silvester K, Knowles S. Lean management systems: creating a culture of continuous quality improvement. *J Clin Pathol* 2013; **66** (8): 638–43.

● Care Quality Commission. *Sherwood Forest NHS Foundation Trust and Kings Mill Hospital Visit and Review*. October 2012. (www.cqc.org.uk/sites/default/files/old_reports/rk5_sherwood_forest_hospitals_nhs_foundation_trust_rk5bc_kings_mill_hospital_20130327.pdf)

● Cross SS, Start RD, Smith JH. Does delay in fixation affect the number of mitotic figures in processed tissue? *J Clin Pathol* 1990; **43**: 597–9.

● Deans ZC, Bilbe N, O'Sullivan B, *et al.* Improvement in the quality of molecular analysis of EGFR in non-small-cell lung cancer detected by three rounds of external quality assessment. *J Clin Pathol* 2013; **66** (4): 319–25.

● Evers DL, Fowler CB, Cunningham BR, Mason JT, O'Leary TJ. The effect of formaldehyde fixation on RNA: optimization of formaldehyde adduct removal. *J Mol Diagn* 2011; **13** (3): 282–8.

● Fisher KE, Cohen C, Siddiqui MT, Palma JF, Lipford EH III, Longshore JW. Accurate detection of BRAF p.V600E mutations in challenging melanoma specimens requires stringent immunohistochemistry scoring criteria or sensitive molecular assays. *Hum Pathol* 2014; **45** (11): 2281–93.

● Franca LT, Carrilho E, Kist TB. A review of DNA sequencing techniques. *Q Rev Biophys* 2002; **35** (2): 169–200.

● Hicks DG, Boyce BF. The challenge and importance of standardizing pre-analytical variables in surgical pathology specimens for clinical care and translational research. *Biotech Histochem* 2012; **87** (1): 14–7.

● Kapp JR, Diss T, Spicer J, *et al.* Variation in pre-PCR processing of FFPE samples leads to discrepancies in BRAF and EGFR mutation detection: a diagnostic RING trial. *J Clin Pathol* 2015; **68** (2): 111–8.

● Keogh B. *Personalized medicine strategy*. NHS England Board Paper: PB.24.09.15/05. September 2015. (www.england.nhs.uk/wp-content/uploads/2015/09/item5-board-29-09-15.pdf).

● Leong KJ, James J, Wen K, *et al.* Impact of tissue processing, archiving and enrichment techniques on DNA methylation yield in rectal carcinoma. *Exp Mol Pathol* 2013; **95** (3): 343–9.

● Lindeman NI, Cagle PT, Beasley MB, *et al.* Molecular testing guideline for selection of lung cancer patients for EGFR and ALK tyrosine kinase inhibitors: guideline from the College of American Pathologists, International Association for the Study of Lung Cancer, and Association for Molecular Pathology. *Arch Pathol Lab Med* 2013; **137** (6): 828–60.

● Maxam AM, Gilbert W. A new method for sequencing DNA. *Proc Natl Acad Sci U S A* 1977; **74** (2): 560–4.

● Nam SK, Im J, Kwak Y, *et al.* Effects of fixation and storage of human tissue samples on nucleic acid preservation. *Korean J Pathol* 2014; **48** (1): 36–42.

● Nicholas MW, Nelson K. North, south, or east? Blotting techniques. *J Inv Dermatol* 2013; **133** (7): e10.

● Nicholson AG. *Dataset for lung cancer histopathology reports*. London: Royal College of Pathologists, 2014 (www.rcpath.org/profession/clinical-effectiveness/clinical-guidelines/cancer-datasets-and-tissue-pathways.html)

● Pareek CS, Smoczynski R, Tretyn A. Sequencing technologies and genome sequencing. *J Appl Genet* 2011; **52** (4): 413–35.

● Qizilbash AH. Pathologic studies in colorectal cancer. A guide to the surgical pathology examination of colorectal specimens and review of features of prognostic significance. *Pathol Annu* 1982; **17** (Pt 1): 1–46.

● Saiki RK, Scharf S, Faloona F, *et al.* Enzymatic amplification of beta-globin genomic sequences and restriction site analysis for diagnosis of sickle cell anemia. *Science* 1985; **230** (4732): 1350–4.

● Sanger F, Nicklen S, Coulson AR. DNA sequencing with chain-terminating inhibitors. *Proc Natl Acad Sci U S A* 1977; **74** (12): 5463–7.

● Sengüven B, Baris E, Oygur T, Berktas M. Comparison of methods for the extraction of DNA from formalin-fixed, paraffin-embedded archival tissues. *Int J Med Sci* 2014; **11** (5): 494–9.

● Singh VM, Salunga RC, Huang VJ, *et al.* Analysis of the effect of various decalcification agents on the quantity and quality of nucleic acid (DNA and RNA) recovered from bone biopsies. *Ann Diagn Pathol* 2013; **17** (4): 322–6.

● Srinivasan M, Sedmark D, Jewell S. Effect of fixatives and tissue processing on the content and integrity of nucleic acids. *Am J Pathol* 2002; **161** (6): 1961–71.

● Ulivi P, Puccetti M, Capelli L, *et al.* Molecular determinations of EGFR and EML4-ALK on a single slide of NSCLC tissue. *J Clin Pathol* 2013; **66** (8): 708–10.

● VanGuilder HD, Vrana KE, Freeman WM. Twenty-five years of quantitative PCR for gene expression analysis. *Biotechniques* 2008; **44** (5): 619–26.

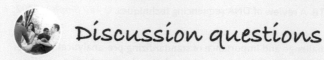

Discussion questions

11.1 Compare and contrast the functions of the main enzymes that play a key role in molecular diagnostics.

11.2 Pre-analytical processing and histopathological analytical pathways have a significant impact on subsequent molecular techniques. How may their adverse effects be minimized?

11.3 Automation has extended the reach of molecular techniques into the routine histopathology laboratory. Discuss.

Answers to the self-check questions and tips for responding to the discussion questions are provided on the book's accompanying website:

 Visit www.oup.com/uk/orchard2e

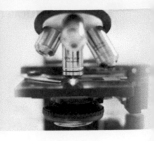

12

Molecular diagnostics in action

Philippe Taniere

Learning objectives

After studying this chapter you should have:

- An understanding of what is the mission of a molecular diagnostic service involved in solid tumour testing.

- An understanding of the complexity of the testing illustrated by examples of diagnostic services that have to face the following challenges:

  - poor quality of samples: small size of specimens; contamination of tumour material by non-tumour cells; degradation of DNA, RNA and proteins by formalin fixation

  - various targets to assess for each sample: gene mutations, chromosome alterations (translocations, amplifications, deletions), protein expression (overexpression, loss of expression) and encompassing requirement to meet

  - quick turnaround time

  - fulfilling laboratory accreditation requirements

  - limited funding.

- A perspective of the author's view on the near future of molecular testing in routine practice.

12.1 Introduction

Histopathology remains the gold standard for the diagnosis of tumours but the histology report now includes the results of supplementary molecular tests (Figure 12.1). The results need to be interpreted by the pathologists in order to issue a final integrated report.

Molecular tests add information on diagnosis, prognosis, and prediction to therapy; targets are chromosomes, genes or proteins.

Cancer Diagnosis Pathway

- Macroscopy
- Microscopy including IHC
- Molecular testing on tissue
  - DNA
  - RNA
  - Proteins

Molecular testing on plasma

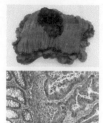

FIGURE 12.1

Full histopathology report includes macroscopic and microscopic description including results of immunocytochemistry to achieve a diagnosis as well as results of eventual molecular tests performed using prognostic and predictive markers. Upper figure: Attribution: Emmanuelm at en.wikipedia. This file is licensed under the Creative Commons Attribution 3.0 Unported license. Lower figure: Copyright © 2011 Michael Bonert (https://commons.wikimedia.org/wiki/User:Nephron). You are free to share and adapt this image as per the CC BY-SA 3.0 (https://creativecommons.org/licenses/by-sa/3.0/legalcode).

Tumours are unstable at the genomic and chromosomal level; this means that there are innumerable alterations within the same tumour which are necessarily not all seen in the same cells. This can be explained by the fact that new alterations can occur at each cell division, once cell cycle controls and DNA repair systems are altered; this is partly what is referred as tumour heterogeneity.

The alterations which are tested in routine practice have been shown, through retrospective or prospective studies or trials, to be clinically relevant; the results of the tests will impact on the patient's management.

Those alterations are clinically relevant only if present in the majority of the tumour cells; they are drivers to tumour development, are maintained throughout tumour progression, and also present in metastatic deposits.

Molecular pathology in tumours has become a proper specialty. There are two main challenges for the setting up of tests and interpretation of the results:

(1) Formalin fixation degrades DNA and proteins.

(2) Any given samples contain a mixture of tumour cells and normal cells (lymphocytes, macrophages, endothelial cells, etc.). So distinguishing the appropriate cell DNA and proteins that are relevant to the analysis is key to the process. It is not possible in routine diagnosis to isolate tumour cells from normal cells by microdissection; this means that DNA extracted from the specimens will be from both tumour and normal cell populations (Figure 12.2).

This will have implications for the selection and the validation of the tests used in routine practice; tests need to be highly sensitive, but not to pick up an alteration present in a minority of the tumour cells (passenger rather than driver for tumour development), rather to detect an alteration within the tumour cells even if those represent a minority of the cell population within the sample (normal cells contain wild type DNA which is also amplified and sequenced during the analysis).

Key Points

Molecular tests need to be highly sensitive to compensate for poor DNA preservation and low tumour/normal cell ratio, not to be able to pick up a mutation present within a minority of tumour cells, which would not be clinically relevant (driver versus passenger molecular alteration).

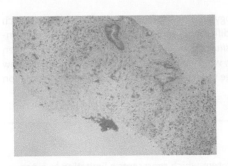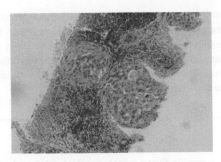

FIGURE 12.2

Two needle core biopsies showing adenocarcinoma. Note the ratio of tumour cells/normal cells is low in both due to the presence of lymphocytes, macrophages and endothelial cells. The ratio is also much lower in the sample on the right; detection of a mutation within the tumour cells would require highly sensitive technology.

In routine practice, molecular pathology diagnostic services need to be able to offer the whole range of techniques needed for patient's management. Nature and number of tests per tumour are guided by clinical relevance. Pathologists play a key role in the prescription of the relevant tests and their final interpretation.

Appropriate management of tissue is crucial; molecular tests are performed following the diagnostic procedure which includes immunocytochemistry. In most of the cases, a single small sample (biopsy, cytology specimen) is available in patients presenting with advanced non-resectable tumours; handling this small fragment in order to be able to apply all required tests remains the pathologist's responsibility. It is a real challenge to be able to obtain sections for H&E stain, sections for ICC, sections for DNA extraction, and sections for FISH on a single biopsy!

SELF-CHECK 12.1

What are the key challenges to setting up molecular tests in histopathology?

Pathologists have made huge progress in the last few years in making accurate diagnosis on very small fragments. Companion diagnostics have been of great help by providing validated and CE marked assays, which reliably work on small and poorly preserved specimens with high sensitivity and high specificity.

Pathologists have also been reactive in changing their practice and adapting themselves to the new needs. A good example is how pathology departments have changed the processing of cytology specimens. Those are more often converted into paraffin blocks or clots which can therefore be processed as histology biopsies in order to be able to apply the same techniques and to archive material.

Obtaining fresh samples of tumour tissue for snap freezing in liquid nitrogen, when possible, represents a precious add-on for molecular testing; DNA, RNA, and proteins would be better preserved in frozen samples, giving more flexibility to perform multiplex testing, up to whole genome sequencing. It seems feasible, and is actually already in place in many centres, at least for banking, to sample surgical resection specimens for snap freezing; it would, however, be more difficult to obtain frozen material in patients with non-operable cancers, for which only biopsies of fine-needle aspirations can be obtained for diagnosis. Histopathology assessment on FFPE specimens is still needed to confirm the diagnosis, so a second biopsy would be needed for freezing.

This would require huge changes in clinical practice and complex pathways to be set up. It remains to be determined if this would be cost effective for patient management.

A compromise would be to find a replacement to formalin for tissue fixation. Several promising alcohol-based fixatives which preserve DNA, RNA and proteins better than formalin are under evaluation. However, the main challenge would be for those fixatives not to induce major changes in tissue morphology following tissue processing for the pathologists to be able to make accurate diagnosis.

All tumour classifications are based on morphology assessment following formalin fixation, which creates specific artefacts; those artefacts will be different if another fixative is used. Also all commercialized assays for immunocytochemistry, *in situ* hybridization, or mutation testing have been validated and accredited on FFPE specimens only, which means that the implementation of a new fixative would imply a universal consensus and huge validation. Changes cannot be made in isolation by any laboratory.

Key Points

Formalin fixation degrades DNA, RNA and protein which represents a limitation to extensive molecular assessment of tumours. Pathologists are likely to be asked to change their practice in the near future by introducing snap freezing of tumour samples, wherever possible.

SELF-CHECK 12.2

What would be the challenges to face in practice to replace formalin by an alternative fixative?

12.2 Molecular pathology diagnostic services: the mission

The duty of molecular pathology diagnostic services is to deliver a wide range of accredited tests (Figure 12.3) within a few working days, on poor quality samples for little amounts of money!

Each tumour type requires a specific panel of tests to be performed, either at the time of diagnosis or at the time of recurrence.

Testing is guided by clinical relevance; this implies a good knowledge of the available treatment options.

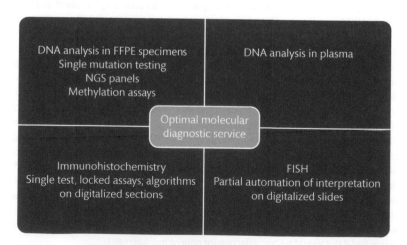

FIGURE 12.3

Optimal molecular diagnostic service. There is a need for a wide range of technologies to be able to deliver the best service, including PCR-based tests in tissue and plasma, and microscope-based tests (brightfield and fluorescence).

12.3 Mutation testing

Mutation testing in routine molecular diagnosis needs to be targeted. The list of genes for which there is strong clinical evidence that testing is helpful for the patient's management is limited.

Furthermore, not all alterations possibly seen in those genes have been clinically validated. This raises the issue of what test should be used for what gene in a specific tumour.

12.3.1 Predictive value of gene mutations in specific tumours

The panel of genes to be tested for single nucleotide variants in a molecular pathology diagnostic laboratory is limited: *KRAS, NRAS, EGFR1, BRAF*. These are the only genes for which testing is mandatory prior to targeted therapy.

KRAS and *NRAS* mutation is a negative predictive marker for anti-EGFR1 monoclonal antibody therapy in colorectal cancers; there are currently two drugs from Merck Serono and Amgene, respectively, which are licensed for *KRAS* and *NRAS* non-mutated tumours (Semrad *et al.*, 2016).

EGFR1 mutation is a positive predictive marker for anti-EGFR1 small-molecule therapy in lung non-small cell carcinoma; there are currently three drugs from Astra Zeneca, Roche, and Boehringer, respectively, which are licensed for *EGFR*-mutated lung cancers (Tan *et al.*, 2016)

BRAF mutation in melanoma is a positive predictive marker for anti-BRAF therapy; there are currently two drugs from Roche and GlaxoSmithKline, respectively, which are licensed in melanoma (Zhang *et al.*, 2015).

Among those genes, only an exhaustive list of mutations has been clinically validated. All four of them have hot spots.

For Food and Drug Administration (FDA) requirements, pharmaceutical companies have developed each targeted drug along a partnership with a companion diagnostic. The assay developed by the latter had to be highly sensitive and specific and accredited, which implies that it had to be as locked as possible (meaning that there should be a minimum of human intervention as possible during the procedure).

In practice, tests have been set up to target a limited number of alterations in each gene for which the drug on trial has been assessed against. It implies that the mutations not assessed by the assay have in theory not been clinically validated. In consequence, using an assay different to the one used during the trial may create some confusion if it does not target exactly the same nucleotide changes as the one used during the trial.

A good example to illustrate this is *EGFR1* mutation testing in lung cancer: the Astra Zeneca drug has been validated with the Therascreen kit and the Roche drug has been validated with the cobas kit; both assays do not exactly target the same panel of alterations; according to FDA rules, Roche drug prescription can only be reimbursed if the tumour has been tested with the cobas kit, etc.

In Europe, licensing and approval by health systems is not so strict; testing for specific alterations needs to be performed by a validating assay according to the laboratory's accreditation standard; this gives more flexibility in practice. This is the reason why it is very important that the molecular report indicates clearly the value of the test: sensitivity and coverage.

Regarding *EGFR* genes, the pathogenic mutations are distributed within exons 18 to 21; not all possible changes found in tumours are covered by the two assays. If direct sequencing is performed in tumours, 13% more mutations will be found than the assays would detect; however, the clinical significance of those is not known yet and needs validation.

One should remember that the great advantage of the real-time PCR based assays from Qiagen and Roche is that they are highly reliable, highly sensitive, and highly specific. In practice, lung tumour samples are small and highly contaminated by normal cells present within the stroma; it is very difficult to obtain larger fragments from very fragile patients. Both assays definitely work in real-life specimens and give a chance in 100% of lung cancer patients to get tumour cells tested for *EGFR* mutation within three working days, those assays convey good comfort to laboratories that they can deliver a good accredited service.

Key Points

During trials assessing a targeted drug against a biomarker, not all mutations potentially present in the gene of interest have been clinically validated.

12.3.2 Other genes tested in practice

Panels available to any diagnostic laboratory also include several genes, which are routinely tested but are not mandatory prior to targeted therapy. Good examples are *KIT* and *PDGFRA* genes which are tested in gastrointestinal stromal tumours (GIST) prior to therapy using tyrosine kinase inhibitors (imatinib, sunitinib, etc.); licensing of those drugs, issued almost 15 years ago, only relied on c-kit protein over-expression. In practice it is now known that some c-kit-expressing GISTs carry no mutation within *KIT/PDGFRA* genes or mutations which convey resistance. Furthermore, some GISTs do not over-express c-kit and do carry good mutations within the genes. It has become routine practice to test GISTs for *KIT/PDGFRA* mutation prior to prescription.

12.3.3 Testing of complex gene changes in practice

Testing for complex alterations such as deletions, amplifications, or translocations require different technologies. In practice, the most validated technique is fluorescence *in situ* hybridization (FISH). There are accredited FISH assays which provide great help, and these are covered in Chapter 11. As for single nucleotide variants, FISH tests have been validated along the various phases of the trials with a companion diagnostic; two good examples are *HER2* amplification in breast and gastric cancers and *ALK* translocation in lung cancer.

However, FISH is labour intensive and requires a high level of expertise; this represents a limitation for its use in routine practice. Laboratories are currently working on making FISH technology cost effective and suitable for higher throughput. The pre-analytical part can be partially automated and new generations of immunostainers are able to accommodate FISH slides within the workflow. Also interpretation could be supported by the use of algorithms applied on digitalized slides. Those will be of great help by making the sophisticated and time-consuming counting and calculation of slides, as required by quality control schemes and guidelines, much easier. Scientist and pathologist expertise will be still required for each test to make the diagnosis of the presence or absence of the specific alteration, but accurate and sophisticated reporting will be facilitated by software packages.

12.3.4 Indirect assessment of complex alterations by immunocytochemistry

The consequences of gene mutations are alterations in the protein structure which could be assessed by immunocytochemistry. Immunocytochemistry represents an alternative to gene or chromosome assessment if validated. Here again clinical validation is essential.

There are a few examples in routine practice which could be mentioned. The historical model is *HER2* assessment through a two-step process which was validated and implemented many years ago when Herceptin was licensed in *HER2*-amplified breast carcinomas. The assumption was that there could not be *HER2* amplification in tumour cells if HER2 protein was not expressed and, inversely, strong membranous expression in tumour cells was correlated to *HER2* amplification. Direct assessment of chromosomes was therefore limited to tumours showing borderline HER2

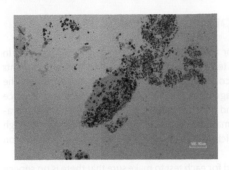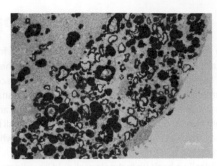

FIGURE 12.4
Lung tumour fine-needle aspiration (cell block prepared following formalin fixation): ALK immunostaining using D5F3 antibody (Ventana) shows diffuse cytoplasmic staining in all the tumour cells.

expression, which helped a lot in reducing the number of tumours to be assessed by the laborious and expensive FISH technology. An FDA-approved assay for protein expression was launched by DAKO (Herceptest) and a few years later, a validated antibody was launched by Ventana (4B5 clone); both tests are still in use.

Another example is ALK assessment in lung non-small cell carcinoma; crizotinib (Pfizer) has been licensed in lung non-small cell carcinomas showing ALK translocation. The companion diagnostic used during the trial was Vysis FISH probes from Abbott. ALK translocation is observed in 3% of lung cancers only. It quickly became apparent that FISH testing was a practical limitation to quick testing on all lung carcinomas and therefore a limitation on all patients receiving the most appropriate treatment.

Immunocytochemistry has therefore become the favoured surrogate to FISH testing in most of the laboratories in Europe. However, strictly speaking, no clinical validation has been undertaken to prove that ALK immunostaining was as accurate as FISH on select patients who would respond to crizotinib. There are two main ALK clones on the market which are used in practice; one has been specifically set up for ALK testing in lung cancers (D5F3 Ventana) (Figure 12.4). In practice, no extensive study has been published yet to demonstrate that replacing FISH by ICC has no consequence on the accuracy of correctly selecting patients who would benefit from crizotinib therapy. The percentage of discrepant cases between both techniques is not known (in particular tumours testing negative by immunocytochemistry and positive by FISH). It is interesting to note that Novartis has chosen Ventana ICC protocol as the gold standard for the validation of its ALK-translocated lung cancer drug.

ALK translocation can also be assessed by looking for transcripts following RNA extraction; however, the exhaustive list of possible transcripts in lung cancer which are assessed by the FISH technique is not known. This will have implications for the relevance of the testing from RNA, for which only a limited number of primers will be included, even if strong data in the literature show that there are hot spots which would represent the vast majority of tumours; when using this technique, there will be a percentage of false-negative cases which scientists and oncologists need to be aware of.

Finally, ALK translocation can be assessed from extracted DNA using deep sequencing technology; this technique would in theory not miss any possible alteration but requires strong validation, bioinformatics analyses, and a larger amount of DNA than the others described above.

Key Points

The assessment is limited to specific alterations in the genes of interest; the significance of a specific alteration can also be different from one tumour type to another: for example, *BRAF* mutation is a predictive marker for anti-BRAF therapy in melanoma and a marker of poor prognosis in colorectal cancer.

12.4 Choosing the appropriate technique

In routine practice the choice of the technique for a specific alteration is always a compromise. In Europe, laboratories have the liberty to choose the technique (which is different to FDA requirements in the United States). Choice should take into account the nature of the specimens expected, the turnaround time needed for efficient clinical management, the platforms which are already in place in the laboratory and scientists are familiar with, and the cost. Tests should be accredited: the laboratory may favour a CE marked IVD assay, which will make the accreditation procedure easier. Although they may decide to validate a homebrew test, which will require more work for the final validation according to ISO criteria.

Ideally, a back-up technology should be validated for each test to make sure that there is no service interruption in case a technical problem occurs; the back-up could also be an agreement with another laboratory to be able to forward samples until any given problem is resolved. Regarding the coverage of alterations for a specific gene, the laboratory may have to compromise between efficiency, accreditation, cost, and clinical relevance.

For example, let's look at *EGFR1* mutation in lung cancer. Anti-EGFR1 drugs are licensed for first-line treatment in advanced lung cancers. It is mandatory that patients do not receive any kind of treatment prior to targeted therapy. Patients with advanced lung cancer are fragile and not fit for aggressive sampling procedures; as a consequence, the only material available will be small bronchial, lung biopsies, fine-needle aspirations, lymph nodes, effusion, or endobronchial ultrasound (EBUS) FNA from mediastinal lymph nodes. As described above, cytology specimens should have been processed as histology specimens, including formalin fixation and paraffin embedding, to be suitable for the testing. One should also keep in mind that samples will reach the molecular laboratory following histology assessments, including immunocytochemistry, which are legitimately needed to confirm the diagnosis and to type the tumour. However, these investigations may well have consumed part of the specimen(s). As a consequence, the technique for *EGFR* assessment should be highly sensitive and quick, as well as reliable and accredited. Real-time PCR would seem to be the technique of choice for many laboratories using commercially available tests. Some laboratories would choose other techniques such as Sanger sequencing, NGS, Sequonom, Pyrosquencing, etc. The inconvenience of real-time PCR assays is that they target a limited number of mutations (around 29 mutations for either Therascreen or cobas assay); of these mutations only those that have been validated clinically will be useful for patient management. Direct sequencing and NGS will cover more mutations within the exons tested but would require more DNA than real-time PCR, which implies that a relatively high number of patients would not have the opportunity to get their tumour tested and therefore miss the chance of being treated with much more efficient treatment. In practice real-time PCR testing can be applied to any specimen; testing could also ultimately be performed on stained sections used for the diagnosis, from which tissue could be used for DNA extraction following removal of the coverslip. The aim is to give any lung cancer patient a chance to benefit from the best treatment.

By contrast, *KIT* and *PDGFR alpha* mutation testing requires sequencing of whole exons, since changes are random within the various exons of either gene. Mutations are distributed within exons 9, 11, 13, and 17 of *KIT* and exons 12, 14, and 18 of *PDGFR alpha*. 85% of GISTs carry a mutation within those two genes. Sanger sequencing or NGS are the techniques of choice; this implies that small biopsies or cytology specimens may not be suitable for testing due to insufficient DNA. A compromise would be to target the two most relevant hotspots for resistance to tyrosine kinase inhibitors, which are, respectively, D842V mutation within exon 18 of *PDGFR alpha* (which conveys full resistance to any type of tyrosine kinase inhibitors) and exon 9 of *KIT* (which conveys relative resistance to imatinib). There are various ways for setting up such targeted assays: homebrew or commercial kits (Pyrosequencing assay from Qiagen), which will be much more sensitive than sequencing.

SELF-CHECK 12.3

What kind of molecular tests could be used to look for *EGFR* mutation in lung cancer and for *RAS* mutation in colorectal cancer?

12.5 **Multiplex gene testing**

The challenge for diagnostic laboratories is to be able to deliver for each tumour type an exhaustive array of molecular tests to determine which of these tests is of clinical value in terms of patient diagnosis, management, and prognostic outcome.

There is limited volume of tissue, which is furthermore often poorly preserved and most of the time formalin-fixed, paraffin-embedded. Furthermore, there are various targets as described above: gene mutations, gene amplification, translocations, protein alterations on both, tumour cells, and surrounding lymphocytes.

It is not reasonable to assume that a single platform will allow the laboratories to deliver the whole testing requirements.

Multiplex testing means grouping the assessment of several targets in a single platform. This can be applied to genes and proteins. However, the techniques allowing multiplex testing should be applicable in real-life samples with a quick turnaround time and should be as reliable as single tests currently in use (i.e. accredited/IVD/CE-marked).

Finally, testing should also take into account the clinical relevance.

There are, in theory, several possible approaches which are not mutually exclusive in routine practice.

12.5.1 **Whole-genome sequencing**

The idea is to screen the whole genome for every tumour; this assessment would include single nucleotide variants and complex alterations. Bearing in mind the innumerable technological challenges, it remains to be determined if this approach would be cost effective.

The main technical challenge is to face the high number of alterations which are present in a tumour; up to 30,000 or more. Not all those alterations would be clinically relevant and the difficulty is to identify which are the key drivers and which are simply the passengers. This implies robust bioinformatics. It is obvious that a large amount of DNA is needed and that formalin fixation represents a huge limitation for this technology due to poor preservation of DNA. The use of frozen tissue represents a complement or an alternative for extensive gene screening. Pathology departments will probably need to be involved in the freezing of samples from surgical resection specimens, also the processing of frozen biopsies in their routine practice. This implies the implementation of liquid nitrogen and −80°C freezer facilities which would need to be resourced. The pathology community should send a clear message to the scientific community that freezing is not a replacement for formalin fixation in routine practice but an add-on for targeted panels using either NGS or real-time PCR.

The validation of panels for genes of various sizes, which would also possibly be tumour-specific, is a realistic approach.

These panels work on formalin-fixed tissues. In practice this approach, which is expanding in the large molecular diagnostic laboratories, allows the validation of various panels adapted to clinical needs. One can imagine that tumours could be assessed in the first instance for a limited number of genes with targeted testing and this will allow first screening for first-line treatment.

There could be a second line of testing, with a wider panel targeting more genes which would help oncologists to plan second-line therapy, including within trials. Those wider panels would probably need to be tumour-specific, including single nucleotide variants, copy number, and translocations.

The smaller panels for first-line treatment would need to be accredited as are the current single gene tests. Several technologies could be used including NGS, real-time PCR, and arrays.

It would, however, be very difficult to get the larger panels accredited according to current standards; those would also need to be upgraded on a regular basis to take into account new drugs on trials, etc.

One more difficulty would be for the laboratories to issue understandable reports on so many alterations bearing in mind that it is likely that not all targets will give satisfactory results. This may lead to a high number of partial failures which would need to be fed back as well. Furthermore, it cannot be expected that the significance of all alterations detected will be understood by everybody. It seems therefore logical to link the molecular results to a list of possible drugs, already licensed or still in trials. Several companion diagnostics have started offering this service (Figure 12.5).

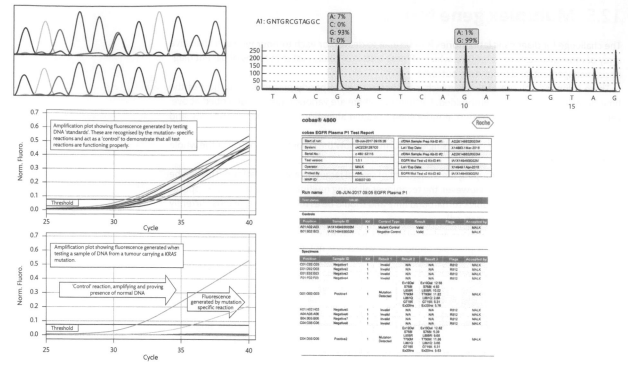

FIGURE 12.5

Mutation testing in routine practice using four techniques and four different ways to interpret the results: Sanger sequencing; pyrosequencing; real-time PCR (off-the-shelf kit; Therascreen assay, Qiagen); real-time PCR, black box assay (cobas, Roche; Idylla, Biocartis).

Key Points

Multiplex gene testing needs to be cost-effective, reliable and accredited before replacing validated techniques; the implementation of panels should be guided by clinical relevance; a two-step process for the assessment of gene alterations in human tumours seems to be appropriate.

SELF-CHECK 12.4

What are the ideal strategies for multiplex tests in molecular pathology?

12.6 Protein assessment

Molecular testing in routine practice does not only include gene alterations assessment, but also protein assessment. This could represent a surrogate or a complement to gene assessment as described above (HER2 and ALK, for example). Protein assessment will also become more and more important in routine testing to assess proteins involved in immune response as either prognostic tests (Immunoscore) or predictive to targeted therapy (PD1/PDL1).

One more level of complexity compared to gene alterations is the need for quantification of both or either number of cells showing the alteration and the intensity of the expression. There will also be a need to assess several proteins to establish a score.

Programmed death 1 (PD1), which is expressed in lymphocytes within the stroma of a tumour, is a validated target for therapy which is very promising; at least five drugs from different pharmaceutical companies are on trial or already licensed for use on various types of tumours. The predictive marker, selected following trials validating the efficiency of the drug in various types of tumours, is the ligand of PD1 or PDL1 which, where present, is expressed mainly in the tumour cells (and also in a variable number of lymphocytes and macrophages). The validated technique for PDL1 assessment is immunocytochemistry; each pharmaceutical company has worked in partnership with a specific clone of PDL1 (Harvey, 2014). As a consequence, there are currently four different PDL1 assays which are currently not cross-validated; a tumour tested with the four assays will show variable patterns, which means that one cannot be used for the other, at least until cross-validation studies have been completed. All assays are locked and fully ready to use on a specific immunostainer with specific guidelines for the interpretation.

In practice this means that a tumour may have to be tested for PDL1 with several assays, each of which will need to be reported respectively. The general agreement among oncologists and molecular pathologists, as well as health systems and commissioners, is that this situation is not sustainable in the long term. Companion diagnostics are currently working on some harmonization strategies of PDL1 assessment but currently with no full guarantee of success.

12.7 Automation of protein assessment

Digitalized pathology offers great potential. Among those is the development of algorithms for interpretation of staining or immunostaining, which is very promising. The validation of this requires lots of work from researchers and/or companion diagnostics before being used in routine laboratories.

There is a real need to use standardized technology for quantification when this precludes the use of specific therapy. All studies show that there is a huge variation and poor reproducibility from one observer to another, which is understandable. The use of algorithms which would have been validated against clinical relevance and would be accredited would be a great improvement. This would be used on brightfield and fluorescence slides. However, there are lots of technical and practical challenges to achieve this. There will be a need for standardization of the paraffin sections, the slides, the staining protocols, the scanners and the algorithms.

12.8 Predictive markers to non-targeted therapy

The majority of advanced malignant solid tumours are still treated with non-targeted chemotherapy; for example, in Caucasian patients, 10% of lung cancers show a mutation within the *EGFR* gene and 3% a translocation with ALK. There is not currently, outside trials, any other targeted therapy to offer.

The mechanism of action of the non-targeted drugs is known. It is also obvious that not all patients respond in the same way to similar chemotherapy. It seems obvious that differences are probably at least in part dependent on the type of molecular alterations present in the tumour cells.

Similarly, to use targeted drugs one could imagine that the assessment of specific alterations within the tumour cells would be helpful to predict which drugs would work. The mechanism of action of the drugs is mainly related to the level of expression in enzymes involved in DNA repair (ERCC1 and platinum-based drugs) or in the transport of molecules into tumour cells (ENT1 and gemcitabine).

There are currently no fully validated tests for any of those markers. The difficulty lies in the fact that testing will require quantification. It is difficult to quantify a level of expression of a gene or a protein within a tumour which includes a variable proportion of tumour cells and non-tumour cells. The genes/proteins of interest will be expressed in the normal cells as well as tumour cells. The validation of robust assays based on the level of expression of the proteins by immunocytochemistry would be extremely helpful in routine practice. The add-on represented by digitization of slides followed by the use of algorithms is also a promising development.

Key Points

Multiplex testing of tumours is not restricted to gene testing but includes protein assessment; it requires the use of various technologies which should all be available in molecular testing centres.

12.9 Reporting

Reporting molecular alterations should include technical details and interpretation of the results to describe the clinical significance. Ideally, this should be seen as supplementary to the primary histopathology report (see Chapter 13).

Diagnostic laboratories should follow various guidelines. It is recommended to describe in detail the technique used, including coverage of alterations and sensitivity. It is also important to mention if tumour burden was assessed, which has implications for the interpretation of the results. Checking a stained section of the tissue to be extracted helps in determining if the technique used would be sensitive enough to detect an alteration in the sample. The assessment can only be semi-quantitative and approximate, and the pathologist is not expected to give an exact count of tumour cells, but rather an estimation of tumour volume and the percentage of the tumour cells among non-tumour cells populating the specimen. It probably makes sense that the assessment is performed in the testing laboratory by the pathologists or biomedical scientists who know about the techniques used for each test. A sample may be suitable for real-time PCR or pyrosequencing testing which are highly sensitive techniques (1–5%) but not for Sanger sequencing which is comparatively less sensitive (10–15%).

12.10 Circulating free tumour DNA

Assessment of specific mutations in plasma rather than tissue is a promising technology which has now become a reality. The idea is that tumour cells release DNA within blood following lysis or necrosis; this DNA is fragmented and the amount is low. There are other technical challenges for the implementation of this technique in diagnostic laboratories. Technically, DNA should be extracted from plasma avoiding contamination by DNA from white blood cells. Samples should be preserved from cell lysis. Plasma should be isolated as soon as possible after sampling if classical EDTA tubes are used; alternatively, specific tubes preserving samples from cell lysis could be used—several types are now available on the market. Techniques of DNA extraction should be set up, manually or on automated platforms, and should ensure that there is no contamination by blood cells.

Testing should use validated highly sensitive techniques. Real-time PCR technology is the technique of choice. Many interesting and promising research projects using NGS have also been conducted. Companion diagnostics are also working on CE-marked IVD assays for specific genes, the first of which have been launched and are targeting *EGFR* mutation for lung cancer patients; Qiagen and Roche molecular have both commercialized a kit which laboratories have started using. It remains to be determined in which clinical scenario(s) this assay will be favoured over tissue assessment; the role of the diagnostic laboratories is to offer both tissue and plasma testing to the oncologists.

One should keep in mind that sensitivity and specificity need to be determined. One has no control on the amount of DNA present in the specimen and there is currently no technique which can distinguish between circulating tumour DNA and other sources of DNA. This implies that the clinical value of the test in terms of sensitivity relies on previous retrospective studies where the presence of the alteration has been confirmed within tumour tissue; it is important to understand the difference between the sensitivity of the technology and the sensitivity for clinical significance. In practice, the clinical sensitivity for the currently available commercialized tests for *EGFR* mutation varies between 65% and 80%, also depending on the stage of the tumours, but they have very high specificity. Digital PCR technology (droplet or BeAMing) offers higher sensitivity but clinical specificity may be compromised (Thress *et al.*, 2015).

As a consequence, reports on *EGFR* mutation testing in plasma need to mention that a negative result will not rule out the presence of a mutation. Nevertheless, the availability of such an assay is definitely a very helpful addition. One can also imagine that such a test could also be helpful for monitoring patients under tyrosine kinase therapy if *EGFR* mutation was detected at the time of diagnosis.

The clinical validation of such assays for *EGFR* and other genes as well as for eventual NGS panels will very much need to take into account the variability in the amount of circulating free DNA in each type of tumour, depending on the histological stage of the tumour. The challenge will be to assess the confidence for a negative result.

Key Points

Circulating free tumour DNA assessment represents a precious addition to tissue testing for specific alterations and is a promising technology to monitor patients under targeted therapy. It cannot be seen, at least currently, as a replacement to tissue sampling, which is needed to confirm diagnosis and to perform protein profiling.

12.11 Accreditation

As in any diagnostic laboratory, molecular pathology diagnostic services need to be accredited. To fulfil ISO standards, any test performed should be accredited. For a homemade assay, the laboratory should provide the evidence that the test was validated according to standard. This requires a huge amount of work; each step of the procedure needs to be documented and the laboratory should be in a position to explain how the assay was validated and is reliable and does what it claims it does. Using CE marker/IVD assays saves time and energy. If used according to the guidelines provided by the company, the laboratory only needs to perform a verification to show that the kit works in the laboratory effectively. This explains why the implementation of a new test in a diagnostic laboratory takes several months in practice even if technology looks straightforward; there is more than the pure technical set-up involved in establishing and incorporating it in a diagnostic repertoire. A new test can only be launched when all documents, including SOPs, validation or verification procedures, have been completed and approved. Once a test is up and running in the laboratory, regular audits and quality control schemes are also required, with performance to be fed back to the users (see Chapter 17).

Key Points

It is important to make the distinction between validation and verification when working on the accreditation of a new test in a routine laboratory.

12.12 Molecular pathology in perspective

Molecular pathology in solid tumours is part of routine assessment of tumours. It should be regarded as a complement to histopathology; panels of tests should be guided by the clinical relevance to be cost effective. Technology moves very fast—it is a tool on which doctors rely to achieve best medical practice; medical practice is, however, not to be guided by the technology. Medicine is an art; delivering molecular profiling in routine practice is supported by the controlled use of various technologies to be used in a cost-effective way and for valid reasons.

Molecular profiling of a tumour requires the assessment of a validated list of specific genes, chromosomes, and proteins. The complexity of the profiling will increase with the further clinical validation of algorithms based on the combination of gene mutations, chromosome alterations and protein alterations (prognostic or predictive value of the combination of a mutation in gene X and down-regulation of proteins y and z in tumour A, etc.). However, there will also be validated systems available on the market for the clinical validation of various molecular profiles which themselves will need to be accredited.

Offering the service will imply being able to cope with high-throughput testing requiring various platforms to issue a single integrated report to be usable in clinics to support patient management; this will require quick turnaround times for both technical assessment and interpretation which can only be achieved by automation at each step. This will apply to tissue or plasma testing or both combined within a single laboratory.

The role of Molecular Diagnostic Laboratories in solid tumour assessment is to deliver the best service to the patients through the oncologists. This service is supported by various technologies which have to be adapted to medical practice. One should keep in mind that technologies are to be used to serve the patient's needs and not the other way around. There is a danger of letting the community believe that any single technology will fulfil all the needs. It is also important to make a clear distinction between research and medical practice.

In practice, for at least the next few years, there will be a need for step process molecular profiling: (1) urgent testing of genes and proteins within a few working days to decide on the most appropriate first-line treatment: assessment of diagnostic, prognostic, and predictive markers for the licensed drugs; (2) second-step testing with the assessment of a wider panel of alterations which requires more tissue and more days to be completed; the latter will be designed to recruit patients within trials.

Routine practice in molecular laboratories in the near future will also include tests to monitor patients under treatment, for which techniques on circulating tumour DNA will be very helpful. Finally, there will be a need at the time of progression under treatment, for various complementary reasons: one of those will be the need to reassess molecular alterations to decide on second-, third-, or more line therapy. New tests will include the screening for secondary alterations in genes which themselves would be targeted by second and further generations of therapy; for example, a lung tumour carrying a mutation within *EGFR* can see an expansion of the secondary mutation *T790M* responsible for progression under first- and second-generation tyrosine kinase inhibitors. There are third-generation tyrosine kinase inhibitors which can be efficient against T790M as well. Testing of progressing tumours for the latter, which is present in 60% of tumours progressing, is mandatory prior to new prescription. The same may apply in the future to look for ALK mutations in tumours carrying ALK translocation which progress under ALK first-line therapy.

One other reason will be to assess tumours for expression of proteins which would have been modified by first-line therapy, such as proteins involved in the immune response (PD1, etc.).

Molecular profiling of tumours requires laboratories to get familiar with various new technologies. However, the aim remains the same for pathology laboratories and involves delivering an efficient and reliable accredited service on a daily basis to all patients.

Furthermore, the other pathology departments also need to implement and accommodate molecular techniques in their repertoire: microbiology, biochemistry, haematology and immunology.

One would think that this is a very exciting time for pathology services which could gain benefit from working together and sharing expertise and equipment, in order to deliver the most cost effective and safest service. High throughput standardized testing, such as whole genome sequencing for rare disorders, inherited disorders, and certain types of tumours would probably be better coordinated in large national screening centres, which would eventually also be responsible for the technical interpretation in an automated way. However, daily testing, guided by the clinical relevance, which will require multiplex testing on multiple platforms within a few working days, would not benefit from centralization, and would appear a little contradictory with the concept of practising personalized medicine.

12.13 Case studies

In order to appreciate the application and value of molecular diagnostics in action, it is necessary to examine some typical examples of the use of this technology in histopathology. The following case studies illustrate the roles played in diagnosis and treatment of gastric (Case study 12.1), breast (Case study 12.2), and colon cancer (Case study 12.3).

CASE STUDY 12.1 *Gastric adenocarcinoma*

A 54-year-old male underwent oesophagogastrectomy for advanced sub-cardia adenocarcinoma (Figure 12.6a).

Histopathology revealed moderately differentiated adenocarcinoma (Figure 12.6b) invading to the sub-serosa (pT3); 12/45 regional lymph nodes contained tumour (pN3a).

The patient was suitable for adjuvant therapy including target therapy. The outcome of the multidisciplinary team (MDT) meeting was to assess the tumour cells for *HER2* amplification (prior to Herceptin therapy).

HER2 assessment was performed by immunocytochemistry (Figure 12.7): staining showed patchy moderate membranous staining in occasional tumour cells amounting to a score of 2+. *HER2* FISH was performed (Figure 12.8) using Vysis probes (Abbott): this revealed *HER2/CEP17* ratio >2 in more than 10% of the tumour cells expressing HER2. The tumour was regarded as positive for *HER2* amplification and the patient was therefore suitable for Herceptin.

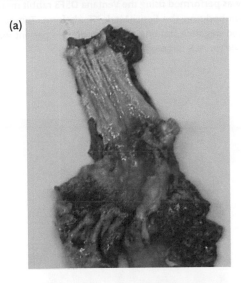

(a)

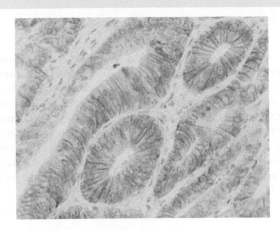

FIGURE 12.7
Tumour cells showing moderate and patchy expression of HER2.

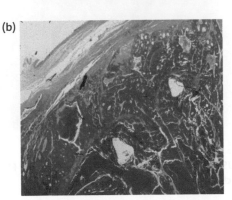

(b)

FIGURE 12.6
Sub-cardia (gastric) adenocarcinoma of intestinal type: a) oesophagogastrectomy specimen; b) section of the tumour (haematoxylin and eosin [H&E] stain).

FIGURE 12.8
FISH showing increase in *HER2* (red signals) copy number with ratio of *HER2/CEP17* (green signals) >2 in more than 10% of cells.

CASE STUDY 12.2 Lung cancer

A 65-year-old female light smoker presented with advanced lung tumour on imaging (Figure 12.9) which was not resectable.

She underwent endobronchial ultrasound (EBUS) and an enlarged mediastinal lymph node was aspirated, and the needle was washed into a transport medium. A paraffin block was prepared from the material following formalin fixation and clotting. Sections from the clot revealed bronchial adenocarcinoma (Figure 12.10). *EGFR* mutation testing and *ALK* translocation testing was requested by the reporting pathologist prior to the MDT meeting.

Epidermal growth factor receptor 1 (*EGFR1*) mutation testing

Sections were prepared from the block; microdissection was performed following marking of an H&E-stained section, and DNA was extracted following a validated protocol. *EGFR1* mutation testing was performed using the Therascreen EGFR RGQ PCR Kit (Qiagen), which screens for the following relevant mutations (coverage >95% of all mutations in the region tested): 19 deletions in exon 19; T790M; L858R; L861Q; G719X; S768I; three insertions in exon 20. Maximum sensitivity of the assay is estimated at 1% mutant allele in a background of wild-type DNA.

Analysis of the *EGFR1* gene showed a missense mutation at nucleotide 2573 (c.2573T>G) which results in substitution of the amino acid leucine by arginine at codon 858 (p.[Leu858Arg]; Figure 12.11), or L858R. This mutation is known to convey sensitivity to anti-EGFR1 small molecule tyrosine kinase inhibitors (TKIs) (EGFR Genbank Accession Number NM_005228.3)

Activin receptor-like kinase (ALK) immunocytochemistry

This was performed using the Ventana D5F3 rabbit monoclonal antibody on the BenchMark XT platform. Tumour cells showed negative staining and therefore the patient was not suitable for ALK targeted therapy.

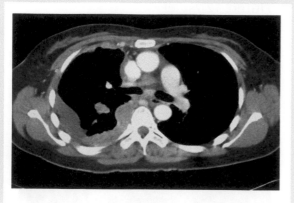

FIGURE 12.9
Computed tomography (CT) scan showing advanced lung tumour.

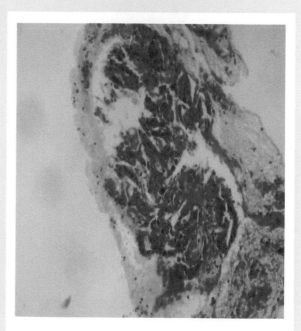

FIGURE 12.10
EBUS FNA specimen; sections from the prepared FFPE block show adenocarcinoma (H&E stain).

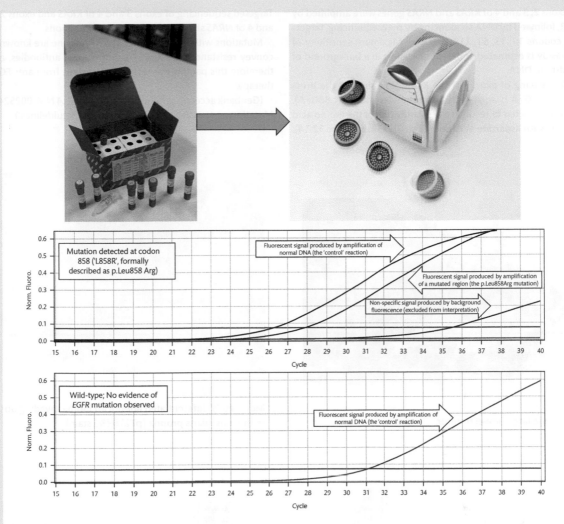

FIGURE 12.11
EGFR1 mutation testing by real-time PCR on the RGQ platform (Qiagen). Tumour shows a mutation within codon 858.

CASE STUDY 12.3 *Colon cancer*

A 76-year-old male underwent left colectomy for adenocarcinoma (Figure 12.12). Histopathology of the resection specimen revealed adenocarcinoma (Figure 12.13) invading up to the sub-serosa (pT2) with 5/15 positive lymph nodes (pN2). Imaging also revealed liver deposits.

The patient was suitable for adjuvant therapy, and *RAS* mutation testing was requested prior to anti-EGFR1 monoclonal antibody therapy.

RAS mutation testing

Histological assessment of sections prepared from the paraffin block selected confirmed the presence of tumour and adequacy for testing (estimated 60–70% tumour nuclei). The selection of areas with tumour for macrodissection was performed with subsequent rehydration, macrodissection, and DNA extraction (QIAamp FFPE Tissue kit)

Exons 2, 3 and 4 of *KRAS* and *NRAS* genes were amplified by PCR, followed by DNA sequencing by pyrosequencing, targeting codons 12, 13, 61, 117, and 146. Maximum sensitivity of the assay is estimated at 5% mutant allele in a background of wild-type DNA.

Sequencing of exon 2 of the *KRAS* gene showed the presence of a G>A base substitution at nucleotide 38 (c.38G>A). This is predicted to result in the substitution of the amino acid glycine with aspartate at codon 13 p (Gly13Asp; Figure 12.14).

Targeted sequencing of exons 3 and 4 of *KRAS* and exons 2, 3, and 4 of *NRAS* showed no evidence of mutations.

Mutations within codon 13 of the *KRAS* gene are known to convey resistance to anti-EGFR monoclonal antibodies, and therefore this patient was unlikely to benefit from anti-EGFR therapy.

(Genbank accession numbers: NM_004985.4 NM_002524.4; Mutation nomenclature according to HGVS guidelines.)

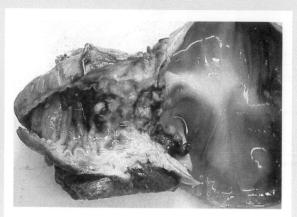

FIGURE 12.12
Stenotic large bowel tumour.

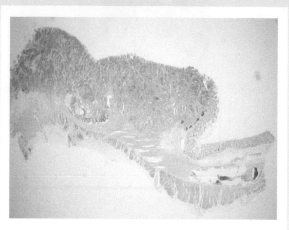

FIGURE 12.13
Moderately differentiated adenocarcinoma invading up to the muscularis propria (pT2) (H&E stain).

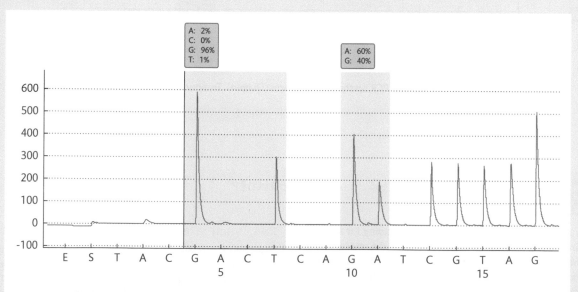

FIGURE 12.14
Pyrosequencing testing reveals a G>A mutation within codon 13.

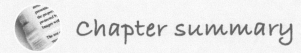

Chapter summary

Molecular pathology is at the forefront of modern laboratory medicine and nowhere is this more apparent than in the role histopathology plays both in the diagnosis and treatment of disease.

Having read this chapter, you should now have an understanding of the molecular diagnostic service and its role in the following:

■ solid tumour testing

■ mutation testing

■ use of immunocytochemistry

■ multiplex gene testing

■ protein assessment and its automation

■ predictive markers

■ circulating free tumour DNA

■ molecular testing in routine practice.

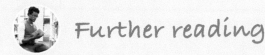

Further reading

● Harvey RD. Immunologic and clinical effects of targeting PD-1 in lung cancer. *Clin Pharmacol Ther* 2014; **96** (2): 214–23.

● Orchard GE, Nation BR eds. *Histopathology*. Oxford: Oxford University Press, 2012.

● Orchard GE, Nation BR eds. *Cell structure and function*. Oxford: Oxford University Press, 2015.

● Semrad TJ, Kim EJ. Molecular testing to optimize therapeutic decision making in advanced colorectal cancer. *J Gastrointest Oncol* 2016; **7** (Suppl 1): S11–20.

● Sorich MJ, Wiese MD, Rowland A, *et al.* Extended RAS mutations and anti-EGFR monoclonal antibody survival benefit in metastatic colorectal cancer: a meta-analysis of randomized, controlled trials. *Ann Oncol* 2015; **26** (1): 13–21.

● Tan DS, Yom SS, Tsao MS, *et al.* The International Association for the Study of Lung Cancer consensus statement on optimizing management of EGFR mutation positive non-small cell lung cancer: status in 2016. *J Thorac Oncol* 2016 May 20.

● Thress KS, Brant R, Carr TH, *et al.* EGFR mutation detection in ctDNA from NSCLC patient plasma: A cross-platform comparison of leading technologies to support the clinical development of AZD9291. *Lung Cancer* 2015; **90** (3): 509–15.

● Zhang W. BRAF inhibitors: the current and the future. *Curr Opin Pharmacol* 2015; **23**: 68–73.

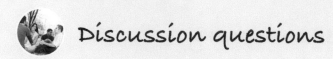 Discussion questions

12.1 How would you define molecular pathology testing in solid tumours in routine practice?

12.2 What are the constraints to validating a molecular test in routine practice, both clinically and technically?

Answers to the self-check questions and tips for responding to the discussion questions are provided on the book's accompanying website:

 Visit www.oup.com/uk/orchard2e

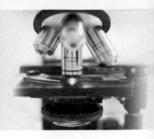

13

Histopathology reporting

Guy Orchard, Chris Ward and Susan Pritchard

Learning objectives

After studying this chapter you should have:

- Developed an understanding of the process and content of a histopathology report, including the supplementary report.

- An understanding of the key microscopic observations seen in the two key areas of histopathology— inflammation and cancer.

- A comprehension of the importance of histopathology reports in the patient management pathway.

- Developed an appreciation of the use of diagnostic datasets and the role of tissue pathways in histopathology.

- An understanding of the value of molecular/genetic information in histopathology reports.

- An understanding of the role of histopathology reporting in research and development.

- An appreciation of the expanding roles for biomedical and clinical scientists in histopathology reporting.

- A knowledge of the current infrastructure of examinations available for advanced involvement in histopathology diagnostics.

13.1 What is a histopathology report?

You will have read something about the histopathology report in Chapter 1. As well as containing all the patient demographical information, the report is divided into specific sections. A histopathology report is a verified document that contains a diagnosis, which is determined following the examination of cells, tissues and sometimes foreign or infectious agents under the microscope. The microscope may not only be the light microscope but may also include the electron microscope (refer to Chapters 14 and 15), or digitalized images from scanned slides. The histopathology report is a highly informative document. In addition to providing information regarding diagnosis it also contains information on tissue sample size, weight, shape, colour and general overall appearances. All of these parameters are recorded broadly under the section of the report termed 'Gross description' or 'Macroscopic description'. The important point about the macroscopic description is that it provides information regarding clinical appearances to the naked eye of any given sample. In medical science there is often a close correlation between the clinical appearance and suspected diagnosis and the pathological confirmatory findings. We call this a clinicopathological correlation. A good example of where this is often key is in dermatology. There are few medical disciplines in which clinical assessments are based largely on the appearance of a lesion to the naked eye. In other words, dermatology clinically does not rely on sophisticated scanning or endoscopic equipment but rather relies on the expertise of the clinician to assess any given lesion with normal visual assessment (at least for the large part).

The second major section of a report is the information based on the pathologist's microscopic assessment of the cells, tissues, etc., formulated following an evaluation under the microscope. In histopathology this part of the report is often highly interpretive and is often composed of free-flowing descriptive text based on the observations of the material assessed. The text highlights what is seen and then continues to draw the reader to a concluding diagnostic statement. This statement is based on the cumulative evidence of both the clinical and pathological findings.

As well as providing diagnostic information on any given sample, the histopathology report plays an important role in cancer treatment pathways and subsequent patient management. The histopathology report can provide information on a wide range of prognostic indicators. All of these, including mitotic index, evidence of tumour cell invasion into blood and lymphatic vessels, will help to determine the treatment regimes, defined following discussions at MDM or MDT meetings. You have already been introduced to the role of MDMs or MDTs in previous chapters and so this concept should not be new to you.

Key Point

The key information in a histopathology report includes:

- Patient demographics (name, date of birth, biopsy date, hospital number).
- Clinical suspected diagnosis and associated patient history.
- Clinicians signature and authorization.
- Macro or gross description.
- Microscopic description.
- Diagnosis ex tumour type/cancer grade (details on how abnormal the cells appear under the microscope and indicators of how rapidly the tumour is likely to grow or spread).
- Tumour size or depth of invasion (metric measurement) often with prognostic significance.
- Tumour margins: There are three outcomes when whole tumours are removed clinically: A) Positive margins, meaning tumour cells remain at the edge of the tissue removed; B) Negative margins, meaning clear or free tumour margins (i.e. there are no cancer cells found at the outer edges and deep margins of the removed tissue); C) Close margins, this indicates that the cancer cells are very close to the margins of the tissue taken.
- Information pertaining to other investigative tests on additional samples taken; this may constitute a supplementary report encompassing such tests that are molecular in nature (e.g. T-cell gene re-arrangement assessments to confirm clonality and confirm cancer).
- Diagnostic code or SNOMED code.
- Histopathologist's signature and details of affiliations/qualifications.
- Departmental contact information.

Histopathologists produce their reports in a variety of ways, utilizing different technologies. Reports can be typed into the laboratory information management system (LIMS) using word processing software. Some histopathologists use voice-recognition systems that interact directly with the LIMS. Reports can also be dictated for transcription by medical secretaries. As a general rule the initial histopathology report is usually issued within 10 working days after the biopsy or surgery is performed. The Royal College of Pathologists have published Key Performance Indicators that state that 80% of all histology reports should be available in 7 working days and 90% within 10 working days. (https://www.rcpath.org/resourceLibrary/key-performance-indicators-in-pathology---recommendations-from-the-royal-college-of-pathologists-.html)

13.2 **The microscopy content of a histopathology report**

Having defined whether any given sample is cancerous or not, there may be reference to a host of other additional tests performed, which can provide evidence of the proposed diagnosis. These additional tests may be special stains, immunocytochemistry (ICC) or molecular-based tests. All of which will provide additional information which cannot be ascertained from simply viewing conventional H&E stains. The final report should include the findings from these additional tests. ICC and molecular assays can often:

- Determine the cell of origin of any given cancer.
- Distinguish among different cancer types (i.e. carcinoma vs melanoma vs lymphoma).
- Help to delineate certain leukaemias from lymphomas.

In additional to the more conventional ICC and molecular tests that may be performed there are a group of molecular-based assays which are broadly characterized under the heading of cytogenetics/karyotypic or perhaps tissue culture methods. These tests are often associated with genetic mutations or are markers of a specific cancer (e.g. Philadelphia chromosome is associated with chronic myeloid leukaemia [CML]). Some examples of these sorts of tests include:

a) Fluorescence *in situ* hybridization (FISH). This method determines the positions of genes. It is used to determine chromosomal abnormalities and to assist gene mapping exercises.

b) Polymerase chain reaction (PCR). This method is used to increase the number of copies of a particular DNA sequence present in a sample.

c) Real-time PCR or quantitative PCR. This can be used to determine copy numbers of particular DNA sequences.

d) Reverse transcriptase PCR (RT-PCR). This method uses copies of specific RNA sequences, which control protein manufacture within the cell.

e) Southern and Western blot hybridization. In the case of Southern blot hybridization, it provides information on specific DNA fragments. In the case of Western blot hybridization, it can provide information relating to specific proteins or peptides.

You will read more about these assays in the molecular chapters that follow this.

Having considered all these options for investigative tests it is still the case that in certain circumstances a definitive diagnosis may not be achieved. In such instances cases are often referred for a second opinion, or indeed referred to specialist centres of excellence for the final confirmation of diagnosis and subsequent patient management.

For further information regarding referral or second opinions refer to the National Cancer Institute (NCI)-designated cancer centres. These centres are open to patients to request second opinions and will provide information on costs and even shipping instructions to have such cases reviewed.

13.3 Reporting datasets and tissue pathways

Histopathological reports for common cancers are prepared according to guidelines produced by Pathological Colleges and Societies around the world. The standards and datasets for reporting cancers help histopathologists to formulate consistent reports. This approach is used to facilitate communication with clinicians to achieve optimal patient management and to improve audit within the pathology service, allow comparison between cancer services, and optimize data collection by cancer registries. The formulation of datasets has driven the move towards 'proforma style' reports, in which pathological parameters associated with the specimen are listed. These types of report replace the more traditional descriptive reports from which it can be difficult to extract information.

There is no doubt that there has been an increasing complexity imposed on diagnostic outcomes and how patient management is subsequently handled. This is principally due to a much closer correlation that now exists between our understanding of the clinicopathological correlations and the use of an ever-increasing plethora of supporting techniques, whether ICC or molecular based or perhaps both. These techniques have enabled us to be more selective and precise about how we classify tumours. Further still, they provide information that enables us to link prognostic outcomes and patient treatment modalities. In brief it is simply no longer sufficient to just diagnose tissue-based disease, but rather there is a demand to qualify these statements with evidence on prognostic indicators such as tumour grade, lymph node and vascular spread, for example. The ever increasing demands for ensuring consistency and reproducibility of assessment of these factors has encouraged the development of 'standardized cancer datasets'. The goal of these datasets is not just to define what are core and non core factors which are relevant to patient management with any given cancer type, but also to include audit criteria as a means to underpinning quality standards. This approach within the United Kingdom is sponsored by The Royal College of Pathologists (RCPath). The RCPath publishes its cancer and tissue datasets on line (www.rcpath.org/piblications/datasets/datasets-TP.htm).

In the USA the College of American Pathologists produces Cancer Protocols and Checklists (http://cap.org/apps/caps.portal?_nfpb=true&pagelabel-home).

Similarly, The Royal College of Pathologists of Australasia produces Structured Reporting Cancer Protocols (www.rcpa.edu.au/Home.htm).

In an attempt to improve end-to-end diagnostic investigations, the UK RCPath publishes Key Performance Indicators in Pathology (www.rcpath.org/rcpath-consulting).

These indicators are there to provide a process of metric assessments of quality standards. They encompass guidance on timeframes and percentage achievement targets. It is these set of standards that are enabling the introduction of ISO 15189 to evolve and replace CPA (UK) Ltd standards by developing a more holistic patient/outcome-based approach.

From a purely logical perspective formalized report structures will enable pathologists to remember to insert necessary data and audit quality standards. Similarly, transcription and reproducibility of reports are effectively easier to maintain. From the clinician's perspective this standardization of format enables them to extract relevant data with ease and consistency.

From the UK, RCPath (Pathology: the science behind the cure) 'Working group on cancer services decisions about authorship of cancer datasets and tissue pathways':

The cancer datasets and tissue pathways must be written with a view to their applicability and implementation in the NHS but as a professional standard the intention is that they should be used by members of the College working outside the NHS.

Royal College of Pathologists UK – EXAMPLE

Dataset for the histological reporting of primary cutaneous basal cell carcinoma

Surname.......................Forenames....................Date of birth...............Sex.......

Hospital.......................Hospital no....................NHS/CHI no...............

Date of receipt................Date of reporting.............Report no....................

Pathologist....................Surgeon...........................

Clinical data

Clinical site: Forehead

Specimen type: Excisional biopsy

Macroscopic description

Size of specimen: Length 20 mm Breadth 12 mm Depth 7 mm

Maximum diameter of lesion: 9 mm

Histological data

Low-risk subtype: Nodular

Or high-risk if present: N/A

Level of invasion*: Dermis

Perineural invasion*: Not identified

Lymphovascular invasion (basosquamous carcinoma only): N/A

Margins:

Not involved (1–5 mm): Peripheral 4 mm Deep 3 mm

Maximum diameter (macroscopic and/or microscopic): <10 mm

TNM pathological (p) stage (AJCC7) pT1

Pathological risk status for clinical management: BCC and stage Low   Margins Low

SNOMED codes T02000 M80903

COMMENTS: none

Pathologist........................... Date.......................

Two main pathology categories that may be reported are:

- Inflammation
- Cancer.

We will now consider the key features of these two distinctive pathological processes.

SELF-CHECK 13.2

What is the purpose of datasets in histopathology reporting?

13.4 Inflammation

Inflammation is the protective response to foreign agents such as microorganisms and facilitates the repair of damaged tissue (Table 13.1). Following minor injury, inflammation is transient and is followed by resolution (i.e. the affected tissue/organ returns to its normal state). However, in some instances the inflammatory response can have harmful effects on the tissue/organ and causes the signs and symptoms of disease.

TABLE 13.1 Common causes of inflammation.

Microorganisms	Bacteria
	Viruses
	Fungi
	Parasites
Physical agents	Mechanical trauma
	Extremes of temperature
	Chemicals
	Radiation (ultraviolet light, radiotherapy)

Inflammation is a complex reaction orchestrated by chemical mediators secreted by a variety of different cells. Initially, there are changes in blood vessels—transient contraction and then prolonged dilatation is followed by the vessels becoming 'leaky'. These events slow the flow of blood and protein-rich fluid escapes from the vessel into the area of damaged tissue. White blood cells (leucocytes) stick to the walls of capillaries and leave the vasculature, migrating to the area of tissue damage. The protein-rich fluid containing leucocytes is called the inflammatory exudate. Inflammation is classified into acute and chronic types.

Acute inflammation is usually of relatively short duration, lasting up to a few days, and is characterized by the accumulation of neutrophils (the principal acute inflammatory cell; see Table 13.2 for other types). Sometimes acute inflammation leads to the formation of pus, which essentially comprises tissue fluid, dead neutrophils and microorganisms. The formation of pus is called suppuration.

TABLE 13.2 Types of inflammatory cells.

Cell type	Nucleus	Cytoplasm	Frequency (% of WBC in blood)	Image
Neutrophil	Segmented, several lobes connected by a fine strand of chromatin	Stains pink with many fine, neutrophilic granules	40–70%	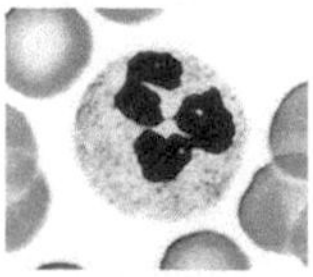 **FIGURE 13.1** (H&E × 1000)
Monocyte	Largest of WBC, unilobar, bean-shaped/notched	Agranular	2–10%	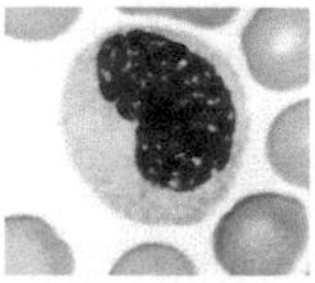 **FIGURE 13.2** (H&E × 1000)
Lymphocyte	Dark purple, compact, rounded nucleus, high nuclear to cytoplasmic ratio	Light blue, agranular	20–45%	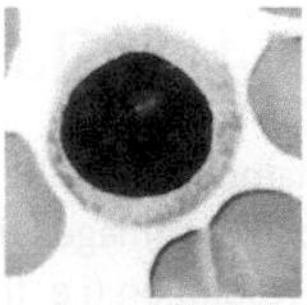 **FIGURE 13.3** (H&E × 1000)

Cell type	Nucleus	Cytoplasm	Frequency (% of WBC in blood)	Image
Plasma cell	Rounded, eccentric, high nuclear to cytoplasmic ratio, heterochromic with 'clock face' appearance	Basophilic, distinct clear perinuclear region of the cytoplasm containing Golgi bodies	Rare	FIGURE 13.4 (Giemsa × 1000)
Eosinophil	Bi-lobed	Numerous large, bright-orange/red granules	1–4%	FIGURE 13.5 (H&E × 1000)
Basophil	Usually two-lobed	Large purple or purplish-black granules that often obscure the nucleus	<1%	FIGURE 13.6 (H&E × 1000)
Mast cell	Rounded, single, low nuclear to cytoplasmic ratio normally	Numerous even-sized granules present that stain with toluidine blue	<1%	FIGURE 13.7 (Giemsa × 600)
Macrophage (produced by differentiation of monocytes)	Rounded or oval, can be multinucleated, low nuclear to cytoplasmic ratio	Large amount of cytoplasm, often contains phagocytosed debris	N/A	FIGURE 13.8 (Giemsa × 1000)

Chronic inflammation is of longer duration and is defined by the accumulation of specialized immune cells such as B and T lymphocytes, plasma cells that secrete immunoglobulin, and macrophages. It occurs due to persistent infections (which can cause delayed hypersensitivity and/or granulomatous inflammatory reaction), prolonged exposure to toxins and autoimmunity. Following removal of the cause of inflammation the body repairs the damaged tissue. The process of repair involves the growth of many new blood vessels and the deposition of fibrous repair tissue, and is termed granulation tissue. Sometimes an excessive amount of fibrous tissue is laid down and this leads to fibrosis, which can impair the function of the tissue/organ.

The clinical signs of inflammation (the cardinal signs) are redness, heat, swelling, pain and loss of function. Redness is caused by increased blood flow to the inflamed tissue. In skin, the increased blood flow warms the skin surface. In addition, inflammatory mediators cause an increase in body temperature (pyrexia). The development of swelling occurs as a result of the accumulation of tissue fluid (oedema). The inflammatory response produces symptoms of pain because there is distortion

TABLE 13.3 Inflammatory processes.

Organ/tissue	Tissues	Inflammation
Brain	Meninges	Meningitis
Mouth	Gum (gingiva)	Gingivitis
	Tonsil	Tonsillitis
Gastrointestinal tract	Oesophagus	Oesophagitis
	Stomach	Gastritis
	Appendix	Appendicitis
	Colon	Colitis
Lung	Bronchi	Bronchitis
	Lung	Pneumonitis (pneumonia)
Breast	Breast	Mastitis
Liver	Liver	Hepatitis
Bladder	Bladder mucosa	Cystitis
Skin	Dermis	Dermatitis
Musculoskeletal system	Tendon	Tendonitis
	Joints	Arthritis

and stretching of the tissues, and inflammatory mediators sensitize pain receptors in the affected tissue. Loss of function is caused by the increasing pain and swelling.

In general, the terms used to describe inflammation affecting different organs and tissues are formulated by adding the suffix 'itis' (see Table 13.3).

CLINICAL CORRELATION

Dermatitis herpetiformis (DH) is an autoimmune blistering disease first described as a clinical entity in 1884 by the American dermatologist Louis Duhring. The name is descriptive in that dermatitis is inflammation of the skin and herpetiformis indicates the group. The lesions are generally small, itchy blisters, often with red plaques, found generally on flexor surfaces such as elbows and knees but also forearms and buttocks. The affected skin is often terribly itchy and blisters will burst on scratching. It commonly affects patients between the ages of 30 and 60 years. The male:female incidence is 3:2. It is rare and within the UK affects approximately one in 15,000. Following this finding, the patient is referred to a gastroenterologist who will test for coeliac disease using antibody blood tests and a confirmatory intestinal biopsy.

CASE STUDY 13.1 Dermatitis herpetiformis

A 38-year-old man presents with a red rash with raised vesicles and blisters on both elbows. The rash itches and the blisters burst when scratched. The man has known coeliac disease for the past 5 years.

A biopsy was taken both of lesional and perilesional skin encompassing a blister and surrounding clinically unblistered skin. The H&E showed subepidermal blister formation with papillary dermal separation (Figure 13.9) with evidence of abundant neutrophil and occasional eosinophils invading the blister area (Figure 13.10). Following direct immunofluorescence assessment of the perilesional skin tissue, granular deposition of IgA within the dermal papillae was seen (Figure 13.11).

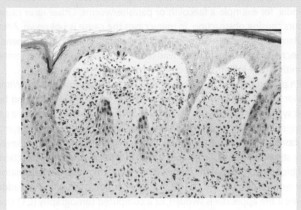

FIGURE 13.9
Subepidermal blister formation (H&E, original magnification ×20).

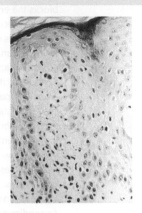

FIGURE 13.10
Abundant neutrophils and occasional eosinophils invading the blister area (H&E, original magnification ×75).

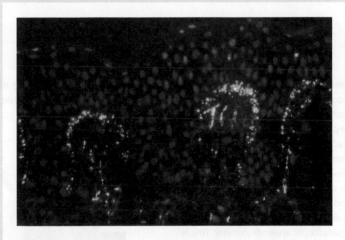

FIGURE 13.11
Granular deposition of IgA within the dermal papillae (indirect immunofluorescence, original magnification ×40).

CLINICAL CORRELATION

Appendicitis is a common condition with approximately 50,000 people admitted to hospital with appendicitis each year in the UK; around one in every 13 people develop it at some point in their life. It can develop at any age, but it is most common in younger people (10 to 20 years old). The appendix is a tubular structure extending from the caecum with no known specific function. It has a lumen which is continuous with that of the caecum, together with (from internal to external aspect); glandular mucosa, muscularis mucosa, submucosa, muscularis propria, subserosa and serosa/peritoneum. Humans can live without an appendix with no consequences.

Appendicitis is inflammation of the appendix. Most cases are thought to occur when something blocks the entrance of the appendix, for example a faecolith or parasite/worms. Other rarer causes include mucosal polyps or tumours causing obstruction. In many cases the cause is unknown. Acute appendicitis consists of acute inflammatory cells (neutrophils) throughout all layers of the appendix wall. This can cause swelling and increased pressure that can lead to the appendix bursting (perforated appendix), and associated peritonitis (acute inflammation of the serosal/peritoneal surface).

Appendicitis typically starts with pain in the middle of the abdomen that may come and go. Within hours, the pain travels to the lower right-hand side, where the appendix is usually located, and becomes constant and severe. Other symptoms include nausea, vomiting, loss of appetite, diarrhoea and pyrexia. It should be noted that appendicitis can be difficult to diagnose unless there are typical symptoms (present in about half of all cases). Pain similar to appendicitis can occur in gastroenteritis, severe irritable bowel syndrome (IBS), constipation, ectopic pregnancy, and in bladder or urine tract infections.

Further tests may involve a full blood count to see the white cell count or to measure inflammatory cell markers, a pregnancy test for women, a urine test to rule out other conditions such as a bladder infection, an ultrasound scan to see if the appendix is swollen, or a computed tomography (CT) scan. Appendicectomy is performed if appendicitis is suspected, due to the risk of perforation and peritonitis, which could cause life-threatening sepsis. This means that some people will have their appendix removed even though it's eventually found to be normal. The procedure is normally performed laparoscopically (keyhole surgery). Open surgery may be necessary when the appendix has already burst or in people who have previously had open abdominal surgery, but this is rare.

CASE STUDY 13.2 *Appendicitis*

A 21-year-old female presented to the emergency department with right lower quadrant abdominal pain, nausea and vomiting of four hours' duration. She has no other symptoms or significant medical history. On examination she has tenderness in the right lower quadrant and is pyrexial. Blood tests show a raised white cell count and raised inflammatory markers. Pregnancy test is negative and urine test normal. An ultrasound scan shows a slightly dilated appendix but is otherwise normal. Her case is discussed with the surgical team and acute appendicitis is the working diagnosis. She is prepared for theatre and consented for a laparoscopic appendicectomy. This is performed later the same day. At operation the appendix looks inflamed with yellowish discoloration of the surface in keeping with localized peritonitis. The appendix is removed and sent for histological examination. The appendix is examined and described macroscopically and dissected. It appears inflamed with a purulent exudate on the surface and swelling of the tip (Figure 13.12). No definite perforation is seen. Examination of the cut surfaces shows no features of neoplasia. A faecolith is present in the lumen towards the proximal part of the specimen. Sections include: tip, resection margin and cross-section (Figure 13.13). The blocks are processed routinely. The H&E slides show appendix wall with severe acute inflammation (Figure 13.14). There are numerous neutrophils seen throughout all layers of the appendix wall together with chronic inflammatory cells including lymphocytes, plasma cells and eosinophils. There is acute peritonitis. There is no evidence of parasites/worms or neoplasia.

The patient goes home two days after surgery and recovers well with no complications. She is seen in clinic four weeks later, histology is reviewed and discussed. No further treatment is required and she is discharged.

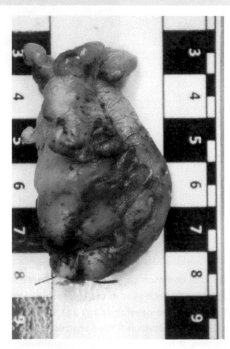

FIGURE 13.12
External appearance of appendix with purulent exudate.

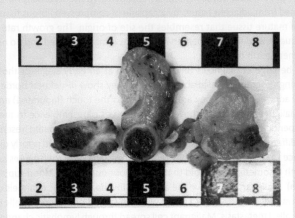

FIGURE 13.13
Cut surface of appendix. These sections are blocked (resection margin, cross-section, and tip from left to right).

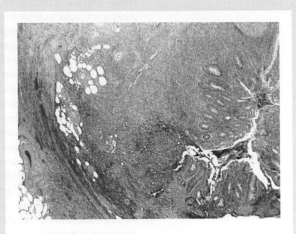

FIGURE 13.14
Appendix with surface ulceration and acute inflammation through all layers of the wall (H&E, original magnification ×100).

SELF-CHECK 13.3

What are the key clinical findings of inflammation?

13.5 Neoplasia

Neoplasia means new growth (Greek: *neo* new, *plassein* to form). A neoplasm has an inherent ability to grow and continues to enlarge unless it is treated. The term tumour is sometimes used instead of neoplasm, but the literal meaning of tumour is swelling. Neoplasms are classified into benign and malignant types depending on their clinical presentation, histological appearance and biological behaviour (see Table 13.4). A general term used for a malignant neoplasm is cancer, a word that is often associated with pain, suffering and death.

TABLE 13.4 Typical features of benign and malignant neoplasms.

	Benign	Malignant
Size	Small	Large
Borders	Well defined	Ill defined
Differentiation	Resembles tissue of origin	Variable
Growth rate	Slow	Rapid
Mitotic figures	Rare	Common
Necrosis	No	Yes
Invasion	No	Yes
Metastasis	No	Yes

Benign neoplasms tend to be small, but large benign neoplasms can occasionally develop because they do not cause symptoms or the patient does not seek medical help. Benign tumours usually have a well-defined edge and are separated from adjacent tissues by a capsule of compressed fibrous tissue. Benign tumours are composed of mature tissue that resembles the site of origin. The growth rate is slow and mitotic figures are infrequent. By definition, benign neoplasms remain localized and do not spread to form new growths at other sites in the body.

Malignant neoplasms tend to be large at diagnosis unless identified at an early stage, or those detected within the many screening programmes available. Typically, they show ill-defined borders because they invade and destroy adjacent tissue. They are often hard to the touch (indurated) and stuck down to adjacent tissues. Malignant neoplasms show varying degrees of resemblance to their tissue of origin and are graded depending on degree of differentiation (i.e. well differentiated [resembles tissue of origin], moderately differentiated [some resemblance to tissue of origin], and poorly differentiated [little or no resemblance to tissue of origin]). They tend to grow rapidly, mitotic figures are usually easily identified and growth is sometimes so rapid that the tumour outstrips its blood supply, leading to necrosis (tumour death). Malignant cells have the ability to invade lymphatic channels or blood vessels, termed 'vascular invasion', and this is associated with the spread of malignant cells to other parts of the body, a process called metastasis. Malignant cell spread through lymphatic channels usually results in the development of lymph node metastases, whereas spread through blood vessels results in metastases to distant organs (e.g. lung, liver, brain and bone).

Neoplasms are classified according to their behaviour and the tissue that they most resemble (histogenesis). All neoplasms share the common suffix 'oma'. Benign epithelial neoplasms can be papillomas (originating from surface epithelium) or adenomas (originating from glandular epithelium). In the case of benign mesenchymal neoplasms, a prefix is used to denote histogenesis; for example, a benign neoplasm of fibrous tissue is called a fibroma. Malignant epithelial neoplasms are termed carcinomas and malignant mesenchymal neoplasms are sarcomas (Table 13.5). However, there are a couple of exceptions where the name suggests a benign tumour but the disease is malignant. Melanomas are highly aggressive malignant skin tumours and lymphomas are malignant neoplasms of the haematopoietic system. For details of the basic neoplastic/malignant cell types see Table 13.6.

It is estimated that one person in three will develop cancer and many die as a consequence of their disease. The vast majority of cancers are diagnosed in elderly patients. Cancers occur in children but they are uncommon. There are over 200 different types of cancer. In the UK the most common cancers are those of breast, lung, colon and prostate. These four cancers account for over half of all new cases each year (breast 15%, lung 13%, bowel 13%, prostate 12%; Cancer Research UK, 2007; http://info.cancerresearchuk.org).

SELF-CHECK 13.4

What are the main benign and malignant types of tumour seen in histopathology?

TABLE 13.5 Classification of benign and malignant neoplasms.

	Benign	Malignant
Epithelial		
Squamous	Squamous cell papilloma	Squamous cell carcinoma
Transitional	Transitional cell papilloma	Transitional cell carcinoma
Glandular	Adenoma	Adenocarcinoma
Mesenchymal		
Fibrous tissue	Fibroma	Fibrosarcoma
Adipose tissue	Lipoma	Liposarcoma
Blood vessels	Haemangioma	Angiosarcoma
Cartilage	Chondroma	Chondrosarcoma
Bone	Osteoma	Osteosarcoma

TABLE 13.6 Basic types of neoplastic/malignant cells.

Cell type	Nuclear features	Cytoplasmic features	Neoplastic conditions	Images
Squamous	Variable, spindle or epithelioid	Variable volume, usually eosinophilic, can be clear, +/– keratinization, intracellular bridges	Squamous cell carcinoma	FIGURE 13.15 (H&E × 200)
Glandular	Variable, rounded, can be very irregular or signet ring cell if poorly differentiated	Variable volume, mucin containing (DPAS positive), can be clear	Adenocar-cinoma	FIGURE 13.16 (H&E × 100)
Melanocytes	Variable, spindle or epithelioid, inclusions, large nucleoli	Often plentiful, eosinophilic +/- melanin (brown) pigment	Melanoma	FIGURE 13.17 (H&E × 200)
Soft tissue cells (variable—fibroblasts, adipocytes, muscle, endothelial)	Variable, most commonly spindle cells, can be epithelioid	Variable, indistinct, eosinophilic, clear cell	Sarcoma	FIGURE 13.18 (H&E × 100)
Haemato-lymphoid cells	Variable from small rounded nuclei to large blasts and Reed–Sternberg (RS) multinucleated cells (arrows in Figure 13.19), heterochromatic	Commonly small volume, in RS cells can be more abundant and clear	Lymphoma (Hodgkin's and non-Hodgkin's), leukaemia (acute and chronic)	FIGURE 13.19 (H&E × 600)

CLINICAL CORRELATION

Malignant melanoma is a highly aggressive and invasive form of skin cancer that can develop from existing moles, although more commonly it arises spontaneously. There are seven common clinical signs of malignant melanoma when assessing moles, including increasing size, changing shape (particularly developing an irregular outline), changing colour (lesions mainly appear to get darker and have uneven pigmentation), loss of symmetry, itching and/or bleeding, and a surrounding inflammatory response. Diagnosis is confirmed with an excision biopsy of the lesion and histopathological evaluation. There are four main types of melanoma: superficial spreading malignant melanoma, nodular malignant melanoma, lentigo maligna melanoma and acral lentiginous melanoma. The most aggressive and invasive form is nodular melanoma as this has no radial growth phase and moves swiftly to a vertical growth phase, invading the tissue both above and below the lesion.

CASE STUDY 13.3 *Malignant melanoma*

An 89-year-old male had focal nodules on his central back. Clinically, the man was well but the suspected diagnosis was a metastatic tumour deposit from an unknown primary.

The H&E revealed a malignant dermal deposit of cells with no involvement of the epidermis (Figure 13.20). On high-power examination of the H&E the cells show pronounced cellular atypia. The nuclei appear to be highly hyperchromatic with prominent nucleoli and evidence of mitoses (Figure 13.21). The deposit was thought to be metastatic in nature and a panel of immunocytochemical markers for carcinoma and melanoma was applied. Cytokeratin stains were negative, but staining for S100 (Figure 13.22), Melan A, tyrosinase, and focally for HMB45 (Figure 13.23) were positive, confirming a diagnosis of metastatic malignant melanoma.

The patient was referred for additional screening and scanning to investigation the source of the primary malignant melanoma lesion.

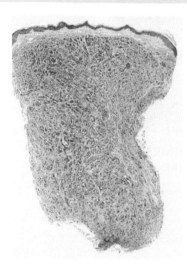

FIGURE 13.20
Malignant dermal deposit of cells with no involvement of the epidermis (H&E, original magnification × 10).

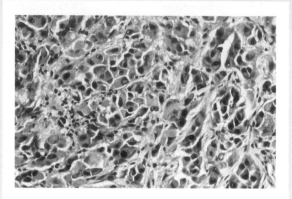

FIGURE 13.21
Nuclei appear to be highly hyperchromatic with prominent nucleoli and evidence of mitoses (H&E, original magnification × 75).

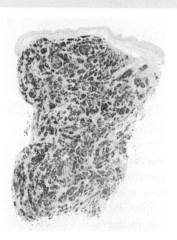

FIGURE 13.22
Staining for S100 (original magnification × 20).

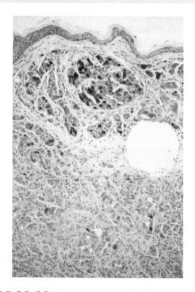

FIGURE 13.23
Focal staining for HMB45 (original magnification × 75).

Breast cancer is the most common cancer in women worldwide, with approximately 1.7 million new cases per year. Survival rates vary from 80% in North America to 40% in low-income countries. The difference in survival is due to the lack of early detection programmes in low income countries resulting in late-stage presentation.

Risk factors include prolonged exposure to endogenous oestrogens (early menarche, late menopause, late age at first childbirth, and oral contraceptive/hormone replacement therapy use), excess alcohol, obesity, and physical inactivity. Breastfeeding has a protective effect. A familial history of breast cancer increases the risk by a factor of two or three. Some mutations, particularly in *BRCA1*, *BRCA2* and *p53*, result in a very high risk for breast cancer. However, these mutations are rare and account for a small portion of the total breast cancer burden.

Breast cancer control involves prevention (promoting a healthy diet, physical activity and control of alcohol intake, avoiding overweight and obesity), early detection (awareness of early signs and symptoms, availability of screening programmes), early treatment, rehabilitation and palliative care.

The most common sign of breast cancer is a lump in the breast. Diagnosis is by triple assessment including physical examination, radiological imaging (mammogram, ultrasound scan +/– MRI scan) and pathology. Pathology is ideally a core biopsy from the lump, providing tissue to allow classification and grading of the carcinoma and the performance of biological studies including oestrogen (ER) and progesterone (PR) receptor ICC and HER2 ICC +/– *in situ* hybridization, which will aid treatment decision making (ER-positive patients will respond to hormone therapies such as tamoxifen and HER2-positive patients can be treated with trastuzumab/Herceptin). Depending on several factors (size of lesion, number of lesions, genetics, breast size, previous radiotherapy to chest wall, and patient choice), the cancer will be excised by wide local excision (WLE) or mastectomy. The aim of both operations is to excise the carcinoma completely and allow for further grading and staging.

Breast cancer can spread to axillary lymph nodes and it is important that these are assessed and treated appropriately to reduce recurrence/systemic spread, but also to minimize overtreatment and side-effects (e.g. lymphoedema of the arm). When a patient is diagnosed with breast cancer the axilla will be examined by palpation and ultrasound looking for any abnormal lymph nodes (enlarged, hard in feel). Fine-needle aspiration, core biopsy, frozen section, PCR, sentinel lymph node (SLN) excision and axillary node sampling are modalities that can be used to assess axillary lymph nodes. If metastases greater than 2 mm are found an axillary node clearance is normally performed.

Additional non-surgical treatments include hormonal therapy, chemotherapy and radiotherapy.

CASE STUDY 13.4 Breast carcinoma

A 64-year-old female presents to clinic with a two-week history of a lump in the right breast. She has no past family history of breast cancer and is otherwise fit and well with no significant past medical history. She has had one screening mammogram five years ago but has not attended screening since. On examination there is a hard, slightly irregular, but mobile lump in the upper outer quadrant of the right breast that is clinically suspicious of cancer. The nipple appears normal. Mammogram and ultrasound show a 14 mm speculate mass consistent with a carcinoma. The axilla appears normal on palpation and ultrasound. A core biopsy is performed under ultrasound guidance and sent to the histology laboratory where it is processed urgently. H&E shows breast tissue infiltrated by sheets of cohesive cells with high nuclear to cytoplasmic ratios, irregular nuclear outlines, vesicular chromatin, prominent nucleoli and easily identifiable mitoses. This is reported as an invasive ductal carcinoma, no specified type,

grade 3. ER and PR are positive and HER2-negative. The case is discussed at the MDT/MDM and a WLE with SLN is planned. This is performed and the specimens are sent for histological assessment. The WLE and SLN are described macroscopically, dissected and appropriate blocks taken. The H&E sections show a 13 mm invasive ductal carcinoma, no specified type, grade 3 (Figure 13.24).

There is no associated DCIS and no lymphovascular invasion. The carcinoma is greater than 5 mm from all resection margins. The SLN is negative for malignancy. A cancer dataset is completed and the report authorized. The patient is again discussed in the MDT/MDM. She has recovered well, went home one day after the operation, and the wound is healing adequately. After reading of the histology report the MDT/MDM felt that post-operative management should include endocrine treatment (as the tumour was ER positive) and radiotherapy (as a WLE was performed). No further surgery is

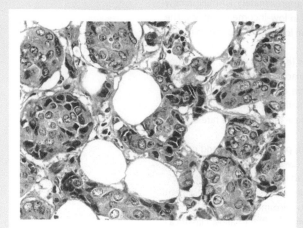

FIGURE 13.24

Invasive ductal carcinoma (grade 3), with no tubule formation, a high degree of pleomorphism and mitoses identified (H&E, original magnification ×400).

necessary. This will be discussed with the patient in clinic and follow up for five years was planned.

CAP dataset:

Surgical Pathology Cancer Case Summary (CAP guidelines)

Protocol web posting date: January 2016

INVASIVE CARCINOMA OF THE BREAST: Complete excision (less than total mastectomy, including specimens designated biopsy, lumpectomy, quadrantectomy, and partial mastectomy with or without axillary contents) and mastectomy (total, with or without axillary contents; modified radical; radical)

Specimen Identification

___ Excision with image-guided localization

Lymph Node Sampling

___ Sentinel lymph node(s)

Specimen Laterality

___ Right

+ **Tumour Site: Invasive Carcinoma**

+ ___ Upper outer quadrant

Tumour Size: Size of Largest Invasive Carcinoma

Greatest dimension of largest focus of invasion >1 mm: 13 mm

Histologic Type

___ Invasive mammary carcinoma of no special type (ductal, not otherwise specified)

Histologic Grade (Nottingham Histologic Score)

Glandular (Acinar)/Tubular Differentiation

___ Score 3 (<10% of tumour area forming glandular/tubular structures)

Nuclear Pleomorphism

___ Score 3 (vesicular nuclei, often with prominent nucleoli, exhibiting marked variation in size and shape, occasionally with very large and bizarre forms)

Mitotic Rate

___ Score 2 (4–7 mitoses per mm^2)

+ Number of mitoses per 10 high-power fields: 11

+ Diameter of microscope field: 0.5 mm

Overall Grade

___ Grade 3 (scores of 8 or 9)

Tumour Focality

___ Single focus of invasive carcinoma

Ductal Carcinoma In Situ (DCIS) (select all that apply)

___ No DCIS is present

Margins (select all that apply)

Invasive Carcinoma

___ Margins uninvolved by invasive carcinoma

Distance from closest margin: 6 mm

Specify margin: Lateral

Lymph Nodes (required only if lymph nodes are present in the specimen)

Total number of lymph nodes examined (sentinel and non-sentinel): 1

Number of sentinel lymph nodes examined: 1

Number of lymph nodes involved: 0

+ Method of Evaluation of Sentinel Lymph Nodes (select all that apply)

+ ___ Haematoxylin-and-eosin (H&E), 1 level

+ **Treatment Effect: Response to Presurgical (Neoadjuvant) Therapy (select all that apply)**

+ In the Breast

+ ___ No known presurgical therapy

+ In the Lymph Nodes

+ ___ No known presurgical therapy

+ **Lymph-Vascular Invasion**

+ ___ Not identified

+ Dermal Lymph-Vascular Invasion

+ ___ No skin present

Pathologic Staging (based on information available to the pathologist) (pTNM) (Note M)

Primary Tumour (Invasive Carcinoma) (pT)

pT1c: Tumour > 10 mm but ≤ 20 mm in greatest dimension

Regional Lymph Nodes (pN) (choose a category based on lymph nodes received with the specimen; immunocytochemistry and/or molecular studies are not required)

Category (pN)

___ pN0(sn): No regional lymph node metastasis identified histologically

+ **Additional Pathologic Findings**

+ Specify: N/A

Ancillary Studies

+ **Microcalcifications (select all that apply)**

+ ___ Not identified

+ **Clinical History (select all that apply) (Note P)**

+ The current clinical/radiologic breast findings for which this surgery is performed include:

+ ___ Palpable mass

+ **Comment(s): none**

13.6 Research and development in histopathology: how does it improve diagnosis?

You will have read about clinical trials in Chapter 1. Here we discuss the importance of the histopathology report to this process.

The NCI is part of the National Institutes of Health and it sponsors clinical trials. The goal of the majority of these trials is to attempt to improve the accuracy and specificity of cancer diagnosis. Clinical trials are vital to improve our understanding of how to improve cancer diagnosis and patient treatment pathways. Any new method or technique that is recommended for general use within a diagnostic setting must have gone through a stringent process of clinical trials and clinical audits to determine whether it is safe to use and also that it is effective and brings improvement to the overall process to histopathological diagnosis.

In order to find cases that are applicable for a given clinical-based trial the histopathology report is the fundamentally most important document to source appropriate patients to review for any proposed trials.

13.7 Extended roles for biomedical and clinical scientists in histopathology

The UK's Institute of Biomedical Science (IBMS) has been working with the RCPath to develop new examination pathways for biomedical and clinical scientists. These currently entail the development of Diplomas of Expert Practice and Advanced Specialist Diplomas in selected areas of histopathology. These examinations are not unique to the UK and are being adopted in different forms internationally. They indicate the changing needs of pathology training and education and of reporting, and offer opportunities in extended roles for biomedical and clinical scientists.

13.7.1 Diploma of Expert Practice (DEP) in Histological Dissection

This is one of the most popular qualifications offered by the IBMS and is run by a Conjoint Board comprising members of The Royal College of Pathologists (RCPath) and IBMS. The DEP in Histological Dissection provides evidence of the attainment of both the necessary scientific and clinical knowledge underpinning the practice of dissection of specimens from categories B & C, with the practical competence required to accurately dissect specimens from these categories within the modules studied. The qualification has five mandatory and eleven optional units.

The mandatory units are:

- Clinical Governance
- General Principles of Dissection
- Surgical Procedures
- Pathological Processes
- Anatomical Nomenclature.

The optional units are:

- Endocrine
- Skin
- Breast
- Osteoarticular and Soft Tissues
- Cardiothoracic
- Gastrointestinal and Hepatobiliary
- Gynaecological
- Genitourinary

- Haemopoietic
- Neuromuscular
- Head and Neck.

In order to undertake the qualification, candidates must be HCPC-registered, be a Member (MIBMS) or Fellow (FIBMS) of the IBMS and have five years' post-registration experience in histopathology. The qualification is assessed through the completion of a portfolio and two written examinations. In the portfolio candidates are required to demonstrate at least two years of current practical experience in the dissection of histological specimens and to provide evidence of case studies, case reviews, audits, training sessions attended and reflection on the learning process. There are two two-hour written examinations. The first examination covers the mandatory units with the second examination covering the optional units.

13.7.2 Diploma of Expert Practice in Mohs Histological Procedures

This is a new qualification that aims to enable successful candidates to undertake a role that involves the evaluation and appropriate tissue handling and processing of Mohs samples, to offer expert professional advice and to participate in the training of biomedical scientists and specialist trainee medical staff in Mohs histological procedures.

The mandatory units are:

- Clinical Governance
- General Principles of Mohs Histological Procedures
- Mohs Tissue Specimens
- Quality Control
- Microscopic Recognition.

The optional unit is:

- Slow Mohs and Immunocytochemistry Procedures.

This examination consists of one written paper, which lasts 120 minutes and covers the five mandatory modules (one question per module), with candidates being expected to answer all questions.

13.7.3 Higher Specialist Diploma

The Higher Specialist Diploma (HSD) is a qualification for biomedical scientists wishing to gain knowledge, skills and competence at a higher level and is designed to be an M-Level qualification.

Those who want to undertake the HSD should be biomedical science practitioners, who have developed skills and theoretical knowledge to a very high standard and are performing an in-depth, highly complex role, and are continually developing clinical, scientific or technical practice and/or have management responsibilities for a section/small department, or be largely involved in research and development.

It requires the completion of a portfolio of experiential learning which needs to include a personal professional profile, evidence of CPD activities undertaken, two essays, two case studies, evidence of a presentation given by the candidate, and reflection on the whole learning process. Once candidates have passed the portfolio they must undertake the examination stage, which involves four papers (Paper 1: Short-answer questions, Paper 2: Generic questions, Paper 3: Discipline-specific questions, Paper 4: Case studies).

13.7.4 Advanced Specialist Diploma (ASD) in Specimen Dissection (Breast and Lower GI)

These qualifications are also run by a Conjoint Board comprising members of the RCPath and IBMS. They aim to enable successful candidates to undertake a role that involves the description, dissection and block sampling of all breast/lower GI pathology specimens, to offer expert professional advice on breast/lower GI pathology dissection and to participate in the training of biomedical scientists and junior medical staff in breast pathology specimen dissection.

The qualification is assessed through the completion of a portfolio, one written examination and a viva voce examination. In the portfolio, candidates are required to demonstrate at least two years of current practical experience in the dissection of histological specimens and to provide evidence of case studies, case reviews, audits, training sessions attended, and reflection on the learning process.

13.7.5 Histopathology Dissection and Reporting (Gastrointestinal Tract and Gynaecological Tract Pathology)

These qualifications aim to provide evidence of the attainment of the necessary scientific and clinical knowledge underpinning the dissection and reporting of gastrointestinal tract/gynaecological pathology specimens.

This is a three-year qualification with candidates expected in each year to submit a portfolio that demonstrates at least 750–1000 reported cases, case reviews, an audit, a case study, MDT meetings attended, multi-source feedback forms and at least 18 work-based assessments (case-based discussion [CbD], direct observation of practical skills [DOPS] and evaluation of clinical events [ECE]).

The examination at the end of Year 1 lasts three hours and is similar to the Year 1 Objective Structured Practical Examination (OSPE) the medical trainees sit, with the overall level designed to recognize scientists close to the end of training, such that they demonstrate an appropriate approach to independent practice.

There are two examinations at end of Year 3. The first, on surgical histopathology, involves a mixture of neoplastic and non-neoplastic material. They will vary in difficulty, from the straightforward to more complex cases requiring more detailed description, differential diagnosis and special techniques, and cases not capable of diagnosis on a single H&E, which should prompt an approach for further techniques, extra blocks and specialist opinions.

The second examination will include four cases in the form of macro-photographs of pathology specimens where candidates will be provided with clinical information and will be asked to prepare their responses to specific questions and to mark on the photographs where they would take blocks.

The second examination will also involve two OSPEs, one of which is conducted face-to-face with two examiners, while the other is a written exercise only. Finally, the examination will include four 20-minute stations that will include long cases that cannot be covered by a single H&E-stained section and either will include more than one H&E slide (e.g. surgical resection) or additional stains (histochemistry or immunocytochemistry).

13.8 Histopathology scientific qualifications in Australia and New Zealand

13.8.1 Australia

In Australia, medical laboratory science comprises the typical distinct professional disciplines, including Anatomical Pathology.

The primary qualification for Medical Laboratory Scientists is a three- or four-year degree in medical laboratory science/laboratory medicine, which is accredited by the Australian Institute of Medical Scientists (AIMS). In the final year of these degree programmes, most students specialize in one or more medical science disciplines. Graduates of these degrees are classified as Medical Laboratory Scientists and are then eligible for professional membership of AIMS.

Fellow

(FAIMS): A Member who has passed the Fellowship Examination according to the guidelines approved by AIMS. The Fellowship is recognized by the Department of Health and Ageing for meeting the requirements for supervision both of large and small multidisciplinary or general laboratories providing comprehensive services (i.e. categories GX and GY). Qualification for Fellowship is by examination in any one of the main pathology disciplines, including in Anatomical Pathology/Histopathology.

Enrolment into the Fellowship programme is open to applicants who have been full Members of AIMS for at least two years and who meet certain other criteria. The Fellowship Programme involves four stages and each stage must be successfully completed before progressing to the next stage.

Member

(MAIMS): A graduate member who has a minimum of two years' postgraduate medical laboratory experience, or member who has passed the AIMS Professional Examination or AIMS Membership Examination, or an applicant with qualifications accepted by AIMS. The AIMS Professional Examination has five sections (Clinical Chemistry, Microbiology, Histopathology/Cytology, Blood Transfusion and Haematology). Upon successful completion of the AIMS Professional Examination, applicants may be eligible for the skilled occupation of Medical Laboratory Scientist and for Professional Membership of AIMS.

Graduate

A member who has completed an AIMS-accredited medical laboratory science degree.

There appears to be no specific examination that is exactly the same as the DEP in Histological Dissection, although the Anatomical Pathology/Histopathology Fellowship examination has some overlap (see a past paper from the examination: www.aims.org.au/documents/item/508).

13.8.2 New Zealand

The New Zealand Institute of Medical Laboratory Science (NZIMLS, www.nzimls.org.nz)is the organization that represents those engaged in the profession of Medical Laboratory Science in New Zealand. Its role is to promote professional excellence through communication, education and a code of ethics to achieve the best laboratory service for the benefit of the patient.

A degree in Medical Laboratory Science (MLS) in New Zealand allows individuals to work as a scientist in diagnostic pathology in NZ and other parts of the world. A Bachelor of Medical Laboratory Science (BMLSc) degree is required for individuals to work as a Medical Laboratory Scientist in a human diagnostic pathology laboratory in New Zealand. It prepares individuals for registration as an MLS with the Medical Sciences Council of New Zealand and allows the individual concerned to hold an Annual Practising Certificate (APC). The vocational pathway to becoming a medical laboratory scientist in NZ (and most other parts of the world) requires students to complete a Bachelor degree in MLSc followed by a minimum period of six months' internship of supervised practice.

Histological Dissection

The NZILMS has developed a memorandum of Understanding (MoU) with the IBMS for its members to access the DEP in Histological Dissection (www.nzimls.org.nz/ibms.html).

The agreed eligibility criteria are:

- Be a Member of the Institute of Biomedical Science. Application will be supported by the NZIMLS.

- Be a NZ-registered Medical Laboratory Scientist with a current annual practising certificate.

- Have a Bachelor of Medical Laboratory Science Degree or equivalent.

- Have five years' post-graduation experience in histopathology.

- Have the NZIMLS approval for their application.

- Have the documented support of their laboratory manager, medical head of department and a named consultant pathologist mentor.

- Have at least two years' current practical experience in the dissection of histological specimens.

It has been agreed that those with the accredited BMLSc and the five years' experience will be able to become a 'Member' of the Institute and therefore access the DEP in Histological Dissection. They will not necessarily have completed anything similar to the Specialist Portfolio but the annual practising certificate provides some assurance that they have developed their skills since the degree.

This is only a limited pilot at present and it will be interesting to see how many actually apply and how well they do with the logbook element of the qualification and the examination. The latter will be the same examination that candidates in the UK sit so they will need to be aware of British issues in relation to clinical governance, for example, which might not be the same as in NZ.

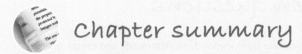

Chapter summary

This chapter will have given you an understanding of the following issues:

- The construction and content of a histopathology report, including the supplementary report.

- The key microscopic cellular and tissue observations seen in the two key areas of histopathology, inflammation and cancer, exemplified in case studies depicting these processes.

- A comprehension of the importance of histopathology reports in the patient management pathway.

- Datasets in pathology reporting and how they are employed and why.

- The value of molecular/genetic information in histopathology reports and how significant these are in supplementary reports.

- An understanding of the role of histopathology reporting in research and development.

- An appreciation of the expanding roles for biomedical and clinical scientists in histopathology reporting.

- The current infrastructure of examinations available for advanced involvement in histopathology diagnostics in Australia and New Zealand.

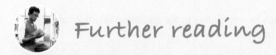

Further reading

- **Allen DC.** *Histopathology reporting. Guidelines for surgical cancer. Tissue pathways and data sets an overview* **3rd edn. Springer Science and Business Media.**

- **Orchard GE, Nation BR eds.** *Histopathology* **1st edn. Oxford: Oxford University Press, 2012 (ISBN 978-0-19-957434-6).**

- **Orchard GE, Nation BR eds.** *Cell structure and function.* **Oxford: Oxford University Press, 2015 (ISBN 978-0-19-965247-1).**

Useful websites

- Australian Institute of Medical Scientists (AIMS) (**www.aims.org.au**)

- Cancer Research UK (**www.cancerresearchuk.org**)

- Institute of Biomedical Science. IBMS Specialist Diplomas (**www.ibms.org>qualifications>> specialist diplomas**)

- New Zealand Institute of Medical Laboratory Science (NZIMLS) (**www.nzimls.org.nz**)

- The Royal College of Pathologists (**www.rcpath.org/resource-library-homepage/publications/cancer-datasets.html**)

- US National Cancer Institute (**www.cancer.gov/about-cancer/diagnosis-staging/diagnosis/pathology-reports-fa**).

Discussion questions

13.1 Explain the key processes and cellular types involved in inflammation and cancer.

13.2 Discuss the importance of the histopathology report and its significance in the patient management pathway.

13.3 The photomicrograph below shows a particular type of chronic inflammation. The section is taken from a white/cream nodule with central cavitation from the lung of an elderly, homeless, frail and malnourished man.

    a)   What is the name given to this type of chronic inflammation?

    b)   What cell types can you see in the photomicrograph?

    c)   What is the most likely cause in this case?

    d)   What other causes can lead to this type of inflammation?

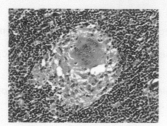

Answers to the self-check questions and tips for responding to the discussion questions are provided on the book's accompanying website:

 Visit www.oup.com/uk/orchard2e

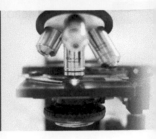

14

Light microscopy and digital pathology

Guy Orchard

Learning objectives

By the end of this chapter you should be able to:

- Describe what is meant by resolution.

- Understand what affects the resolution of a microscope.

- Identify the various components of a microscope and describe their function.

- Understand the steps required to ensure that microscope illumination is set up according to the principles of Koehler illumination.

- Understand the principles of image formation.

- Describe the principles and application of darkfield illumination.

- Describe the principles of polarization microscopy.

- Understand and describe the phase contrast microscope.

- Understand the principles of fluorescence microscopy.

- Describe the application of the various forms of light microscopy in the field of biomedical science.

- Understand the concept of digital pathology.

- Appreciate the mechanisms behind 'virtual' microscopy.

14.1 Introduction

The light microscope is perhaps the most widely used instrument in the field of biomedical science. You will already have read about 'What is histopathology' and you will also have an understanding of the key objectives of the science behind it. In real terms, the light microscope is to the histologist what the scalpel is to the surgeon and a paintbrush is to an artist. Its contribution to our knowledge and understanding of pathological processes is without parallel.

The earliest optical instrument used for aiding the observation of small objects was the simple magnifying lens—these have been used for centuries. The Romans created glass in the first century AD and documents described the observation that objects appeared larger when viewed through pieces of glass that were thicker in the centre than at the edge. These simple lenses were termed 'burning' or magnifying glasses. Magnifying lenses were not used routinely until the thirteenth century, when they were put into metal frames and used as spectacles. However, it wasn't until the sixteenth century that people started to assemble glass lenses so that distant objects could appear to be closer or for small objects to appear bigger. It is believed that the earliest compound microscope was developed in England and was, in fact, an altered telescope.

In the late sixteenth century, Zaccharias and Hans Janssen (father and son) modified a telescope and by using two lenses—one at the eyepiece of the microscope (ocular) and one close to the sample (objective)—could significantly increase the size of the sample being viewed (up to approximately nine times). The lenses were held in an extending tube which could be used to change the magnification of the instrument. However, this instrument had limited use because the quality of the glass lenses used was not very good.

In the 1700s, a Dutchman, Antonie van Leeuwenhoek, developed high-quality glass from which he created very highly ground and polished lenses which produced a lens with very high **magnification** for the time (×270 compared to the ×20-30 of the early compound microscopes). His microscope consisted of a single lens mounted in a brass plate. The sample was held on a sharp point in front of the lens (which could be focused) and the whole instrument was held close to the eye. With this instrument he made very detailed observations of many microscopic objects including bacteria, red blood cells, and various animals swimming in water.

It was also in the seventeenth century that creation of the compound microscope was attributed to Robert Hooke. He realized that the use of lenses with a very short focal length could result in increased magnification. This led to the use of double convex lenses, which not only increased magnification, but also increased the resolution of the compound microscope. He used his compound microscope to describe the structure of cork and first used the term 'cell', which he then identified in other plant tissues. He also observed and gave detailed drawings and descriptions of other microscopic structures including bird feathers, the foot of a fly, and bee stingers.

Development of the microscope did not progress further until the nineteenth century, when research and subsequent developments in optical theory by Ernst Abbe (in particular) and glass technology and design by Otto Schott were introduced, which in turn led to the ability of microscope companies to create microscopes with greatly increased resolution and magnification.

14.2 Scientific principles behind light microscopy

The principle behind the light microscope is to provide a magnified image of the sample of interest such that we can see what is happening to our samples at a scale which our eyes alone could not perceive. It is not enough, however, simply to provide a large image of a specimen, as a simple magnifying lens would. Biomedical scientists are typically interested in quite small and fine detailed structures so it is important that the microscopic image contains sufficient resolution of fine detail.

In the following section you will learn about the factors involved in producing a high-quality microscope image and understand how they affect the final image. We then go on to discuss the structural features of the microscope and the impact that these can have on final image quality.

14.2.1 Resolution

Resolution can be defined as the smallest distance that can be distinguished between two points. In mathematical terms, the resolution can be represented by the formula $R = 0.6\,\lambda/NA$, where R is resolution, λ is the wavelength of the radiation and NA is the numerical aperture of the lens.

The numerical aperture can be described as a numerical representation of the light-gathering capacity of a lens and is represented by the formula $NA = n \sin \alpha$, where n is the refractive index of the medium between the glass coverslip and the front lens of the objective, and α is the angle between the outermost ray of light that enters the front of the objective lens and the optical axis of the objective lens. If the medium between the coverslip and objective is air then the maximum theoretical NA is 1.0. However, this is not possible in practice because the lens would have no working distance from the object. If, however, we substitute oil or water for the air then the theoretical NA is increased to 1.3–1.51. In practice, the theoretical values cannot be attained and in air the best possible NA is approximately 0.95 and in oil approximately 1.5.

14.2.2 Light and wave forms

Light emitted from a single source can be regarded as a series of waves travelling in straight lines in all directions. The length of the wave, termed the '**wavelength**', gives the light its colour. White light consists of a spectrum of wavelengths ranging from short ultraviolet through to long infrared light. Monochromatic light has a single wavelength. The amplitude of the wave represents the brightness of light—the larger the amplitude the brighter the light emitted. It is important to understand these two elements of the light waveform in order to understand the effect that they have on any image viewed under a microscope (Figure 14.1).

When light passes through air it travels in a straight line. If, however, it strikes a different medium (e.g. glass) the light is retarded and refracted at the air/glass interface, resulting in light of different wavelengths being refracted or deviated to a variable amount (see **Refractive index**). This refraction is best seen when light passes from air into a glass prism and out again into air. The white light is refracted to produce a spectrum of the component colours (Figure 14.2). The prism acts to slow down the light waves, with shorter wavelengths (e.g. blue) travelling more slowly than longer wavelengths (e.g. red). This causes the white light to split into its component colours.

Wavelength

The distance (measured in the direction of propagation) between two points in the same phase in consecutive cycles of a wave.

Refractive index

A numerical measure of a substance's ability to deviate light rays.

SELF-CHECK 14.1

How is resolution defined?

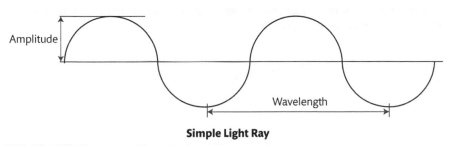

Simple Light Ray

FIGURE 14.1
Annotated waveform.

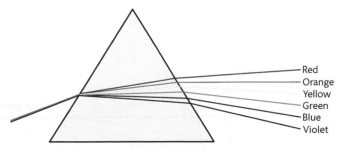

FIGURE 14.2
Diagram of prism to show spectrum of light.

14.3 Image formation and lens defects

Focal point

The point at which a lens brings all of the light passing through to a common focus.

When parallel light rays passes through a lens they are refracted and brought to a common focus, called the **focal point**. The distance between the centre of the lens and the focal point is called the focal length.

14.3.1 Chromatic aberration

Chromatic aberration

The inability of a lens to bring light of different wavelengths to a common focal point.

Chromatic aberration is the inability of a lens to bring light of different wavelengths to a common focal point, resulting in a fuzzy image with multiple coloured fringes. This is due to the fact that different wavelengths are refracted to different degrees, as seen in a simple prism illustrated in Figure 14.2. Short wavelength light is brought to a shorter focal point than longer wavelength light. The effect is shown in Figure 14.3, and results in coloured fringing in the image.

14.3.2 Spherical aberration

Spherical aberration

The inability of a lens to bring light passing through different parts of the lens to a common focus.

Spherical aberration is the inability of a lens to bring light passing through its periphery to the same point as light passing through the central part of the lens. It is caused by the fact that the lens refracts the light to different degrees depending on the curvature of the lens and the angle at which light enters the lens (Figure 14.4). This defect is usually overcome when the lens system is corrected for chromatic aberration.

Both spherical and chromatic aberration create significant deterioration in image quality, but both can be corrected by the use of different glass additives and the combination of lenses with different curvature and shape.

14.3.3 Astigmatism

Astigmatism

The inability of a lens to bring light passing through one part to the same focal point as light passing through another part.

Astigmatism can be described as the inability of a lens to bring light passing through one part to the same focal point as light passing through another part. It results in a distorted, unsharp image and is best illustrated when viewing a lattice. Astigmatism is perhaps the least important lens aberration as correction of either chromatic or spherical aberration usually results in the elimination of astigmatism. However, in electron microscopy astigmatism plays a much more important role in image quality and will be dealt with more fully in Chapter 15.

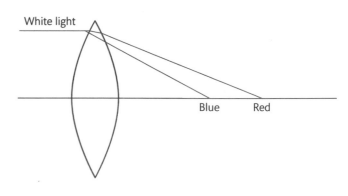

FIGURE 14.3
Diagram of lens defect producing chromatic aberration.

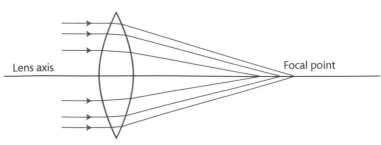

FIGURE 14.4
Diagram of a lens showing spherical aberration.

14.4 Components of the compound microscope

While the main components of the microscope have changed little since the mid-nineteenth century, there have been significant improvements made in lens quality in recent years which has resulted in greatly improved image quality. Much emphasis has also been placed on the ergonomic design of microscopes in order to provide the user with the most comfortable working position. The main components of the microscope are shown in Figure 14.5, and their functions are described in the following sections.

14.4.1 Light source

All microscopes require a reliable light source. In early designs this light source was the sun, using a mirror to reflect its rays into the microscope condenser. As optics improved it became obvious that this form of illumination was totally inadequate. The next form of light source to be used was the tungsten filament lamp fitted with a variable rheostat which would allow adjustment of brightness. Tungsten filament bulbs create considerable heat in use and may need cooling in order to be used safely. Most modern microscopes use low-voltage halogen light sources which give a much brighter, intense light without the heat generated by tungsten filament lights. One drawback of using halogen lamps is that the colour of the light changes with the voltage applied to the bulb. Low voltages result in a warm colour temperature (orange-yellow light), while higher voltages result in a colder colour temperature (blue light). While the eye adjusts easily to this change in light temperature, devices such as digital cameras cannot display the colours in the sample correctly unless the user adjusts the 'white point' of the image (through either an automatic or manual camera setting) to enable a camera image with the correct colour rendition to be recorded.

Very recently the development of high-intensity white light-emitting diode (LED) units has allowed their use in microscopes. These have several advantages over halogen lamps. First, they have a very long life (typically many thousands of hours) which reduces the running costs of the microscope. Second, they produce light of a uniform colour temperature, regardless of the intensity at which the

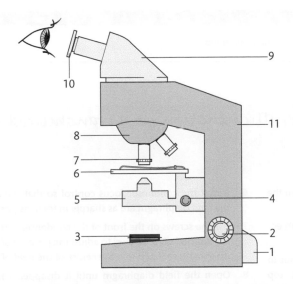

1. Lamp for transmitted light illumination
2. Focus control
3. Field diaphragm for transmitted light
4. Condenser focus control
5. Condenser with aperture diaphragm
6. Specimen stage
7. Objective
8. Objective nosepiece
9. Binocular tube
10. Eyepiece
11. Microscope stand

FIGURE 14.5
Schematic diagram of a simple microscope.

LED is operated. This is of particular benefit in digital image recording as the user does not have to keep adjusting the white balance setting of the camera. The third benefit is that LEDs produce very little heat so there is very little chance of heating the specimen and causing the creation of condensation between the coverslip and the sample.

14.4.2 Condenser

The purpose of the condenser is to focus the light produced by the lamp onto the specimen, giving maximum and even illumination. In its simplest form, the substage condenser consists of one or two lenses with vertical adjustment which allows vertical focusing of the light in order to compensate for varying thicknesses of microscope slide. It is vital for optimal illumination to be able to align accurately the axis of the condenser with the objective lens and to be able to adjust the size and brightness of the cone of light hitting the specimen. The condenser mount is fitted with adjusting screws to move the condenser in the x–y axis so that it can be centred, and an iris diaphragm to adjust the light cone.

In order to obtain the best illumination on the specimen it is possible to set the condenser in two ways: critical illumination and Koehler illumination. Each has its advantages and applications in biomedical science.

Critical illumination relies on focusing the light source directly on the specimen using the substage condenser. It is a very effective way of ensuring that the maximum level of illumination reaches the specimen. This is particularly necessary for high-magnification objectives with short working distances, but with low-magnification objectives it results in very uneven illumination. Microscopes with critical illumination tend now to be low-cost educational microscopes.

Koehler illumination requires the condenser to be set in such a way that light reaching the specimen illuminates over a wide area without variation in intensity and evenness. This form of illumination is particularly necessary when recording photographic images in order to ensure even illumination across the whole field. The following section describes how to set up Koehler illumination on a transmitted light microscope (see Method 14.1).

SELF-CHECK 14.2

How do we correct for chromatic aberration?

METHOD 14.1 *Koehler illumination on a transmitted light microscope*

1. Switch on the microscope light source and fully open the condenser aperture diaphragm.

2. Place a stained slide on the stage and put the 10× objective into place.

3. Ensure that light is diverted to the eyepieces (and not to the camera port). If your condenser has a swing-in top lens then this should be swung into the light path. Adjust the condenser height so that the top lens is close to the specimen slide.

4. Focus the specimen using the coarse and fine focus controls.

5. Close the field diaphragm so that it is visible in the centre of the eyepiece field.

6. Adjust the condenser focus control so that the edges of the field diaphragm are as sharply in focus as possible.

7. Use the screws on the front of the condenser carrier (usually knurled silver screws) to adjust the position of the field diaphragm so that it is in the centre of the field of view.

8. Open the field diaphragm until it disappears from the field of view.

9. Remove an eyepiece and close the condenser aperture diaphragm so that it is approximately 70% open. This is done to provide a balance between sample contrast and resolution of the image details. You can adjust this further if necessary.

10. Replace the eyepiece and then observe the sample as required.

14.4.3 Stage

The stage is the rigid flat surface on which the sample sits immediately above the condenser. Most stages incorporate sample clamps attached to mechanical manipulators which allow accurate and easy movement of the sample under observation. Vernier scales are incorporated in the mechanism, which makes it possible to return to the same area of the specimen with ease.

SELF-CHECK 14.3

When setting up Koehler illumination, what objective magnification should I use?

14.4.4 Stand

The body stand of the microscope is the rigid structure on which all other components are fitted. It provides a sturdy, vibration-free base for the various attachments. It incorporates the coarse and fine focus of the microscope, which allows very fine vertical movement of either the stage or the objective lens, depending on the manufacturer. Above the stage, the stand has a nosepiece for holding between three and seven objectives of various magnification. The nosepiece is able to rotate, allowing the correct objective lens to be brought into the light axis.

14.4.5 Objective lens

The objective lens is perhaps the most important component of the microscope and is most responsible for the ultimate quality of the image. There are numerous types of objective lens, each with specific uses and qualities. Selection of objective lens is determined by the function to which the microscope is to be put.

14.4.6 Objective lens types

Achromatic

Achromatic lenses are the simplest form of corrected lens available and are corrected for chromatic aberration in two wavelengths (colours) only, with spherical aberration corrected only for one wavelength. They have a relatively low numerical aperture, which permits a good working distance and depth of field. The best image quality in this type of lens is seen through the lens axis, as there is blurring at the periphery, which makes them unsuitable for colour photomicrography.

Semi-apochromatic or fluorite

When the mineral fluorite is incorporated into the lens glass it allows the construction of lenses with improved numerical aperture and increased image resolution. They are compensated for chromatic aberration in up to four wavelengths, although spherical aberration is still present, but they provide superior performance over simple achromats.

Apochromatic

The best quality of lens is represented by the apochromat. It is corrected for up to seven wavelengths and exhibits no spherical aberration or astigmatism.

These lenses provide the highest numerical aperture with the highest resolution. The working distance of these lenses is usually very short in high-power **apochromatic** objectives but this is used to advantage by the addition of high refractive index immersion oil or water between the specimen and the objective lens. As described previously, this has the effect of increasing numerical aperture, thereby increasing the potential resolving power of the lens. With this type of lens it is possible to achieve numerical apertures in excess of 1.4 with full colour correction.

Apochromatic

A lens corrected for up to seven colours and represents the best quality of lens available.

14.4.7 Observation tube

Above the nosepiece is the observation tube which consists of either a binocular or trinocular attachment. Binocular tubes are used for conventional observation, while a trinocular tube allows the attachment of a camera for simultaneous viewing and image recording.

Until the 1980s microscopes had a fixed tube length (defined as the distance between the nosepiece and the eyepiece seat). This tube length played an important part in the measurement of the final magnification of the microscope and was standardized to 160 mm by the Royal Microscopical Society in the nineteenth century. During the 1980s infinity-corrected optical systems were introduced by the major microscope manufacturers. Here the focused image leaving the lens is not brought to a focal point but rather remains parallel at the same focal plane to infinity, with no change in magnification. A tube lens is then introduced into the light path and this lens brings the light rays to a point of focus at the intermediate image plane. Infinity-corrected optical systems have enabled manufacturers to vary the tube length without any alteration to magnification, and so allowed the introduction of optical accessories into the optical path (e.g. fluorescence illuminators, multi-discussion systems, and the development of ergonomic microscopes).

14.4.8 Eyepiece

Eyepiece

The lens situated at the observation tube of a microscope used to view the magnified image of the specimen.

The **eyepiece** is the last lens system through which the image passes. It magnifies the intermediate image formed by the objective and tube lens and allows a virtual focused image to fall on the eye of the observer. Some eyepieces are capable of accommodating a measuring graticule that can be used for quantitative and accurate measurement of images. Modern microscopes are fitted with widefield, flatfield and high focal point eyepieces especially designed for spectacle users.

To see online videos demonstrating 'How to set up a light microscope' and 'How to maintain a light microscope', log on to www.oxfordtextbooks.co.uk/orc/fbs

14.4.9 Ergonomics

The introduction of the infinity-corrected microscope has allowed the development of more ergonomic microscope designs. The binocular tubes of microscopes have been redesigned to include options to alter the viewing height, viewing angle and/or provide lateral adjustment of the eyepieces. These different adjustments enable the viewing position to be altered to accommodate microscope users of different heights.

Consideration of ergonomic design should not be limited to just the viewing height and angle of the eyepieces; rather it should include the entire microscope design, including positioning of the focus control, height adjustment of the stage controls (so that users do not have to keep their arms lifted to adjust the stage position), and the use of different materials to make controls non-slip and comfortable to use for long periods of time.

This focus on ergonomics has meant that manufacturers are now designing ergonomic microscope stands on which all the major controls (i.e. lamp intensity control, focus and stage controls) are located within fingertip reach of each other. In this way, the microscopist can concentrate on the sample and not have to look away from the eyepieces in order to make the slightest adjustment to the microscope, or suffer from discomfort when using the microscope for long periods of time. Figure 14.6 illustrates one of the latest ergonomic microscopes. With this instrument the eyepiece viewing height and angle of observation are adjustable, the stage controls are height-adjustable, and all major controls are within fingertip reach of each other.

14.5 Contrast techniques

The most important consideration for the observation of biological material using a microscope is how to introduce sufficient contrast to view the sample.

When looking at large specimens through a dissecting microscope, it is usually possible to see sufficient detail by adjusting the contrast through varying the illumination alone. However, when viewing

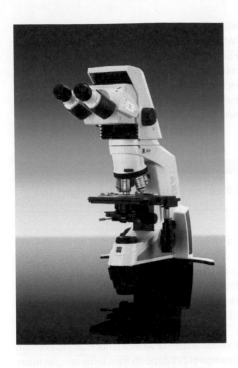

FIGURE 14.6
Carl Zeiss Axio Lab.A1–a modern ergonomic microscope for routine biomedical science applications. (Image courtesy of Carl Zeiss Microscopy)

smaller samples with a compound microscope the most straightforward way of introducing contrast is to use a chromogen. Stains such as haematoxylin and eosin (H&E) introduce contrast by means of adding colour to the sample. We then are able to distinguish differences in tissue types and different disease states through morphological changes.

The specificity of stains can be greatly increased by the use of immunocytochemistry. Here it is possible to stain particular molecules so that they can be visually identified and their distribution throughout a tissue detected.

Sometimes it is not possible to stain with chromogenic compounds, such as when looking at living cells or where no stains are sufficiently specific. In this case we must use a microscope which utilizes a different contrast technique. In the following section we discuss different microscope types for various common applications in biomedical science. This will give you an introduction to alternative methods available to visualize different specimen types.

14.6 Phase contrast microscope

Light is a waveform and the wavelength determines the colour of the light and the amplitude determines the brightness.

When two rays of light originate from the same source they are termed **coherent**. They are in phase with each other and their amplitudes coincide, and as a consequence they are able to combine to form a ray with amplitude twice the height of the original, thus resulting in a brighter ray. If, however, the two rays become out of phase then they are able to interfere with one another. If the degree of interference is half a wavelength then this would result in extinction of the ray. This phenomenon can be utilized in the phase contrast microscope by illuminating the samples with a cone of light produced by an annular stop positioned in the brightfield substage condenser. This cone of light then passes through the sample, which is positioned at the focal point of the cone. Light leaving the sample enters the objective lens of the microscope which has a phase plate fitted. The phase plate consists of a disc of glass with a ring etched into it, which corresponds exactly with the shape and size of the annulus. The depth of the etching is critical and represents the depth required to retard the light rays passing through the full thickness of the phase plate by quarter of a wavelength when compared with the light passing through the etched ring. This retardation, while resulting in interference, does not in itself produce the desired increase in contrast. The sample is responsible for producing this effect. Tissue will

Coherent rays
Light rays which are in phase with one another, of the same amplitude and wavelength.

also retard light by approximately quarter of a wavelength, with the combined specimen and phase plate retardation resulting in the total interference. When light passes through a sample, some light is scattered and passes into the objective lens in the normal way and passes to the eye of the observer through the unetched part of the phase plate. When the unaltered rays are focused with the retarded rays they combine to form the real image of the specimen. Subtle changes in refractive index within the sample are seen as varying degrees of brightness in the image against a dark background. If set up correctly, a good phase contrast microscope should be able to distinguish differences in refractive index of less than 5% with ease.

SELF-CHECK 14.4

In a phase contrast microscope, by how much does the phase plate retard the rays of light?

It is vitally important when setting up a microscope for phase contrast to ensure that the annulus and the phase plate are exactly aligned, and it is usual to utilize an auxiliary microscope to view the back focal plane of the objective. This allows the operator to view the phase plate and to align it with the annulus with great accuracy, using adjusting screws fitted in the condenser. In practice, each objective lens and phase plate has a matching annulus fitted into a rotating disc set into the base of the substage condenser. Each annulus can be adjusted and set individually to match its objective. Figure 14.7 illustrates the light path in a phase contrast microscope.

Phase contrast microscopy is used extensively in biomedical science when it is necessary to examine unstained tissue samples. Examples include the examination of cell deposits from urine samples in the microbiology department from patients suffering from urinary tract infection; for counting platelets in haematology; and for assessing sperm motility and viability in andrology laboratories. Phase contrast microscopy is also used extensively to examine tissue culture samples *in vitro* and to identify the cellular component of such samples.

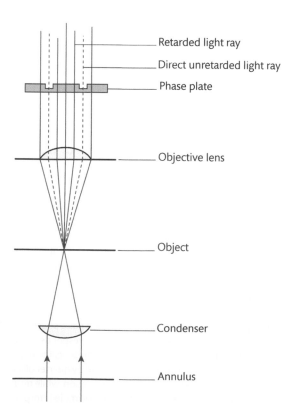

FIGURE 14.7
Diagram of the light path in a phase contrast microscope.

14.7 Polarization microscope

Light emitted from a single source can be regarded as electromagnetic waves, the amplitude of which represents brightness and the wavelength as the colour. This waveform is emitted and vibrates in all directions. Polarized light, however, only vibrates in a single direction. Certain crystals are capable of producing plane polarized light by splitting incident rays entering the crystal into two components which are refracted by the crystal in two different planes. This phenomenon is termed **birefringence.**

If we place two similar polarizing crystals so that their plane of polarization is parallel to each other then any light entering the first would be capable of passing through the second crystal. However, if we rotate the second crystal through an angle of 90° then the light would not exit from the second crystal and would result in light extinction.

The polarization microscope makes use of this phenomenon and allows us to examine and measure substances which are capable of polarizing light. It has a polarizer filter situated within or below the substage condenser, which causes the specimen to be illuminated by plane polarized light. A second polarizing filter (or **analyser**) is situated between the objective lens and below the eyepiece. Typically, one of these polarizing filters is capable of being rotated through 180°. In use, the two filters are orientated so that their planes of polarization are at right angles, resulting in light extinction. Any specimen containing a birefringent substance will appear to rotate the light so that it is able to pass through the analyser and appear bright against a dark background. This form of microscope is particularly useful in the examination of body fluids that may contain crystals (e.g. urine and joint fluid). One particular example of use in biomedical science is for the identification of uric acid crystals when diagnosing cases of gout. Gout crystals are strongly birefringent, while pseudogout crystals (calcium pyrophosphate crystals) are weakly birefringent. By altering the orientation of the crystals it is also possible to distinguish between the two crystal types. When parallel to the polarizer direction the gout crystals are yellow (pseudogout crystals are blue). When the crystals are orientated perpendicular to the polarizer, gout crystals are blue while pseudogout crystals are yellow. This effect is demonstrated well in Figure 14.8. Polarizing microscopy also can be useful in detecting the artefactual presence of, for example, starch grains (Figure 14.9).

Another major application of the polarization microscope is in the diagnosis of amyloid diseases. Typically, a renal biopsy is taken and the tissue stained with Congo red. Normal tissue is stained a light red colour while amyloid stains a dark red colour. When polarized light is used, amyloid glows a characteristic green colour and this is used to highlight its presence.

Birefringence
The ability of a substance to split a ray of light into two components: the ordinary and extraordinary ray.

Analyser
Polarizing filter placed in the light path fixed within the body of the microscope. It is used in conjunction with a substage polarizer.

SELF-CHECK 14.5

What is meant by birefringence?

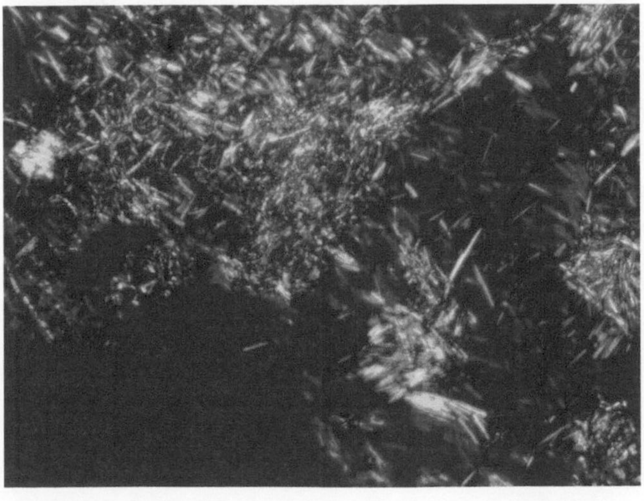

FIGURE 14.8
Photomicrograph of gout crystals.

(a) 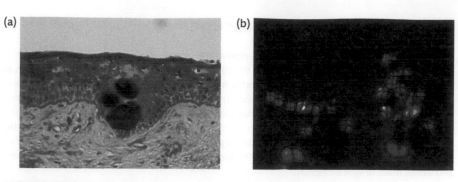 (b)

FIGURE 14.9
a) Starch grains on a section of skin (periodic acid Schiff [PAS], original magnification ×60);
b) Starch grains from (a), visualized using cross-polarizers. Note the characteristic Maltese cross appearance. Starch grains as an artefact on a tissue section most notably come from the starch that may be used as a 'lubricant' in some surgical gloves. This appearance is regarded as a 'fingerprint' identification for starch grains microscopically (original magnification ×40).

14.8 Darkfield microscope

Brightfield illumination will in itself provide only minimal contrast in the biological samples as there is insufficient variation in optical density to produce contrast, and therefore unstained samples are virtually invisible. In order to overcome this problem it is usual to introduce contrast by staining with coloured dyes. This principle has been covered extensively in earlier chapters. However, when it is necessary to examine samples in the 'living' state, staining may result in death and disruption of the sample, so alternative methods of illumination are needed.

The simplest method of introducing contrast to unstained samples is to use oblique light. The effect of doing this is to increase refraction, while at the same time creating a decrease in direct illumination. Unstained samples thus appear bright against a dark background. The darkfield condenser was developed so that this effect could be created in a more controlled way.

The darkfield condenser consists of a parabolic mirror placed in the substage condenser, which only allows light to reach the specimen stage at a very acute angle as illustrated in Figure 14.10. When no specimen is present on the microscope stage no light passes through to the objective lens. When a

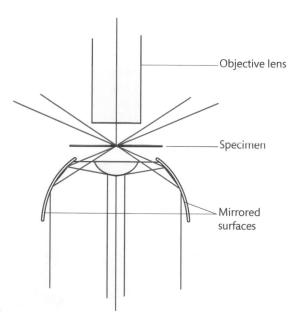

Objective lens

Specimen

Mirrored surfaces

FIGURE 14.10
Light path in darkfield illumination.

sample is placed on the stage the small variations in refraction created by the specimen result in light being collected by the objective and this makes the sample appear bright against the dark background.

In biomedical science, one of the most common applications of darkfield microscopy is for the identification of the bacterium *Treponema pallidum*, the causal agent of syphilis. It is a spirochaete that moves in a characteristic corkscrew fashion. The darkfield microscope permits this very small organism (less than 0.2 µm in diameter and 6–20 µm in length) to be visualized, due to the gain in resolution. Darkfield microscopy allows the biomedical scientist to examine fresh samples of exudate from the sores of patients suspected of having syphilis, and identify the characteristic motility of the *T. pallidum* spirochaete.

14.9 Fluorescence microscope

Certain substances when illuminated with high-energy light of a short wavelength will re-emit light of a longer, low-energy wavelength. This phenomenon is termed fluorescence and it is utilized in the fluorescence microscope. The resolution of the microscope relies on the wavelength of the light. Short wavelength ultraviolet light is outside the visible spectrum for humans so its use to improve resolution is limited. Its use in the fluorescence microscope does, however, allow us to visualize very small quantities of biological components in tissue samples.

Some substances are autofluorescent (i.e. they exhibit primary fluorescence), while some substances need to have fluorochromes added to produce secondary fluorescence. Examples of substances that exhibit autofluorescence are vitamin A and some porphyrins. Various dyes exhibit fluorescence and these can be used to demonstrate specific cellular components.

There are two types of fluorescence microscope, transmission and incident, and their use depends on the desired mode of illumination.

In the transmission fluorescence microscope the light source is beneath the specimen, as in conventional light microscopy, while for incident light fluorescence microscopy (also known as epifluorescence) the specimen is illuminated from above and the viewer sees visible light transmitted from the specimen. Virtually all modern microscopes equipped for fluorescence make use of epifluorescence so only these microscopes will be considered in this section.

14.9.1 Incident light fluorescence microscope

As the fluorescent light emitted from a fluorochrome is emitted in all directions it is possible to illuminate the specimen from above (epi-illumination) and to collect the incident light directed back into the objective for observation by the user. This is the basis of epifluorescence microscopy.

In operation, the excitation light passes from the lamp and through the excitation filter, which allows only light of a specific wavelength range to pass through. The filtered excitation light then is reflected by a dichroic mirror into the microscope objective. A dichroic mirror is a very precise filter that reflects light of specific wavelengths while permitting light of longer wavelengths to pass through. A fluorescence filter set is designed so that the excitation light is reflected into the microscope objective. The excitation light then illuminates the sample and excites the fluorochrome. The fluorochrome then emits light of a longer wavelength. This emitted light passes into the objective and passes through the dichroic mirror, which is able to transmit light of a longer wavelength than that of the excitation light. The light then passes through an **emission filter**, which ensures that only the wavelength range of the fluorochrome emission is allowed to pass to the observer and so enable observation of a bright coloured image against a dark background. A simplified diagram of the light path in an epifluorescence microscope is shown in Figure 14.11.

14.9.2 Fluorescence light sources

Fluorescence microscopes traditionally require light sources that produce a high level of ultraviolet light, which neither tungsten nor halogen lights are able to do. For this purpose the best source has been the high-pressure mercury vapour arc lamp. However, this requires a special lamp holder and power supply and in use generates a significant amount of heat.

Mercury vapour lamps are unstable when hot and this requires safety protocols to be implemented in the laboratory to reduce the likelihood of bulb breakage and hence reduce the chances of users being exposed to mercury vapour. In addition to not handling the bulb when it is hot, the lamp unit

Barrier (or emission) filter

A filter used in the fluorescent microscope which is capable of only transmitting the light wavelength range emitted by a particular fluorescence dye.

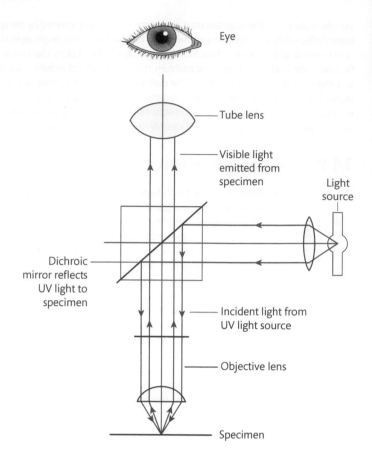

FIGURE 14.11
Diagram of incident light fluorescence microscope (simplified).

should only be switched on from cold and then left to run for approximately 30 minutes before being switched off again. It is also important not to touch the glass envelope of a mercury lamp as grease deposits can make the glass liable to break. Mercury lamps have a finite life (up to 300 hours, depending on wattage) and so it is imperative that the bulb running time is recorded (most mercury lamps have a time counter built in to the power supply unit) and that the manufacturer's safe lifetime limits are followed. Provided that these safety considerations are followed then the mercury lamp is a perfectly safe light source for routine fluorescence microscopy.

Mercury vapour lamps

- The mercury vapour lamp contains mercury gas at a high pressure in a glass envelope. The lamp should always only be handled when cold and handled gently so as not to break the glass.

- Monitor the length of time that the mercury lamp has been used. Do not exceed the manufacturer's stated lifetime—if the time is exceeded you run the risk of the lamp exploding and mercury vapour being released into the laboratory.

- Before changing a mercury lamp, ensure it has been switched off for more than 30 minutes.

- Do not touch the glass of the replacement mercury lamp. If you do, then fingerprints should be wiped off as per the recommendations given by the lamp manufacturer.

- Allow the mercury lamp to cool down for at least 30 minutes before switching it back on.

- Do not dispose of mercury lamps in the waste bin. Use a specialist disposal service (your organization should have a specific disposal contractor).

In recent years there have been a number of technological developments aimed at making fluorescence microscopy easier to use and more economical. Apart from the safety considerations of the traditional mercury vapour arc lamp, there are two further drawbacks: first, the lamp must be aligned correctly by the user to ensure maximum field coverage and even field illumination; and second, the lamp has a limited lifetime of between 100 and 300 hours depending on the lamp wattage.

The first technological advance to address these problems was metal halide light sources. These use a lamp which, while utilizing mercury vapour, has an extended lifetime of up to 2000 hours. The lamp is contained in a unit with the power supply and is precentred so there are no alignment issues. The light is then delivered into a liquid light guide attached to the microscope via a suitable collimating adapter. The use of the light guide ensures that the illumination field is extremely homogenous due to the scrambling effect in the light guide. These metal halide sources commonly include an iris diaphragm, which can be closed to reduce the intensity of the fluorescence (thus overcoming another problem associated with mercury vapour arc lamps). Collimating adapters are available for many recent microscope models from the major manufacturers and therefore these light sources can be used to upgrade existing fluorescence microscopes and enhance their performance.

The second technological advance now in common use for fluorescence microscopy is the use of light-emitting diodes (LEDs). In recent years the output power of LEDs has increased to the point that they can now be used to excite fluorescence dyes. In addition, developments in LED production have led to the availability of many different LED modules producing different wavelengths that are suitable for the excitation characteristics of commonly used dyes. Light-emitting diodes have the key advantages that they have a very long lifespan (typically many thousands of hours), they can be switched on and off extremely quickly without increasing the chance of early failure, and the output intensity can be adjusted easily and reproducibly. The LED fluorescence sources are available either integrated into new microscope stands or as upgrade units for existing fluorescence microscopes.

Fluorescence microscopy is used routinely in biomedical science for the study of autoimmune states in skin and kidney diseases (using **immunofluorescence** techniques) and also through the use of fluorescence *in situ* hybridization (FISH) probes in cytogenetic and histopathology studies to examine changes in the genome (e.g. chromosome rearrangements, gene amplifications and deletions) and thereby diagnose certain diseases. An example of this is the diagnosis of breast cancers involving the *HFR2/neu* gene. In 15–20% of breast cancers there is amplification of this particular gene, which can be identified by the use of a suitable FISH probe kit. If there is amplification of this gene then the patient may respond to treatment with the drug trastuzumab (Herceptin). Figure 14.12 is of a breast tumour showing high amplification of the *HER2/neu* gene (red signals).

Immunofluorescence
A method employing the fluorescence microscope to identify the presence of specific antigens within tissue samples using fluorescence-labelled antisera.

FIGURE 14.12
Breast tumour showing amplification of the *HER2/neu* gene (red signals). The nuclei of the cells are stained with DAPI (blue regions) and a marker for chromosome 17 is shown by the green signals.

14.10 Confocal microscopy and optical sectioning

When a sample is illuminated by a fluorescence light source, fluorescent molecules throughout the sample are excited and give off light at the emission wavelength. With thick samples (e.g. tissue sections) this fluorescence from molecules above and below the plane of focus results in an image which appears hazy and has a large amount of background fluorescence that reduces the clarity of the microscope image. In addition to the aesthetic drawbacks, this can cause issues if small signals are to be identified (e.g. counting FISH signals in the diagnosis of breast cancer using *HER2/neu* probes). The signals of interest are extremely small and so can be masked by the much brighter background. Therefore, various technologies have been developed which aim to remove the out-of-focus light and provide a clean fluorescence image of only the light from the required plane of focus or optical section.

One of the most frequently used technologies for the acquisition of 'clean' fluorescence images is the confocal laser scanning microscope. Here, the excitation light is provided by a laser of a specific wavelength, which is scanned very quickly over the region of interest in the sample. The laser is focused on the focal plane of interest and the emitted fluorescent light is detected by a photomultiplier detector. Before the light reaches the photomultiplier, it passes through a pinhole which only permits light from the focal plane to pass to the detector. In this way, the confocal microscope captures only an image from the optical section of interest and light from other focal planes is blocked.

The confocal microscope is an expensive instrument and is not used routinely in histopathology; however, it has extensive applications in research where high-quality images are required.

Other technologies are also available which can be used to obtain a fluorescence image with the out-of-focus light removed. These include software-based deconvolution algorithms and structured illumination systems. These methods do not require the use of such complex microscope hardware as the confocal laser scanning microscope and so are cheaper and easier to use.

14.10.1 Deconvolution

Three-dimensional (3D) deconvolution is a software-based approach to generating a set of images that have removed the out-of-focus light, which would normally blur a fluorescence image. In fact, the deconvolution algorithms work on a stack of images at different focal planes and the algorithms act to assign the photons to the plane of focus from which they came. It is this reassignment of light to the correct plane which acts to optically 'deblur' the fluorescence image.

Software deconvolution relies on a stack of images being captured with precise and even Z-spacing, requiring the use of a high-quality motorized focus drive on the microscope. The step size between image planes must be calculated for the objective being used in order for the data to be captured correctly. Once an image stack is acquired, the image data are deconvoluted by software routines in a suitable image processing software package. The deconvolution algorithms require much data to be analysed and processed, so require a powerful computer in order for the images to be deconvoluted quickly. As such, the drawback of deconvolution is that it requires time—both to capture a correct dataset and then to run the deconvolution algorithms on the image data. However, it creates a true optically deblurred image of the sample, so could be said to give the most accurate representation of a fluorescent specimen.

14.10.2 Structured illumination

There are several commercially available semi-confocal systems that enable the user to capture a clean optically sectioned image from a standard fluorescence microscope. These systems rely on the principle of structured illumination. Typically, a fine regular pattern (e.g. a grid) is superimposed on the sample and viewed by the camera—by moving the patterned structure across the sample, and by acquiring several images, the entire image area can be sampled. Software packages then analyse the images to look for contrast between the grid and the sample—areas with high-contrast differences are taken to be image data from the optical section, while areas with low-contrast differences are taken to be from outside the optical section. By removing the light from the low-contrast areas of the sample (i.e. out-of-focus light) an optically sectioned image is generated. Advantages to this approach are that

TABLE 14.1 An overview of the different microscope types and their most common uses.

Sample type		Drawbacks	Comments
Upright brightfield	Stained slides (e.g. H&E or ICC).	Only usable for non-living samples.	Most commonly available microscope.
Upright darkfield	Unstained cells, particularly where high resolution is required.	For high resolution/ magnification an oil immersion condenser is required.	Generally only used for specialist tasks (e.g. identification of *Treponema pallidum* spirochaetes).
Upright phase contrast	Unstained cells/tissues.	Can only be used with samples mounted on a slide.	Useful when combined with fluorescence for identification of cell/tissues. Also used for cell counting (e.g. andrology applications).
Inverted phase contrast	Unstained cells/tissues.	Usable with low magnifications.	Generally used for checking cell cultures in flasks/counting chambers.
Upright fluorescence	Cells/tissues stained with fluorochromes or with immunofluorescence-labelled probes.	Specialist dyes and more complex microscope required.	Can give very high specificity with staining only of the cells or cell component of interest. Generally very high contrast of signal to background, which aids diagnosis.
Confocal microscope	Cells/tissues stained with fluorochromes or with immunofluorescence-labelled probes.	Specialist dyes and complex microscope required. Ongoing running costs have to be considered.	Gives a high-quality image of fluorescent samples without out-of-focus blur.
Multiheaded microscope	Generally stained slides.	Expensive and large amount of space may be required. High light requirements so generally suited only for brightfield microscopy.	Good for discussion purposes as all observers see the same image as the main observer. LED pointers can be used to highlight specific regions of interest. Less technical knowledge needed than with other discussion options.
Slide-scanning microscopes	Stained slides (some scanners will work with fluorescence).	Cost and large data storage requirements. Image quality can vary if slides are not stained and prepared uniformly.	Very good for dissemination of slides across different locations for discussion and remote diagnosis. Ability to look in detail at specific areas and then 'zoom out' to examine the entire specimen is a very useful feature.

optically sectioned images can be generated relatively quickly (focal stacks are not required) and on relatively standard fluorescence microscopes (only standard fluorescence light sources are required).

As the method relies on the projection of a structure onto the sample, it requires relatively good contrast between the fluorescence signal of the labelled areas and the background (i.e. high signal-to-background ratio).

For a summary of different types of microscopy, see Table 14.1.

14.11 Alternative microscope designs

So far in this chapter we have described upright microscopes which are designed for looking at samples mounted using conventional glass slides and coverslips. There are times when such microscopes cannot be used because either the sample is too large or because the sample cannot be mounted on a glass slide. We then need to use other microscope designs which are more suited to the task in hand.

14.11.1 Inverted microscope

The inverted microscope is particularly suited to observing living samples such as cell or tissue cultures. These are typically grown in culture flasks or dishes (typically made of relatively thick plastic—approximately 1 mm thick). The inverted microscope allows the specimen to be examined from below, enabling the microscopist to see the culture on the growing surface without disturbance. These microscopes have a large stage which is capable of accommodating tissue culture flasks or

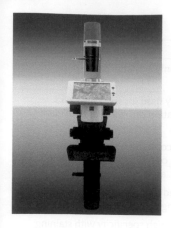

FIGURE 14.13
A recent inverted microscope for cell culture observation. This Carl Zeiss Primo Vert Monitor has an integrated camera and display screen in place of binocular eyepieces. This permits easy observation of samples in flow cabinets. (Image courtesy of Carl Zeiss Microscopy)

Petri dishes. The objective lens and condenser are designed to work at considerably longer working distances than in a conventional upright microscope, which allows the use of thick plastic sample vessels. Generally, these microscopes include phase contrast illumination to view the unstained samples, and higher grade instruments include epifluorescence to give the instrument maximum flexibility. Typically, inverted microscopes are used to examine cell cultures and ensure that growth is healthy (see Figure 14.13).

14.11.2 Dissection or stereo microscope

As with the inverted microscope, the dissection of stereo microscope is designed specifically for the examination of low surface structures at low magnification. Illumination is from the top of the specimen and viewing is via a pair of objective lenses with long working distance set at approximately 7° to the vertical, giving good stereoscopic vision with a large depth of focus. They are used extensively in materials sciences and the electronics industry, but have a wide application in biomedical science as a dissection microscope, allowing for very fine manipulation of samples.

Stereo microscopes are commonly used to visualize renal core biopsies to identify the presence of glomeruli. The tissues containing glomeruli may be processed for subsequent immunofluorescence observation or the glomeruli may be dissected out for subsequent scanning electron microscopy.

14.12 Sharing the microscope image

It is increasingly important to be able to share the information from the microscope with other observers. They may be in the same location as the microscope or, increasingly, in a different city or even another country. To permit the sharing of microscope images, various options are now used commonly to cope with the different requirements of users. These technologies range from multiple binocular heads attached to a single microscope, through to automated microscopes that can automatically scan hundreds of slides and then provide a digital representation of the slide to be accessed anywhere in the world via the internet.

14.12.1 Multidiscussion microscope

With the development of infinity corrected optics, manufacturers have been able to develop multi-headed microscopes designed specifically for teaching and discussion purposes. It is important that the light source is capable of producing an adequate light intensity for all viewers but the use of high-powered halogen lamps, together with suitably placed neutral density filters, results in identical illumination intensity for all observers. In addition, multidiscussion systems include a coloured pointer which allows the main observer to point out areas of particular interest to the other observers. With this type of microscope it is possible for more than 20 individuals to view simultaneously (Figure 14.14).

14.12.2 Digital image capture

It is now common for digital cameras to be fitted to microscopes in order to provide a permanent record. This can be particularly valuable when viewing sections where the staining is not permanent (e.g. immunofluorescence). There are a number of digital camera options available for microscopy and these vary in terms of cost, image quality, and suitability for different microscopy techniques.

The simplest (and cheapest) solution is to connect a standard 'point and shoot' digital camera, such as one that would be used for standard photography. Dedicated adapters for different cameras and different microscopes are available commercially. While this is a low-cost solution, there are a number of drawbacks to this approach.

First, these cameras have integrated lenses designed for imaging the world at large, so, when attached to a microscope, the connecting adapter has to include optics to ensure that a flatfield image can be recorded. These extra optics can introduce aberrations (reducing image quality) and can also cut light to the camera, resulting in longer exposure times to record an image and hence increase the

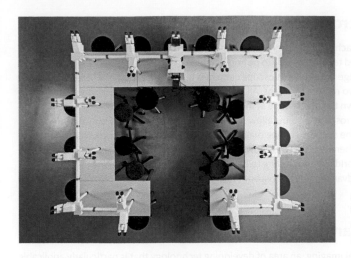

FIGURE 14.14
A multiheaded microscope for 20 observers. (Image courtesy of Carl Zeiss Microscopy)

likelihood of 'noisy' images. Second, if you attach these cameras to a microscope it can be difficult to check the image focus because the small liquid-crystal display (LCD) screens make it very difficult to ensure a sharpness of focus. Third, these camera models are replaced very quickly by manufacturers. If a camera fails then quite often the replacement model will require a different camera adapter, thus increasing the overall cost. The use of digital cameras with interchangeable lenses (D-SLR) gets around the drawbacks of points one and three, but the second drawback remains and leads many people to opt for purpose-designed microscope cameras.

Dedicated microscope cameras interface directly with the microscope via a special adapter, and use the high-quality optics of the microscope to deliver the image to the sensor—this results in the best image possible. There are a large number of different cameras available, most of which are connected directly to a computer, and software is used to display the live image. This enables accurate image composition, maximum focus sharpness to be achieved, and adjustment of image parameters such as exposure and colour balance. Once an image is captured by the software it is very easy to add scale bars, make measurements, and add annotations to the images. The stored images can then easily be added to patient records, used for referral diagnoses, added to presentations, and used for publication.

A large number of digital microscope cameras are available and each has specific technologies that lead to a particular camera being suited to specific tasks. The merits of each type of camera are not covered in this chapter but the key areas to consider and discuss with a technical representative are:

- *Microscopy requirements* (e.g. brightfield and/or fluorescence). Fluorescence microscopy results in much lower light levels reaching the observation system, so more sensitive cameras are required. In addition, long camera exposure times can result in the generation of electrical 'noise' in a camera, and specific cooling technologies are available to reduce this noise and improve fluorescence image quality.

- *Resolution and pixel size*. What are the images to be used for? If images are to be used for reports and presentations then it is not necessary to have a camera with multiple megapixels. Pixel size is directly related to light-gathering ability, which can have an effect on exposure times and image quality.

- *Use of camera* (e.g. documentation or discussion system). Depending on the use of the camera, the speed of the live image refresh rate may be very important. If the camera is to be used as part of a projection system for discussion or teaching purposes then it is important to have a fast live image on screen so that one can move smoothly around the sample as if one were looking down the microscope.

More recently, new microscopes have been released by some of the manufacturers which do not have eyepieces and instead have integrated cameras and display monitors (Figure 14.12). These eyepieceless microscopes can be useful in the teaching and discussion arenas.

14.12.3 Telemicroscopy

Digital camera systems attached to the microscope, together with recent developments in computer network links, have enabled telemicroscopy to be implemented in biomedical sciences (Figure 14.15). At its simplest, the live image from the microscope camera is broadcast as part of a video conference between participants at two remote locations. All conference participants are able to view the image as if they were looking down the microscope at the same location.

More advanced telemicroscopy systems allow a user to connect remotely to a motorized microscope and move around the section, change magnification, adjust the microscope illumination and focus the sample. The real benefit is that this allows a specialist to give an opinion on a sample located on the other side of the world, without having to have the sample physically to hand.

However, these more advanced telemicroscopy systems are now being superseded by slide-scanning technologies.

14.12.4 Slide scanning

As a development of digital imaging, an area of developing technology that is particularly applicable to histopathology is slide digitization. There are a number of slide scanners available which range from simple brightfield scanning systems through to those capable of scanning slides stained with multiple fluorescent dyes and capable of automatically analysing slides for different tasks. Some slide scanners have slide loading mechanisms included and so can scan hundreds of slides in one operating cycle. All that is required is for an operator to load the slides and then start the scan. The operator can walk away and the slides will be digitized and the images uploaded to the slide image database automatically.

Currently, one problem that is holding back the widespread rollout of slide scanning in routine histopathology is the issue of data storage. A single digitized slide could be several gigabytes in size, so, when multiplied by the number of slides produced in a year by a laboratory, the storage requirements become vast. While storage costs are continually falling, currently they remain at a level where it is not economically viable to scan every slide. However, these systems are being used to create libraries of teaching slides for education and also for scanning slides for remote secondary diagnosis by specialists in the pathology of rare diseases.

Over the next few years, as scanning speeds and data storage technologies develop further, it is likely that slide-scanning systems will become adopted into routine pathology workflows. Coupled with advanced image analysis routines, it is likely to speed up the diagnosis of disease. In addition to speeding up the analysis of microscope slides, it will also add standardization to the process.

A further benefit of remote diagnosis, compared to telemicroscopy, is that a digital slide can be disseminated easily via the internet to several specialists. It does not require an operator to be stationed at the microscope to load slides for the remote observer and so is a much more efficient way of allowing others to provide an opinion on the tissue section.

Digital image microscopy or 'virtual' microscopy technology will now enable us to employ increasingly sophisticated computer-based software packages that will enable increased precision (reproducibility).

Algorithms can be used to automate the manual counting of cells or structures. This may lead to reduced human error and ultimately improved accuracy of diagnosis. The advent of these new developments means that defined reference values will need to be established to ensure that control, consistency and accuracy are maintained. The interpretation and validation of these captured images will remain largely with the pathologist. It is also clear that a change in how these new tools are used will require training and developmental needs for pathology reporting staff. In a sense, it indicates the need to develop the abilities not only to use analogue, but also digital skills to interpret disease states. There is, however, a recognized risk that in order for these new tools to work optimally, there is clearly a need to ensure that automatic image capture, analysis and transfer of such data is standardized. When this is achieved, digital pathology will become fully integrated into pathology/laboratory-based information management systems and finally the overall operational environment for patient management and clinical care.

The primary challenges for digital pathology include the need to ensure:

- Improved quality of overall patient care.
- Increased efficiency for pathology performance.

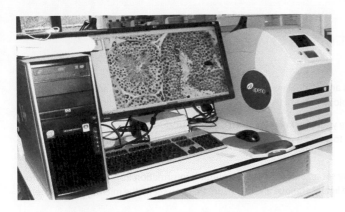

FIGURE 14.15
Digital telemicroscopy system.

- Reduced costs overall.
- Decreased reliance on less-efficient manual glass slide storage management.
- Reliable data capture and storage with the abilities to ensure secure data libraries of pathology images.
- Secure and reliable data transfer capabilities to enable multisite interaction and discussion.

SELF-CHECK 14.6

What is digital pathology and what are the main benefits of its widespread use?

14.13 The future

Currently, one area of rapidly emerging technology in light microscopy is the production of systems with enhanced resolution—so-called 'super resolution' systems. These are being deployed in cutting-edge research projects and are used to look at molecular interactions of proteins. It is very unlikely that these systems will be seen in histopathology in the near future, but it is possible that the knowledge gained from the use of these systems will have an impact on the diagnosis and treatment of disease in the future.

One area likely to have a big impact on the working practices of the biomedical scientist in the very near future will be the deployment of slide-scanning systems. Currently, the scanning speed and image storage requirements are holding back the widespread adoption of this technology. As we are all aware, the data storage capacity of computers continues to increase, and it is not difficult to contemplate a time in the near future when all laboratories will have access to large data storage facilities, so this will not be a limiting factor for digital slide creation. It is also likely that scanning speeds and image quality will continue to increase to the point where all slides generated by a laboratory can be scanned quickly and stored at a resolution which permits rapid and accurate diagnosis. The adoption of virtual microscopy systems will allow easier collaboration between laboratories and specialists across the world and should bring great benefit to the patient. This will maintain the microscope's position as one of the most important tools used routinely by biomedical scientists, and facilitate collaboration with other scientists.

Pathology is now entering the realm of personalized medicine. This means that the patient management pathway is now closely linked and tailored, according to the input from ongoing pathology testing and review. This brings new challenges and increased expectation for pathology staff and patients, respectively. It also puts the emphasis on accuracy and precision of the tissue-based diagnosis. This is paramount when quantification of biomarker expression is to be reviewed. Ultimately, this will translate into alterations in patient treatment across the wider clinical spectrum that is the hallmark of personalized medicine. Digital pathology or virtual microscopy will have an increasing role to play in the development of personalized medicine and also in our abilities to use generated data in research and development in translational science.

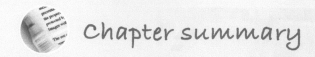

Chapter summary

- The light microscope is an essential instrument in a biomedical laboratory and is used in many disciplines within pathology.

- Contrast is vital to seeing your specimen. Contrast can be introduced in many ways—optically and chemically. Remember to select a contrast technique which is relevant to the question you are asking.

- The microscope must be set up correctly to get optimum information from your sample. Before utilizing any transmitted light technique always ensure that you set up the microscope for Koehler illumination.

- Digital pathology represents an exciting new development and offers the latest tool in the armoury of the histopathology laboratory. Its role will become increasingly significant in the patient management pathway and will play an influential role in personalized medicine procedures for the future.

Further reading

- Bradbury S, Bracegirdle B. *Introduction to light microscopy*. Royal Microscopical Society Microscopy Handbooks 42. Oxford: Bios Scientific Publishers, 1998.

- Lacey AJ ed. *Light microscopy in biology: a practical approach*. Oxford: Oxford University Press, 1999.

- Murphy DB. *Fundamentals of light microscopy and electronic imaging*. New York: Wiley-Liss, York 2001.

Discussion questions

14.1 What factors are important in producing a high-quality microscope image?

14.2 What techniques and microscopes could be used to examine unstained samples? Give examples of different samples and the microscope and/or technique used to visualize different samples.

14.3 Describe how you would set up a microscope for Koehler illumination.

14.4 Describe with a diagram how an epifluorescence microscope works, and what its uses are in a biomedical laboratory.

Answers to the self-check questions and tips for responding to the discussion questions are provided on the book's accompanying website:

 Visit www.oup.com/uk/orchard2e

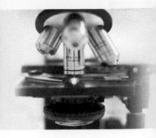

15

Electron microscopy

David N Furness

Learning objectives

By the end of this chapter you should be able to discuss:

- Why the resolution of an electron microscope is greater than the resolution of a light microscope.

- The main types of biomedical electron microscopy.

- The various components of the two main types of electron microscope and their function.

- Aberrations seen in electron microscope images and how they are overcome.

- How images can be recorded.

- The specific preparatory requirements for samples requiring electron microscopy.

- The application of transmission and scanning electron microscopy in the field of biomedical science and examples of their use in pathological evaluation.

15.1 Introduction

Microscopy is a means to examine objects smaller than can be seen using the natural optical capacity of the human eye. Because tissues are made of microscopic units, i.e. cells, and extracellular macromolecular matrices that help bind them together, the study of both normal tissues and the pathological changes that accompany them in disease or injury is dependent on microscopy. There are, of course, several different kinds of microscopy and related histological techniques reviewed in this volume. Electron microscopy allows higher magnification than other types of microscopy and is responsible for the discovery and detailed description of most subcellular organelles. This chapter describes electron microscopy, specifically covering the principles of how electron microscopes work and the differences between light and electron microscopes. The requirements for fixation, processing and, where needed, sectioning of tissues for electron microscopy will be highlighted. Finally, case studies will be given of how electron microscopy is used in diagnostic histopathology.

A video demonstrating the concepts of sample preparation, insertion and imaging in the electron microscope for examination can be found on the book's accompanying website: www.oup.com/uk/orchard2e

15.2 General introduction to electron microscopy

Electron microscopes (EMs) are important diagnostic tools able to screen human tissues at very high magnification. This type of microscope uses electrons to illuminate a specimen and create an enlarged image; as will be explained below, they have much greater resolving power than light microscopes and as a result can be used to achieve much higher magnifications. There are types of EM that can magnify specimens up to two million times, although most diagnostic EMs magnify to approximately 500,000 times. Although it is theoretically possible to make a light microscope with optics capable of high magnification, the lack of resolving power in even the best such optical systems limits their effective magnification to ×1000. The reason for this is not the physical construction of the microscope but the limit imposed by the physics of light and its interaction with lenses.

There are two main kinds of EM, the transmission EM and the scanning EM. The main difference between these two types of microscope is that TEM is used to look at sections of samples, or naturally very thin/small samples, whilst SEM is used to image the surface and so can handle bulky samples of a size that is only limited by the microscope sample chamber size, although typically, samples are only a few millimetres across. A comparison of imaging by light microscopy, SEM and TEM of equivalent samples is shown in Figure 15.1.

Both kinds of EM are relatively large pieces of equipment and generally stand alone in small, specially designed rooms. Most TEMs will stand over two metres in height and two metres in width. SEMs are generally not as tall but still occupy a substantial floor space. Both types are heavy and TEMs may require floor reinforcement. Most commonly, they are located in a basement laboratory where vibration is minimized and local electrical fields need to be monitored prior to installation to ensure that they do not interfere with imaging. Anti-vibration mountings may be required, depending on local conditions, as vibration can affect the operation of the microscope. Separate pumping units, compressor tanks, power supplies and water chillers also have to be housed in close proximity to these microscopes.

Trained personnel are required to operate EMs. As will be seen, they operate at high voltages, under high vacuum, and using many electrical systems. Damage can easily be done to the instrument or the sample if the operator is not fully trained in its use.

New EMs are expensive (£200,000–300,000) and require maintenance contracts to ensure they run efficiently. Along with the need for trained operators, this generally makes EM an expensive service to provide. However, there are multi-user units in research laboratories that can offer the service for a trained EM pathologist to use, which can reduce the costs considerably compared with a dedicated pathology unit.

(a) 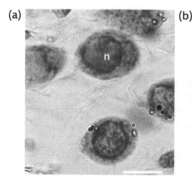   (b) 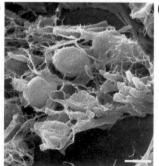   (c)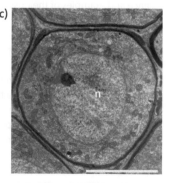

FIGURE 15.1
Comparative microscopy of nerve cells. a) Wax section of the spiral ganglion of the cochlea stained using the Nissl method to show the cytoplasm and nucleus of the nerve cell. b) SEM of a dewaxed spiral ganglion section, dried and coated with gold. The nerve cell surfaces are seen but little detail inside them. c) TEM of an ultrathin section of a spiral ganglion nerve cell. A considerable amount of detail is visible, even at low magnification. n = nucleus. Scale bars: a, b = 10 μm, c = 5 μm.

An EM can be used to examine the surfaces or internal structures of biological materials such as microorganisms, cells or tissues. This is the main use for them and is the area to be discussed in this chapter. Other things that can be examined by EM include metals and crystalline structures, and the elemental composition of samples. EMs can be used in manufacturing (e.g. the production of silicon chips) or in forensics for examining samples such as gunshot residues. In quality control, EMs can be used to look for stress lines in engine parts or simply to check the ratio of air to solids in ice cream.

15.2.1 Why can electron microscopes magnify objects more than a light microscope?

All microscopes are designed to reveal details in objects that are too small to be visualized clearly with the naked eye. The critical property of a microscope is its resolution: this is defined as the smallest gap that can be observed between two objects in a sample and this establishes the amount of detail that can be seen. No matter how much magnification is applied, if the gap between two objects is too small to be resolved, the image will look fuzzy and unclear. As discussed in the chapter on light microscopy, resolution can be calculated by the equation $R = 0.6\ \lambda/NA$, where R is resolution, λ is the wavelength of the radiation and NA is the numerical aperture of the lens (see Chapter 14). Whilst NA is critical in this calculation, lenses can be manufactured to have very small NAs, so clearly the ultimate limiting factor is the wavelength of the illumination used.

In a light microscope where the NA may be 1.4 and the wavelength of light may be 500 nm, maximum resolution will be about 200 nm. This means that if the gap between structures is less than 200 nm it is difficult to visualize them as separate items. This does not preclude the observation of objects smaller than 200 nm, however. If a sub-resolution object is labelled with a fluorescent dye, for instance using an immunocytochemical technique, it can be visualized as a light source. Modern developments in fluorescence microscopy using specialized laser-based optical techniques derived from confocal microscopes have produced new, super-resolution microscopes where resolutions down to 50 nm or less can be achieved. At present, these very specialist microscopes are not readily available to the pathologist and are even more expensive to buy and maintain than EMs. Thus EMs remain the best way to achieve resolutions sufficient to visualize the ultrastructure of cells and tissues. As the limiting factor in the system is the wavelength of the light used in the microscope, to achieve better resolution, and thus be able to see smaller objects, illuminating radiation of a shorter wavelength needs to be used.

Electrons are sub-atomic particles that possess dual particle–wave natures. They can be generated from a filament of wire carrying a current and condensed into a beam that can be made to accelerate by means of a high voltage. In 1924, De Broglie used the mathematical equation $\lambda = 0.1\sqrt{150/V}$, where λ is the wavelength of the radiation and V is the accelerating voltage, to show that electrons in a beam accelerated by 60,000 V have wavelengths of 0.005 nm, higher voltages producing shorter wavelengths. In practice, in a modern TEM using 100 kV, the wavelength achieved, given the complex engineering of an EM, is about 0.2 nm. This wavelength is 1000× shorter than the 200 nm wavelength of visible light and thus has the potential to allow far better resolution of very fine detail. In an SEM, resolution is determined by the width of the electron beam at focus. With modern technology, this can get down to 0.5 nm in very specialist devices.

In using electrons for microscopy, however, there are a number of difficulties to be overcome. Firstly, unlike light waves, electrons cannot travel far in air; secondly, glass lenses cannot be used to focus an electron beam since the glass would simply stop the electrons. It is thus necessary to evacuate the microscope column to a sufficiently high vacuum that will allow the beam to pass down it, and to focus the beam and the image formed requires electromagnetic lenses. These factors dominate the design of an EM.

Key Points

Using an accelerated electron beam in an appropriately designed microscope has enabled subcellular elements to be examined and visualized.

Why does the use of electrons allow cellular organelles to be visualized in great detail?

15.3 Design of transmission electron microscopes

The two kinds of EM have some similarities, but also differ in a number of ways, and there are some specialized versions in addition to this. Generally, though, the TEM can be seen to be analogous to a compound light microscope with objective lenses and eyepieces designed to form an image after light passes through a thin sample or section (see Box 15.1 for an overview of how a TEM works). The SEM is more analogous to a zoom microscope or dissecting microscope where a whole object (e.g. such as a piece of tissue or an insect) is placed on a stage and viewed by reflected light. These analogies are not perfect and there are hybrid versions as well, but they serve to illustrate the principal differences.

15.3.1 Electron source

A stream of accelerated electrons is generated by an 'electron gun' at the top of the microscope column. By passing current through a tungsten wire filament, a cloud of thermionically emitted electrons can be generated (negatively charged particles produced by heat energy). This cloud of electrons is concentrated and controlled by placing the tip of the filament a carefully determined distance from a cathode shield (the Wehnelt cap) on which a negative charge has been applied. This filament and cathode shield assembly is in turn placed a carefully controlled distance away from an anode plate in the column to which a positive charge is applied (Figure 15.2). The difference in voltage between the cathode and anode is the accelerating voltage of the microscope. Alternative forms of electron generation are becoming increasingly common, such as cold field emission, which produces a more stable beam allowing higher resolution.

This combination of electron cloud generation and charged plates attracting or repelling the negative charge has the effect of producing an accelerated stream of electrons from the electron gun. Most EMs offer a choice of accelerating voltage for use in different situations. In TEMs these are usually from 30 kV to 120 kV. Choice of accelerating voltage can be influenced by a variety of factors, for example:

- Image contrast will decrease as the accelerating voltage increases.
- Image penetration and brightness will increase as the accelerating voltage increases.
- The phosphor screen works more efficiently at higher accelerating voltage (80–100 kV).
- Chromatic aberration (caused by variations in the wavelength of the electrons) decreases with increasing accelerating voltage due to a reduction in inelastic scattering of the incident beam by the specimen.
- The electron gun becomes more sensitive to unwanted particles or vapour in the column as the accelerating voltage increases; this means that more care in the maintenance and operation of the EM has to be taken when selecting higher voltages.

Taking the above factors into consideration, higher voltages are usually selected for use in diagnostic TEM. Commonly, 80–120 kV are used in many institutions and produce images with good resolution, contrast and brightness. If more contrast is required from a sample then an accelerating voltage of 60 kV could be used. Alternatively, if more brightness or penetration is required from a sample then a voltage of 120 kV could be used.

15.3.2 Electromagnetic lenses

The electromagnetic lenses in an EM serve the same purpose as the glass lenses in the light microscope. The strong axial magnetic field generated by passing electrical current through copper wire coils (electromagnetic lens) is able to change the path of the electrons in a beam. The pathway of electrons passing through in the lens is helical, allowing the electron paths to converge or diverge in a

(a)

(b)

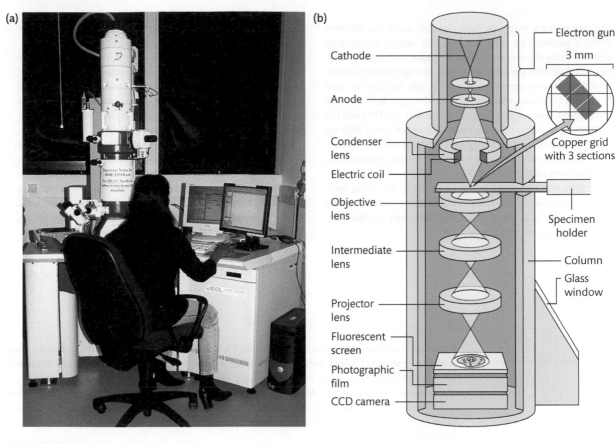

Electron gun

Cathode

3 mm

Anode

Condenser lens

Copper grid with 3 sections

Electric coil

Objective lens

Specimen holder

Intermediate lens

Column

Glass window

Projector lens

Fluorescent screen

Photographic film

CCD camera

FIGURE 15.2
a) An example of a typical TEM and b) a cutaway diagram of a TEM column showing the design and the electron beam path.

way that produces the same effect as light being refracted through a glass lens. Thus electromagnetic lenses behave in a similar way to glass lenses and also suffer from aberrations or defects, such as spherical or chromatic aberrations, in a similar way (see Chapter 14).

BOX 15.1 Overview of how a transmission electron microscope works

Electrons are used as the illuminating energy source in the TEM. These electrons are produced by passing an electrical current through a tungsten filament, much like the filament found in a light bulb. The current heats the filament and results in the emission of electrons that form a cloud around the tip of the filament. This is thermionic emission. The filament is housed in a biased cathode shield, called the Wehnelt cap, at the top of the column. The Wehnelt cap has a small hole at its tip. As the Wehnelt cap is held at a negative charge, the

electrons are repelled and move through the hole. Below the Wehnelt cap is an anode plate, also with a hole in it. The anode plate has a positive charge compared to the Wehnelt cap. This positive charge will attract and accelerate the electrons from the filament down the column as a beam much of which then passes through the hole in the anode plate (see Section 15.3.1).

The electron beam travels down the column through a condenser lens assembly. The lens is a soft iron core surrounded by coils of copper wire through which a current is passed.

This generates a magnetic field through which the electron beam is passed. The magnetic field will deflect the electron beam. Varying the amount of current passed through the copper wire will alter the strength of the lens and therefore alter how much the electron beam is deflected. This can be used to change both magnification and focal length. Unlike a light microscope, there is only one objective lens in a TEM and the current through this lens sets magnification of about 100× up to about 350,000× depending on the model of microscope. The condenser lens assembly focuses the electron beam onto the specimen (see Section 15.3.2).

Samples are introduced into the column by mounting them into a metal holding rod. This rod is placed in an air lock on the side of the column. Once the air lock has been pumped out, the sample is eased into the column.

Objective lenses then form a primary image that is further magnified by the projector lens system.

The final image is visualized on a fluorescent screen (see Section 15.3.6). Below the screen is a camera system that can be used to photograph the sample. More commonly now, a digital camera is used to capture images, which can be seated in the same place as the photographic plate, or mounted on the side of the column (see Section 15.3.9).

As the passage of electrons is blocked by molecules in the air, the entire microscope column is held to a high vacuum (see Section 15.3.7). The column also needs to be cooled by water, as the diffusion pump that maintains the high vacuum, the generation of the electron beam, and the electromagnetic lenses all produce considerable amounts of heat that will affect the performance of the EM (see Section 15.3.8).

15.3.3 Chromatic aberration

A glass lens can produce coloured fringes around the edge of the lens due to the slightly different focal lengths for red and blue light. This can be corrected in the light microscope by compound lenses that have complementary refractive indices or by using monochromatic light.

Chromatic aberration in the EM is produced by slight variations in the energy of individual electrons within the electron beam. Any variance in the accelerating voltage of individual electrons or variance in the current applied through the lens coils will produce variation in the focal length of individual electrons through the lens.

Prevention of chromatic aberration in the EM is achieved by tight control of the stability of the high-voltage supply to the electron gun and of the electrical power supply to the objective lens. A stable power supply should limit or prevent most variation in the energy of individual electrons.

15.3.4 Spherical aberration

Spherical aberration is the failure of a lens to focus all incident beams from a point source into a point. This is usually due to the outer part of a lens having a different strength from the inner part. In a glass lens this is corrected at the same time as is chromatic aberration by using a compound lens combining lenses of complementary properties.

In the EM this can only be corrected by using apertures or 'round holes' that only allow electron beams to pass through that have crossed the central axis of the lens. This avoids or selects out the electrons that have been adversely influenced by the edges of the lens.

15.3.5 Astigmatism

Any asymmetry of the magnetic field within the electromagnetic lens will produce astigmatism of an image. This occurs when a point image has two focal lines due to different lens strengths in two directions at right angles to each other. This aberration is generated during manufacture of the magnetic lens and can be corrected by applying a compensating field to a level where the resolution of the image is no longer affected. Build-up of dirt in the lens through use will also affect the circularity of the lens and produce a varying astigmatism. For this reason, of all the aberrations seen in an EM, astigmatism must be checked for and corrected on a regular basis on each specimen to ensure a well-focused image. Groups of stigmator coils surrounding the lens allow it to be corrected electromagnetically to compensate for the astigmatism.

15.3.6 Viewing screen

The viewing screen is a phosphor screen at the base of the microscope column designed to visualize the electron beam. Without a viewing screen, the electron beam is invisible to the eye and no image can be observed. When electrons hit the phosphor screen, individual particles in the screen fluoresce to produce visible light of varying intensities that are determined by the electron transparency of individual parts of the sample. Where no electrons hit the screen, no fluorescence is seen. In this way, the 'shadow image' of the specimen can be examined.

The viewing screen can be observed by the microscopist through a thick glass window at the base of the column, allowing the operator to see the large fluorescent screen. The latter is usually flat with respect to the orthogonal of the electron beam so that the image is undistorted. However, there is usually a central portion in the viewscreen that can be raised to a 45° angle (in some models, there is a separate small screen that can be brought into the path of the beam). The observer can look at this small screen using a pair of binoculars, and so focus the microscope.

A high-quality screen can also be imaged with a digital camera to allow live imaging on a computer monitor and acquisition of images through appropriate software.

15.3.7 Vacuum system

The electron beam can only pass down the microscope column if the stream of electrons is not impeded. Any gas molecules (i.e. atmospheric air) will interfere with and block the passage of electrons and prevent an image being formed. To stop this occurring, the microscope column must be maintained under a vacuum less than 10^{-5} torr. This is often achieved by a combination of rotary and diffusion pumps. Modern EMs may use turbo pumps or ion pumps as an alternative.

Awareness of this vacuum requirement is necessary as it places operational requirements on examining samples in the EM. For example:

- When switching the EM on and off, time must be allowed for the necessary vacuum to be achieved before an electron beam can be generated.

- A specimen has to be introduced into the microscope column via an airlock so air is not introduced into the column.

- Specimens must be dehydrated thoroughly before entry into the column otherwise water or liquid molecules will be drawn off by the strong vacuum and may contaminate the column with charged particles that can subsequently interfere with electron beam generation. Contamination created this way can:
    - reduce the life of the filament in the electron gun
    - become positively or negatively charged and inappropriately attract the electron beam, producing unwanted flickering/movement of the beam
    - create distortion of the image by astigmatism
    - cause deposition of material on the section, obscuring the detail.

15.3.8 Cooling system

The electromagnetic lenses will generate heat as a by-product of their action. This heat can produce instability in the action of the lenses and can also produce thermal expansion of metal components around the lenses, which can adversely affect the generation of a well-focused image. To prevent these undesired effects the lenses are water-cooled. This is simply achieved by passing water pipes around and through the electromagnetic lenses. Water is pumped through these pipes continuously via a cooling unit that chills the circulating water to a predetermined temperature (usually 18–20°C).

15.3.9 Recording images

Permanent images of the sample under investigation may need to be generated. This can be important because:

- These images provide a record of what was seen when the sample was examined—this can be accessed whenever necessary and the same information can be seen, which is of value when previous patient results need to be reviewed.

- Permanent images can easily be looked at by many people in locations away from the EM (e.g. when cases need to be reviewed by external experts or by groups).

- Permanent images are a good source of illustration of normal cellular structures and specific pathological features.

15.3.10 Photographic imaging

Most EMs manufactured prior to the year 2000 had a photographic plate camera assembly directly beneath the phosphor screen. This screen has a smaller screen within it that can be lifted to expose the photographic plate containing a negative sheet. When the electrons forming the image (previously seen on the phosphor screen) hit the negative sheet, the silver halide grains react with the electrons and record the image. This negative sheet then must be chemically processed before it is used to produce a photographic print (micrograph).

Key Points

To *expose* a negative sheet or photographic paper means to allow silver halide grains in the sheet to react with light, capturing the image on the medium. In an EM, electrons impinge directly on the negative and interact with it to produce silver grains in a similar way.

When the negative sheet or photographic paper is *developed* the silver grains that have reacted with light or electrons are converted to a permanent black metallic silver. In a negative, the image can be seen in which the black and white parts of are reversed, and when projected onto photographic paper and developed, the negative is reversed to a positive.

The negative or photographic paper is then *fixed* to remove all unexposed, unreacted silver halide grains to prevent further reaction with light, which would gradually destroy the image.

Until the negative sheets or photographic paper have been fixed and developed they are stored in light-tight cassettes or handled in a room illuminated by a safelight (i.e. darkroom). A safelight gives out a defined spectrum of light that will not react with the silver halide crystals in the negative film or paper. The type of safelight required is dictated by the type of negative film or paper used.

Photographic negatives (micrographs) produce high-quality images. However, there are many drawbacks to them, making their use less popular nowadays. For example:

- Developing and printing takes time (up to 24 hours) to produce a set of photographic prints once a sample has been examined in the EM—this is a significant additional delay.

- Developing and printing requires chemicals that can present a health and safety hazard, and needs safety assessment and control.

- There are a decreasing number of manufacturers of sheets suitable in size for TEM—this means it is expensive and the long-term supply must be in doubt.

- Digital images are now necessary for publication, and they also lend themselves to rapid transfer via the internet if they need to be sent to another centre for a second opinion. Digitizing negatives is an extra layer of complication and can result in loss of detail.

15.3.11 Digital imaging

An increasing number of EMs now use digital imaging to produce a permanent record. Digital cameras produce an image that can be stored directly on a hard drive and are ready for assessment and examination immediately. They are of a high quality and are more than adequate for diagnostic purposes, although the resolution is less than photographic negatives. The quality of digital images is dictated by the quality of the camera system (see also Box 15.2). The more pixels the camera uses to capture the image, the better the final image. Currently, typical digital camera systems use between one and 16 megapixels.

Digital cameras can be mounted on the side of the column, entering beneath the specimen but above the viewing chamber. These camera systems use a smaller fluorescent screen that enters the electron beam and directs the image produced to the camera lens.

Alternatively, a digital camera can be mounted at the bottom of the column, usually in place of a traditional photographic plate camera assembly. In these camera systems the camera lens receives the electron image by raising the fluorescent screen previously used for photographic exposure.

The image captured by the digital camera is displayed on a computer monitor. This can be viewed as a live image and it will move if the specimen is moved. In most systems this live image will then be integrated into a final image. Integration is where multiple frames of the same region are overlaid to produce a final image of better quality—one that is sharper and clearer. This image can then be stored as a file on a hard drive, server or disk. The resolution can also be improved by auto-montaging, where the digital imaging software controls the microscope to move the sample around and take a sequence of overlapping images. The software will then stitch the images together to provide a large-format image which can be resampled to high resolution in appropriate photographic software. Once a digital image has been acquired, it is possible to measure organelles and ultrastructural features or annotate the images.

BOX 15.2 Some things to consider about digital images

It is not considered appropriate to manipulate an image prior to evaluation and assessment for diagnostic purposes. For example, if an image has had its contrast altered or blemishes removed then there is a potential for diagnostic information to have been lost. It is therefore advised that only raw data are presented for diagnostic evaluation.

The quality of the image is only as good as the quality of the components used in its production. Camera quality has been mentioned. The result will be poor if the image is then printed on ordinary printer paper by a standard printer. Using good-quality photographic printer paper in a good-quality printer will produce far superior results.

Storage of digital images must be considered. The images can take up a lot of storage space and this space must be secure and backed up. Consideration must be given to image security, and how easily digital images may be lost or corrupted. Regardless of the storage method, one must ensure that a reliable back-up system is available (i.e. images can be recovered from back-up servers or portable discs). This is of particular importance for the storage of diagnostic images.

SELF-CHECK 15.2

The passage of electrons is blocked very easily. What impact does this have on the design of the EM?

15.4 Design of scanning electron microscopes

Scanning EM is much less commonly used for diagnostic histopathology, as it is generally limited to viewing only the surface of samples and tells us little about internal structure. Nevertheless, it has an enormous role to play in biological and biomedical research, as well as other materials applications, so it is useful here to briefly summarize how it works.

In a TEM, the electrons of the primary beam pass through the sample, which must be very thin and stained with heavy metals to improve the contrast. An image of organelles and cellular detail is produced with this technique. In an SEM, the electron gun is generally very similar to that of a TEM, but lower accelerating voltages tend to be used, from as low as 0.5 kV to 30 kV. In contrast to TEM, SEM produces images by detecting secondary electrons emitted from a surface due to excitation by the primary electron beam (see Figure 15.3). The electron beam is scanned across the surface of a sample in a raster pattern, and detectors build up an image by mapping the emitted electrons with beam position. Larger whole samples can be imaged by SEM (e.g. entire cells or hair shafts). The lower voltage is better as it reduces the penetration of the sample by the beam, important when trying to image the surface. Clear visual information can then be generated about the surface of a cell or tissue; for example, are there any processes extending from the cell? Is the cellular organization of a tissue normal from an external point of view?

The size of samples requiring SEM examination is determined by the mounting platform in the microscope and the entry door size (which can allow very large samples to be put in). The sample is fixed as for TEM and then gently dehydrated so that the cellular surface is not damaged or destroyed. This can be achieved using alcohol and acetone followed by critical point drying (a technique that overcomes drying damage caused by the surface tension of fluids) or by chemical dehydration in substances such as hexamethyldisilazane (HMDS). The sample should then be coated with a thin layer of metal (e.g. gold or palladium), which keeps the sample dehydrated and also improves the emission of secondary electrons from the tissue surface. The image is recorded by direct acquisition into a PC. Again, as with TEM, this digital acquisition method has gradually replaced photographic film.

(a)

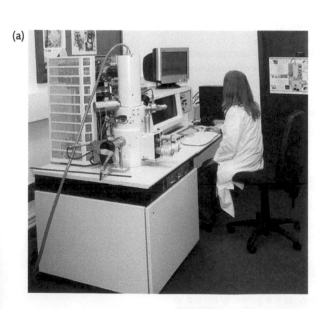

(b)

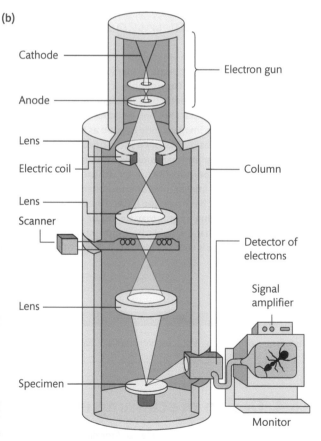

FIGURE 15.3
a) An example of an SEM and b) a cutaway diagram of an SEM column showing the design and the electron beam path.

15.5 Specific tissue preparation for TEM

Preparing tissue for light microscopy and EM is very similar. Each requires aldehyde fixation, dehydration and embedding. For TEM as for LM, this is followed by sectioning and subsequent examination of sections by some form of illumination. However, there are also some significant variations between preparing tissues for light and EM. For SEM, tissue preparation starts similarly but diverges from that for TEM (Figure 15.4).

15.5.1 Fixation

Tissues to be examined in the EM require good fixation to ensure that ultrastructural detail is adequately preserved. A solution of 1–5% glutaraldehyde in a suitable buffer is still considered to be the best primary fixative available for this purpose. Glutaraldehyde contains two aldehyde groups whereas a common related fixative, formaldehyde, contains one aldehyde group. Thus glutaraldehyde will cross-link protein molecules in tissues better than formaldehyde. This is usually combined with a post-fixation solution of osmium tetroxide, which acts on and stabilizes lipid and phospholipid molecules. This combination of the glutaraldehyde acting on proteins and osmium acting on lipids produces a good ultrastructural fixative. Alternative fixation regimes are sometimes used for EM (see Method 15.1 box).

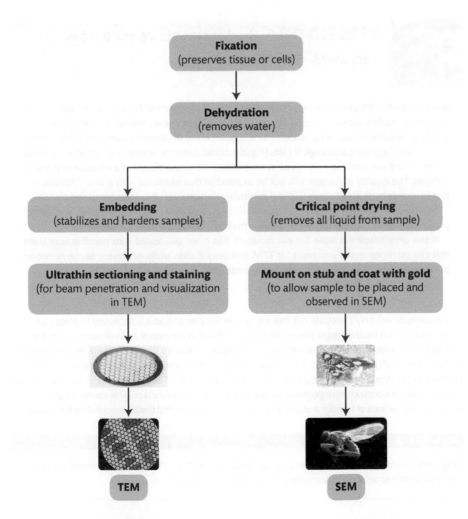

FIGURE 15.4
Tissue preparation for SEM is similar initially but diverges from that for TEM.

METHOD 15.1 Summary of specific tissue preparation for TEM

Tissues requiring TEM need to be suitably fixed to preserve good ultrastructural detail. Glutaraldehyde solutions remain the first choice for diagnostic samples, but they do present significant health and safety concerns (see Health & Safety 15.1). Other fixatives can be used for TEM in specific circumstances (see Method 15.2).

Once tissues have been fixed, they require processing into a support medium suitable for the production of the very thin sections required for examination in the TEM. This involves a secondary fixation stage, dehydration through alcohols, a clearing agent, and impregnation by the support medium. The support medium used for EM is a plastic resin as this provides more support to the tissues than paraffin wax (see Section 15.5.2).

Once tissues have been processed to resin, sections can be prepared from the blocks. Tissue sectioning is performed using a specially designed microtome able to produce the very thin sections required for TEM. Sections are cut at 80-90 nm using a glass or diamond knife, floated out on a waterbath and then mounted on a grid (see Section 15.5.4).

Contrast is introduced to the tissue section by staining with heavy metal solutions. Contrast is necessary to allow visualization of the cellular organelles in the EM (see Section 15.5.6).

METHOD 15.2 Alternative fixation regimes for TEM

A solution of 1–5% glutaraldehyde in buffer is the 'gold standard' for optimum fixation and should be the fixative of choice where possible. However, there may be occasions when the use of glutaraldehyde is not possible. For example, if the decision to carry out TEM is taken after other diagnostic histological tests (e.g. tinctorial stains or immunocytochemistry) have been carried out, and the only tissue available may be already fixed in a solution of formaldehyde. The quality of fixation will not be as good as that obtained with glutaraldehyde but this formaldehyde-fixed tissue will still produce adequate results when examined by TEM.

In situations where the use of glutaraldehyde is prohibited due to its health and safety concerns, solutions of freshly made paraformaldehyde can be used successfully.

If the only tissue available for examination has been processed into paraffin wax then this can be reprocessed into resin for TEM, but only if absolutely necessary as the resulting preservation of ultrastructure is often very poor (see Case studies 15.1 and 15.4).

Glutaraldehyde will only penetrate 1–2 mm into tissue samples and so it is necessary to place only very small pieces in this fixative (larger pieces will remain unfixed in the centre and will continue to degrade through the process of autolysis). Needle biopsy material is suitable for this, or tissue pieces must be sliced carefully into small pieces (1–2 mm^3). It is necessary to be very careful when selecting these small tissue pieces to ensure the diagnostic features of importance are included. For example, in kidney disease, have you sampled renal cortex where glomeruli are found and not renal medulla only? In cancer diagnosis, have you sampled the area of tumour and not an area of remaining normal tissue surrounding the tumour?

SELF-CHECK 15.3

Why are formaldehyde-based fixatives a second choice for TEM? Think about chemical composition and what happens when formaldehyde solutions are stored.

15.5.2 Processing

Once a tissue sample has been fixed adequately it can be processed (embedded) in a suitable support medium. Tissue processing for EM has many similarities to processing tissues for light microscopy.

As noted earlier, only small pieces of tissue can be fixed for TEM because of the limitations of the penetration of glutaraldehyde. The support medium will also only penetrate tissue pieces by 1–2 mm. The tissue sample is first washed in a buffer to remove traces of fixative. This buffer traditionally was a cacodylate formulation, but it contains arsenic, and this has now made its use less popular. Currently phosphate buffers are used more commonly. The tissues are then dehydrated through a series of graduated ethanols and several changes of absolute ethanol, and then they may be immersed in a clearing agent. Suitable clearing agents could include acetone or propylene oxide and provide a link between the alcohol and the support medium selected.

Support media used for TEM are variations of liquid plastic resins. These will impregnate tissues thoroughly and, when polymerized (converted to the solid state), will allow very thin sections of the tissue to be cut. Sections of tissue for examination by TEM need to be extremely thin to allow the electron beam to pass through so that the ultrastructure of the cell and its organelles can be visualized. Sections for light microscopy are usually cut at 4 μm, while sections for TEM are cut around 0.09 μm (90 nm). It is this requirement for such extremely thin sections that dictates the use of a hard plastic resin as the support medium. The paraffin wax used in light microscopy does not provide sufficient support to allow such ultrathin sections to be cut.

There are many different variations of resin available and the selection of which to use will be influenced by the tissue to be processed and the purpose of the ultrastructural investigation. Simple examination of the ultrastructure of tissue (the main use of TEM) will require an araldite or epoxy resin. These are the most widely used and they are excellent for morphological studies, have good cutting properties, and are stable under the electron beam. These resins are not suitable for most immunocytochemistry purposes as they are hydrophobic and will not allow water-based solutions (e.g. antibody preparations) to penetrate and reach cellular components.

The resin is formed by mixing the resin base with a hardener and an accelerator. The purpose of the accelerator is to hasten the conversion of the liquid resin to a fully polymerized (hardened) resin. The hardness of the araldite/epoxy resin used will need to be varied according to the hardness of tissue to be impregnated. For example, bone samples will require a harder polymerized resin than samples of kidney. The hardness of the resin is altered by varying the amount of plasticizer in the resin mix. Suppliers of resins will provide premeasured resin components in the form of kits that are very easy to use and avoid the potential inaccuracies of measuring the component parts. These kits can be purchased to produce soft, medium or hard block consistencies.

An example of a standard processing schedule for TEM suitable for diagnostic tissue samples is given in Method 15.3.

SELF-CHECK 15.4

Why are tissue blocks for EM impregnated with resin and not wax?

HEALTH & SAFETY 15.1

Certain chemicals used in the processing schedule for EM pose significant health and safety concerns that need to be fully understood and assessed before use. Appropriate control measures for these chemicals need to be implemented and used on every occasion to ensure the welfare of all involved in the process:

- *Aldehyde solutions*: workers can be exposed to aldehyde solutions such as formaldehyde or glutaraldehyde through inhalation or skin contact. Health effects include, but are not limited to, the following:
  - throat and lung irritation
  - asthma and difficulty breathing
  - nasal irritation

— sneezing

— wheezing

— burning eyes and conjunctivitis

— contact and/or allergic dermatitis.

■ Aldehyde-containing solutions should always be handled in a controlled environment such as a safety cabinet, extraction bench or aldehyde-approved fume extraction hood. Gloves and personal protective equipment such as aprons or laboratory coats should be worn to protect against skin exposure.

■ *Osmium tetroxide*: this is an acute poison and is capable of causing serious illness or death very quickly. It is toxic if inhaled, swallowed or absorbed through the skin. Long-term exposure can cause permanent damage to the eyes, including blindness. Contact can lead to allergic skin or respiratory reactions. When handling osmium tetroxide, wear safety glasses and use protective gloves. Work in a well-ventilated area such as a fume cabinet or similar extraction facility. Ensure any spills are cleaned up without delay.

■ *Liquid resin*: all resins when in the liquid form have the capacity to irritate the respiratory system and produce or aggravate allergic skin conditions. They should be handled in a well-ventilated area such as a fume cabinet or similar extraction facility. Gloves resistant to resin should be worn, along with personal protective equipment such as aprons or laboratory coats. Ensure any spills are cleaned up without delay. Hazards associated with resin use are considered to be removed once the resin has polymerized and therefore hard resin blocks are safe to handle. Safe handling, storage, spillage and disposal of all the above chemicals need to be risk-assessed, and safe procedures/protocols put in place before these chemicals are handled. Do not use these chemicals before you are fully familiar with their safe use.

METHOD 15.3 Processing schedule for transmission electron microscopy

- Dissect aldehyde-fixed tissue into 1 mm³ pieces and orientate if necessary—muscle fibres should be cut into rectangular blocks (approx 3 mm long by 1 mm diameter) with the muscle fibres running longitudinally along the length of the rectangle.
- Wash in a phosphate buffer: 2 × 10 minutes.
- Secondary fixation in 1% osmium tetroxide at 4°C: 60 minutes.
- Wash in a phosphate buffer: 2 × 10 minutes.
- Dehydrate through a series of graduated alcohols (50%, 70%, 90%, absolute [×3]): 10 minutes each.
- Impregnate with several changes (×3) of a clearing agent (acetone or propylene oxide): 10 minutes each.
- Slowly impregnate with liquid resin:
  · 50% liquid resin/clearing agent at 37°C: 30 minutes
  · 100% liquid resin at 37°C: 60 minutes
  · 100% liquid resin at 37°C: 60 minutes.
- Embed the tissue in suitably shaped and sized moulds labelled to allow identification.
- Polymerize the tissue blocks at a temperature suitable for the resin (usually 70–80°C) and for a length of time suitable to produce hard blocks (approx. 16 hours, usually overnight).

15.5.3 Immunocytochemistry on ultrathin resin-embedded sections

There may be situations in which it would seem desirable to use antibody labelling techniques to identify specific morphological features at the ultrastructural level.

In this technique, tissue is fixed appropriately and processed into a hydrophilic resin (see Fixation and Processing later in this Section). Sections are then prepared and an antibody labelling technique applied to the section. The labelling techniques are similar to those used on paraffin wax sections (see Chapters 6 and 7) except that the final antibody layer applied to the section is usually labelled with colloidal gold rather than a coloured label. Colloidal gold is a solution of gold particles of a uniform and defined size, and different sizes can be obtained from suppliers. The gold particles completely block the electron beam and will act as a label for the antibody bound to the tissue. Immunogold labelling for two different antigens is illustrated in Figure 15.5. The gold appears as small, round, black particles.

This technique is not widely used in diagnostic histopathology because it is difficult to reconcile the need for good ultrastructural morphological preservation (fixation) while maintaining tissue antigenicity. Therefore, immunoelectron microscopy techniques are largely confined to research institutions.

If immunocytochemistry is to be attempted on ultrathin sections then fixation, processing and resin selection must be considered.

Fixation

Glutaraldehyde tends to alter antigenic sites in the tissue more than paraformaldehyde, reducing the effectiveness of the immunocytochemical technique. Therefore, a compromise is made that provides both reasonable ultrastructural preservation and good antigenicity so that antibodies still bind. Many fixatives use varying proportions of a solution of paraformaldehyde, with or without other additives, but fixative choice must be determined on an individual basis. Osmium tetroxide should also be avoided as a secondary fixative as this, too, will affect antigenic sites in the tissue.

Processing

Once preserved in a suitable fixative, the tissue will need to be dissected into 1 mm³ pieces and processed through graduated ethanols, as previously described. The instructions supplied with the resin selected should be studied and followed carefully because the hydrophilic resins used for ultrastructural immunocytochemistry usually only require the tissue to be dehydrated as far as 70% alcohol before being impregnated with the resin. The tissue should not be treated with clearing agents such as acetone or propylene oxide.

(a)
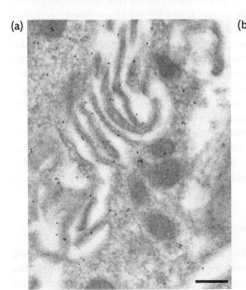
(b)
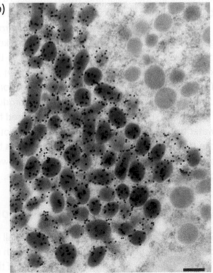

FIGURE 15.5
a) Immunogold labelling of a membrane protein in the hearing organ (cochlea). The particles of gold can be seen lying on the membrane. b) Immunogold labelling of insulin granules in pancreatic tissue. Scale bars A = 100 nm, B = 200 nm. (Image b Courtesy Tracey de Haro)

Resin selection

Hydrophilic resins must be used to allow water-based antibody solutions to penetrate the resin and bind with tissue elements. Hydrophobic resins used for standard transmission EM (e.g. araldite CY212) are less suitable for immunocytochemistry. This resin will not permit penetration of water-based solutions into the section and the processing of tissues into this resin will destroy or irreversibly block antigenic sites. Several hydrophilic resins available commercially are suitable for immunocytochemistry (e.g. the acrylic resins LR White and LR Gold or Lowicryl). LR White and LR Gold are blends of hydrophilic and acrylic monomers that penetrate tissue rapidly because of their low viscosity. LR Gold is cured (polymerized) by ultraviolet light in the cold, while LR White can be cold-cured, using an accelerator, or heat-cured. Lowicryl is a highly cross-linked acrylate- and methacrylate-based embedding medium designed for use over a wide range of embedding conditions, but embedding is performed using frozen tissue and resin infiltration at low temperature. If these resins are to be used then care must be taken with the processing of tissues prior to impregnation. Consult the data sheet or information provided by the resin manufacturer for advice about suitable processing schedules.

SELF-CHECK 15.5

Why are tissues fixed in glutaraldehyde and processed into araldite resin generally not suitable for immunoelectron microscopy?

15.5.4 Sectioning

To examine tissue by TEM, very thin sections must be cut from the resin-embedded blocks. These sections must be thin enough to allow the electron beam to interact with, and pass through, the cellular constituents of the tissue to produce the shadow image seen on the fluorescent screen. If the sections are too thick then the electron beam will be blocked and no image will be seen.

Thin sections are prepared on an ultramicrotome (Figure 15.6), which is very similar in principle to the rotary microtomes used to cut paraffin wax sections. There are, however, some important differences.

Ultramicrotomes use glass or diamond knives to cut tissue sections

The steel knives used in a rotary microtome to cut paraffin wax blocks are not sharp enough to produce good-quality sections of the thinness required for examination in the TEM. Glass knives are broken along the molecular line, which produces a far sharper knife edge and allows thinner sections to be cut. Diamond knives can also be made with a sharp edge, by grinding and polishing the diamond.

Glass knives are produced in the laboratory from a glass strip carefully scored and broken into triangular pieces by a commercial machine. These knives have to be used quickly because the knife edge degrades as the molecular structure adapts to the break, making the knife unsuitable for use. Glass knives can only be used to cut a limited number of sections before the quality of the knife edge is lost. This means that a new knife should be used for each block cut. Glass knives are cheap and easy to produce, however, and are suitable for the production of semithin and ultrathin sections.

Diamond knives (Figure 15.6) are purchased from suppliers and are permanently mounted into a water trough. The diamond knife edge does not suffer the degradation seen with the glass knife and can be used hundreds of times before it needs to be replaced. Such knives are particularly suited to the preparation of serial ultrathin sections. However, diamond knives are very expensive and should only be used by experienced ultramicrotomists.

Waterbaths are mounted directly onto the knife

Sections cut on an ultramicrotome are so small and thin that they cannot be handled as you would paraffin wax sections. By mounting a waterbath onto the knife, the sections are cut and immediately float on water without having to be handled. If there is a need to manipulate the sections then a fine

(a)
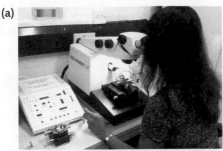

(b)
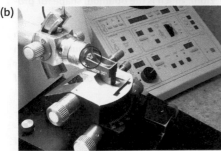

(c)
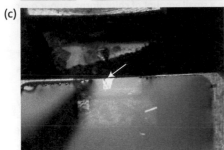

FIGURE 15.6
a) An ultramicrotome in use. The resin block is being trimmed with the aid of the microtome's binoculars. b) The location of the diamond knife after alignment to the block face. c) The cutting edge of a diamond knife viewed down the microtome binoculars, with a gold-coloured section that has just been taken floating on the surface of water in the knife's waterbath. The area in c is within the ring in b.

mounted filament (e.g. an eyelash that is glued onto the end of a cocktail stick) is ideal. When the resin sections float on the surface of the water, the overhead light illuminating the waterbath is refracted through the sections and is split into its constituent colours depending on the thickness of the section. Therefore, the thickness of each section can be assessed by its colour (blue/green 0.5 µm, gold 90 nm) when floating on the surface of the water (Figure 15.6).

Optical binoculars are mounted directly above the sectioning area

Sections cut on an ultramicrotome are so small that the cutting stage needs to be magnified to allow the operator to see the cutting operation and the sections being produced. This optical binocular system also includes various light sources to provide overhead fluorescent illumination and also a backlight source to aid alignment of the block to the knife. A typical cutting process is detailed in Method 15.4.

SELF-CHECK 15.6

At what thickness are ultrathin sections cut, and why is this important?

15.5.5 Choice of grids

Ultrathin tissue sections, when cut, must be picked up and supported by something that will allow the electron beam to pass through. Glass and plastics will block the path of the electron beam and so no image will be seen on the fluorescent screen. Traditionally, sections are picked up on copper, aluminium or nickel grids with a line spacing designed to allow a varying percentage of the electron beam to pass through (Figure 15.4). Choice of grid type is largely down to personal preference, but immunogold procedures require the use of nickel grids.

METHOD 15.4 Cutting protocol

- Lock the resin block into the ultramicrotome.
- Secure a new glass knife into the knife holder and lock it so that the knife is very close to the face of the resin block.
- Advance the knife in small amounts (1 μm each) and trim away the excess resin from the surface of the block until the resin-embedded tissue is exposed.
- Replace with a new knife mounted with a waterbath. Fill with clean distilled water until the fluorescent light is seen to reflect on the surface of the water.
- Cut 6–8 semithin survey sections by advancing the block to the knife by 0.5 μm each time. The sections should appear blue/green in colour.
- Transfer each section to a drop of distilled water on a glass slide. Dry the section by placing on a hotplate.
- Stain with 1% toluidine blue in 1% borax for approximately 30 seconds. Wash off with distilled water and allow the slide to dry. Coverslip and mount using a DPX mountant.
- Examine using a light microscope to identify the area of interest.
- Compare the surface of the resin block with the toluidine blue-stained section and cut away the excess resin and tissue with a sharp new steel blade, leaving only the area of

interest in a raised plateau. This should ideally be cut in the shape of a trapezium, which is the optimum shape for production of a ribbon of sections.
- Replace the glass knife with a new one, again mounted with a waterbath, or with a diamond knife with in-built waterbath if you have one. Fill the bath with clean, fresh distilled water until the fluorescent light is seen to reflect on the surface of the water.
- Using the motorized advance, cut a ribbon of ultrathin sections (10–12 sections) at a thickness of 90–100 nm. The sections should appear gold when floating on the surface of the water. Wave a small amount of chloroform vapour over the sections (this can be done using a cotton bud dipped in the chloroform). This results in them spreading out flat.
- Inspect the sections for quality, as any scratches, scores or imperfections will be magnified in the EM. Change glass knives and recut as necessary.
- Pick up the ultrathin sections onto a grid. This is achieved by holding the grid in a pair of fine-tipped forceps and immersing the grid under the surface of the water. Lift the grid out of the water at an angle of 45° underneath the ribbon, allowing the sections to fall across the centre of the grid.
- Allow the grids to dry in a dust-free environment.

There are slot and spot/hole grids of different sizes, which need to be coated with a thin film of plastic (e.g. formvar) before use. They can be tricky to use as the sections must be mounted accurately along the slot or spot, but they have the advantage that all of the tissue section can be examined in the microscope.

The most common choice of grid is a mesh grid, composed of a mesh of copper bars across the grid that offer support to the tissue section. Grids are available with mesh sizes and bar widths. More bars and wider grid bars offer more support to the section, which can be of benefit for fragile tissues, but they obscure more of the tissue section from view (the electron beam is blocked by the copper grid bars). In some grids up to 50% of the tissue section is unavailable for examination. A good compromise between tissue support and availability of the section for examination is to use a 200 mesh grid with thin grid bars.

SELF-CHECK 15.7

Why do we not pick up ultrathin sections on a glass slide?

15.5.6 Staining

In order to visualize cellular components in the TEM the tissue must be 'stained' to impart contrast. Heavy metal solutions are used commonly as they bind to cellular components and selectively block the electron beam. Double staining with uranyl and lead solutions is often employed as they are easy to prepare and use and they produce reliable results. Uranyl salts bind with nucleic acids and proteins, while lead salts are thought to bind with the osmium tetroxide bound to phospholipids in the cell.

Many variations of uranyl acetate can be used. Both alcoholic and aqueous solutions of varying concentration have been used successfully but probably the most widely employed is saturated uranyl acetate in 50–70% ethanol solution. Aqueous solutions tend to require longer staining times and are prone to producing a precipitate on the tissue section.

There are also many variations of lead stain that can be used, including aqueous lead hydroxide and alkaline solutions of lead salts. The alkaline lead solutions tend to stain faster and are less likely to produce contamination than are aqueous lead hydroxide solutions. By far the most commonly used lead stain is the lead citrate method published by Reynolds (see Method 15.5).

When staining with uranyl and lead salts, care must be taken at all times to prevent contamination and precipitation on the tissue section. Uranyl salts are photolabile so exposure to light will cause deposition of uranyl crystals on the tissue section. Lead salts will react with the smallest amount of carbon dioxide to form insoluble lead carbonate. This produces a fine precipitate on the tissue section. These contaminants and precipitates cannot be seen by the naked eye but they appear immense under the EM. In order to prevent this contamination, always:

- use spotlessly clean equipment when staining
- rinse in ultrapure water or cooled freshly boiled distilled water
- stain grids with uranyl salts in the dark
- stain grids with lead salts in the presence of sodium hydroxide pellets to remove carbon dioxide from the surrounding air.

HEALTH & SAFETY 15.2

- All lead stains are cumulative poisons.
- Uranyl stains are radioactive and toxic.

When using or handling these solutions, care must be taken to work cleanly so you do not expose yourself or others around you unintentionally to the staining solution. Only make up small volumes of the solution that will be used within a reasonable amount of time (e.g. 50 mL, and store in a suitable, preferably airtight container). Solutions should be centrifuged or filtered before use. A 50 mL syringe is a convenient storage vessel as it remains airtight as the solution contained within reduces through use, and it can have a filter attached. Dispensing droplets of solution from the syringe is also easy to achieve, while limiting exposure to yourself. Wear gloves and a laboratory coat when staining grids or preparing the solution, and work in a fume cabinet or hood. Wash used glassware in water before sending for washing. The solutions and staining procedure should be risk-assessed by the local institution prior to use and a method of safe working written. Ensure that you have read and understood these assessments before following the staining protocol.

 ## METHOD 15.5 *Lead citrate*

Reynolds' lead citrate: Mix 1.33 g lead nitrate and 1.76 g sodium citrate with 30 mL distilled water in a 50 mL flask. Mix for 30 minutes to ensure complete conversion of lead nitrate to lead citrate. Add 8 mL N sodium hydroxide and make up to 50 mL with distilled water. The resulting colourless solution is stable for six months in a stoppered bottle and should be centrifuged or filtered through a 0. 25 μm Millipore filter before use.

An alternative to Reynolds' lead citrate that can be made up quickly and used on the day of staining is to dissolve 0.1–0.4 g of lead citrate directly into 10 mL of distilled water by the addition of concentrated NaOH (typically it will take 250 to 500 μL of 4 N NaOH to completely dissolve the lead citrate).

A typical staining method is given in Method 15.6.

If the ultrathin sections fall off the grid during staining then adherence can be improved by drying the sections on the grid for longer or at higher temperature. Place the grids to be stained in a 60–70 °C oven for 10–20 minutes and then continue with the staining protocol.

SELF-CHECK 15.8

Why are heavy metals used as stains for EM?

15.6 Preparation for SEM

Although the primary diagnostic form of EM used is TEM, it is worth considering, briefly, how samples are prepared for SEM. The fixation is typically the same, glutaraldehyde followed by osmium tetroxide at similar concentrations and durations. As it is primarily the surface that is to be observed, penetration of the tissue by the fixatives is less important, so larger pieces can be used. In addition, the SEM allows for larger samples to be placed in the vacuum chamber.

After fixation, samples for SEM are dehydrated, as for TEM, but they do not need to be sectioned. Thus, after osmification, they are dehydrated in a graded ethanol series and all liquid removed. The removal of liquid is typically performed using critical point drying. In this method, the sample is placed into a pressure chamber connected to a cylinder of liquid carbon dioxide. The chamber is then sealed, and the CO_2 introduced at high pressure so that it remains liquid. Over a period of time, the CO_2 is exchanged several times, replacing the ethanol, and the chamber is heated up to 34 °C which is just above the critical point of CO_2 where it turns to gas without boiling. The liquid is gently vaporized, minimizing distortion, although there can be significant shrinkage in this process.

Once dry, the sample is mounted on aluminium stubs designed to fit into the particular make of SEM and coated with a layer of gold (typically) in a sputter coater, in order to make sure the sample emits enough electrons to form a good image. The coater has a vacuum chamber in which the sample on its stub is placed, then the air is evacuated and replaced with a low pressure atmosphere of argon. The chamber also contains a gold target in its top. By applying a high voltage from the floor of the chamber to the gold target, ionized argon bombards the target, displacing gold atoms which are deposited on the sample. The sample can then be imaged in the SEM.

This basic technique can be modified in various ways to produce higher quality results depending on the resolution of the SEM (the gold can be seen as 'crazy-paving' in high resolution SEMs), for example by using platinum/palladium coating or an osmium impregnation technique which eliminates the need for sputter coating.

Scanning electron microscopy can be combined also with immunogold for labelling of surface antigens. In this case normal gold coating cannot be used, and it is best to use a different kind of detector to image the samples, which increases the contrast between gold particles and other coatings.

METHOD 15.6 *Staining method using saturated uranyl acetate in 50% ethanol and Reynolds' lead citrate*

- Gently rinse grid in 50% ethanol.
- Float grid, section down, on a droplet of freshly filtered saturated uranyl acetate in 50% ethanol formed on a sheet of dental wax for 4–8 minutes (the exact time should be evaluated by the user). Cover with a box or place wax sheet in the dark to prevent precipitation.

- Gently rinse grids in 50% ethanol.
- Gently rinse grids in six changes of ultrapure water or freshly boiled, cooled distilled water for 30 seconds each.
- Float grid, section down, on a droplet of freshly filtered lead citrate solution formed on a sheet of dental wax in

a covered plastic box for 2–4 minutes (exact time should be evaluated by the user). Place a few pellets of sodium hydroxide in the box to prevent precipitate contamination.

- Gently rinse grid in six changes of ultrapure water or freshly boiled, cooled distilled water for 30 seconds each.

- Carefully blot grid dry with filter paper—avoid touching the section.

- Store stained grids in a labelled gridbox until examined.

15.7 Case studies/applications

Although the EM can be used to examine many different structures (e.g. metals, crystals and large molecules), this section will demonstrate some of the major uses of the EM in diagnostic histopathology.

15.7.1 Tumour diagnosis

In the early days of the EM in 1939 it was thought that the high magnification and improved resolution would prove invaluable in facilitating the diagnosis of difficult tumours. This has not proved to be the case as molecular techniques and immunocytochemistry have been shown to be of much greater value. Nonetheless, EM still has a limited role in tumour diagnosis, particularly in poorly differentiated tumours where other techniques fail to provide a definitive diagnosis. The value of EM here is that it can identify organelles present in low numbers and this may indicate the nature of the tumour cells. To do so requires identifying structural features that enable the tissue type to be characterized. (Examples of epithelial and neural tissue characteristics are given in Figures 15.7 and 15.8.)

It can be seen that the demonstration of specific organelles in tumour cells can give an indication of the lineage of the tumour, but not a specific tumour diagnosis. This has a limited value in diagnosis but can be of benefit in those tumours that are proving difficult to identify by, for example, immunocytochemical means. However, EM can be of great value in the diagnosis of some tumour types.

In Case study 15.1, organelles identified as pre-melanosomes were observed in the tumour cells. Pre-melanosomes are the precursors of melanin formation. The granules have not differentiated sufficiently to produce the melanin that would be identified by Masson Fontana staining. No other organelles have this particular structure or appearance so observation of their presence identifies the tumour as a malignant melanoma.

(a)
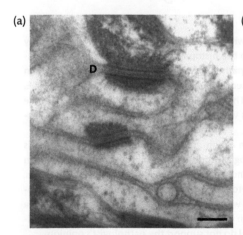
(b)
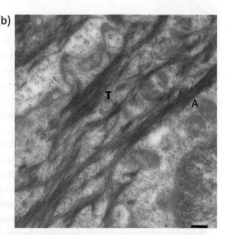

FIGURE 15.7

Characteristic ultrastructural features only seen in epithelial cells. a) Desmosomes (D) and b) tonofilament bundles (T) are seen in large numbers in squamous epithelia only and define this type of cell. If a sample of tumour cells is examined in the EM and well-formed desmosomes and bundles of tonofilaments are seen then it is likely that the tumour is epithelial in origin. Scale bars: a = 50 nm, b = 400 nm. (Courtesy Tracey de Haro)

(a) 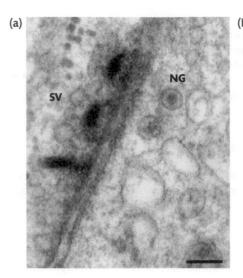   (b)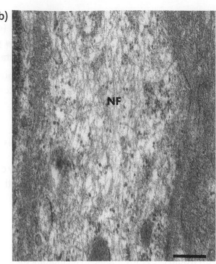

FIGURE 15.8

a) Neurosecretory granule (NG), and b) neurofilaments (NF). These are features usually only seen in neural-type cells in the non-neoplastic state. If these neural organelles are seen in tumour cells then this would indicate that the tumour cells are neural in origin. Scale bars: a = 100 nm, b = 400 nm. (Courtesy Tracey de Haro)

Carrying out EM on this tumour enabled a specific diagnosis to be made, which tinctorial stains and immunocytochemistry alone failed to achieve. A specific diagnosis allows the patient to receive appropriate targeted therapy and prognostic information about the malignancy.

CASE STUDY 15.1 *Malignant melanoma*

A 55-year-old man was admitted to hospital with enlarged tonsils. The tonsils were surgically removed, fixed in formaldehyde and sent to the histopathology department for examination. When the tonsils were dissected by the pathologist a firm white mass was found within the tissue. A sample of this mass was processed to paraffin wax, a section stained with H&E, and sent to the pathologist for assessment. The pathologist identified the tissue within the section to be a malignant tumour. The cells were pleomorphic, spindle-shaped and contained numerous mitoses.

The pathologist thought that this could be a high-grade squamous malignancy which is an epithelial tumour. To confirm, the pathologist requested special stains including Masson Fontana to demonstrate melanin pigment and also a range of immunocytochemical tests. The immunocytochemistry included pan-cytokeratin markers (a positive result would indicate epithelial differentiation). These tests were not helpful as most markers produced a negative result. The negative pan-cytokeratin would indicate that the tumour was not epithelial in origin. Results of the antibody panel do not support the pathologist's opinion.

EM was requested but the only tissue available was already fixed in formaldehyde. Although it was accepted that the ultrastructural preservation would be less than ideal, this formaldehyde-fixed tissue was processed to resin for EM. Examination of sections of this tumour revealed particular ultrastructural features that proved to be diagnostic for malignant melanoma. See Figure 15.9.

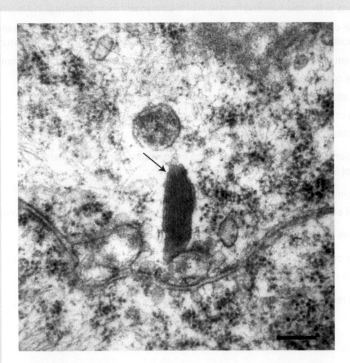

FIGURE 15.9
A pre-melanosome (arrow) in the cytoplasm displaying its characteristic internal structure. Scale bar = 100 nm. (Courtesy Tracey de Haro)

15.7.2 Renal disease

A major use for the EM is in the evaluation of renal disease. Patients suspected of having renal disease will undergo clinical evaluation and assessment. Most will then go on to have a renal biopsy. Together with the clinical evaluation, this biopsy will give a definitive diagnosis of the renal disorder or will stage the progression of the disease.

After the biopsy is taken the tissue is usually immediately divided into three pieces: one is fixed in formaldehyde for evaluation by light microscopy, the second is quickly frozen in liquid nitrogen for immunofluorescence studies, and the remaining piece is fixed in glutaraldehyde for EM.

The piece fixed in formaldehyde is processed to paraffin wax. Sections are taken for H&E staining and tinctorial stains such as methenamine silver, Congo red and PAS (see Chapter 5 on tinctorial stains). Sections can also be taken for immunoperoxidase demonstration of tissue-bound immunoglobulins. The piece of tissue frozen in liquid nitrogen can provide unfixed frozen sections for immunofluorescent demonstration of tissue-bound immunoglobulins. The piece of tissue fixed in glutaraldehyde is processed to resin and sections prepared for examination in the EM.

The glomerulus is the principal structure of the kidney to be examined in detail by the EM. It is composed of a capillary wound up into a ball, held together by mesangial cells and contained within a connective tissue covering known as Bowman's capsule (Figure 15.10) (for further details refer to *Cell structure and function* [Chapter 12] in the *Fundamentals of Biomedical Science* series). The capillary walls, consisting of basement membrane lined by endothelial cells and covered by epithelial cells, are examined for alterations from the 'normal' state.

Features of interest in renal disease include:

- alterations to the thickness (increased or decreased) of the basement membrane (e.g. in diabetes or thin membrane nephropathy)

- alterations to the structure and formation of the basement membrane (e.g. in Alport's disease)
- presence of antibody/antigen immune complexes within the basement membrane and their exact location (e.g. systemic lupus erythematosus [SLE] or membranous glomerulopathy)
- effacement or flattening of the epithelial cell foot processes (e.g. minimal change glomerulopathy)
- presence of tubuloreticular bodies within the endothelial cells (e.g. SLE)
- reduplication of the basement membrane in transplant nephropathy
- sclerosis or fibrosis of areas of the glomerulus
- interposition of mesangial cells.

The mesangium (Figure 15.10) is also examined for variations from the normal state.
Features of interest include:

- increase in mesangial cell numbers (cellular proliferation)
- presence of antibody/antigen immune complexes within the mesangium (e.g. IgA nephropathy).

Other features of interest within the glomerulus might include:

- presence of abnormal structures/proteins (e.g. amyloid)
- abnormal storage of products within cells (e.g. Fabry's disease).

Examples of renal pathology are given in Case studies 15.2 and 15.3.

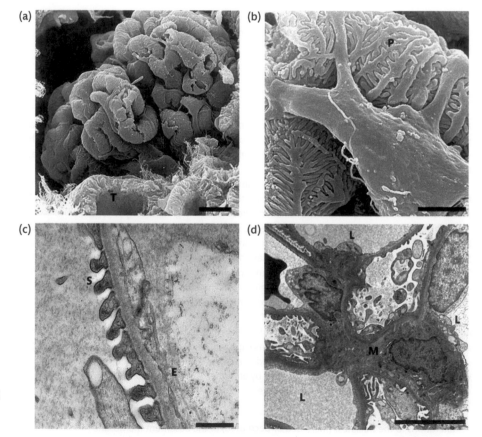

FIGURE 15.10
Ultrastructural features of the glomerulus from Bowman's capsule. a) SEM of a glomerulus stripped from its Bowman's capsule. Tubules can also be seen (T). b) Detail of the tubule surface in SEM. Epithelial cells called podocytes (P) and their 'finger-like' projections can be seen. c) TEM illustrates the slits between the podocyte processes (S). The endothelial cells (E) have a flattened appearance on the inner aspect or lumen of the capillary loop. d) Glomerular mesangium. Mesangial cells and matrix (M) lying between several capillary loops (L). Scale bars: a = 10 µm, b = 1 µm, c = 500 nm, d = 5 µm. (a and b: courtesy Peter Furness; c and d: courtesy Tracey de Haro)

CASE STUDY 15.2 *Membranous glomerulopathy*

A 37-year-old woman presented to the nephrologists with hypertension (blood pressure 172/108 mmHg) and oedema of the legs. She was found to have blood and protein in her urine. Her creatinine clearance was low at 58 mL/min and a 24-hour urine collection revealed 9.7 g protein. The woman underwent a renal biopsy to determine the nature of her condition.

Examination of an H&E-stained section revealed thickened capillary loop basement membranes and a silver stain of a similar area demonstrated spike formation. These features would suggest that there may be deposition of immune complexes within the glomerulus. This was supported by the results of immunofluorescent staining which demonstrated the presence of significant amounts of IgG in the glomeruli.

Examination of the glomeruli by EM confirmed that the glomerular basement membrane was thickened by discrete, well-demarcated, electron-dense immune complexes lying under the epithelial cells (sub-epithelial deposit). The epithelial cells overlying these deposits had effaced and lost their foot processes (Figure 15.11). This picture is quite different from normal where the basement membrane is uniform in thickness and the epithelial cells form well-defined foot processes and filtration slits (see Figure 15.10).

The clinical presentation and features seen in the renal biopsy support a diagnosis of idiopathic membranous glomerulopathy. The pathogenesis of this condition is not fully understood. It is suggested that a likely pathogenesis for idiopathic or primary membranous glomerulopathy involves an autoimmune disease in which circulating autoantibodies

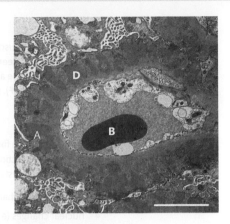

FIGURE 15.11
Glomerular basement membrane (A) containing sub-epithelial electron-dense deposits (D). A red blood cell can be seen lying within the capillary lumen (B). Scale bar = 5 μm. (Courtesy Tracey de Haro)

with specificity for determinants on visceral epithelial cells develop. The autoantibodies cross the glomerular basement membrane and form immune complexes *in situ* in the sub-epithelial zone.

Muscle biopsy

Examination of muscle biopsies by TEM remains an important part of the histological assessment of muscle disorders. Although abnormal features can be identified by TEM, none is specifically diagnostic for muscle disorders. The features seen in the muscle by TEM must be considered with all other histological tests and clinical information before a diagnosis can be made. Normal skeletal muscle ultrastructure, such as sarcomeres, a myocyte nucleus and the sarcoplasmic membrane, is shown in Figure 15.12.

Muscle biopsies can be taken from any of the muscle groups in the body, including those of the eye, but will often be taken from the larger and easily accessible muscles (e.g. quadriceps). The biopsy is taken and a piece snap-frozen in isopentane suspended in liquid nitrogen. This preserves the enzymes in the tissue and permits their demonstration by histochemical techniques. A second piece of muscle will be allowed to relax and is then fixed in glutaraldehyde for examination by TEM.

Sections are prepared from the frozen muscle tissue and stained with H&E. Other frozen sections are stained with Gomori's trichrome and PAS with diastase (see Chapter 5). Histochemical techniques for cytochrome oxidase, succinic dehydrogenase and NADH are carried out to illustrate the enzyme activity in the muscle tissue, as this is known to alter with different muscle disorders. Histochemistry for ATP and immunocytochemistry are carried out to demonstrate muscle fibre type and muscle membrane proteins. Alterations to the accepted 'normal' patterns of staining help to inform the diagnostic process.

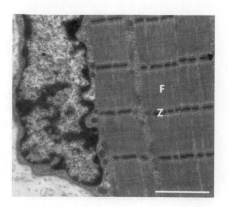

FIGURE 15.12
Normal skeletal muscle. Typical sarcomere formation can be seen with the dark bands of the 'Z-band' (Z) and the actin and myosin filaments running between (F). Scale bar = 5 μm. (Courtesy Tracey de Haro)

The piece of muscle fixed in glutaraldehyde is processed and then embedded such that the fibres run longitudinally in sections taken from the resin block.

Features of interest include:

- mitochondrial changes (e.g. size, shape and internal cristae structure)

- nuclear changes (e.g. location or presence of inclusions)

- alterations in muscle fibre structure (e.g. disruption of z-bands)

- disruption to the order of muscle fibres (e.g. an outer ring of fibres circling at 90° around the inner fibres)

- abnormal product storage (e.g. glycogen or lipid).

However, since ultrastructural features are not of themselves diagnostic, the value of TEM here is to add supporting evidence to be considered with the results of all other techniques and clinical information.

CASE STUDY 15.3 *Myofibrillar myopathy*

A 59-year-old woman presented with a two-year history of waddling gait with weakness in her legs and a tendency to fall easily and often. The woman had a strong family history of heart problems. On examination she was found to have generalized muscle wasting with proximal and distal weakness. An electromyogram (EMG) was reported as myopathic. The woman had a mild sensory loss in her toes, winged scapulae, and paravertebral muscle wasting.

An open muscle biopsy was performed on the woman's right thigh and a piece of skeletal muscle was sent promptly, unfixed and wrapped in a saline-soaked piece of gauze to histopathology. On arrival in the laboratory the tissue was frozen in cooled isopentane and stored in liquid nitrogen for histological and histochemical analysis. A piece of tissue was also immersed in 4% buffered glutaraldehyde for TEM.

Examination of an H&E section showed some variation in fibre size, with occasional small angular fibres present. There was no evidence of necrosis, inflammation or regeneration. Immunocytochemical studies showed no abnormality of fibre type. A Gomori trichrome stain demonstrated areas within the fibres that were more darkly stained than the surrounding myofibrils, indicating an accumulation of protein in the fibres. A COX/SDH histochemical stain showed occasional COX-negative fibres, suggesting a reduction in oxidative enzymes in certain muscle fibres.

EM was performed on the muscle sample after selecting a suitable area for examination from the toluidine blue-stained survey sections. This demonstrated concentric laminate whorls in the subsarcolemmal space of the fibres (Figure 15.13).

The age of the patient and the symptoms, presented together with the histochemical and ultrastructural findings, led to a tentative diagnosis of myofibrillar myopathy.

Myofibrillar myopathies can be hereditary or occur sporadically (spontaneously) and encompass a number of disorders frequently associated with involvement of the heart muscle. The hallmark of myofibrillar disease is the abnormal accumulation of protein in the muscle fibres, which causes progressive weakness. These accumulations are often seen as inclusions on EM. Various types of inclusion have been described, including spheroid bodies, sarcoplasmic bodies, cytoplasmic bodies and granulomatous material.

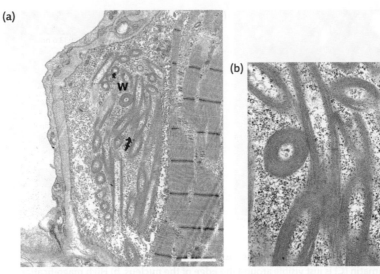

FIGURE 15.13
a) Concentric whorls (W) lying beneath the sarcoplasmic membrane of the muscle fibre.
b) High magnification of the concentric whorls showing the structure of these inclusions.
Scale bars: a = 5 μm, b = 2.5 μm. (Courtesy Tracey de Haro)

15.7.3 Other tissues

All tissue types can be examined by EM (e.g. bone samples, cell preparations, sperm, viruses and bacteria). Some may need specialized preparation techniques, but all can provide information that may aid the diagnostic process or inform the cellular response to a particular stimulus.

CASE STUDY 15.4 *Human papillomavirus in skin*

A 23-year-old patient presented to the dermatologists with a raised, pigmented area on the dorsum of the right little toe. This area was painful, dark blue/grey in colour and associated with subungual hyperkeratosis (hard skin under the toe nail). The dermatologist removed the entire raised area and sent it for histopathology to identify the nature of the lesion.

This tissue was sampled and processed to paraffin wax for light microscopy. An H&E-stained section was prepared and examined. The sample consisted of large amounts of keratin formed from abnormally keratinizing superficial squamous cells. No normal epidermis or dermis was seen. The abnormal squamous cells contained slate-grey intranuclear inclusions and similar cytoplasmic inclusions. The exact nature of the cellular change was unclear, but might have indicated a viral infection.

A small piece of the formalin-fixed tissue was selected for EM. It was accepted that formalin fixation was not the most appropriate for EM and would produce lower quality ultra-structural detail (see Section 15.5.1); however, it was considered that the information provided would aid the diagnostic process.

The tissue was processed to resin and survey sections stained with toluidine blue confirmed that the sample contained keratinized tissue only, with no recognizable epidermis or dermal tissue. Multiple nuclei with a 'glassy' appearance were identified and these were selected for detailed ultra-structural examination.

EM of the tissue confirmed that most of the nuclei present in the sample contained large, organized viral arrays. These had overtaken the majority of the nuclear area in most nuclei. Viral particles were also identified in the cytoplasm. The individual viral particles are round in shape and have a diameter of 30–35 nm (Figure 15.14).

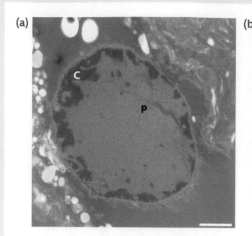

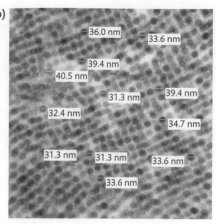

FIGURE 15.14

a) An epidermal nucleus containing numerous arrays of viral particles (P). The remaining nuclear chromatin (C) is just visible around the edge of the nucleus. b) High magnification of viral arrays indicating the diameter of individual viral particles. Scale bar: a = 2 μm. (Courtesy Tracey de Haro)

The results confirmed the patient's sample to contain human papillomavirus (HPV). The size and the shape of the particles seen by EM are consistent with the known features of HPV. The clinical presentation and symptoms experienced by the patient are also consistent with this diagnosis.

CASE STUDY 15.5 *Virus identification*

A number of residents of a residential home for the elderly became unwell with sickness and diarrhoea over a short period of time. In order to determine the cause of the outbreak, stool samples were taken for analysis.

Each stool sample was mixed with sterile water and allowed to stand. The fluid was then centrifuged to remove debris. A drop of the resulting fluid was placed onto a sheet of dental wax. A formvar-coated carbon grid was then floated, formvar side down, on the surface of the fluid for one minute. This allowed the viral particles to adhere to the formvar surface. The excess fluid was then tapped off and the grid floated, formvar side down, on a drop of 2% phosphotungstic acid for 30 seconds. The grid was allowed to dry before examination in the EM.

Examination of the grids prepared from each resident showed that an adenovirus was present in each sample and was responsible for the outbreak (Figure 15.15).

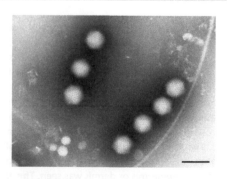

FIGURE 15.15

Adenovirus particles showing external structure. Scale bar = 100 nm. (Courtesy Dr Alan Curry)

15.7.4 Ciliopathies

Cilia are present in numerous tissues and organs of the body. They are found lining the nasal epithelium, bronchial passages, fallopian tubes and in many other places. A diagnosis of ciliopathy is given in Case study 15.6. Cilia form the motile tail of sperm. The structure of the sperm tail is similar to the structure of nasal cilia and sperm motility problems, for example causing infertility, will be seen as a direct result of alterations to the internal structure. The sperm tail, like the nasal cilium, is made up of an axoneme containing nine outer microtubule doublets arranged around two single central microtubules (a 9 + 2 formation). Alterations to this arrangement can be the result of genetic abnormalities or occur following infection, trauma, pathology or an immunological response. This structural alteration results in sperm that are non-motile or only poorly motile, leading to fertility issue in the male affected. TEM assessment of sperm is of clinical importance in assessing the presence of abnormalities of the structure of the sperm tail and in establishing potential causes of the abnormality with a view to managing fertility issues successfully.

CASE STUDY 15.6 Nasal cilia evaluation

A three-year-old girl developed respiratory problems and bronchiectasis rapidly after birth, which required oxygen therapy in a special care baby unit. Subsequently, she suffered a constant cough that was dry and non-productive, with a day and night wheeze. She had no rhinorrhoea or ear infection, and no known allergies. There was no relevant family history but the parents were first cousins.

On investigation, a chest X-ray showed dextrocardia and situs inversus (a condition in which there is complete transposition [right to left] of the thoracic and abdominal organs). A sweat test was normal, ruling out cystic fibrosis, and immunoglobulin testing was unremarkable. It was decided to carry out a nasal brush biopsy to investigate the ciliated epithelium.

A specially designed brush was inserted carefully into the nose and rubbed along the surface of the back of the nasal cavity. The brush was then withdrawn and washed in tissue culture medium. This dislodged the sampled respiratory epithelium into the medium. A special video camera allowed the movement of the cilia found on the respiratory cells to be recorded. This examination demonstrated that the nasal cilia were not beating with a normal rhythm or pattern. They appeared stiff and were only seen to twitch. A normal beat

pattern would see the cilia beating rhythmically in time with each other in a pattern similar to fields of corn moving in a wind. The beat frequency was recorded as 1.1 Hz (normal beat frequency: 13–16 Hz).

A sample of the respiratory epithelium was also fixed in glutaraldehyde and processed for EM. Ultrastructural examination of the cilia present on the respiratory cells clearly demonstrated a morphological abnormality. Both the inner and the outer dynein arms (dynein is an ATPase required for movement of the microtubules that form the axoneme, which provides motility) were missing from all cilia examined (Figure 15.16).

This morphological abnormality, with its associated functional deficit, supports a diagnosis of primary ciliary dyskinesia (PCD), also known as Kartagener's syndrome. In this disorder a genetic mutation produces the morphological abnormality in the cilia. This in turn produces a functional deficit that results in failure of mucociliary clearance from the lungs, leaving the sufferer prone to respiratory infection and other associated problems. As similar ciliary bodies are found in the Fallopian tube and sperm, fertility can also be affected in those who have PCD. There is also a known association between PCD and situs invertus.

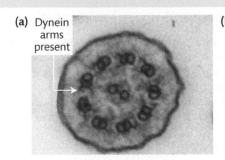
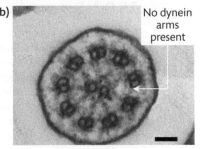

(a) Dynein arms present

(b) No dynein arms present

FIGURE 15.16

a) Normal nasal cilium with inner and outer dynein arms arrowed. b) Abnormal nasal cilium showing the absence of dynein arms (arrow). Scale bar = 50 nm. (Courtesy of Tracey de Haro)

15.8 Other applications

15.8.1 Scanning electron microscopy in diagnosis

The place for SEM in diagnosis is somewhat limited. In histopathology, it is more useful in understanding the disease process, for example, in animal models of various disorders and in translational medicine. An example is given in Figure 15.17. This shows the effects of a gene mutation in a protein vital for function of the sensory cells of the inner ear. These cells have a precisely organized bundle of stereocilia on their apices. Malformation of this bundle has been demonstrated in a number of different hearing loss conditions. In this case a mutation in a gene known to cause Usher Syndrome (deaf-blindness) in people is demonstrated to have affected the bundle organization in a mouse model.

Despite the clinical limitations, there are some diagnostic applications for SEM. As noted earlier, renal damage can be identified where podocytes are effaced. Also, hairs are easily examined by SEM, for example in children suspected of suffering from Menkes kinky hair syndrome. In this disorder there is an absence of copper uptake from the small intestine, which results in a deficit of copper-dependent enzymes in the mitochondria. This produces, among a range of other symptoms and problems, short, brittle, wiry hair. If a sample is examined by SEM it is possible to demonstrate apparent knots or localized thickening of the hair shaft. Presence of these features would lend support to a diagnosis of Menkes kinky hair syndrome.

Corneal samples can be examined by SEM to demonstrate the irregular growths produced on the surface of the cornea due to infection by *Acanthamoeba castellani*, for example. It also has illustrative value in, for example, demonstrating cilia on respiratory epithelia, cells binding to arterial shunts, or even insects and small parasites.

(a) 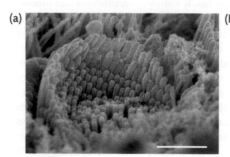 (b)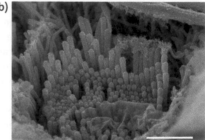

FIGURE 15.17
Stereocilia bundles in sensory cells of the inner ear in normal mice and in Usher syndrome mouse models viewed by SEM. a) The precise bundle organization is evident in this normal neonatal mouse. b) A mouse with a mutation in an orthologous gene for Usher syndrome. The bundle is somewhat disorganized. Scale bars = 1.5 μm.

15.8.2 Energy dispersive X-ray microanalysis

Energy dispersive X-ray microanalysis is an extension to either SEM or TEM. When samples are bombarded by the electron beam then X-rays are emitted. The energy of these X-rays is a characteristic of the element that emitted them, so, by analysing the X-rays produced, the element can be identified. The technique is generally limited to analysing elements of a high atomic number, the range of which is dependent on the type of energy dispersive equipment used.

To allow this technique to work, the sample must be uncoated, or coated with carbon and not gold or palladium (as used in SEM).

Examples of the value of energy dispersive X-ray analysis include:

- identification of foreign bodies in tissue samples (e.g. identifying elements within granulomas)
- analysis of the composition of items such as bladder or renal stones to aid treatment and prevention of recurrence
- identification of a specific type of asbestos body in lung tissue.

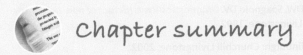

Chapter summary

Having worked through this chapter you should:

■ Have an understanding of what electron microscopes are and what makes them different from light microscopes both in their construction and function.

■ Have an awareness of fixation and processing requirements for maintenance of ultrastructural detail, and how these need to be varied to adapt to specific needs.

■ Understand how tissue is prepared safely for examination.

■ Have knowledge of the small but vital role electron microscopy plays in the diagnostic process and how this complements other histological techniques.

Further reading

● Carpenter S, Karpati G eds. *Pathology of skeletal muscle* 2nd edn. New York: Oxford University Press, 2001.

● Cheville NF. *Ultrastructural pathology. An introduction to interpretation*. Iowa: Iowa State University Press, 1994.

● Dickersin GR. *Diagnostic electron microscopy. A text/atlas* 2nd edn. London: Springer, 2000.

● Doane FW, Anderson N. *Electron microscopy in diagnostic virology: a practical guide and atlas*. Cambridge: Cambridge University Press, 1987.

● Eyden B. *Organelles in tumor diagnosis: ultrastructural atlas*. New York: Igaku-Shoin Medical Publishers, 1996.

● Ghadially FN. *Diagnostic electron microscopy of tumours* 2nd edn. Oxford: Butterworths, 1985.

● Ghadially FN. *Ultrastructural pathology of the cell and matrix* 4th edn. London: Hodder Arnold, 1997.

● Ghadially FN. *Diagnostic ultrastructural pathology. A self-evaluation manual* 2nd edn. Chichester: Elsevier, 1998.

● Horne RW. *Virus structure*. London: Academic Press, 1974.

● Jennette JC, Olson JL, Schwartz MM, Silva FG. *Heptinstall's pathology of the kidney* 5th edn. Philadelphia: Lippincott, Williams & Wilkins, 1998.

● Kierszenbaum AL, Tres LL. *Histology and cell biology. An introduction to pathology* 2nd edn. Chichester: Elsevier, 2002.

● Madeley CR, Field AM. *Virus morphology* 2nd edn. Edinburgh: Churchill Livingstone, 1988.

● Maunsbach AB, Afzelius BA. *Biomedical electron microscopy. Illustrated methods and interpretations*. London: Academic Press, 1999.

● Mobberley MA. Electron microscopy in the investigation of asthenozoospermia. *Br J Biomed Sci* 2010; **67** (2): 92–100.

● Orchard G, Nation B. *Cell structure and function*. Oxford: Oxford University Press, 2015.

- Papadimitriou JM, Henderson DW, Spagnolo DV. *Diagnostic ultrastructure of non-neoplastic diseases*. Edinburgh: Churchill Livingstone, 1992.

- Weedon D. *Skin pathology*. Edinburgh: Churchill Livingstone, 2002.

Useful websites

- Association of Clinical Electron Microscopists (**www.acem.org.uk**)
- Society for Ultrastructural Pathology (**http://sup.ultrakohl.com**)

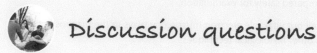

Discussion questions

15.1 Glutaraldehyde is the 'gold standard' fixative for electron microscopy.

    a) Why is this?

    b) If it is such a good fixative, why is it not used for light microscopy?

    c) Can other fixatives be used in electron microscopy?

15.2 Why do samples for electron microscopy have to be so small and what difficulties can this introduce to interpretation?

15.3 Electron microscopy is a vital part of the evaluation of renal disorders. Why is this the case?

15.4 What could electron microscopy add to the work-up of a sample of lung tissue from a patient whose chest X-ray shows a mass?

Acknowledgements

The author is grateful to Tracey de Haro, author of this chapter in the first edition.

Answers to the self-check questions and tips for responding to the discussion questions are provided on the book's accompanying website:

 Visit www.oup.com/uk/orchard2e

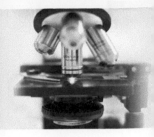

16

Mortuary practice

Ishbel Gall

Learning objectives

After studying this chapter you should be able to:

- Describe the five functions which may be fulfilled by a mortuary and post-mortem facility.
- List the naturally occurring processes which occur after death.
- Understand the work of the Human Tissue Authority (HTA) and how it impacts on the mortuary.
- Understand which Acts and Regulations affect the work and what can be done in the mortuary.
- Understand the difference between consented, or authorized, post-mortem examinations and those instructed by legal process.

16.1 Introduction

The word mortuary, according to the universal dictionary, is defined as a place where dead bodies are kept or prepared prior to burial or cremation. In many cases these bodies are those of former patients who will have undergone laboratory investigations to define a disease process. The mortuary deliveries the last point of care for pathology and can be the final stage of the patient care pathway.

This chapter outlines the functions of a mortuary and the work that is carried out by **Anatomical Pathology Technologists (APTs)**.

16.2 The mortuary

16.2.1 Mortuary function

A mortuary and post-mortem facility fulfils five functions, which may not all be provided at one site. These five functions are:

- The receipt and storage of the deceased.
- Facility to investigate cause and/or circumstances of death by performing a post-mortem examination of the deceased.

Anatomical Pathology Technologist
A healthcare scientist who specializes in mortuary practice and has trained in that field.

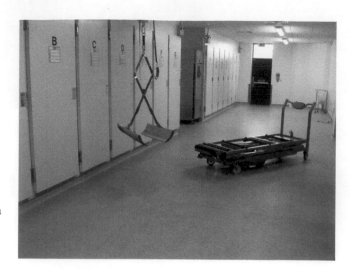

FIGURE 16.1
Mortuary reception area showing refrigerators and manual handling equipment.

- Facility to enable demonstration of post-mortem findings to clinical staff and allow teaching.
- Facility to allow the viewing and/or identification of a body, if requested or required.
- Provide facilities for relatives or next of kin when visiting the mortuary to view or identify a deceased.

The most basic of functions for any mortuary is adequate body storage facilities. The deceased should be refrigerated as soon as possible after death to delay deterioration of the tissues. Some disease processes lead to the body deteriorating more quickly, so cooling the body to below 6°C in as short a time as possible is important. Body storage designs vary, with some being individual spaces within a tall unit and others being large refrigerated rooms with space for wheeled trolleys (Figure 16.1). Whichever design is favoured, there must be adequate space to accommodate the deceased at the busiest times of year. Refrigerator temperature should be monitored so that any malfunction is noticed promptly. All mortuaries should have lifting and moving equipment compatible with their chosen storage design, which keeps manual handling by staff to a minimum.

In modern mortuaries there should be **bariatric** refrigerators, which are much wider than regular refrigerators; these are necessary to accommodate the growing number of larger deceased who may need to be stored. In mortuaries where Coroner- or Procurator Fiscal-instructed post-mortems are carried out there is a requirement for a body storage freezer where the deceased may be kept long-term if required.

Mortuaries may be run by the NHS, local authority or by a private company. The NHS has a duty to provide appropriate accommodation for deceased patients, and local authorities (LAs) have a duty to provide similar facilities for deaths within the community. Many NHS mortuaries also provide accommodation and a post-mortem service for those deaths which fall under the jurisdiction of the Coroner or the Procurator Fiscal service. Small hospitals or LAs may buy the mortuary storage service from another NHS facility or LA, or a private company.

In other countries the regulations regarding mortuary provision differ, and in some countries such as Australia and the United States of America each state has its own laws.

Many mortuaries also provide a facility which enables post-mortem examinations to take place. The size and type of facility will depend on the population of the area served, the type of post-mortem carried out and the post-mortem rate. Children's hospitals and maternity hospitals may have separate mortuaries or share a facility with another hospital. It is important that any mortuary which provides a post-mortem examination service for babies and children is equipped to cope with the specialized needs of these cases. **Prenatal, perinatal and paediatric pathology** is a specialty within histopathology requiring specialist training. Mortuaries should provide separate storage facilities for babies and children.

A post-mortem facility will, as a minimum, have one post-mortem table in a purpose-built room which has good lighting, running water and an electrical system compatible with the wet environment

Bariatric

Pertaining to obesity and weight problems.

Prenatal, perinatal and paediatric pathology

A specialty within pathology which covers the unborn baby and placenta, the neonatal period, childhood and young adulthood.

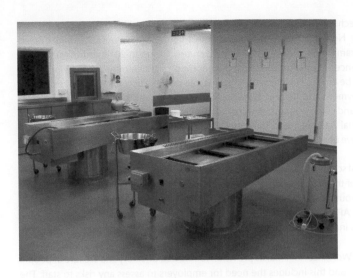

FIGURE 16.2
Post-mortem room with refrigerators.

(Figure 16.2). In the main, mortuaries are much larger with many tables and a separate suite where 'increased-risk' or forensic post-mortem examinations may be carried out. As services are becoming more centralized within each area, this is becoming more common. Smaller mortuaries are being closed and used as satellite body storage only.

Within the post-mortem room will be an area set aside for organ dissection where fixtures and fittings, usually of high-grade stainless steel composition, will be easily cleaned. A sealed off viewing area with two-way communication will allow the post-mortem examination to be viewed by those with a legitimate interest, such as clinical staff, medical students and police officers, without them entering the post-mortem room.

Many mortuaries have facilities which can be used for families to visit the deceased and/or carry out a formal identification. Viewings may be carried out with the deceased in the same room or sometimes they are carried out with the deceased behind a glass panel. The latter is more usual in suspicious deaths or if the deceased has suffered severe trauma. Modern facilities should have a bright, pleasant viewing area with neutral décor, and also be non-denominational. If requested, religious objects such as a copy of the Holy Bible may be laid out. Family members often wish to spend some time with the deceased individually so a waiting room with a toilet for visitors to use is important and again this should be decorated in neutral colours. Disabled access is important as often relatives may be elderly or require assistance. If police statements are to be taken, it is useful to have a small interview room adjacent to the viewing area especially for this purpose. If the viewing area is used for all ages of deceased, from prenatal to adult, then appropriate furnishings and equipment should be used to lay them out. A baby or a **fetus** should be placed in a Moses basket or cot, and children should be placed on an appropriately sized bier. Adults need something large enough for their height and weight. For viewings it is useful to have a selection of gowns or nightclothes for adults and clothes for children or babies, as this is much more pleasing than a paper hospital gown. Babies and children often have their own clothes, which should always be used if possible.

Fetus
A non-viable pregnancy up to 23 weeks and 6 days' gestation showing no sign of life on delivery.

16.2.2 Mortuary staff

Most mortuaries are run by a Mortuary Manager or Senior Anatomical Pathology Technologist, but others fall under the control of the histopathology laboratory manager. The job of an **Anatomical Pathology Technologist** (APT) is diverse and can include many different roles, varying from assisting in post-mortem examinations, to removing tissue for transplant, to talking to relatives of the deceased. Generally, APTs are responsible for the day-to-day maintenance and running of the mortuary as well as care of the deceased. There is a great deal of administrative work and many legal aspects to the job, as well as a need for anatomical knowledge and a good understanding of health and safety and infection control.

Anatomical pathology technologists gain their qualifications over a period of time, which combines practical skills with theory. New qualifications were approved by the *Modernising Scientific Careers Practitioner Training Programme Education and Training Scrutiny Group* in 2014 and the first Level 3 Diploma Course commenced soon after. Although the educational programme is still being developed, ultimately there will be an APT Healthcare Science degree qualification. Qualifications can only be gained when in employment and there is greater emphasis on practical assessment than previously. Training is modular and covers areas such as risk assessment, Control of Substances Hazardous to Health (COSHH), manual handling, and infection control, as well as anatomy and physiology. Post-mortem standards have been developed and these are the minimum level at which APTs will be required to work.

Occasionally, biomedical scientists may have to go to the mortuary either to collect tissue (i.e. for a frozen section) or as part of their learning programme within the department, so it is important that they are knowledgeable about basic mortuary practice. Anyone visiting the mortuary will need to take instruction from the senior APT regarding health and safety issues, especially those involving personal protective equipment; this includes clinical staff, relatives, healthcare scientists and other visitors to the mortuary.

The Health and Safety at Work Act 1974 makes provision for the health, safety and welfare of people in the course of their work, and this includes the need for employers to assess any risks to staff. The Control of Substances Hazardous to Health (COSHH) Regulations 2002 require that employers assess the risks from exposure to hazardous substances, including pathogens, and implement any measures necessary to protect workers from any risk as far as is reasonably practicable.

Mortuary staff should undergo a comprehensive health check by the NHS or LA occupational health department prior to their employment, which ensures they are adequately protected against the most common pathogens. A COSHH assessment will determine the risk from pathogens, and staff should be offered pre-exposure immunization. A comprehensive guide to immunization is available in The Department of Health Green Book, which can be found online. It is regularly updated by the Department of Health to reflect current needs.

https://www.gov.uk/government/collections/immunisation-against-infectious-disease-the-green-book

16.3 Death and decomposition

Death **verification** is performed by a competent trained person, usually a registered medical practitioner but sometimes this can be a paramedic or senior nurse. Once blood has stopped circulating, there are no breath sounds and the pupils do not react to light then the person is usually dead. Exceptions such as hypothermia may need to be excluded.

From this point onwards the body starts to decompose, albeit usually slowly, but factors such as disease process, body size, ambient temperature and humidity may affect the process. Autolysis is the breakdown of tissues and cells caused by chemicals and enzymes inside the body. Putrefaction is caused by bacterial breakdown of tissue and often starts in the abdomen, especially around the caecum.

Rigor mortis is the contraction of the muscles after death caused by a chemical reaction due to depleted oxygen levels. Rigor mortis onset is usually a few hours after death, becoming most pronounced around 12 hours after death, and it may last up to 72 hours after death. Livor mortis or hypostasis is the post-mortem discoloration of the body areas closest to the ground, caused by red blood cells settling under the effect of gravity. Parts of the body in contact with the ground, frequently the shoulder blades and buttocks, do not show this due to pressure on the blood vessels. Onset can be as little as half an hour after death occurs.

It is therefore important that patients who die in hospital are laid on their back in a natural position as soon as possible after death in order to minimize discoloration to the face and hands. The pattern of hypostasis can be a good indication of whether or not a body has been moved after death in cases where there is any suspicion of foul play.

The **decomposition** process can be slowed by placing the deceased in a cool place. The most effective way of doing this is by refrigeration at around 5 °C. Many hospitals operate a policy of ensuring that patients who die are in the mortuary refrigerated accommodation, where practicable, within six hours of death. This is very important where tissues for donation, or research, may have to be retrieved in the mortuary. The decomposition rate is also affected by the cause of death and certain disease processes can accelerate the process.

What method is used to slow decomposition of the deceased?

16.4 Certification

Once death has been verified there is the question about whether or not a Medical Certificate of Cause of Death (MCCD), commonly called a death certificate, can be issued. If the death is expected and the medical history well documented then in most cases the deceased's doctor will issue the MCCD.

Although life can be pronounced extinct by a trained, competent professional, the MCCD can only be issued by a registered medical practitioner.

There are laws that need to be observed and sometimes the death will need to be reported to the **Coroner** or, in Scotland, the **Procurator Fiscal**. Reasons for reporting a death vary slightly between the two legal systems, but one obvious reason is that the doctor is unable to issue the MCCD as they do not know why the patient died.

Deaths where the cause may be known but has to be reported are suicide, industrial disease or death after trauma, including fractured neck of femur, which is very common in older people. The fracture itself may not be the cause of death, but the patient may develop bronchopneumonia or a deep vein thrombosis (DVT) as a result of being immobilized. Often in these cases the medical practitioner will be instructed to issue the MCCD as the cause of death is clear, there are no suspicious circumstances, and it is not in the public interest to investigate the death further.

As well as the MCCD, medical practitioners may be required to complete forms that allow cremation to take place. In England and Wales there are 13 different forms recognized by cremation authorities but not all of them are required, as some relate to stillbirths and another set pertain to cremation of body parts. **The Cremation Regulations 2008**, which are amended regularly, legislate about the documentation required so that cremation can take place. Other forms may require to be completed if the deceased is to be moved out of the Coroner's jurisdiction or abroad.

Cremation in Scotland is governed by The Cremation (Scotland) Regulations, which have also been amended several times. Most recently, on 13 May 2015, the Certification of Death (Scotland) Act 2011 was introduced. One of the main changes is the establishment of the Death Certification Review Service, which is run by Healthcare Improvement Scotland. The review service checks on the accuracy of a sample of MCCDs. Once the death has been registered a Form 14 is issued and the deceased can be buried or cremated (Table 16.1). Permitting future potential disposal methods, such as **resomation**, have been included in the Act.

In other parts of the world the post-mortem examination process is subject to different legislation; for example, in Australia each State (Victoria, New South Wales, Queensland, West Australia and South Australia) and the two Territories (Northern Territory and Australian Capital Territory) each have their own Coronial Acts and legislations for consented post-mortem examinations (e.g. Human Tissue Act [NSW] or Transplant and Anatomy Act [SA]). The legislation is broadly the same, requiring the next of kin to provide consent, which is usually in writing, although verbal consent may be accepted in some states.

This has to be presented to a Designated Officer, who is usually a hospital administrator acting as the 'gatekeeper' to ensure that the necessary consent has been obtained and that it is legal to perform the post-mortem examination. Consent may be provided for a full examination, but the next of kin may specify body parts or regions not to be examined. Most consent forms divide consent for the post-mortem examination and consent for research and/or teaching. Retention of whole organs, such as the brain or lungs, will usually require further consent. Some large hospitals have a specialist team to assist with the process of obtaining consent, and information packs for staff and relatives are made available. Currently, few hospital post-mortem examinations are performed; a large hospital of 1000–2000 beds might only carry out around 50 cases each year, many of which will not be full post-mortem

Coroner

A doctor or lawyer responsible for investigating deaths under certain circumstances who can also order a post-mortem examination of the body if necessary.

Procurator Fiscal

A qualified lawyer who is responsible for prosecuting crime in Scotland; they also investigate sudden and suspicious deaths and can order a post-mortem examination.

The Cremation Regulations 2008

These came into effect on 1 January 2009 to modernize and consolidate all previous regulations, replacing the Cremation Regulations 1930 as previously amended.

Resomation

Also known as alkaline hydrolysis, resomation is a water-based chemical process using strong alkali in water at temperatures of up to 180°C under high pressure to safely and rapidly reduce the body to ash.

TABLE 16.1 Cremation forms required under current legislation.

Form number	Name of form	Scottish equivalent
Form Cremation 1	Application for cremation of remains of deceased person	A Form
Form Cremation 2	Application for cremation of body parts	AA Form
Form Cremation 3	Application for cremation of stillborn baby	Stillbirth A Form
Form Cremation 4	Medical certificate	Form 14
Form Cremation 5	Confirmatory medical certificate	Form 14
Form Cremation 6	Certificate of coroner	Form E (Procurator Fiscal)
Form Cremation 7	Certificate following anatomical examination	Form 14
Form Cremation 8	Certificate releasing body parts for cremation	Form N
Form Cremation 9	Certificate of stillbirth	Form 8
Form Cremation 10	Authorization of cremation of deceased person by medical referee	N/A
Form Cremation 11	Certificate after post-mortem examination	N/A
Form Cremation 12	Authorization of cremation of body parts by medical referee	N/A
Form Cremation 13	Authorization of cremation of remains of stillborn child by medical referee	N/A

examinations. Most sudden deaths in hospitals are referred to the Coroner, and most Coronial Acts include wide statements such that if a clinician suspects a death may in any way be a consequence of a complication of treatment it must be referred.

In the USA there are two medicolegal systems for death investigation in operation, the Coroners' system and the Medical Examiners' system. Within these over 2000 separate death investigation systems operate across the country.

In states using a coroner system, coroners are elected officials and do not need to be registered medical practitioners, the exceptions being Kansas, Louisiana, North Dakota and Ohio. Should a post-mortem examination be warranted, the coroner will often consult with a pathologist or forensic pathologist.

Medical Examiners (MEs) are usually appointed and are registered medical practitioners, although they may not be required to have special training in pathology or forensic pathology.

Terminology differs from state to state, with some having county MEs who are not always pathologists, but in some states (e.g. Kentucky) the term 'medical examiner' is synonymous with 'forensic pathologist'.

The Model Post-Mortem Examinations Act in 1954 described a foundation to develop ME systems, and subsequently issues of education, training, funding and legislation have been addressed in a 1968 National Research Council Committee on Forensic Pathology, and a 2003 Institute of Medicine Workshop.

Many organizations, such as the National Association of Medical Examiners (NAME) and American Academy of Forensic Sciences (AAFS), are trying to improve death investigation and to address issues including education, training and funding.

Consented examination legislation varies from state to state, and consent forms vary in length between one and eight pages, but all address similar issues as in other countries.

SELF-CHECK 16.2

What document is required to register a death in the UK, and who can issue this document?

16.5 **Other documentation**

16.5.1 Identification

Where possible, all deceased should arrive in the mortuary with appropriate identification (ID) attached to them. Exceptions will be where a deceased has been found in the community or has died shortly after arrival in hospital. In these cases, identification should include the place of death, or where they were brought in from, the date and time of death or verification of death, and any known circumstances (e.g. road traffic collision [RTC]).

It is important that ID is more than just a name and date of death, as many people have similar names and this could lead to confusion. As a gold standard, patients who die in hospital should be identified with their full name, hospital number, date of birth, date and time of death, and the ward name or number, as well as the consultant's name. This gives several pieces of information that can be checked to verify identity.

This can be compared to a laboratory sample acceptance policy and booking in of samples once they arrive in the laboratory. It is very important that samples are not mixed up leading to misdiagnosis. When two people with the same name, or similar names, are in the mortuary this must be highlighted and extra checks made before any procedures are carried out or the deceased is released to the family or funeral director.

16.5.2 Infection

All deceased persons are an infection risk but if there is any known specific risk then this should be indicated on an infection notification sheet accompanying the deceased. For patient confidentiality, the nature of the infection should not be disclosed, but rather the infection category, route of infection and what precautions need to be taken by those who come into contact with the deceased. Sometimes it is not known if the deceased is an infection risk but lifestyle may dictate a potential higher risk, so this should be taken into account when handling the deceased. As a rule, **Standard Infection Control Precautions (SICPs)** should be taken whenever in contact with the deceased.

Infections are caused by pathogens (microorganisms) that can cause harm to the human body. Pathogens include bacteria, fungi, parasites, protozoa and viruses. Some pathogens are more hazardous than others so they have been classified by the Advisory Committee on Dangerous Pathogens (ACDP) into four categories according to the potential risk (Table 16.2).

This categorization does not take into account any additional risk a pathogen may pose to someone with underlying disease, **immunocompromised** persons, or those who are pregnant. Allergenic properties of pathogens have also not been taken into account.

> **Standard Infection Control Precautions (SICPs)**
> Previously known as Universal Precautions, SICPs are the basic infection prevention and control measures necessary to reduce the risk of transmission of infectious agents.
>
> **Immunocompromised**
> Having an immune system that has been impaired by disease or treatment.

TABLE 16.2 Categories of pathogen.

	Risk	Example
Category 1	An organism that is most unlikely to cause human disease.	Any organism not classified by ACDP
Category 2	An organism that may cause human disease and might be a hazard but is unlikely to spread to the community. Effective prophylaxis or treatment is usually available.	*Clostridium tetani* *Streptococcus pyogenes*
Category 3	An organism that may cause severe human disease and present a serious hazard. It may present a risk of spread to the community. Prophylaxis or treatment is usually available.	Tuberculosis Hepatitis B HIV
Category 4	An organism that may cause severe human disease and present a serious hazard. It may present a high risk of spread to the community and there is no effective prophylaxis or treatment available.	Ebola virus Lassa fever

When handling the deceased there are four main sources of infection that APTs and those coming into contact with the deceased have to protect themselves against:

- blood and other body fluids, such as saliva and pleural effusion
- waste products: faecal material and urine
- aerosols caused when moving the deceased or opening the body
- direct contact from the skin.

Routes of infection:

- inoculation: needlestick injury caused by sharps (needle, lancet etc.)
- ingestion: usually from eating contaminated food but also by poor hand hygiene
- inhalation: airborne infection caused by aerosol or splashes
- contact: direct contact with a body, fluids or excreta or indirectly via contaminated surfaces such as a telephone or table
- across the surface of the eye, usually by splashing.

If the deceased has a Category 3 infection then they should be placed in a body bag. Category 4 infections are not routinely dealt with in the UK and specialist precautions are required depending on the pathogen. These cases should be dealt with using the most up-to-date information from the UK government's Public Health England (www.gov.uk/government/organisations/public-health-england) or Health Protection Scotland (www.hps.scot.nhs.uk/).

16.6 **Post-mortem examinations**

Post-mortem examinations are either carried out under the direction of the Coroner or Procurator Fiscal, or with consent, or authorization, of the next of kin or nominated representative of the deceased.

The post-mortem service across the United Kingdom was investigated thoroughly in the wake of several 'organ scandals' starting in Bristol in 1998 when it came to light that hearts had been retained at post-mortem examinations carried out following surgery. Another scandal at Alder Hey emerged when it was revealed, at an official inquiry into heart surgery at Bristol, that a store of children's hearts was also held there.

Following these two revelations, it was also found that Birmingham's Diana Princess of Wales Children's Hospital and the Alder Hey Children's Hospital, in Liverpool, had been harvesting organs and tissues from babies who had died. These incidents led to a national inquiry into post-mortem practice and the publishing of several reports.

In January 2001, the official Alder Hey report, The Royal Liverpool Children's Inquiry, also known as the Redfern Report, was published and in July 2001 the Bristol Royal Infirmary Inquiry report was also published. Other reports, including the Isaacs Report and, in Scotland, The Review Group on Retention of Organs at Post-Mortem, led by Professor Sheila McLean, published a three-part report. All these inquiries and reports led to a major review of legislation.

The **Human Tissue Act 2004** replaced the Human Tissue Act 1961, the Anatomy Act 1984 and the Human Organ Transplants Act 1989 in relation to England and Wales, and the corresponding Orders in Northern Ireland; the **Human Tissue (Scotland) Act 2006** is an Act of the Scottish Parliament and is the equivalent in Scotland regarding the handling of human tissue. NHS Quality Improvement Scotland published *Standards for Management of Post-mortem Examinations* in 2003 and subsequently reviewed all NHS organizations in Scotland that carried out post-mortem examinations. National authorization for post-mortem examination forms and associated booklets were brought into use in Scotland in 2006.

In England, Wales and Northern Ireland the Human Tissue Authority (HTA) regulates and licenses organizations, including mortuaries, that store and use human tissue. There are nine Codes of Practice but the ones that are applicable depend on the work carried out within each mortuary. In particular, Code of Practice 3 pertains to post-mortem examinations. Many mortuaries have more than one licence.

Each licensed establishment has to nominate a Designated Individual, who will supervise the activities being carried out under licence. The Designated Individual is often a pathologist or the mortuary manager and they have to ensure compliance and practice within the scope of the licence(s) held. There is also a Licence Holder who oversees the licence; this is usually a corporate body such as an NHS trust rather than a named person.

Post-mortem examinations, whether authorized or instructed, must be carried out on premises with the appropriate licence(s). There are currently no national post-mortem forms but a template is provided which should be used on which to base local forms.

SELF-CHECK 16.3

Which of the HTA Codes of Practice is most relevant to mortuaries?

16.6.1 Post-mortem examinations carried out under instruction from a legal authority

If the post-mortem is instructed then no consent or authorization is required from the family or legal representative. The legal system in England, Wales and Northern Ireland employs the coroners' system, which has been in its current form since the late nineteenth century. The coroner is appointed by the local authority and is either medically or legally qualified, occasionally both.

In Scotland the Procurator Fiscal is a legally qualified public prosecutor who, when a death is reported to them, has a responsibility to identify if any criminal action has occurred and, where appropriate, prosecute.

Many deaths reported to either authority are those where a medical practitioner is unwilling, or unable, to issue a Medical Certificate of Cause of Death (MCCD). This can be due to the death being sudden, unexplained or as a result of trauma or an unlawful act.

The **Coroners and Justice Act 2009** received Royal Assent on 12 November 2009 and aims to deliver more effective, transparent and responsive justice and coroner services, but has not as yet been fully implemented.

It is up to the coroner or Procurator Fiscal to decide whether to instruct a post-mortem examination or allow the medical practitioner to issue the MCCD. In Scotland the Procurator Fiscal may instruct the pathologist to examine the deceased externally, and, with access to the medical history and knowledge of the circumstances surrounding death, issue the MCCD on that basis. This is known as 'view and grant'.

Ordinarily, the pathologist will be instructed to carry out a full post-mortem examination to establish the cause of death. This may involve taking small samples of tissue for histological examination as well as swabs or fluid samples for microbiology and biochemical analysis.

Where there has been foul play, or there is a suspicion that a crime has been committed, a full forensic post-mortem examination may be instructed. In the coroners' system this involves asking a Home Office Pathologist to carry out the examination. This is called a forensic post-mortem examination and may involve many people being present at the post-mortem examination.

Although the basic principles of the examination are the same, there may be many extra samples and swabs taken for forensic examination. Often the deceased will be subjected to a full body X-ray or scan prior to the examination, as well as dental X-ray if required. Scenes of Crime Officers (SOCOs) will take photographs and may be required to take fingerprints, hair samples and fingernail clippings for analysis, depending on the circumstances.

In Scotland the Procurator Fiscal would attend the examination and the post-mortem would be carried out by two pathologists.

Post-mortem examinations carried out under instruction do not allow for tissue to be retained unless it is for diagnostic or forensic purposes, and the family or legal representative of the deceased must be informed and given a choice regarding tissue disposal. This is covered by the respective Human Tissue Acts.

Certain faith groups object in principle to post-mortem examination and request a non-invasive examination, but these are not widely available, relatively costly and often inconclusive. Some coroners will utilize imaging techniques but the family may have to pay for this service and a full post-mortem examination might have to be carried out subsequently to establish the cause of death.

A case study in which imaging would not have confirmed the cause of death can be found later in this chapter (see Case study 16.1).

SELF-CHECK 16.4

Who has the legal power to instruct a post-mortem examination in the UK?

16.6.2 Post-mortem examinations with consent or authorization (medical interest post-mortem examinations)

A comparatively small number of post-mortem examinations are carried out in hospital mortuaries with the agreement of the family. The number of consented post-mortem examinations has fallen considerably since the late 1990s and the only area where workload has remained relatively constant is in paediatric and perinatal centres.

There are many reasons for this sharp decline in numbers, but much can be attributed to the organ retention inquiries mentioned previously. Scanning techniques such as magnetic resonance imaging (MRI) and computed tomography (CT) have advanced so that medical practitioners feel less need for examination after death to confirm diagnosis. Post-mortem pathology is also less widely taught to undergraduate medical students, and therefore the merit of the post-mortem examination is less widely understood.

Essentially, the post-mortem examination is to confirm the known cause of death, but it can be a tool to assist clinicians' understanding of the particular disease process and the impact of any medical intervention. Occasionally something will be found at post-mortem which may warrant the death being reported to the appropriate authority, but this is relatively rare.

If a post-mortem examination is to be requested, the person seeking to gain consent must have a good knowledge of the post-mortem examination procedure and what it entails. This may mean that it is a senior member of the clinical team or possibly an APT or pathologist. Some centres employ nursing or bereavement staff to carry out this role, but it is important they have attended post-mortem examinations and know the post-mortem procedure in order to answer any questions from relatives. It is also important that if a limited post-mortem is being carried out, the limitations will not exclude pathology important to a full diagnostic report.

A post-mortem examination will normally include the removal of small samples of tissue from the organs for histological examination. These are postage stamp-sized pieces of tissue a few millimetres thick. These will often be placed in cassettes in a pot of **fixative** in the mortuary. This fixative is usually formalin, a 10% solution of formaldehyde. Small samples are best as they will 'fix' more quickly.

Where special staining may be required, small samples may be taken fresh straight to the histopathology laboratory so that this can be undertaken as soon as possible before the tissue has autolysed (see Case study 16.2)

Swabs and fluid samples, as well as X-rays, photographs and samples for DNA testing, may also be required, and this has to be explained to the person giving consent. All these samples are purely for diagnostic purposes and will form part of the medical record of the deceased. If it is thought that any organ(s) might be required to be retained to complete the post-mortem fully then separate consent for this must be gained. Commonly, it is the brain and lungs that are retained from an adult, but other organs may be of interest depending on the cause of death. If there is consent to retain organs then these must be specified on the consent form, along with an agreed method for their disposal.

Usually there are three options available:

- organ(s) to be returned to the body prior to the funeral
- organ(s) to be returned to the family after all diagnostic tests have been completed
- organ(s) to be disposed of respectfully by the hospital.

The first option is not entirely satisfactory as the organ may not be fixed properly and inevitably there will be some delay to the funeral. The second option may cause some distress to the family as it may

Fixative

Fixative preserves the tissue by stopping autolysis and putrefaction, keeping tissue from further deterioration after death. Formalin fixes permanently and causes tissue to shrink slightly and harden, but it retains its three-dimensional structure.

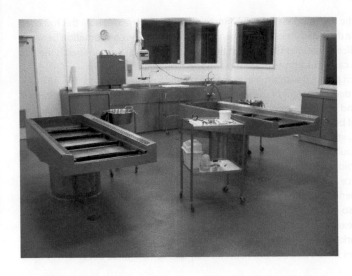

FIGURE 16.3
Post-mortem tables and ancillary equipment.

be some time before the organ(s) are returned to them for disposal. Funeral directors may also charge for disposing of tissue. Hospitals must have a comprehensive procedure for respectful tissue disposal, which can be made available to any relative who enquires.

16.6.3 Post-mortem preparation

Experienced APTs will know what equipment and personal protective equipment (PPE) is required prior to the examination. An assessment of information from the available medical history, lifestyle and circumstances surrounding death will allow a risk assessment of each post-mortem examination prior to its commencement. As a minimum, PPE should include a complete change of clothing into 'scrubs' or a protective suit and a waterproof apron which should be long enough to reach below the top of a pair of waterproof boots. Long hair should be covered by a cap and the arms should be covered, either by a long-sleeved apron or waterproof oversleeves. Eye protection, preferably in the form of a full face visor, and good fitting gloves should also be worn. In certain cases a face mask is desirable. The senior APT should ensure that everyone in the post-mortem room complies with health and safety legislation before entering the room (Figure 16.3).

Many APTs and pathologists have a preference for particular instruments but there are basic requirements for any post-mortem examination. A PM40 is the bladed knife used in most mortuaries for evisceration. A scalpel is often used for dissection of the organs along with a selection of scissors and a long-handled knife. Dissection also requires a pair of forceps, and a blunt-ended probe is useful. A metal ruler is required for measurements as it is easily cleaned. A weighing scale for the organs and a dissection bench is needed as well as bowls or basins for the organs. A marker board mounted on the wall above the dissection bench or waterproof dictation system is helpful for the recording of any weights or volumes. Cellulose sponges and receptacles for samples should be readily available along with a bin for disposing of any sharps. The post-mortem room should have adequate lighting above the post-mortem table and the dissection area. Ventilation should comply with the latest guidance.

The APT may wish to prepare a sheet of labels with the details of the deceased prior to the post-mortem examination so that when samples are taken they can be labelled quickly to avoid any mistakes.

16.6.4 Post-mortem procedure

Post-mortem examinations usually follow a set routine regardless of whether they are instructed or consented. The examination starts by the pathologist and APT checking the consent or instruction to establish what is to be done. The identification of the deceased, if known, is then confirmed and checked against the paperwork. If there is any discrepancy between the paperwork and the identification attached to the deceased then the examination should not proceed until this has been verified. If the identity of the deceased is not known then there will need to be corroboration between the pathologist and the police or coroner's officer that the deceased about to be examined is the one to whom the instruction to carry out a post-mortem examination pertains.

The examination will then proceed with a full external examination of the deceased. The APT usually has weighed and recorded the height of the deceased prior to the examination. The pathologist will note the age, gender and build of the deceased, and whether this is in keeping with the available information. Distribution of body hair should also be noted.

Starting at the head, the external description will include the hair colour and length and record the facial features. The head should be palpated carefully through the hair to identify any wound that may be hidden from view. Eye colour and the diameter of the pupils are recorded and the conjunctivae are checked for signs of jaundice and **petechial haemorrhage**. Prosthetic eyes should be recorded but left *in situ*. The mouth is opened and the dentition is checked for its state and whether it is natural or false. The tongue should also be checked for bite marks, which are commonly found in epilepsy. The body and limbs should be examined and any medical intervention, such as surgical scars or bruising associated with needle marks, noted. It should also be noted whether these are old or new. Non-medical bruising and injuries should also be recorded. This may take some time to document in cases of extreme trauma.

Fingers should be examined for injury, **clubbing** and the length and state of nails noted. Similarly, the toe nails should be examined. Amputated or missing limbs or digits need to be recorded. Areas and extent of hypostasis and rigor mortis should also be noted. It is important that the back is examined to exclude any trauma or pathology (e.g. abscess). Many mortuaries have a form to simplify this examination, which includes a diagram of a human body on which injuries and other information can be recorded. Other forms for individual body parts are sometimes used when there has been extreme trauma or when the body has been fragmented.

The pathologist may wish to swab any wounds for possible infection and take blood samples at this stage. Fluid samples need to be taken as early as possible in the examination to avoid contamination, as well as deterioration of the sample as the decomposition processes continue.

Once the external examination is complete and the pathologist and APT are satisfied then the internal examination can proceed.

If the post-mortem has been consented the consent may now dictate how the examination proceeds, as there may be limitations to permission for the examination.

Pathologists and APTs have their preferred methods of **evisceration,** but there are two main methods of removing the internal organs once the initial incisions have been made.

One method involves the removal of all the organs in a single block; this is known as the Letulle or Rokitanski method. The second method commonly used in the UK is the 'en bloc' method described by Ghon. This method involves removing the abdominal and thoracic organs in four distinct blocks, as follows:

- lungs and heart, along with the tongue, thyroid, oesophagus and trachea
- jejunum, ileum and colon (the small and large intestine)
- stomach, liver, spleen, pancreas and duodenum
- adrenal glands, kidneys, ureters, bladder and gonads.

The internal pathology may dictate that one method is preferred over another in a particular case, so APTs and pathologists should be proficient in both methods and adapt their technique to suit the individual case.

These methods are described in great detail in many pathology textbooks, together with specialized techniques such as exposing the middle ear, removing the spinal cord, and sampling nerves.

Once the organs have been removed from the thoracic and abdominal cavities, the brain should be removed (only if there is permission in consented examinations). Some pathologists like to start by examining the brain, so this may have been done after the external examination.

In order to examine the brain an incision is made in the scalp as posteriorly as possible so that it will not be seen after reconstruction. The incision should start behind the right ear, curve upwards to the midline and then downward to end behind the left ear. The scalp is reflected forward to expose the skull and posteriorly the scalp is reflected back towards the neck.

Petechial haemorrhage

Small pinprick haemorrhages that may indicate asphyxia.

Clubbing

Clubbing is an increase in the soft tissue under the proximal nail plate of the distal part of the fingers or toes. Its causes are varied and may be hereditary, incidental or a sign of underlying disease.

Evisceration

Literally 'to empty the organs or disembowel', it is removal of all the organs for examination.

Using a scalpel, the temporalis muscles can be incised posteriorly and reflected forward; this will help with reconstruction after the brain has been removed. With a scalpel, mark a guide line on the skull from behind the right ear upwards over the frontal bone, keeping the line away from the frontal sinus, and then sweep back down behind the left ear. A mark should then be drawn posteriorly between the ends of the first mark crossing above the external occipital protuberance.

Using an **oscillating saw**, one which moves backwards and forwards rapidly rather than in a continuous circle, the skull should be opened taking care not to saw too deeply and cut the meninges. Once the skull has been sawn through a skull key can be used to loosen the skull cap. The dura mater (the outer layer of the **meninges**) must be opened carefully and the brain can be exposed and removed carefully.

In order to remove the brain, the carotid arteries, optic nerves, pituitary stalk and cranial nerves will have to be cut and the tentorium cerebelli carefully incised to expose the cerebellum. Once this has been done the vertebral arteries, final cranial nerves and the spinal cord can be cut and the brain lifted from the cranial vault. The brain should be weighed and then examined or fixed as quickly as possible as it is no longer being supported by the cerebrospinal fluid in which it is surrounded. To fix the brain, it should be suspended in a large container of formalin. It can be suspended by the basilar artery, and by 'floating' in fixative it retains its natural shape.

After careful examination of the inside of the skull, the head should be reconstructed as soon as possible to stop the scalp from drying out and shrinking. The cranial vault should be packed with appropriate material and the skull cap fitted; the notches at the temporal bone should stop the bone from moving. The temporalis muscles can be reflected posteriorly to their original position and this will help keep the skull cap in place while the scalp is taken back over the bone and the incision sewn up.

The pathologist will dissect all the major organs and these will be weighed and the weights recorded (Table 16.3). Often this is the job of the APT.

While the organs are being removed, the presence of any fluid in the pleural or abdominal cavities should be noted. Fluids should be described and the volumes recorded. The pathologist may wish to sample these fluids; if so, they should be put into sterile universal containers as soon as possible to avoid contamination. While evisceration is taking place, it is important that the APT or pathologist record any obvious abnormalities or pathology.

There may be adhesions or a tumour mass that may require the evisceration technique to be altered for an individual case. Adhesions may be as a result of previous surgery and in the abdomen especially require extreme care in order not to puncture the intestine. It should be noted if any tissue has been surgically removed prior to death (e.g. appendix or gall bladder). If urine is required, this should be taken from the bladder *in situ* prior to its removal.

Fluid and tissue samples can be tested for signs of infection, drug or alcohol levels, toxins and other chemical imbalances that may have contributed to the cause of death.

If the death has occurred in hospital, it is possible that the laboratories may already have ante-mortem samples which may be of use. It is important to note exactly when these samples were taken in any post-mortem report.

Meninges
Three layers of membranes that cover the central nervous system.

TABLE 16.3 Average organ weights: variations are seen between different populations, and the individual height and build should also be considered.

	Male	Female
Heart	320–360 g	280–340 g
Lungs	360–570 g (Right) 325–480 g (Left)	340–550 g (Right) 305–460 g (Left)
Liver	1400–1600 g	1400–1600 g
Brain	1100–1600 g	1000–1500 g
Kidney (left usually larger than right)	125–170 g	115–155 g

CASE STUDY 16.1 Deep vein thrombosis and pulmonary embolism

Patient details

- 48-year-old male
- Generally fit and healthy
- No other known medical issues
- One-week history of chesty cough

- Pleuritic pain in left lower chest area
- Not responding to amoxicillin
- Admitted to hospital with increased SOB on exertion

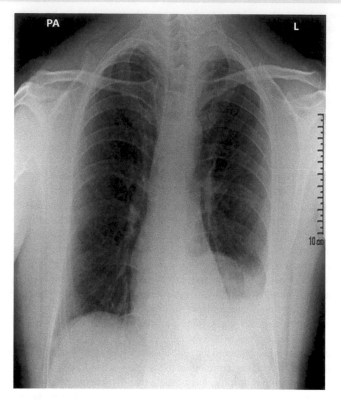

FIGURE 16.4
Posterior–anterior chest X-ray. The rest of the film looks clear and the heart and mediastinal contours are normal. A diagnosis of pneumonia was made.

Posterior–anterior chest X-ray with no previous films for comparison. Opacification of the left lower zone and the diaphragm cannot be seen. The rest of the film looks clear and the heart and mediastinal contours are normal. A diagnosis of pneumonia was made (Figure 16.4).

- Prescribed further antibiotics.
- Discharged home with new prescription as he does not wish to stay in hospital as he feels stressed.
- Three days later found dead at home.
- GP willing to issue MCCD as 'pneumonia' but family wish this clarified by a post-mortem examination (Figures 16.5–16.7).

Post-mortem findings

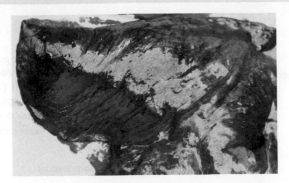

FIGURE 16.5
Infarcted lower lobe of left lung.

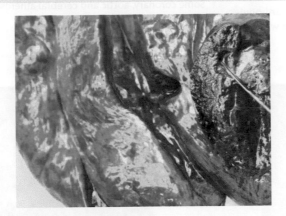

FIGURE 16.6
Bisected lower lobe of the right lung. The radiological interpretation of pneumonia was in the infarcted left lower lobe.

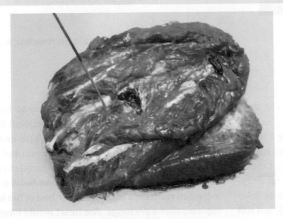

FIGURE 16.7
Deep vein thrombosis (DVT) in veins of the calf muscle.

CASE STUDY 16.2 Post-surgery fat embolism

Patient details

- 70-year-old female
- Elective third revision of right total hip replacement
- No co-morbidities
- Intra-operation hypotension
- Five hours post-op reduced consciousness
- ECG showed 'classic' S1, Q3, T3
- Cardiac arrest

During the operation there were no major complications; she received 1000 mL fluid and her oxygen saturation remained above 98%. Unfortunately, five hours after the operation her condition deteriorated and ultimately she suffered a cardiac arrest. After 35 minutes of attempted cardiopulmonary resuscitation (CPR) and drug therapy she was pronounced dead.

Commonly a large embolus associated with pulmonary artery obstruction can lead to acute right ventricular dilatation producing an S wave in lead I and a Q wave in lead III. T-wave inversion in lead III may also be present, producing the S1, Q3, T3 pattern.

The doctor is willing to write the MCCD but the family would like a hospital post-mortem examination to confirm the diagnosis.

Summary of findings on examination

- No evidence of pulmonary thromboembolism.
- 'Heavy' lungs are slightly oedematous but there is no sign of infection.
- Some coronary, aortic and cerebral atherosclerosis but not enough to have caused death.
- No obvious coronary thrombus.

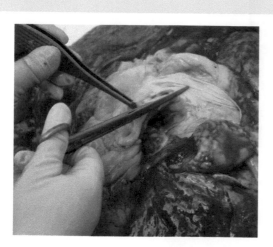

FIGURE 16.8
Checking blood vessels for signs of emboli.

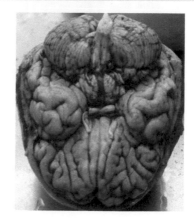

FIGURE 16.9
Normal appearance of brain on removal, with no obvious infarct or thrombus.

As the diagnosis was embolism (Figure 16.8), the pathologist decided to take fresh tissue samples from the lungs, kidneys and brain (Figure 16.9) for immediate analysis. Using a frozen section technique and a stain specifically for fat (Oil red O), the sections were processed in the histopathology laboratory. Oil red O staining identified numerous foci of fat droplets in the small alveolar capillaries and in the small arterioles of the lung (Figure 16.10) and kidney (Figure 16.11), but not in the brain.

The fatal demise of this patient is likely to have occurred as a result of fat emboli, a known complication arising from the long bone surgery. The presence of these emboli within the small capillaries of the lung would have caused a vasoconstrictive response from the vessels and reduced oxygenation of the blood. This in turn would lead to right heart strain due to the increased resistance in the vascular bed of the lung, which also explains the heavy lungs. The heart would have been made to work harder due to the hypoxia.

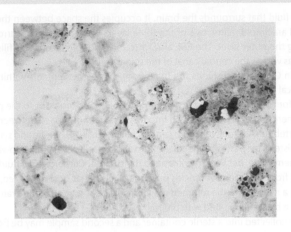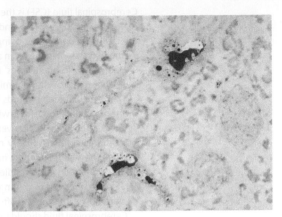

FIGURES 16.10 & 16.11
Fat emboli detected by Oil red O staining.

The presence of fat emboli, blood loss and narrowing of the coronary vessels by atheroma would have reduced the oxygenation to the heart muscle, causing episodes of myocardial ischaemia and precipitating a presumable fatal dysrhythmia and death.

16.6.5 Common samples at post-mortem

Blood

Blood is usually collected from one of the large veins such as the jugular vein in the neck or the femoral vein at the top of the thigh. Heart blood is sampled only when it is not possible to obtain any samples elsewhere.

Blood can be collected in sterile universal containers for most analyses, but if alcohol or glucose levels are to be tested then blood should be collected into a container containing potassium oxalate and sodium fluoride.

Blood samples can also be collected in anaerobic and aerobic blood culture bottles which are sent to the microbiology laboratory. Tubes containing ethylenediaminetetraacetic acid (EDTA) may also be used to collect blood as the EDTA binds with calcium ions to prevent coagulation.

Urine

Urine can be obtained in various ways before and after the abdomen has been opened. Most commonly it is collected once the abdomen has been opened but prior to organ removal. It is easiest with two people, one to keep the bladder exposed and clear from the intestine while the other can make a small incision in the bladder wall and use a syringe to sample the contents.

Urine in plain tubes can be used to test for unknown drugs or poisons, and in particular substances of abuse. Urine is also useful for alcohol analysis and, as with blood samples, should be collected in a specimen tube containing potassium oxalate and sodium fluoride.

Cerebrospinal fluid

Cerebrospinal fluid (CSF) is the fluid that surrounds the brain. It occupies the space between the pia mater, closest to the brain, and arachnoid mater, two of the three layers of meninges that surround the brain, the dura mater being the outer layer. The CSF also surrounds the spinal cord and fills the ventricular system in the brain as well as the central canal of the spinal cord.

Essentially, the brain 'floats' in CSF and it cushions the brain from sudden movements within the skull as well as providing chemical stability.

There are different methods for collecting CSF, the first being a lumbar puncture prior to the post-mortem examination. This is where a needle is introduced into the subarachnoid space between the laminae of the lower lumbar vertebrae. Alternatively, fluid can be collected using a needle and syringe from the cerebellomedullary cistern by passing a needle anterosuperiorly (forward and upwards) through the atlanto-occipital membrane, between the atlas and the occiput. Cerebrospinal fluid can also be collected with a needle from the lateral ventricles once the skullcap has been removed, and can also be removed by putting a needle into the foramen magnum just before or once the brain has been removed, but this will often be contaminated with blood.

Cerebrospinal fluid should be collected into a sterile container and a second sample may be frozen for later analysis.

Vitreous humour

Vitreous humour is the soft, transparent gel-like substance that fills the eyeball between the lens and the retina. It can be sampled by puncturing the sclera with a sterile needle and syringe. Ideally, the needle should be introduced laterally at the corner of the eye and around 5 mL of fluid should be re-moved. The eyeball will collapse when the vitreous is removed so best practice is to leave the needle *in situ* and place the contents of the syringe in a sterile container. The syringe is then filled with saline, reconnected to the needle, and the correct volume of fluid returned for a natural looking eyeball.

Vitreous samples are useful where a body has been exposed to heat, or if putrefaction is beginning to occur. This specimen may be especially useful for biochemistry tests as well as glucose, alcohol and heroin levels.

Stomach contents

If analysis of stomach contents is required, it is best collected from the unopened stomach once it has been removed from the body. It is important to remember to clamp the oesophagus (entrance to the stomach) and duodenum (exit and first part of the small intestine) so that no contents are lost. It is important that a representative sample of all the stomach contents is taken. In cases of suspected overdose all the stomach contents should be examined and if individual capsules or tablets can be seen then these should be picked out and sent for analysis.

16.6.6 Other post-mortem samples

Bile

Bile from the gall bladder may sometimes be used for drug analysis especially to establish morphine levels.

Brain

Brain tissue, usually a small cube frozen at the earliest opportunity, can be used where volatile gas is thought to have played a part in the death. Volatile gases such as butane (lighter fuel) can be inhaled and brain tissue analysis is the best way of establishing whether this contributed to the death.

Liver

A small cube of liver, usually from the right lobe so as not to be affected by bile or stomach contents, can be taken to investigate certain poisons.

Lung

A small piece of lung, usually taken from the apex of the lung, may be used to investigate death involving gases or volatile substances. This should be put in a sterile container and refrigerated prior to analysis. Lung can also be sent for microbiological analysis.

Hair

Hair may be used in the investigation of death related to drug abuse, especially opiates and methadone. Hair grows at the rate of approximately 1 cm/month so information concerning the deceased's drug abuse, chronic or otherwise, can be established. Ideally, hair should be plucked from the head; however, if it is cut then the proximal end should be tied for easy orientation prior to being sent for analysis. As blood circulates in the hair follicle any drugs present become incorporated in the hair matrix during growth. Once incorporated, the drug becomes fixed in the hair and remains as the hair grows. Hair is washed with shampoo and solvent prior to analysis to remove environmental contaminants. Gas and mass spectrometry both may be used in hair analysis.

Nail and bone

Chronic metal poisoning, especially arsenic and lead, may be confirmed by small samples of nail and bone.

16.7 Reconstruction

One of the most important parts of the post-mortem examination is the reconstruction of the deceased. It is generally accepted that the deceased should look as good as, if not better than, before the post-mortem examination.

All the organs removed should be replaced within the body cavity unless there is permission for their retention. Organs should be placed in a sealed viscera bag to prevent seepage. The neck and pelvic areas should be packed with absorbent material where necessary and the breast plate replaced over the chest in alignment with the ribs to give a good shape. The APT should then sew up the incisions that have been made. Any small marks can be sutured using cosmetic thread and subcutaneous stitches. Superglue can also be used to seal small holes such as those caused by cannulae so that there is no blood leakage. Once the body has been reconstructed satisfactorily, any blood or fluids should be washed off and the body dried. Hair should be washed and dried as necessary. Often it is easiest to suture scalp wounds when the scalp is reflected, especially if the hair is long or very thick.

Ensuring that the identity bracelet is still *in situ* and legible, the deceased can be redressed in a shroud and/or sheet, placed in a body bag if necessary and returned to the refrigerator.

In paediatric and child cases special care must be taken with reconstruction as often the family may wish to pick up or hold their child.

16.8 Disinfection

After the post-mortem examination it is important that the post-mortem room and all the instruments used are cleaned to a high standard. While it is possible to use disposable instruments, in most cases this is prohibitively expensive and usually is only employed in increased-risk cases such as suspected transmissible spongiform encephalopathy.

Each mortuary should have a rigorous and robust protocol for disinfection and sterilization of instruments, and most have moved on from washing by hand in a sink. Ideally, after rinsing, the instruments should be placed in an ultrasonic bath to loosen any material which may adhere to difficult-to-reach area of scissors and the teeth of the saw blades. Instruments should then be washed in a washer-disinfector that achieves a temperature of at least 85°C. Once washed, the instruments should be dried thoroughly before being placed in an autoclave. Some machines will dry instruments after washing. These processes will ensure that at the next post-mortem examination there is no cross-contamination when the instruments are used subsequently.

The post-mortem room should be thoroughly cleaned; this includes all work surfaces, the post-mortem room table(s) and the floor. There are many different disinfectants available but most mortuaries will use one or two in order to keep chemical storage and risk of chemical reaction or deactivation to a minimum.

Phenolics and aldehydes have gradually been replaced by more modern cleaning agents that potentially are less harmful to those coming into contact with them. These chemicals can be absorbed by the skin and mucous membranes and are highly irritant to users. Many people who used them previously became sensitized and had to wear full PPE subsequently.

Alcohol is mainly used for disinfecting the skin and occasionally for pieces of equipment in the post-mortem room. However, its main use is as a hand sanitizer in public areas and for cleaning items such as computer keyboards and telephones in the mortuary office. Alcohol is effective against some bacteria and viruses but not fungi or bacterial spores.

Chlorine-releasing agents continue to be used in many mortuaries and are effective against viruses including hepatitis B and human immunodeficiency virus (HIV). They are also deemed to be effective against prions so are used in suspected TSE cases. Unfortunately, chlorine-releasing agents are very corrosive and therefore use is limited usually to spillages on the floor and the cleaning of sponges. Stainless steel surfaces can be cleaned but need to be washed down immediately to prevent damage. Rubber boots can also be damaged if left in contact with the agents for too long.

Quaternary ammonium compounds and halogenated tertiary amines are modern chemicals commonly used in the modern mortuary as they are considered safer to use and are effective against most common pathogens. Non-corrosive, non-staining and safe to use on most surfaces within the mortuary, they are increasingly replacing the older types of disinfectant.

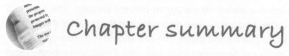 Chapter summary

Mortuary function

- The mortuary has many functions the most basic of which is body storage.
- There are many different laws which govern what can and cannot be done in each mortuary.

Natural processes after death

- As soon death occurs the body is starting to break down.
- Natural decomposition processes can be slowed by cooling the body to around 5°C.
- Some disease processes will hasten the deterioration of the body as will external factors such as temperature and humidity.

Post-mortem examinations

- Post-mortem examinations can be agreed to by the family or instructed by a legal process.
- In England, Wales and Northern Ireland the Coroners' system is used whilst in Scotland the Procurator Fiscal implements the laws around death.

- Post-mortem examinations must be carried out in premises licensed by the HTA in England & Wales.

- Tissue cannot be retained at post-mortem without the full knowledge and usually the consent of the next of kin.

- Retained tissue must be disposed of by a route agreed by the family and the authority retaining the tissue.

After the post-mortem

- Reconstruction of the deceased is very important.

- Cross-contamination can be minimized by thorough cleaning and disinfection of the post-mortem room and equipment.

- Samples should be stored correctly and sent to the correct laboratory as soon as possible.

 Further reading

- Crown Office and Procurator Fiscal Service. *Death and the Procurator Fiscal*. Edinburgh: COPFS, 2008 (www.procuratorfiscal.gov.uk).

- Department of Health. *Immunisation against infectious disease*. London: DH, 2006 (www.dh.gov.uk/en/Publichealth/Immunisation/Greenbook/index.htm).

- Health and Safety Executive. *Safe working and the prevention of infection in the mortuary and post-mortem room*. London: HSE, 2003b (www.hse.gov.uk/pubns/books/mortuary-infection.htm).

- NHS Estates. *Facilities for mortuary and post-mortem room services* 3rd edn. Health Building Note 20. London: NHS Estates, 2005. ISBN 9780113227150.

- Procurator Fiscal Service. *Reporting deaths to the procurator fiscal. Information and Guidance for Medical Practitioners*. Crown Office and Procurator Fiscal Service 2014.

Useful websites

- Association of Anatomical Pathology Technology (www.aaptuk.org)

- Human Tissue Authority (www.hta.gov.uk)

- Information on the coroner (www.justice.gov.uk)

- The Cremation (England & Wales) Regulations 2008 (www.legislation.gov.uk/uksi/2008/2841/contents/made)

- The Cremation (Scotland) Regulations (www.legislation.gov.uk/ssi/2003/301/contents/made)

- The Royal College of Pathologists (www.rcpath.org)

- UK Government Information. When a Death is Reported to the Coroner (www.gov.uk/after-a-death/when-a-death-is-reported-to-a-coroner)

Discussion questions

16.1   What are the advantages of an invasive post-mortem in diagnosis of cause of death or incidental pathologies?

16.2   What checks would you carry out as a minimum before commencing a post-mortem examination?

16.3   Why is it important to have access to the clinical history and/or circumstances of death prior to commencing a post-mortem examination?

Answers to the self-check questions and tips for responding to the discussion questions are provided on the book's accompanying website:

 Visit www.oup.com/uk/orchard2e

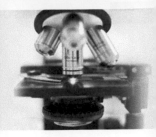

17

Essentials of laboratory management

Sue Alexander and Patricia Fernando

Learning objectives

By the end of the chapter you should:

- Have a practical working knowledge of all aspects of work involved in laboratory management and how these interact within a clinical governance framework in histopathology.

- Be able to participate in managing quality management systems, as applied to your laboratory, including audits.

- Appreciate the role that quality control (QC) and quality assurance (QA) and quality improvement play in the maintenance of quality standards.

- Be able to identify risks and be able to control/reduce the risks to staff and patients.

- Be conversant with all relevant legislation and accreditation requirements, as applied to histopathology.

- Be aware of the options for management qualifications and training and qualifications for staff in specific departmental roles.

17.1 Introduction

Good laboratory management is a difficult concept to define absolutely, being made up of many different component parts, but it is essential to the smooth running of a modern histopathology laboratory. It is incumbent on all laboratory staff to take responsibility for the safety of themselves and others (Health and Safety at Work Act 1974), but it falls to the laboratory management to implement systems to assess risk and ensure there is safe practice (risk management). However, it is the systems that ensure good quality that reap the most benefits in the workplace, both to staff and patients, and these quality management systems will be described in more detail for a histopathology laboratory working within a clinical governance framework (Figure 17.1a).

Accreditation and regulation bodies have played a large part in the introduction of quality management systems. This is intended to ensure that accreditation with standards for diagnostic laboratories derived from ISO 9000 laid down by the International Organization for Standardization (ISO), based in Geneva, is achieved and maintained. Accrediting organizations such as Clinical Laboratory Accreditation (UK) Ltd (CPA) and the United Kingdom Accreditation Service (UKAS) have encouraged a programme of maintenance of laboratory quality and continuing improvement against these standards (Burnett, 2002).

There are comparable bodies and programmes operating in many other countries. In the USA it refers to the College of American Pathologists Accreditation Program (CAP Accreditation); its principles ensure consistent practice and its two-year cycle and model of peer-based inspections are designed to go well beyond regulatory compliance and help laboratories to achieve the highest standards that address quality, efficiency and safety.

The National Pathology Accreditation Advisory Council (NPAAC), which is a ministerially appointed council, originally established in 1979 by a statutory instrument known as an Order in Council, updated in 2003, plays a key role in ensuring the quality and safety of pathology services and is responsible for the development and maintenance of standards and guidelines for pathology practices in Australia. The National Association of Testing Authorities, Australia (NATA), conducts audits against these standards and guidelines, and, when determining access to the Medicare Benefits Scheme, these audit assessment reports are considered by the Department of Human Services.

(a)

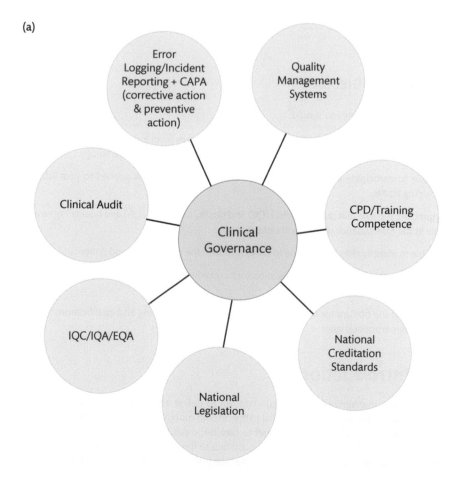

FIGURE 17.1A
Diagram illustrating the components of a clinical governance framework.

(b)

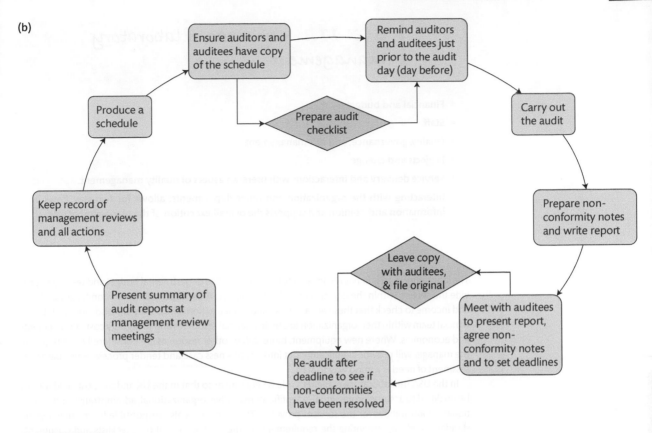

FIGURE 17.1B
Audit process flowchart.

In addition to defined standards for laboratories undertaking histological investigations on human tissue samples, there are also national laws governing the use of tissue samples, and compliance with such laws and regulations is required, being assessed in a similar way to laboratory standards. In the UK, the Human Tissue Authority issues licences for post-mortem work, anatomy, public display of bodies and tissues, and, where it is undertaken, research work. There is a cost associated with registration and assessment with all these bodies: it should also be borne in mind that an assessment visit may result in a requirement for departmental resources to be made available to address specific deficiencies.

In addition to external assessments, the quality performance of laboratories is continually assessed and compared to other similar laboratories to complete the quality assurance process via interlaboratory comparison schemes (Figures 17.1a and 17.1b).

17.2 **Roles in laboratory management**

The role of the laboratory manager is to be in day-to-day charge of the effective, efficient, economic and quality assured delivery of the laboratory service to the service users (see Box 17.1). This means patients as well as the direct users of the service (i.e. clinicians and other medical professionals). The skills and competences of the manager need to be diverse and extensive; it is likely that the manager will need to undertake a range of training in order to acquire and develop skills. The manager also needs to be forward-thinking, open to change, adaptable, and both willing and able to keep up to date with developments in management and the science and technology used in delivering their service.

BOX 17.1 Key areas of laboratory management

- Financial and budgetary.
- Staff.
- Quality, governance, and risk management.
- Projects and change.
- Service delivery and interactions with users: an aspect of quality management.
- Interacting with the organization and other departments: allows for two-way flows of information and opinion and supports the overall execution of the management role.

The laboratory manager has responsibility for managing the departmental budget and seeking to provide the service within the constraints of the budget. It is their responsibility to monitor expenditure and income to check that these are accurate, and to take action if not. They will also work with the financial team within their organization to obtain financial resources and to identify cost improvements and economies. Where new equipment, more staff or other resources are considered to be required, the manager will provide significant input into any business case and tender process. A risk-based assessment of need is a good way to start.

In the USA the laboratory manager's role is very similar to that in the UK and the post-holder must be qualified to assume professional, scientific, consultative, organizational, administrative and educational responsibilities for the services provided. The manager is also responsible for maintaining the standards and implementing the requirements of the CAP accreditation checklists and documenting compliance, and must have the authority to fulfil these responsibilities effectively. The manager should ensure that the laboratory is staffed with a sufficient number of personnel to perform quality laboratory procedures, lines of authority within the laboratory are defined, and individuals who work in the laboratory fulfil their responsibilities and interact effectively with one another.

17.2.1 Laboratory and procurement processes

Purchasing equipment, information technology systems, goods and services is no longer a simple matter. Procurement law applies in the UK, for example, and hospitals usually have their own procurement department to ensure that all requirements of the law are met and to provide guidance to managers over procurement processes. Procurement departments frequently take a lead in negotiating prices and contracts, and overseeing tender processes where it is necessary to tender for the required item or contract. In Australia the Public Governance, Performance and Accountability Act 2013 provides a framework for the proper expenditure of public resources by corporate and non-corporate entities, and this Act is supplemented by local government and state rules. In the USA, procurement law is complex; the overarching legislation is the Federal Acquisition Regulation, 48 C.F.R. (FAR), which applies to government bodies and specific defined independent bodies. A number of other Acts are in place to ensure fairness of competition and transparency.

The purpose of all these laws is to seek the best price for the best goods and services, preventing favouritism, nepotism or influence via inducements, leading to fair and open competition. Having established a supplier and contract, the manager is responsible for ensuring that the department practises good stock control and management. ISO 15189:2012 includes clauses covering both the selection of suppliers and monitoring their performance, plus clauses on reagent management (see Case study 17.1). Bulk purchasing can lead to better prices but this must not be countered by careless use of stock such as allowing items to go out of date. Stock management must be assessed and reviewed to ensure a balance of purchasing and use. A contract could stipulate that reagents must be delivered with a specific shelf life, for example.

17.2.2 Roles of the manager

The manager is responsible for the selection, recruitment and induction of non-medical staff. Thereafter they ensure that appraisals and monitoring of these staff take place, although they may not necessarily appraise all staff individually. This activity can be delegated to other staff who have been trained appropriately. Also, the supervision of staff may be delegated to others involved with the day-to-day running of sections of the department. Section leaders are usually experienced senior biomedical scientists who supervise staff (both qualified and support) within their area. They take responsibility for a specific section of departmental work during the day, but will liaise with the manager if issues arise that are beyond the scope of their capability and/or knowledge. It is important to set boundaries for all staff and establish at which point a more senior staff member must become involved. Section leaders will frequently participate in the planning of new developments related to their area of expertise (Totty, 2003). When serious staff issues need to be addressed, such as capability, disciplinary action and management of absence, this will involve the manager working alongside other organizational departments such as human resources and occupational health.

Appraisals are usually carried out annually and objectives set in line with trust or departmental objectives. Appraisals should be positive experiences, with successes and achievements acknowledged, and no surprises with regard to negatives. Capability, performance and disciplinary issues must be raised as they occur and not wait for the appraisal or annual review. Feedback (360 degree), from and to senior and junior staff and at the same level as the appraisee, and where relevant from other departments, can all be invited to provide feedback relevant to their relationship and reporting lines. The appraisal needs to be a two-way open discussion.

Review dates may be set after three or six months to ensure progress is being made—a form of performance management. Job descriptions, previously evaluated by Agenda for Change (AfC), are reviewed and Knowledge and Skills Framework (KSF) levels are evaluated. A personal development plan (PDP) is put in place to support the individual in achieving the agreed objectives. These objectives should link personal development and training, departmental needs and objectives, and the objectives of the host organization. Continuing professional development (CPD) requirements such as those audited by the Health and Care Professions Council (HCPC) in the UK and supported by the Institute of Biomedical Science and The Royal College of Pathologists CPD schemes, often referred to as continuous personal and professional development (CPPD), should also be discussed.

Laboratory management meetings are held regularly to take decisions about how to deal with issues as they arise. Often, a histopathologist will take responsibility as clinical lead and work with the laboratory manager to run the department. Laboratory meetings should be open, supportive forums to disseminate information, discuss developments and changes, include review of quality objectives and performance indicators, allow staff to make suggestions for improvements, and cover any general points of discussion. The head of department and manager will appoint other pathologists and biomedical scientists as deputies to assist them in various specific roles (see Box 17.2)

BOX 17.2 Key roles in laboratory management

- **Training Officer**, coordinating the training and development of all staff.
- **Health and Safety Officer**, taking a lead on risk management.
- **Quality Manager**, overseeing the quality management system.

The manager is responsible for ensuring that the department adheres to the requirements of national legislation and applicable guidelines and standards, including current quality standards (see Section 17.3).

Science and technology are continually moving forward with new methods, equipment and techniques becoming available. Additionally, organizations and pathology services are increasingly engaged in implementing changes and/or running projects. These changes can range from amendments to standard operating procedures, to putting a new instrument into service, to implementing a new laboratory information system.

The manager needs to determine the level of impact of the change and as a result the approach to its introduction. A formal project-based approach is useful for larger changes in order to ensure a structured and documented plan from which to work. Changes to staff work patterns or terms and conditions of employment will require input from human resources and trades unions.

To undertake their role successfully, managers will need to liaise with various individuals and will require strong communications skills, diplomacy and political awareness. The ability to engage with service users, other departments in the organization, and key individuals should not be underestimated.

17.3 Quality management systems and clinical governance

Quality management is a method used to ensure that all the activities necessary to design, develop and implement a product or service are effective and efficient with respect to the system and its performance. In histopathology, there are many steps, both manual and automated, in the production of a diagnostic histopathology report, including processing fixed tissue and staining cut sections, all of which must be controlled separately (Totty, 2000). This extends to the production of the final histopathology report, which must conform to the highest degree of diagnostic accuracy possible.

Cases, especially cancer cases, are discussed at multidisciplinary team (MDT) meetings, during which the pathology and radiology findings are discussed with the clinical team looking after the patient. Sometimes a diagnosis may need to be altered in light of further clinical information. Review of complex or difficult cases in this forum provides additional expert information if an unusual or unexpected report is issued, and provides an opportunity to audit the entire diagnostic process before further treatment or surgery is undertaken (see Box 17.3).

BOX 17.3 Quality management system

The quality management system (QMS) is overseen by a quality manager and includes:

- quality policy
- quality manual
- quality objectives
- quality control
- quality assessment
- quality improvement
- document control
- maintenance of audit calendar.

17.3.1 Quality standards for medical laboratories

Medical laboratory standards in the United Kingdom have been set and assessed by Clinical Pathology Accreditation (UK) since 1992. Initially, enrolment on the scheme was voluntary but over time it became a requirement of the Department of Health that all medical laboratories would enrol. CPA (UK) also assessed laboratories issuing material for external quality assessment (EQA) schemes using similar standards with some modifications. The medical laboratory standards have been revised over time, with a particularly significant change in the version published in 2003, which was more aligned with ISO 15189. The CPA (UK) standards were also adopted by a number of other countries.

In 2009, CPA (UK) became a wholly owned subsidiary of the United Kingdom Accreditation Service (UKAS) and a transition period began, moving towards assessment of laboratories against the internationally recognized standard ISO 15189:2012 (Medical Laboratories–Requirements for quality and competence) and for CPA-accredited EQA providers to ISO/IEC 17043:2010 (Conformity Assessment–General requirements for proficiency testing). Assessment remains in the format as used by CPA (UK)–a peer-review system supported and coordinated by an assessment manager with UKAS observation–but will involve an annual assessment element in order to comply with ISO 17011, the international standard governing national accrediting bodies. As ISO 15189: 2012 is an international standard it can be applied to many countries.

In the United States of America, standards were first determined under the Clinical Laboratory Improvement Amendments (CLIA) regulations of 1988, entitled 'Standards and Certification: Laboratory Requirements'. These regulations established quality standards for the laboratory testing of human specimens including blood, other body fluids, and tissues for the purposes of diagnosis, prevention or treatment of disease, or health assessment. This latter point is not explicitly described in ISO 15189:2012. The CLIA 1988 regulations were first published in 1992, phased in during 1994, and amended in 1993, 1995 and 2003.

The American Association for Laboratory Accreditation holds 'Deemed Status' awarded by the Centers for Medicare and Medicaid Services (CMS) for the accreditation of clinical testing laboratories to the requirements under CLIA. The organization offers options for approaching accreditation including ISO 15189:2012 as well as to CLIA requirements. An assessment team approach is taken with assessors matched to the repertoire.

The College of American Pathologists Laboratory Accreditation Program accredits the full range of laboratory test disciplines, again using a peer-review model and customized checklists. This accreditation programme inspects a range of laboratories from major medical centres to laboratories in local physician offices. The accreditation cycle runs on a two-year basis and also encompasses animal testing as well as human testing.

In Australia there are several organizations involved in standards covering laboratories undertaking medical sample testing. The National Pathology Accreditation Advisory Council (NPAAC) sets standards and requirements that laboratories must meet in Australia in order to be accredited providers of Medicare rebateable services. This is the Australian government service providing free or subsidized elements of healthcare to eligible individuals.

The National Association of Testing Authorities (NATA) is the authority responsible for the accreditation of laboratories, inspection bodies, calibration services, producers of certified reference materials and proficiency testing scheme providers throughout Australia. For medical testing, it refers to ISO 15189. It is also Australia's compliance monitoring authority for the OECD Principles of Good Laboratory Practice. Standards Australia is an independent, not-for-profit organization, recognized by the Australian government as the peak non-government standards body in Australia. Standards Australia develops internationally aligned Australian Standards and is the Australian member of ISO and IEC.

Assessments to ISO 15189:2012 (there is a new revision coming as there were some minor translation discrepancies, but to all intents and purposes it is the same) are carried out by an assessment team that will include a team leader from UKAS or NATA plus volunteer technical experts who will undertake the assessment of the laboratory and clinical aspects of a department. It is also common for a UKAS observer to be part of the team to ensure that all procedures are carried out appropriately and professionally. The standard states what is expected of laboratories in terms of a quality management system and technical and clinical competence to deliver the tests described within the scope of the assessment. It does not specify how this should or must be achieved, leaving laboratories free to determine their own approaches appropriate for their local situation. Laboratories must define their practices and procedures and then provide evidence that they are working to these and are in conformance with the requirements of ISO 15189:2012 and any relevant associated regulations, documents and standards.

A **quality manager** may be based within the histopathology laboratory or may be shared with other pathology disciplines. They implement the quality management system and work with the clinical and laboratory teams to embed it in the department. They should report to someone other than the laboratory manager to ensure that quality remains high on the laboratory's agenda.

The **quality policy** is a standalone document and must be read and understood by all employees. It describes the service provided and the department's commitment to the provision of high-quality pathology services to patients, together with a commitment to continual quality improvement.

Quality objectives are established in consultation with users and are reviewed regularly to ensure that they are appropriate and that the needs and requirements of users are met; they may change if the objectives of the organization change or as a result of comments obtained from a user survey or complaint. The concept not just of corrective action, but also preventive action to avoid errors, incidents and complaints needs to be embedded in daily life.

Key quality indicators are determined to identify underpinning critical elements of laboratory practice. If these indicators are substandard, all or part of the service may be put in jeopardy.

The **quality manual** describes the scope, purpose, organization and management of the histopathology laboratory, and acts as an index to how each quality standard is met. It includes an organizational chart to show how the department fits into the structure of the host organization and in the pathology committee structure, including a list of laboratory meetings. The document can be used for the induction and training of new staff in the principles of a pathology quality management system and its contribution to clinical governance and patient safety. All staff must read and understand the quality manual. The scope of the quality manual and adherence to national standards and legislation supports a culture of clinical governance. Many histopathology laboratories have used various approaches (e.g. Lean, Six Sigma) to become more efficient and improve the service they deliver to patients.

Quality control comprises internal processes that need to be carried out at every stage in the process, such as daily routine checking of the quality of standardized control sections stained (e.g. haematoxylin and eosin [H&E]) and examined using a light microscope (Bancroft and Gamble, 2007). These processes should be documented as evidence of internal quality control (IQC).

Sections can vary in thickness and often appear darker if the section is slightly too thick, making cellular detail difficult to discriminate under the light microscope. The length of fixation in formalin will also affect staining, especially as speed is often perceived to be important, and there is a temptation to 'hurry' this essential step and compromise quality for the sake of a short turnaround time. Similarly, different processing schedules also affect the final appearance of the stained section.

For these reasons, control sections are used and follow the standard operation procedures (SOPs) to maintain the workload of the laboratory. A tissue block of stomach is often used as a control because gastric cells show various staining patterns using the H&E method. A control section should be put through the automated stainer and checked under the light microscope each day before routine work is allowed on the machine (see Method 17.1). If staining results on the controls are found to be substandard, appropriate reagents must be replaced and the staining rechecked by a senior member of staff. This is a form of audit. The stained section should be labelled with date, time, and the staff initials, and stored for future reference. At times of high workload, or if solutions need to be changed, a second control section should be used and the process repeated.

METHOD 17.1 *Automated staining*

It is especially important to use control sections, which are validated for use with a particular technique (according to requirements or equivalent) when staining a section by hand, as each time you follow a method you will tend to obtain a slightly different result. Some workers would argue that having the flexibility to increase haematoxylin staining by decreasing differentiation can be advantageous in certain pathological conditions and when photomicrography is required. Automated procedures are very common in today's pathology laboratories and the majority of workload is undertaken with these processes. Automated staining machines have, to a large extent, standardized the staining process and have made results more consistent; however, there are variables that need to be controlled, such as:

- ready-made reagents
- reagent management
- pH of water
- room temperature
- effective lifespan of a prepared solution
- solution usage.

All special stains require a positive control to be stained alongside a test section (sometimes even mounted on the same slide as the test section) to ensure the method works correctly, and is particularly important when the test section is negative. This type of control section must be used when staining for infectious agents (e.g. tubercle bacilli), and they should be dated and filed alongside the test case, in case future review is required.

In immunocytochemistry, both negative and positive controls are required. The positive control will contain the appropriate antigen, while the negative control will act as a test for non-specific staining, due to interference in the technique. Positive controls should not contain too much specific antigen (i.e. they should show low antigen expression) to control the sensitivity as well as the specificity of the technique, and ideally the antigen should be spread evenly throughout the section. Reagent substitution controls omit the primary antibody, replacing it with buffer, to ensure the correct antigen is stained. Ideally, control sections should be mounted on the same slide as the test section to ensure identical exposure to the same reagents.

Tissue sections can act as their own internal control if they contain both normal and tumour areas (e.g. lymphocytes), but it is preferable to have a known positive external control so that performance can be reviewed over a period of time. Some tissues can act as a control for several different techniques (e.g. tonsil). Control blocks can be created from several different tissues (which are validated) and then used to test new antibodies for cross-reactivity, and therefore be able to quality control several different antibodies and staining techniques (see Case study 17.1).

SELF-CHECK 17.1

What are you carrying out if you review microscopically a number of control sections to identify trends in method performance? How may deteriorating performance be addressed?

SELF-CHECK 17.2

a)   Which tissues would you choose to put in a multi-tissue control block?
b)   Is each new control block validated before use against the test?

Quality assurance can be internal (IQC) or external (EQA) where the performance of one laboratory is compared to others and encompasses all aspects of the process. External quality assessment schemes (e.g. UK NEQAS for Cellular Pathology Technique or UK NEQAS for Immunocytochemistry and *In Situ* Hybridization) are generally used for this purpose and issue regular reports on the laboratory's performance. The UK NEQAS Steering Committee for Technical EQA schemes ensures the needs of the participants are being met. Individual pathologists participate in diagnostic EQA schemes appropriate for the specialist diagnostic area (e.g. breast, hepatology, neuropathology, etc.), but regional general histopathology EQA schemes are considered sufficient in many routine diagnostic areas (e.g. dermatopathology), and also provide an educational element.

CASE STUDY 17.1 *Reagent management*

Do you have to record the batch number of all reagents you use every day? Reagent management (according to ISO 15189) is a detailed documentation process which will be completed every day with routine procedures, and will consider the following:

- **Carry out a risk assessment to decide on the frequency of recording reagent data, such as:**
  - weekly
  - only when reagents are changed
  - only when solutions are made up for use.

- Ensure traceability in case of problems with the method.
- Check the reagent is being stored at the correct temperature. If stored in a refrigerator or freezer, is the temperature being recorded regularly?
- Use suitable controls (validated according to ISO standards) to monitor the performance of the reagents (IQC).

Technical EQA schemes are either selective, which means that stained material is submitted to the scheme for expert assessment, or distributive, in which case standardized unstained sections are circulated for staining by different methods, depending on laboratory repertoire, and returned for expert assessment. Material selected randomly from the laboratory archive can also be assessed for the quality of fixation, processing, embedding and cutting. Methods used are submitted with the stained slides and the best scoring methods are made available to help participants improve their technique (www.kneqascpt.org.uk). This process occurs quarterly, typically to ensure that quality of work is monitored, which is especially important when using predictive or prognostic markers such as HER2 (www.ukneqasiccish.org). Three low marks trigger a local report and the offer of assistance from the scheme organizer. Substandard performance is reported to the National Quality Assurance Advisory Panel (NQAAP) and must be declared to UKAS on annual re-application.

Quality improvement is required as an inherent aspect of a quality management system, and quality objectives are set to ensure continued service quality improvement is achieved. Quality and/or performance indicators are used to monitor that this has occurred.

Document control for all laboratory SOPs, policies and documents is best achieved using a commercial, password-controlled, web-based software package, although hard copies may be printed for use at the bench. Documents must be identified uniquely and dated with the revision number and date of next review, as well as other information as required by ISO 15189 or its equivalent. The author can send documents electronically to other members of the team for review and authorization, and each member of the team can be notified by email of a revision.

Quality management tools are used by the quality manager to provide evidence that the QMS is working satisfactorily. Audit is a useful tool and involves the collection and objective evaluation of evidence to see if the criteria set are fulfilled. An audit schedule is planned by the quality manager so that the full scope of laboratory activities is subjected to audit over a one-year period, and must include an audit of the QMS itself. There are several types of audit that can be carried out.

- **Vertical audit** takes a single recent specimen number or worksheet and looks across all aspects of the processes involved, including at all the supporting documentation. A vertical audit covers the information given to users before they submit a specimen, transportation of the sample to the laboratory, and all pre-examination, examination and post-examination procedures involved until a report is received by the requestor.

- **Horizontal audit** looks at a single process or aspect of work such as staff training logs or instrument maintenance records.

- **Witness audit** looks at a process, usually a technique, and comments on the way it is carried out, compared to the written standard operating procedure, and whether or not the members of staff involved have a good understanding of the procedure. It assesses their competence to carry out a task.

- **Annual management review** is carried out every year to review the quality policy, establish progress against the previous year's quality objectives, and set new quality objectives for the coming year. All senior staff should attend and report on internal audits carried out within their area of responsibility. ISO 15189 specifies agenda items to include in the review.

- **Performance monitoring** frequently includes reviewing specimen turnaround times over a specific time period, comparing them to figures for the previous period and years. It may also include a review of IQC or EQA results and looks at error logging or the reasons for repeat testing (see Case study 17.2). An action plan can be put in place and monitored regularly for improvement. Other ideas for performance indicators can be found in the College of American Pathologists Q Probe programme.

- **External reviews** are carried out by external agencies that visit the department and can be useful in identifying areas for improvement, especially if the external inspectors are looking at the processes from multiple perspectives (e.g. Good Laboratory Practice) as well as national standards.

- **Regulatory bodies** may also visit the department and make recommendations against national standards and regulations. These include the Medicines and Healthcare products Regulatory Agency (MHRA), Human Tissue Authority (HTA) and the Care Quality Commission (CQC) in the UK, the US Food and Drug Administration, and the Therapeutic Goods Administration in Australia.

CASE STUDY 17.2 Dealing with poor performance

What actions would you take if your NEQAS results showed 'poor performance'?
Regular review of NEQAS results at departmental meetings.

- **Identify the 'root cause' of the problem:**
  - look back at previous results/controls
  - find out who carried out the test
  - identify training needs
  - was the SOP followed appropriately?

- **Prepare an action plan of remedial work and timelines.**

- **If all else fails, ask for help from another centre that scored well. Follow 'best method' SOPs and compare results.**

Non-conformity or non-conformance arises when a laboratory fails to achieve a particular standard either in internal or external audit.

Corrective action is put in place to rectify the immediate problem and steps are taken to determine and apply preventive action to ensure the event does not occur again.

An **action plan** is drawn up with details of the action to be taken which must be regularly monitored:

- by whom?
- by when?

Preventive action aims to ensure that a non-conformity, error or other adverse event does not recur.

17.4 Clinical governance

Clinical governance intends to provide the best possible patient care in a safe environment within a clinical governance framework. It ensures that systems are in place and functioning properly to govern and monitor the quality of clinical practice, so that clinical practice is reviewed and improved as a result. For example, biomedical scientists are regulated by the Health and Care Professions Council (HCPC) and must meet the required standards to maintain registration. Laboratory managers can check the status of each qualified member of staff on the HCPC website.

Clinical audit relates to an audit carried out specifically on a clinical aspect of work and can be scheduled or unscheduled. An idea for an audit may arise from many sources including a complaint or an incident. Organizations have different formal procedures for registering and approving audits. Progress is reviewed at regular audit meetings and may include the need to re-audit to ensure that improvement is maintained. Audits may be set against known national standards (e.g. minimum datasets for cancer reporting) to assess pathologist reporting standards, but may also give useful information about the performance of the surgeon.

An **audit cycle** (Figure 17.2a) and **audit loop** (Figure 17.2b) describe the steps required to complete a cycle of quality improvement (Crombie et al., 1993).

SELF-CHECK 17.3

Suggest some titles for clinical audits in histopathology, and prepare an audit plan.

FIGURE 17.2A
An audit cycle.

(a)

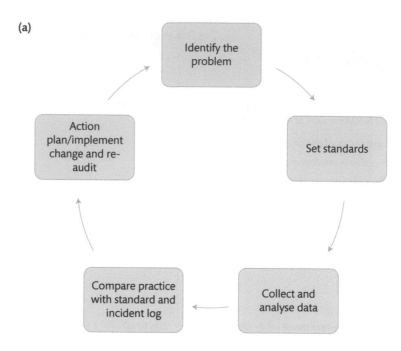

FIGURE 17.2B
The audit loop.

(b)

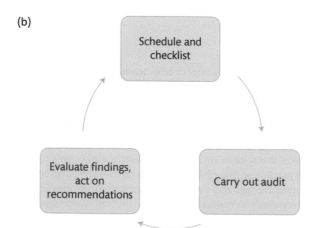

- If non-conformities are found, these need to be cleared as soon as possible.
- Once cleared, it is necessary to establish whether this has made a difference to the area that was audited (i.e. has it been improved; does it now meet the required standard?)
- The best way to establish this is to re-audit (i.e. close the audit loop).

Post-mortem, also known as an **autopsy,** is the examination of a body after death. The aim of a post-mortem is to determine the cause of death, but can also be used as a form of clinical audit, providing useful information for the trust on clinical practice. Post-mortems are carried out by pathologists, who are specialized doctors in understanding the nature and causes of death. They can either be authorized by the coroner (because the cause of death is unknown, or following a sudden, violent or unexpected death) or consented to by the family or through a hospital doctor (to find out more about an illness or the cause of death or to further medical research and understanding). A coroner is usually a lawyer or a doctor who is responsible for investigating deaths in certain situations, with a minimum of five years' experience. The purpose of a post-mortem requested by a coroner is to find out how someone died and decide whether an inquest is needed, and consent (permission) from the family is not required. Hospital post-mortems can only be carried out with consent and by hospital doctors (see Chapter 16).

Some reports have been compiled using these data by the National Confidential Enquiry into Patient Outcome and Death (NCEPOD) (www.ncepod.org.uk).

Clinical benchmarking: participation in a national benchmarking scheme is a way that the laboratory can demonstrate its performance against similar laboratories across the country. Data are submitted annually and the details of the analysis should be discussed and fed back to staff. Areas for improvement may be identified and data extracted and used to support business cases for resources (Galloway and Nadin, 2001).There are some caveats relating to benchmarking schemes; for example, no two laboratories are absolutely comparable and data may not always be available in the precise format the benchmarking scheme requires. Membership of a formal benchmarking scheme will usually incur a cost.

Cross reference
See Chapter 16, Mortuary practice, for further discussion of post-mortem examinations.

17.5 Risk management

Risk management is recognition that risks exist in the workplace. Factors that contribute to risks need to be identified and steps then taken to eliminate them (preventive actions), or at least minimize risks to patients and staff. All staff must be trained in incident reporting and understand their responsibilities for safe working practices (e.g. wearing personal protective equipment [PPE] when working with chemicals or biological hazards). Unscheduled health and safety inspections may be carried out by the Health and Safety Executive (HSE) across the organization if poor practice is suspected (www.hse.gov.uk). **Risk assessment** is a proactive approach to investigating hazards and their potential severity. This is usually performed using a standard format document to describe the issues, current controls, if any, and the potential outcome if the risk is not mitigated. Depending on the severity of the risk assessed, it may need to be added to the organization's formal risk register for the attention of senior management. Corporate risk registers are reviewed periodically with progress on actions taken recorded. Risks may include possibility of injury, impact to the service, financial loss, adverse publicity or potential for litigation.

Incident reporting is not undertaken simply to satisfy legal requirements or to comply with healthcare standards, but to ensure lessons are learned from mistakes and errors when they occur in order to prevent them from happening again. Incidents can be subject to the same procedure as nonconformities in an audit (i.e. initial corrective action is recorded and further preventive action needed to prevent the incident from happening again is then recorded in the form of an update or incident review) (Francis, 2013).

A **root cause** is a fundamental cause which, if resolved by preventive action, will eradicate or significantly contribute to the resolution of an identified problem or adverse event, either within the local department or more widely across the organization.

The underlying root causes of many incidents are system failures. The immediate cause may involve an individual failure (often an individual in a poorly designed system). It is recognized that individuals will make mistakes—people are only human. Minimizing error therefore focuses on improving systems not punishing individuals, and when investigating incidents the question is not 'Who is to blame?' but 'What went wrong?' and 'What can we learn?'

Root cause analysis investigation involves gathering the data to establish the cause of an adverse event. This may require input from a number of individuals and may involve a formal investigation meeting, depending on the severity of the event. Knowing how far back to go in order to investigate the incident fully may be difficult. Root cause analysis maps information on a timeline, identifies contributing factors, analyses their impact and determines the root cause(s). Based on this, investigators can generate solutions and implement and monitor progress. A simple approach to root cause analysis is the five 'Whys', starting with the event or incident discovered and then asking 'why?' repeatedly, tracking back along the pathway that has developed to the original precipitating factor (see Box 17.4).

BOX 17.4 Examples of common issues identified by root cause analysis

- **Adherence to policies and procedures**
  - SOP not followed.
- **Organizational and strategic**
  - lack of leadership
  - lack of safety culture.
- **Communication factors**
  - handover arrangements
  - ineffective MDTs
  - lack of escalation of problems.

- **Working conditions**
  - staffing issues
  - workload pressures
  - noisy, disturbed environment.
- **Education and training**
  - use of temporary staff
  - poor supervision
  - lack of induction training.

CASE STUDY 17.3 Inconsistent specimen labelling

You receive a sample with a request form: details do not match with the specimen pot details. What actions would you take?

- Refer to relevant pathology SOP. Document what you have done on the laboratory information system. Complete an incident form/error log.
- Inform the senior in charge and take advice and alert the rest of the team.
- Consider if the sample can easily be repeated.
- Take steps to contact the clinician to identify sample.
- Follow up incidents to see if the same ward/area is involved and offer training. Inform the relevant pathologist a mismatch case is received and hence the delay in processing the specimen.

Error logging is a useful way of documenting the reasons why a specimen has been delayed or has to be repeated (e.g. essential information is missing from the specimen container at booking in and the junior doctor has to be bleeped to identify that it came from the patient identified on the request form). Otherwise a note may be made on the final report; for example, 'the specimen cannot be guaranteed to be from that patient'. The number of errors of this type should be reviewed periodically to ensure there are no particular trends that need to be addressed, as mislabelling or missing vital information on a request form can lead to unnecessary delays to treatment as well as causing anxiety to the patient awaiting a diagnosis.

Likelihood	Insignificant (1)	Minor (2)	Moderate (3)	Major (4)	Catastrophic (5)
Rare (1)	1	2	3	4	5
Unlikely (2)	2	4	6	8	10
Possible (3)	3	6	9	12	15
Likely (4)	4	8	12	16	20
Certain (5)	5	10	15	20	25

FIGURE 17.3
Risk rating matrix.

If a specimen is lost or mislaid after being received in the department this incident is very serious and therefore a formal incident report must be written. The relevant staff and the team must be informed; the paperwork is the same as error logging, but more detailed, and senior management will be involved.

17.5.1 Risk assessment

To contribute to good governance and risk management (Figure 17.3 and Table 17.1), and to prevent errors, incidents and accidents, the following list indicates a range of points that are constantly changing in the workplace and which need to be considered from a risk management point of view:

- New and expectant mothers.
- New techniques.
- New hazards.
- Change in health of employee.
- Have there been any changes in working practice?
- Are improvements still required?
- Receipt of complaints/suggestions.
- Has there been a trend of similar incidents?

In summary, in managing risk a manager must:

- Take an integrated approach.
- Have staff in defined roles and responsibilities.

TABLE 17.1 Evaluate risk and decide on actions.

Risk rating	Risk	Action required	Review
1–4	Low (Green)	Accept risk (manage routine procedures).	Every three/six months by risk officer.
5–10	Medium (Yellow)	Management action required. Cost funded locally.	Every four weeks/three months by risk officer. Quarterly review at SDU/clinical governance meeting.
12–25	High (Red)	Senior management action required. High risk identified. Re-evaluate risk management and develop greater controls.	Every two/three months by risk officer. Quarterly review at local SDU/clinical governance meeting.

- Continuously strive to improve patient safety.
- Identify, assess and minimize risk.
- Use risk assessments to inform investment.
- Encourage open and honest reporting of incidents.
- Identify incident trends and use this to inform change.
- Use root cause analysis methodologies to investigate incidents.
- Report to key stakeholders.
- Foster an open culture, share information and learning.

17.6 Dealing with complaints

Complaints are usually received via the organizational complaints department or the Patient Advice and Liaison Service (PALS), or equivalent, in a UK hospital and forwarded to the laboratory manager. There may be an independent investigator appointed or the manager may be asked to investigate. Practices vary between organizations. In any case the manager will be involved in the root cause analysis investigation to ascertain if the complaint is true and should be upheld and to determine why the complaint came to be raised, that is, what was the cause for the complaint. A summary of all pathology complaints is discussed at the most relevant departmental forum(s). Complaints will also be recorded within the organization and discussed at clinical governance and risk management meetings. Written feedback is given to the complainant to summarize the results of the investigation and to explain the corrective actions introduced. This may need to be followed up by further correspondence or a face-to-face meeting, as required.

17.7 Human Tissue Act

The Human Tissue Act 2004 established that the wishes of the individual are paramount and made consent the fundamental principle underpinning the lawful removal, storage, use and disposal of any human tissue from the living or deceased (see Box 17.5). The Human Tissue Act 2004 covers England, Wales and Northern Ireland. It established the Human Tissue Authority (HTA) as the body to produce codes of practice for the use of human tissue for scheduled purposes. The HTA aims to create an effective regulatory framework for the removal, retention, use and disposal of human tissue and organs in which the public and professionals have confidence, as it was recognized that more donations would be needed for research and to teach pathologists in autopsy techniques and surgeons in surgical techniques in the future (www.hta.gov.uk). It also carries out inspections (see Box 17.6).

BOX 17.5 What is human tissue?

- **Human body or body parts.**
- **Whole organs.**
- **Tissue blocks and slides.**
- **Cells.**
- **Biological fluids.**
- **Proteins, nucleic acids, etc.**

Consent is always required for human tissue taken from the deceased but is not required for human tissue taken from the living if it is to be used anonymously (or coded to make sure patient or participant information is not identifiable) in an ethically approved research project (see Case study 17.4); or if the tissue samples were obtained before 1 September 2006 (when the Human Tissue Act came into force). Human tissue (scheduled purpose) can be used for the following:

- obtaining scientific or medical information about a living or deceased person which may be relevant to any other person (including a future person)
- research in connection with disorders, or the functioning, of the human body
- transplantation
- clinical audit, education, teaching, public health monitoring and quality assurance.

Consent should be obtained in accordance with the:

- HTA Code of Practice on Consent (Code 1)
- Human Tissue (HT) Act (Part 1) 2004.

However, it:

- is different depending on whether the human tissue is obtained from the living or the deceased
- relates only to material taken after 1 September 2006 (when the Act was introduced)
- does not apply to 'existing holdings' from the living or the deceased before 1 September 2006.

The flowchart shown in Figure 17.4 summarizes the current situation for consent requirements if human tissue is needed for research.

Consent should be obtained from a living person, as long as they are competent to do so (Mental Capacity Act 2005). If a person's wishes were not made known prior to death, consent should be obtained from persons in 'a qualifying relationship' (i.e. this person may not necessarily be the spouse). To qualify as obtaining 'informed consent', the person seeking consent must provide sufficient information to enable the person giving consent to make a decision. They should be able to explain clearly any risks, benefits and alternatives to treatment and have a procedure in place should the person

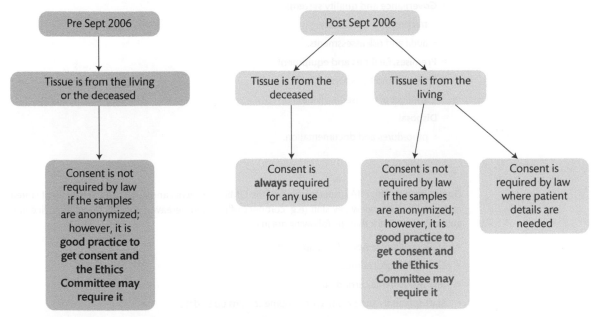

Note 1. Use of any human tissue for research requires Ethical Approval
2. Consent is obtained with reference to the Mental Capacity Act (2005)

FIGURE 17.4
Flowchart to show consent requirements that must be satisfied in order to use human tissue for research.

change their mind. Recent studies show that 80% of people would agree to donate leftover samples if asked, and many are willing to provide one-time general consent for research and rely on the decisions of ethics committees with regard to the projects in which the samples are used.

There are five HTA licences that institutions can apply for, but most post-mortem services based in a histopathology department have a Pathology HTA Licence. A **designated individual** (DI) is trained and appointed to lead the licence for the trust, but other people working on licensed premises and carrying out licensed activities do so under the direction of the DI or a person designated by the DI.

SELF-CHECK 17.4

Who should be the designated individual?

The DI needs a direct link with the trust board for support with issues via a governance structure (e.g. Human Tissues Committee reports to Clinical Governance Committee). The DI must be able to effect change (i.e. have managerial capability) and needs time allocated within their substantive role, included in their job plan and stated in their job description.

BOX 17.6 Human Tissue Authority inspection

The HTA inspection is risk-based and may depend on additional conditions. It can be scheduled, random or unannounced and is focused on:

- Consent
- Governance and quality systems
  - tracking and traceability
  - audit and risk assessments.
- Premises, facilities and equipment
  - storage and transport
  - conduct of licensed activities.
- Disposal
  - procedures and documentation.

During the visit, the HTA inspectors review the QMS documents and audit the traceability of stored material. They interview key staff (e.g. coroner's officer and bereavement officer), offer advice and guidance, and check that the following are in place:

- SOPs regularly reviewed and updated.
- Complaints procedures.
- Risk assessments carried out.
- Staff appraisals and personal development plans up to date.
- Reference to organizational procedures (e.g. data protection).
- Investigate incidents and review actions—corrective and preventative actions.
- Service level agreement (SLA) with coroner.
- Agreements with visiting pathologists.
- Tissue bank transfer agreements/materials transfer agreements.

- Service level agreements or contracts with couriers and other organizations.
- Check documentation (e.g. freezer maintenance records).
- Knowledge of HTA and evidence of training in HTA.
- HTA licence displayed.
- Audit trail of retained blocks and slides.
- Information about transplant operations.
- Annual report.

CASE STUDY 17.4 Use of human tissue

I want to use specimens of human tissue/blood for an MSc project. What do I need to do to ensure I comply with the Human Tissue Act?

- Gain ethical approval for your project via the local Research & Development Department.
- Refer project proposal to a pathology advisory committee (or equivalent) to check scientific content.
- Check patient consent covers use of the sample for research (not needed if taken prior to September 2006). Approach a human tissue bank that issues samples anonymously for research. Submit paperwork and sign 'tissue transfer agreement'.
- Return samples at the end of the project (or when the ethical approval expires) for storage or respectful disposal.

17.8 Training and qualifications

The IBMS offers managers options for training and qualifications. The Certificate of Expert Practice runs annually and is an online, self-directed 12-week programme supplemented by discussion forums, assessed work and an examination. The course is supported by tutors who are experienced managers. The Higher Specialist Diploma in Leadership and Management is a portfolio-based approach to gaining a qualification. The candidate compiles a set of required evidence and once this has been assessed and deemed to be complete and at a suitable level, the candidate may progress to the examination element.

Other options for management qualifications include those offered by universities and business schools, face-to-face and online, which lead to certificate, diploma and Masters.

A Certificate of Expert Practice is also available both in Quality Management and in Training. Useful training courses for health and safety officers include those offered at several levels by the Chartered Institute for Environmental Health, The National Examination Board in Occupational Safety and Health, and the Institution of Occupational Safety and Health, which is a Chartered body for health and safety professionals. Similarly, the Chartered Quality Institute is empowered to make its own awards relating to quality management and offers membership at varying levels in the same way as the IBMS.

Where staff are working in new extended roles (e.g. advanced practitioner biomedical scientists), appropriate training and assessment by suitably skilled and competent individuals is essential. This training must be clearly defined and documented.

The IBMS also offers a range of appropriate qualifications including the Higher Specialist Diploma (HSD) in Cellular Pathology, the Advanced Specialist Diploma (ASD) in Specimen Dissection in Breast Pathology and in Lower GI Pathology, with ASD qualifications in Urology and Female Genital Tract under development. Both ASD qualifications require that candidates must have completed the

Diploma of Expert Practice (DEP) in Histological Dissection, including in the appropriate optional module, before the ASD can be undertaken.

The DEP in Histological Dissection requires the completion of a portfolio of evidence and accompanying training logbook, which must show evidence of two years of current practice. The logbook requires the completion of the mandatory units and then as many of the optional units that the individual may wish to take (typically three or four). Candidates also have to sit and pass two two-hour examinations.

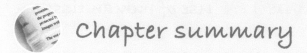

Chapter summary

You should now have an overview of the main management issues encountered in a diagnostic histopathology laboratory and understand how quality management and clinical governance work together to provide more effective and safer patient care.

- The laboratory manager works within their own team and within the framework of their host organization to manage the delivery of a quality, timely and relevant service repertoire.

- Relevant legislation and accreditation standards have helped to improve the service offered to users, and quality improvements are based on their needs and requirements, as identified in user surveys.

- Internationally defined standards provide the opportunity for laboratories to meet a set of common quality parameters recognized around the world giving credibility to their operation.

- Service users are not only clinicians and healthcare professionals, but also the patients when consulting healthcare professionals.

- Effective quality management systems are essential to reassure the government and the public that they can depend on the reports produced by the laboratory and that this will be achieved within a professional and open culture.

- Staff are the main resource in any laboratory and they need to receive adequate training and support to carry out their role to the best of their abilities, and their performance will be subject to regular review.

- Risks to staff and patients must be recognized and controlled. Where incidents do occur they must be fully investigated to identify the root cause(s) to ensure they never happen again.

- Performance and productivity must be measured and monitored, both internally and externally, and action plans put in place where targets are not being met.

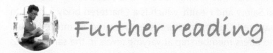

Further reading

- **Alexander S. Climbing the management qualification mountain: the road to the MBA.** *The Biomedical Scientist* 2015 April; **59** (4): 216–17.

- **Bancroft JD, Gamble M.** *Theory and practice of histological techniques* 6th edn. Edinburgh: Churchill Livingstone, 2007.

● Burnett D. *A practical guide to accreditation in laboratory management*. London: ACB Venture Publications, 2002.

● Carter P. *Independent review of NHS pathology services*. London: Department of Health, 2008.

● College of American Pathologists. Q Probe Program.

● Crombie IK, Davies HTO, Abraham SCS, Florey CDuV. *The audit handbook*. Chichester: Wiley, 1993.

● Darzi A. *High quality care for all*. London: Department of Health, 2008.

● Francis R. *The Mid Staffordshire NHS Foundation Trust Public Inquiry, 2013* (www.midstaffspublicinquiry.com/sites/default/files/report/Executive%20summary.pdf).

● Galloway M, Nadin L. Benchmarking and the laboratory. *J Clin Pathol* 2001; **54** (8): 590–7.

● Totty BA. Histopathology under the microscope. *The Biomedical Scientist* 2000 October; **44** (10): 932–3.

● Totty BA. Advanced practice in histopathology. *The Biomedical Scientist* 2003 May; **47** (5): 491.

Useful websites

- www.ukas.com/services/accreditation-services/clinical-pathology-accreditation
- www.hpc-uk.org
- www.hse.gov.uk/pubns/law.pdf
- www.hta.gov.uk
- www.ukneqas.org.uk
- www.ibms.org
- www.institute.nhs.uk/quality_and_value/lean_thinking/lean_six_sigma.html
- www.ncepod.org.uk/reports.html
- www.rcpath.org
- www.ukneqasiccish.org
- www.cap.org/web/home/lab/accreditation
- www.health.gov.au/npaac
- www.nata.asn.au
- www.standards.org.au
- www.a2la.org/appsweb/Clia.cfm

 # Discussion questions

17.1 How would you encourage a quality culture within your laboratory?

17.2 What are the possible consequences if your laboratory loses CPA accreditation?

17.3 What systems need to be in place to ensure compliance with the HTA 2004?

Answers to the self-check questions and tips for responding to the discussion questions are provided on the book's accompanying website:

 Visit www.oup.com/uk/orchard2e

Glossary

Acid reflux: The clinical condition in which gastric acid is released into the oesophagus.

Affinity: A measure of the binding strength between an epitope and its specific antibody binding site.

Anaemia: A condition in which a person has a low level of haemoglobin in their blood. This can be due to the presence of fewer red blood cells than normal, or an iron deficiency state.

Analyser: A filter placed in the light path fixed within the body of the microscope. It is used in conjunction with a substage polarizer.

Anatomical Pathology Technologist: A healthcare scientist who specializes in mortuary practice and has trained in that field.

Antacids: A type of medication that helps to control the level of acid in the stomach.

Antibody: Proteins belonging to the immunoglobulin (Ig) group that arise in the blood of immunized humans and animals. There are five main subgroups (IgG, IgA, IgM, IgD and IgE), which collectively form the basis of the body's humoral immune response mechanism.

Antibody dilution: Determined by antibody titre evaluation. Antibodies may be provided with recommendations for dilution or may be provided as ready-to-use (RTU) reagents. This should be viewed as a guide only, as antibody dilution may not be optimal and will depend on a host of variables.

Antibody label: A compound, usually an enzyme such as peroxidase, attached to the final linking complex, which reacts to allow the visualization of a final reaction product at the site of the antigen–antibody reaction.

Antibody sensitivity: A measure of the relative amount of antigenic epitope that a given ICC method is able to detect. The greater the sensitivity of any given ICC technique, the smaller will be the amount of antigenic epitope that may be detected.

Antibody specificity: A definition of the characteristics of an antibody to bind selectively to a given antigenic epitope. Specificity ultimately defines the labelling selectivity of any given antibody. It is important to remember that this is an absolute definition. Antibodies, when compared for labelling profiles, should not be stated to be more specific than each other. They may be more selective but not more specific.

Antigen or antigenic epitope: Antigen is the protein that interacts with an antibody complex. The epitope indicates the binding components that may be involved in this interaction.

Antigen retrieval: A series of techniques that permit the controlled unmasking of antigenic epitopes, following the fixation of tissue and prior to subsequent demonstration of final reaction products with labelled antibodies. Conventionally, this relies on the application of heat (HIER) using a waterbath, microwave oven, or pressure cooker in conjunction with selective buffer systems, or the application of proteolytic enzyme digestion procedures using enzymes (e.g. chymotrypsin or protease).

Antibody titre: The highest dilution of an antibody that results in the maximum intensity and specificity of the final reaction product with minimal background staining.

Apochromatic: A lens which is corrected for up to seven colours and represents the best quality of lens available.

Astigmatism: The inability of a lens to bring light passing through one part to the same focal point as light passing through another part.

Asymptomatic: Without clinical signs or symptoms. Early cancers often grow unknown to the patient.

Avidity: The combining strength of an antibody with its antigen is directly related to both the affinity of the antibody–antigen interaction and the valency of the antibody and antigen.

Bariatric: Pertaining to obesity and weight problems.

Barrier (or emission) filter: A filter used in the fluorescence microscope which is capable of only transmitting the light wavelength range emitted by a particular fluorescence dye.

Birefringence: The ability of a substance to split a ray of light into two components: the ordinary and extraordinary ray.

Broad-spectrum cytokeratin: A solution of a number of monoclonal antibodies to cytokeratins. The purpose of a broad-spectrum cytokeratin in diagnosis is to label all tissues that express cytokeratins. This can be useful in the identification of a carcinoma or the extent of invasion.

Chlorocarbons: Chlorocarbons are organic compounds consisting of carbon-based molecules with chlorine and hydrogen. Once they were commonly used but this is declining due to environmental and health considerations.

Chromatic aberration: The inability of a lens to bring light of different wavelengths to a common focal point.

Chromogen: A compound that interacts with the final antibody–antigen complex to facilitate visualization of the final reaction product at the site of the antibody–antigen interaction. Examples include diaminobenzidine tetrahydrochloride (DAB) or alkaline phosphatase.

Clarke's fixative: An alcohol and glacial acetic acid solution that provides rapid fixation but poor tissue penetration. This fixative is ideal for fixing fresh sections adhered to a slide.

Cluster of differentiation (CD): This represents the characterization and subsequent classification of human leucocyte antigens. The cluster number relates to different antibodies that have been found to have the same specificity as defined by at least two or more antibody-based techniques.

Coherent rays: Light rays which are in phase with one another, of the same amplitude and wavelength.

Coroner: a doctor or lawyer responsible for investigating deaths under certain circumstances who can also order a post-mortem examination of the body if necessary.

Cytokeratins: These are structural cytoplasmic proteins expressed in epithelial tissue. Cytokeratins are divided into around 20 categories based on molecular weight.

Decomposition: The biological and chemical change that a body undergoes after death where organic substances are broken down into simpler forms of matter.

Differentiation: The removal of excess dye from tissue to provide a good balance/contrast of stained and unstained elements to aid identification.

E-cadherin: A cell adhesion molecule.

Ethics: Ethics is the branch of medicine that deals with establishing the rights and wrongs of clinical practice. Sometimes known as medical ethics, the values expressed as right and wrong are not static, and public opinion about what is acceptable does change over time. Biomedical practitioners need to be sensitive to these changes.

Evisceration: Literally 'to empty the organs or disembowel' it is removal of all the organs for examination.

Eyepiece: The lens situated at the observation tube of a microscope used to view the magnified image of the specimen.

Fetus: A non-viable pregnancy up to 23 weeks and 6 days' gestation showing no sign of life on delivery.

Fixative: Preserves the tissue by stopping autolysis and putrefaction, keeping tissue from further deterioration after death. Formalin fixes permanently and causes tissue to shrink slightly and harden, but it retains its three-dimensional structure.

Focal point: The point at which a lens brings all of the light passing through to a common focus.

Haematoma: A localized collection of blood outside a blood vessel. This may be spontaneous in the case of an aneurysm or caused by trauma.

Heat-induced epitope retrieval (HIER): The use of heat in automated ICC platforms, microwave ovens, pressure cookers or waterbaths to recover antigen reactivity in formalin-fixed, paraffin wax-embedded tissue.

Hyaluronic acid: An ionic, non-sulphated glycosaminoglycan distributed widely throughout connective, epithelial and neural tissues (e.g. synovium and synovial fluid, skin, aorta, umbilical cord, cartilage and bone).

Immunocompromised: Having an immune system that has been impaired by disease or treatment.

Immunofluorescence: A method employing the fluorescence microscope to identify the presence of specific antigens within tissue samples using fluorescence-labelled antisera.

Lean technology: Lean technology is the concept derived from the manufacturing industry. It is the process of analysing the steps of the process to ensure the most efficient work patterns. Within tissue processing this is the concept of reducing batch size to the smallest number possible with the aim of ensuring work moves progressively through the laboratory without any waiting steps.

Lymphoma: A lymphoid neoplasm which is distinguished from leukaemia by cellular proliferations involving discrete tissue masses in lymph nodes, secondary lymphoid organs such as the spleen, or extranodal such as the stomach. Leukaemias usually involve widespread involvement of circulating tumour cells in the bone marrow and circulating bloodstream.

Lypsochromatic dyes: Dyes that are more soluble in the substance to be demonstrated than in the substance they are prepared in. For example, Oil red O staining solution is worked up in 60% aqueous isopropyl alcohol, the solution of which is about at the point of saturation. However, the dye is much more soluble in cellular lipid. Lypsochromatic solutions should always be filtered before use.

Magnification: The process of enlarging something only in appearance, not in physical size.

Meninges: Three layers of membranes that cover the central nervous system.

Mesothelioma: A cancer of mesothelial cells that line internal body cavities. Most cases of mesothelioma are related to exposure to asbestos.

Metalloprotease: A protease enzyme whose catalytic mechanism involves a metal.

Microtome: Tissue sections are prepared on a machine called a microtome. This word comes from the Greek micro – small, and tome – cut.

Monoclonal antibodies: These are the product of a single clone of chimaeric cells formed from an antibody-producing B cell and a myeloma cell line, and are immunologically identical and will react with the specific epitope to which they are raised.

Neuroendocrine carcinoma: This includes Merkel-cell carcinoma. Merkel cells are cells of neuroendocrine origin present in the epidermis of the skin. Merkel-cell carcinoma is a serious form of cancer and patients may have a very poor prognosis Also, small-cell neuroendocrine carcinoma may arise in different organs, in particular the lung.

Peltier plate: A bimetallic strip through which an electric current is passed. The electric current causes one side of the bimetallic strip to cool; this is known as the Peltier effect.

Petechial haemorrhage: Small pinprick haemorrhages that may indicate asphyxia.

Polyclonal antibodies: These are produced by different antibody-producing cells and as such will be different in terms of how they recognize the various epitopes to which they are raised.

Prenatal, perinatal and paediatric pathology: A specialty within pathology which covers the unborn baby and placenta, the neonatal period, childhood and young adulthood.

Procurator Fiscal: a qualified lawyer who is responsible for prosecuting crime in Scotland; they also investigate sudden and suspicious deaths and can order a post-mortem examination.

Prostate-specific antigen (PSA): A protein secreted by the prostate. When the gland is enlarged, inflamed and/or malignant the level of PSA is seen to rise above the normal reference range. The normal PSA reference range in healthy men under 60 is 0–3 ng/mL, rising to 0–5 ng/mL in men over 70 years of age. A raised PSA level will trigger further investigation by biopsy.

Proteolytic enzymes: Examples include trypsin, chymotrypsin, pronase (now rarely used) and protease.

Proton pump inhibitors: Reduce the amount of acid the stomach produces.

Refractive: A numerical measure of a substance's ability to deviate light rays.

Resolution: The smallest distance that can be distinguished between two points.

Resomation: Also known as alkaline hydrolysis, it is a water-based chemical process using strong alkali in water at temperatures of up to 180°C under high pressure to safely and rapidly reduce the body to ash.

Spherical aberration: The inability of a lens to bring light passing through different parts of the lens to a common focus.

Standard Infection Control Precautions (SICPs): Previously known as Universal Precautions, these are the basic infection prevention and control measures necessary to reduce the risk of transmission of infectious agents.

The Cremation Regulations: The Cremation Regulations 2008 came into effect on 1 January 2009 to modernize and consolidate all previous regulations, replacing the Cremation Regulations 1930 as previously amended.

Topical: Treatment applied directly to the lesion.

Verification of death: This is different from certification, in that someone who is competent and trained but not a registered medical practitioner can verify death. Only a registered medical practitioner can certify death.

Wavelength: The distance (measured in the direction of propagation) between two points in the same phase in consecutive cycles of a wave.

Abbreviations

Some common abbreviations in use in histopathology

ABC	avidin–biotin complex
ACADM	medium-chain acyl CoA dehydrogenase
ACDP	Advisory Committee on Dangerous Pathogens
AfC	Agenda for Change
AIDS	acquired immune deficiency syndrome
ALCL	anaplastic large cell lymphoma
ALL	acute lymphoblastic leukaemia
APAAP	alkaline phosphatase–anti-alkaline phosphatase
APR	abdominoperineal resection (of rectum)
APT	anatomical pathology technologist
AR	anterior resection (of colon)
BMZ	basement membrane zone
BSE	bovine spongiform encephalopathy
CAP	College of American Pathologists
CD	cluster of differentiation
cDNA	copy/complementary DNA
CEA	carcinoembryonic antigen
CGIN	cervical glandular intraepithelial neoplasia
CI	colour index
CIN	cervical intraepithelial neoplasia
CISH	chromogenic in situ hybridization
CJD	Creutzfeldt–Jakob disease
CLL	chronic lymphocytic leukaemia
CML	chronic myeloid leukaemia
COPFS	Crown Office Procurator Fiscal Service
COSHH	Control of Substances Hazardous to Health
CPA	Clinical Pathology Accreditation (UK)
CPD	continuing professional development
CPPD	continuing personal and professional development
CPT	cellular pathology technique
CS	caesarean section
CSA	catalysed signal amplification
CSF	cerebrospinal fluid
CT	computed tomography
DAB	3,3 diaminobenzidine tetrahydrochloride
DI	designated individual
DNA	deoxyribonucleic acid
dNTP	deoxy nucleotide triphosphate
DPAS	diastase periodic acid Schiff
DVT	deep vein thrombosis
EBV	Epstein–Barr virus
EDTA	ethylenediaminetetraacetic acid
EGFR	epithelial growth factor receptor
EM	electron microscopy
EMA	epithelial membrane antigen
EPOS	enhanced polymer one-step staining
EQA	external quality assessment
EQC	external quality control
ER	estrogen (oestrogen) receptor
ERCP	endoscopic retrograde cholangiopancreatography
FACS	fluorescence-activated cell sorting
FCF	for colouring food
FFPE	formalin-fixed, paraffin wax-embedded
FISH	fluorescence in situ hybridization
FITC	fluorescein isothiocyanate
FOB	faecal occult blood
FS	frozen section
GCDFP-15	gross cystic disease fluid protein 15
GLP	good laboratory practice
HBV	hepatitis B virus
H&E	haematoxylin and eosin
HCC	Healthcare Commission
HCPC	Health and Care Professions Council
HCV	hepatitis C virus
HIER	heat-induced epitope retrieval
HIV	human immunodeficiency virus
HLDA	human leucocyte differentiation antigen
HPV	human papillomavirus
HSE	Health and Safety Executive
HTA	Human Tissue Authority
HVG	haematoxylin and van Gieson
IBD	inflammatory bowel disease
IBMS	Institute of Biomedical Science
IBS	irritable bowel syndrome
ICC	immunocytochemistry
Ig	immunoglobulin
IHC	immunohistochemistry

IMF	immunofluorescence		PET	positron emission tomography
IMS	industrial methylated spirit		PPC	personal protective clothing
IPA	isopropyl alcohol		PPE	personal protective equipment
IQA	internal quality assurance		PR	progesterone receptor
IQC	internal quality control		PSA	prostate-specific antigen
ISH	*in situ* hybridization		PTAH	phosphotungstic acid haematoxylin
ISO	International Organization for Standardization		QA	quality assessment
KSF	Knowledge and Skills Framework		QC	quality control
LA	local authority		QD	quantum dots
LBC	liquid-based cytology		QIPP	Quality, Innovation, Productivity and Prevention
LCA	leucocyte common antigen		QMS	quality management system
LLETZ	large loop excision of the transformation zone		RBC	red blood cell
LIMS	laboratory information management system		RCPath	The Royal College of Pathologists
LMP-1	Epstein–Barr virus latent membrane protein 1		RFLP	restriction fragment length polymorphism
LSAB	labelled streptavidin–biotin		RIDDOR	Reporting of Injuries, Diseases and Dangerous Occurrences Regulations 1995
LSCS	lower segment caesarean section			
MALT	mucosa-associated lymphoid tissue		RNA	ribonucleic acid
MCAD	medium-chain acyl CoA dehydrogenase		RT	reverse transcriptase
MCCD	Medical Certificate of Cause of Death		RTA	road traffic accident
MDT	multidisciplinary team		RTC	road traffic collision
MHRA	Medicines and Healthcare products Regulatory Agency		RTU	ready to use
			SCC	squamous cell carcinoma
MM	malignant melanoma		SCLC	small cell lung carcinoma
MRI	magnetic resonance imaging		SEM	scanning electron microscopy
mRNA	messenger RNA		SISH	silver *in situ* hybridization
MSB	Martius scarlet blue		SOCO	Scenes of Crime Officer
NCAM	neural cell adhesion molecule		SOP	standard operating procedure
NCEPOD	National Confidential Enquiry into Patient Outcome and Death		StABC	streptavidin–biotin complex
			SUI	serious untoward incident
NHL	non-Hodgkin's lymphoma		*Taq*	*Thermus (Thermophilus) aquaticus*
NHS	National Health Service		TCC	transitional cell carcinoma
NQAAP	National Quality Assurance Advisory Panel		TCR	T-cell receptor
NSCLC	non-small cell lung carcinoma		TEM	transmission electron microscopy
NSE	neuron-specific enolase		TSE	transmissible spongiform encephalopathy
NST	no special type		TTF-1	thyroid transcription factor-1
PALS	Patient Advice and Liaison Service		TURB	transurethral resection of bladder
PAP	peroxidase–antiperoxidase		TURP	transurethral resection of prostate
PAS	periodic acid Schiff		UK NEQAS ICC & ISH	UK National External Quality Assessment Scheme for Immunocytochemistry and *In Situ* Hybridization
PCD	primary ciliary dyskinesia			
PCR	polymerase chain reaction			
PD	person designated		UKAS	United Kingdom Accreditation Service
PDP	personal development plan		UK NEQAS	United Kingdom National External Quality Assessment Scheme
PECAM-1	platelet endothelial cell adhesion molecule-1			
			ZN	Ziehl–Neelsen

Index

Note: *b*, *f* and *t* denote *box*, *figure* and *table*